Advances in Plastic Surgery

Advances in Plastic Surgery

Editor: Archer Queen

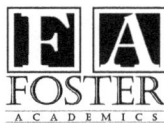

FOSTER
ACADEMICS

www.fosteracademics.com

www.fosteracademics.com

FA
FOSTER
ACADEMICS

Cataloging-in-Publication Data

Advances in plastic surgery / edited by Archer Queen.
  p. cm.
Includes bibliographical references and index.
ISBN 978-1-63242-808-0
1. Surgery, Plastic. 2. Surgery, Plastic--Technique.
3. Transplantation of organs, tissues, etc. I. Queen, Archer.
RD118 .A38 2019
617.95--dc23

Foster Academics,
118-35 Queens Blvd., Suite 400,
Forest Hills, NY 11375, USA

ISBN 978-1-63242-808-0 (Hardback)

Contents

Permissions

List of Contributors

Index

Preface

A surgical specialty concerned with the alteration, restoration or reconstruction of the human body is known as plastic surgery. There are two main categories of plastic surgery, namely, reconstructive surgery and cosmetic surgery. Hand surgery, the treatment of burns, craniofacial surgery and microsurgery are classified as reconstructive surgery. It is concerned with the reconstruction or the improvement in the functioning of any specific body part. Cosmetic surgery deals with the improvement of the appearance of a body part. Some of the common techniques and procedures of plastic surgery include autotransplantation, allotransplant, xenotransplantation, etc. Different approaches, evaluations, methodologies and advanced studies on plastic surgery have been included in this book. It provides significant information of this discipline to help develop a good understanding of plastic surgery and related fields. As this field is emerging at a rapid pace, the contents of this book will help the readers understand the modern concepts and applications of the subject.

After months of intensive research and writing, this book is the end result of all who devoted their time and efforts in the initiation and progress of this book. It will surely be a source of reference in enhancing the required knowledge of the new developments in the area. During the course of developing this book, certain measures such as accuracy, authenticity and research focused analytical studies were given preference in order to produce a comprehensive book in the area of study.

This book would not have been possible without the efforts of the authors and the publisher. I extend my sincere thanks to them. Secondly, I express my gratitude to my family and well-wishers. And most importantly, I thank my students for constantly expressing their willingness and curiosity in enhancing their knowledge in the field, which encourages me to take up further research projects for the advancement of the area.

Editor

Surgical Treatment of 55 Patients with Pressure Ulcers at the Department of Plastic and Reconstructive Surgery Kosovo during the Period 2000–2010: A Retrospective Study

Shkelzen B. Duci,[1] Hysni M. Arifi,[1] Mimoza E. Selmani,[2] Agon Y. Mekaj,[3] Musli M. Gashi,[4] Zejn A. Buja,[1] Vildane H. Ismajli,[1] Adem N. Kllokoqi,[1] and Enver T. Hoxha[1]

[1] Department of Plastic and Reconstructive Surgery, University Clinical Center of Kosovo, Pristina, Kosovo
[2] Dentistry Faculty, University Clinical Center of Kosovo, Pristina, Kosovo
[3] Department of Neurosurgery, University Clinical Center of Kosovo, Pristina, Kosovo
[4] Department of Emergency Center Kosovo, Pristina, Kosovo

Correspondence should be addressed to Shkelzen B. Duci; xeni978@hotmail.com

Academic Editor: G. L. Robb

Objective. The objective of this study is to determine the incidence of PUs, the distribution of PUs, common injuries contributing to the occurrence of PUs in patients admitted to the Department of Plastic and Reconstructive Surgery Kosovo for surgical interventions of PUs, localization of PUs in body, the topical treatment of pressure ulcers before surgical intervention, the methods of surgical interventions, number of surgical interventions, duration of treatment, complications, and mortality. *Materials and Methods.* This study includes 55 patients with PUs treated surgically in 2000–2010 period in the Department of Plastic and Reconstructive Surgery Kosovo. The data were collected and analyzed from the archives and protocols of the University Clinical Center of Kosovo. Data processing was done with the statistical package In Stat 3. From statistical parameters arithmetic median and standard deviation were calculated. Data testing is done with χ^2-test and the difference is significant if $P < 0.05$. *Conclusion.* Despite preventive measures against PUs, the incidence of Pus remains high.

1. Introduction

Pressure ulcers (PUs) are defined as localized injury to the skin or underlying tissue usually over bony prominence, as a result of pressure, or pressure in combination with shear or friction [1, 2]. Pressure ulcers are almost a serious, secondary complication of spinal cord injury that has the potential to interfere with physical, psychological, and social well being and to impact overall quality of life [3]. PUs are classified by the level of visible tissue damage, where stage I PUs exhibit nonblanchable erythematic (i.e., redness) on intact skin, stage II PUs are partial thickness ulcers, and stages III and IV ulcers involve full-thickness damage [4]. They are believed to occur from combination of extrinsic forces such as pressure, shear, and friction and intrinsic factors such as

age, malnourishment, and consciousness level that influence a person's tissue tolerance [5, 6]. Previous studies have identified the following factors as increasing the likelihood of developing a pressure ulcer: immobility, admission to the ICU, malnutrition, incontinence, hypoalbuminemia, spinal cord injury, stroke, reduced level of consciousness, fractures and/or major orthopedic procedure, advanced age, trauma, decreased perfusion, poor wound healing, inadequate nursing care, and chronic illness [7–10].

Contributing risk factors increase the patient's susceptibility to a complex etiology that causes PUs [11].

Debridement of pressure sores often results in extensive soft tissue defects that cannot be closed primarily and are further associated with increased risk of flap ischemia, wound dehiscence, and deep infection [12]. Numeral surgical methods have been used to correct these defects, including skin grafting [12, 13], local flaps [12, 14], muscle flaps [12, 15], and free flaps [12, 16].

2. Objective

The objective of this study is to determine the incidence of PUs in our population, the distribution of PUs, common injuries contributing to the occurrence of PUs in patients admitted to the Department of Plastic and Reconstructive Surgery Kosovo for surgical interventions of PUs, localization of PUs in the body, the topical treatment of pressure ulcers before surgical intervention, the methods of surgical interventions, number of surgical interventions, duration of treatment, complications and mortality.

3. Materials and Methods

This is a retrospective study that included 55 patients with 72 defects caused from PUs treated surgically in 2000–2010 period in the Department of Plastic and Reconstructive Surgery Kosovo. The data were collected and analyzed from the archives and protocols of the University Clinical Center of Kosovo. This research project was approved by the Regulation and Ethical Standards Commission. In this study we included patients with PUs stages III and IV who underwent surgical interventions, and we excluded the patients who underwent topical treatments of small wounds without surgical intervention. Data processing was done with the statistical package In Stat 3. From statistical parameters arithmetic median and standard deviation were calculated. Data testing is done with χ^2-test and the difference is significant if $P < 0.05$.

4. Results

In this study PUs were predominant in male patients with 42 cases or 76.3% with only 13 cases or 23.6% in female patients (Table 1). The incidence of pressure ulcers was noted to be higher in the age group 30–39 with 20 cases or 36.3% followed by children where the children are considered up to the age 19 years old by WHO with 10 cases (18.1%), 20–29 years 9 cases (16.3%), 40–49 years 5 cases (9%), 50–59 years 5 cases (9%), 60–69 years 2 cases (3.6%), and over 70 years 4 cases (7.2%). The average age of patients was 34.8 years (Table 1). We found that patients with spinal cord injuries had the highest incidence of PUs with 48 cases, followed by patients with cerebral injuries 3 cases, orthopedic traumatic injuries with 3 cases, and 1 case with congenital anomaly of spinal cord. From 48 patients with spinal cord injuries 37 patients or 77% were male and 11 patients or 22.9% were female; from 3 patients with cerebral injuries 2 patients were male and 1 patient were female; from 3 patients with orthopedic traumatic injuries 2 patients were male and 1 patient was female, in addition to 1 case (male) with congenital anomaly of spinal cord. Distribution of PUs in years had the following features: 2002 and 2003 are the years where the incidence of PUs was the highest with 7 cases (12.7%); 2005 with 6 cases (10.9%); 2001, 2006, 2007, and 2008 with 5 cases

TABLE 1: General characteristics of patients with PUs.

	No ($n = 55$)	%
Gender*		
Male	42	76.3
Female	13	23.6
Age groups (years)		
Children	10	18.1
20–29	9	16.3
30–39	20	36.3
40–49	5	9
50–59	5	9
60–69	2	3.6
70+	4	7.2
Mean ± SD	34.8 ± 10.0	
Range	1 –79 years	

*Significant by gender (χ^2-test = 15.3, $P < 0.001$).

(9%); 2004, 2009, and 2010 with 4 cases (7.2%) and 2000 with only 3 cases (5.5%). In terms of body localization of pressure ulcers, the most frequent localization was the sacral region with 41 cases (74.5%). Other localizations had the following distribution: the trochanteric region with 12 cases (21.8%), ischia region 11 cases (20%), femoral region 3 cases (5.4%), occipital region 2 cases (3.6%), malleolar region 2 cases (3.6%), and calcaneal region 1 case (1.8%) (Table 2). Topical treatment of the wounds before surgical intervention was mostly performed with wound dressing with povidone iodine solution and silver sulfadiazine ointment. For coverage of defects caused by PUs 20 musculocutaneous flaps, including V-Y flaps and transposition (36.3%) usually to cover defects over sacral region and 18 cutaneous local flaps (32.7%); 12 small defects are closed with direct closure (21.8%); in 12 cases cutaneous grafts (21.8%) were used, and in 10 cases fasciocutaneous flap of tensor fascia lata for reconstruction of trochanteric region (18.1%) (Figures 1, 2, 3, and 4) (Table 2). Forty-five cases underwent surgical intervention only once, while 7 cases had two surgical interventions. Three cases required surgical intervention because of partial necrosis of the flaps and dehiscence (Table 3). Duration of treatment ranged from 8 to 178 days. The mean hospitalization was 63.6 days. Four cases were complicated with necrotizing fasciitis and sepsis from which two cases died (3.6%) [3].

5. Discussion

PUs are serious health problem [17, 18]. They cause pain and distress in the affected individuals. Their treatment is very costly for the health care system and the society [17, 19]. In this study PUs were predominant in male patients with 42 cases or 76.3% with only 13 cases or 23.6% in female patients (Table 1). The highest incidence of pressure ulcers was noted in the age group from 30 to 39 years old with 20 cases or 36.3% followed by children (children are considered up to the age 19 years old by WHO) with 10 cases (18.1%), 20–29 years 9 cases (16.3%), 40–49 years 5 cases (9%), 50–59 years

TABLE 2: Localization of PUs and surgical methods used for treatment of defects caused by Pus.

	No (n = 72)	%
Localization by the regions		
Sacral region	41	74.5
Trochanteric	12	21.8
Ischia	11	20
Femoral	3	5.4
Occipital	2	3.6
Malleolar	2	3.6
Calcaneal	1	1.8
Surgical methods		
Musculocutaneous flaps	20	36.3
Cutaneous local flaps	18	32.7
Direct closure	12	21.8
Cutaneous grafts	12	21.8
Fasciocutaneous flaps TFL*	10	18.1

*TFL-tensor fascia lata.

TABLE 3: Duration of hospitalization, number of surgical interventions, complications, and morbidity in patients with pressure ulcers.

	No (n = 55)	%
Number of surgical interventions		
1 time	45	81.8
2 times	7	12.7
3 times	3	5.4
Complications		
Necrotising fasciitis	4	7.2
Morbidity (sepsis)	2	3.6
Duration of hospitalization (days)		
Range	8–178 days	
Mean ± SD	63.6 ± 10.0	8–178 days

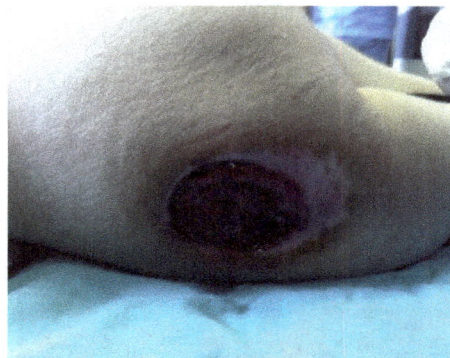

FIGURE 1: Pressure ulcer in 16-year-old patient with spinal cord injury in trochanteric region after topically treatment of the wound.

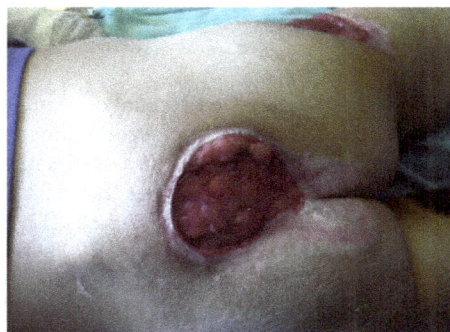

FIGURE 2: Pressure ulcer in the same patient in sacral region after topical treatment.

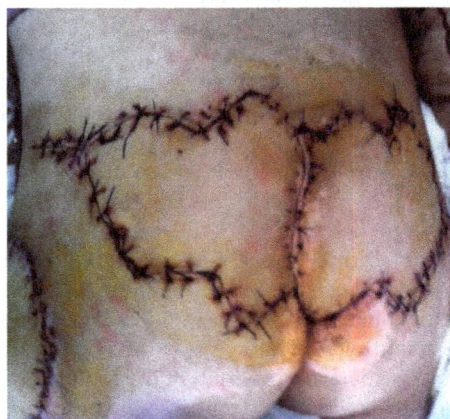

FIGURE 3: Sacral defect covered with two musculocutaneous advancement flaps.

5 cases (9%), 60–69 years 2 cases (3.6%), and over 70 years 4 cases (7.2%). We found that PUs had the highest incidence in patients with spinal cord injuries with 48 cases, followed by patients with cerebral injuries 3 cases, orthopedic traumatic injuries with 3 cases, and 1 case with congenital anomaly of spinal cord. Out of 48 patients with spinal cord injuries 37 or 77% of them were male and 11 patients or 22.9% were female. Two out of 3 patients with cerebral injuries were male and only one patient was female (all cases are associated with coma after severe cerebral injury). Two out of 3 patients with orthopedic traumatic injuries were male (1 with amputation of right extremities and another associated with fracture of pelvic bone) and 1 patient was female (with septic arthritis associated with head necrosis of femoral bone), with 1 case with congenital anomaly of spinal cord (myelomeningocele). The most important finding which was not noted in other studies is the predominance of the young age 31–40 years with 20 cases; the average age of patients in our study is 34.8 years. A similar study of 60 patients with PUs by Schiffman et al. reported that average age of patients in their study was

73.1 [20]. This high incidence of PUs was noted in patients with spinal cord injuries and also the predominance of young age in our country probably results from a couple of factors. After 1999, our country emerged from the war and many deadly weapons still remain in the hands of our citizens; therefore spinal cord injuries by firearms were very frequent. Detailed history and physical examination showed that 18

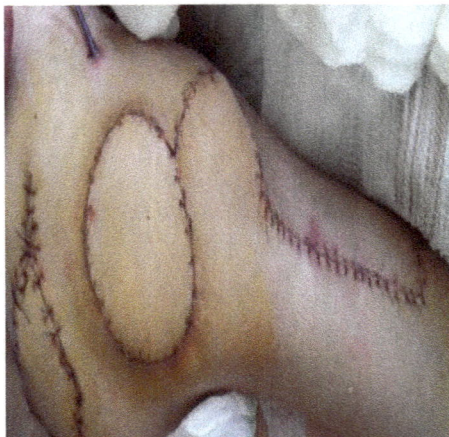

FIGURE 4: Right trochanteric defect covered with TFL flap.

cases or 32.7% of these patients had spinal cord injuries from firearms. Traffic accidents were the second most common cause of spinal cord injuries. Distribution of PUs in years had the following features: 2002 and 2003 are the years where the incidence of PUs was the highest with 7 cases (12.7%); 2005 with 6 cases (10.9%); 2001, 2006, 2007 and 2008 with 5 cases (9%); 2004, 2009, and 2010 with 4 cases (7.2%); and 2000 with only 3 cases (5.5%). Body localization of pressure ulcers has the following features: the most frequent localization was the sacral region in 41 cases (74.5%). Other localizations had the following distributions: the trochanteric region with 12 cases (21.8%), ischia region 11 cases (20%), femoral region 3 cases (5.4%), occipital region 2 cases (3.6%), maleolar region 2 cases (3.6%), and calcaneal region 1 case (1.8%). In other similar studies conducted by Nogueira et al. in 46 patients with spinal cord injuries the sacral region had the most frequent localization with 17 cases, followed by heel region with 8 cases and gluteus region with 5 cases [21]. Topical treatment of the wounds before surgical intervention usually is done with wound dressing of povidon iodine solution and sulfadiazine ointment. Our department is not fully equipped with modern technology for treatment of PUs such as wound closure device of vacuum-assisted closure techniques, topical application of growth factors, and health care products designed for local pressure distribution. Therefore depending on the local status of the wound we determine which of the following dressings (povidon iodine solution and sulfadiazine ointment) will be used for treatment of these wounds. Also some patients are followed in the operating room for debridement of necrotic tissue before the surgical intervention in order to prepare pressure ulcers for surgical closure. For coverage of defects due to PUs 20 musculocutaneous flaps, included V-Y flaps and transposition (36.3%) usually to cover defects in the sacral region, 18 cutaneous local flaps (32.7%) are used; 12 small defects are closed with direct closure (21.8%), in 12 cases cutaneous grafts (21.8%) were used, and in 10 cases fasciocutaneous flap of tensor fascia lata for reconstruction of trochanteric region (18.1%). In pressure ulcers over sacral and trochanteric regions (30 cases) 20 musculocutaneous and

10 fasciocutaneous flaps were used. The operative treatment was done with complete pressure ulcer excision, removal of dead and necrotic tissue, lavage with hydrogen peroxide, and achievement of hemostasis. Bone debridement and contouring are performed with rongeurs and rasps and the final procedure was placement of drains. In 5 cases after reconstruction of defects in sacral region with transposition flaps cutaneous grafts were used to cover this defects together with flap. From 18 cutaneous local flaps 10 flaps were transposition, 6 rotation, and 2 V-Y flaps and were used to cover small defects caused by pressure ulcer. In 6 cases together with transposition local cutaneous flaps were used and cutaneous grafts to cover this defects while in 6 cases with reconstruction of defects with rotation flaps also cutaneous grafts were used. In 12 cases with small defect were closed with direct closure of the wound. Forty-five cases underwent surgical intervention only one time and they do not have postoperative complication of the flaps while 7 cases had two surgical interventions from which 5 cases after direct closure because of dehiscence of the wounds and 2 after reconstruction of defects with cutaneous local flaps because of partial necrosis of flaps, and 3 cases had three surgical interventions from which 2 after direct closure because dehiscence of wound and 1 after reconstruction of defects with cutaneous local flaps because of partial necrosis of flap. Another important finding in our study, which is not noted in other studies, is the hospitalization of patients in our department ranged from 8 to 178 days. The mean hospitalization was 63.6 days. Alderden et al. in their study in 87 patients with PUs found that the mean of hospitalization was 37 days [22]. This difference in our study compared with other studies done for PUs probably results from some reasons. Our department is the only department in our country that treats the patients with PUs from debridement of the wound, local treatment and preparation of patients for surgical interventions and their postoperative care. Thereupon the treatment of patients with PUs in our department had a long stay hospitalization. Four cases are complicated with necrotizing fasciitis and sepsis from which two cases died (3.6%). Detailed history taking and physical examination showed that in most of these patients infection would spread from sacral and trochanteric region down towards the femoral region all the way to the knee level and was complicated with necrotizing fasciitis and sepsis. Major factor contributing to high mortality in these patients is considered delayed referral by primary care services. If patients are referred late, mortality remains significantly high (despite radical debridement of wounds and systemic antibiotic therapy two cases died and two cases survive the disease in our study).

6. Conclusion

Management of pressure ulcers lies mainly in its prevention. Despite preventive measures against PUs, the incidence of PUs remains high. In our study population the incidence of PUs was very high in patients with spinal cord injuries caused by firearms, where vast majority of injuries were noted in the 2000–2010 period. The average age of patients with PUs was 34.6. In 1999, our country emerged from war; however a lot of deadly weapons still remain illegally in the hands of our citizens. As a consequence the number of spinal cord and other injuries causing pressure ulcers is much higher as compared to the other neighboring countries. Once pressure ulcers develop their course, there are variety of treatment modalities. Topical treatment of the wounds before surgical intervention usually is done with wound dressing of povidon iodine solution and sulfadiazine ointment. Our department, in cooperation with the Ministry of Health, should make effort to secure other modern devices for treatment of PUs such as vacuum-assisted closure techniques, topical application of growth factors, and health care products designed for local pressure distribution and to organize special training courses for use of these devices. We used musculocutaneous flaps to cover sacral defects, whereas fasciocutaneous flaps of TFL were used in trochanteric region. The use of cutaneous local flaps for coverage of defects and direct closure in 10 patients was accompanied with partial necrosis of flaps and dehiscence of the wound. Based on this study we can conclude that the use of cutaneous local flaps and direct closure is not appropriate option for these defects. Subsequently flaps should routinely be utilized for these complicated defects. Four cases are complicated with necrotizing fasciitis and sepsis from which two cases died (3.6%).

Spread of infection was noted from sacral and trochanteric regions towards the femoral region all the way down to the knee level and was complicated with necrotizing fasciitis and sepsis. Major factor contributing to high mortality in this patient population is delayed referral by primary care services. As a consequence we need to organize special training programs for practitioners in primary care services through which they will be familiarized with PU pathology, treatment, and complications. The involvement of families and other medical professionals is essential for successful treatment of PUs.

Authors' Contribution

S. Duci is the designer of paper, H. Arifi, M. Selmani, and A. Mekaj analyzed and interpreted the data and V. Ismajli and M. Gashi analyzed the data and were major contributors in writing the paper. Z. Buja, A. Kllokoqi, and E. Hoxha reviewed and statistically analyzed the data. All authors read and approved the final paper.

Acknowledgments

The authors thank the archive and all the staff of the Department of Plastic Surgery for their technical support.

References

[1] L. J. Cowan, J. K. Stechmiller, M. Rowe et al., "Enhancing Braden pressure ulcer risk assessment in acutely ill adult veterans," *Wound Repair and Regeneration*, vol. 20, pp. 137–148, 2012.

[2] Pressure Ulcer Stages Revised by NPUAP, *National Pressure Ulcer Advisory Panel*, Press Release, Washington, DC, USA, 2007.

[3] M. A. Regan, R. W. Teasell, D. L. Wolfe, D. Keast, W. B. Mortenson, and J. A. L. Aubut, "A systematic review of therapeutic interventions for pressure Ulcers after spinal cord injury," *Archives of Physical Medicine and Rehabilitation*, vol. 90, no. 2, pp. 213–231, 2009.

[4] B. M. Bates-Jensen, H. E. McCreath, V. Pongquan, and N. C. R. Apeles, "Subepidermal moisture differentiates erythema and stage I pressure ulcers in nursing home residents," *Wound Repair and Regeneration*, vol. 16, no. 2, pp. 189–197, 2008.

[5] M. M. Metassan, "Pressure ulcers in the medical wards of RIPAS Hospital: incidence and risk factors," *Brunei International Medical Journal*, vol. 7, no. 3, article 157, 2011.

[6] R. M. Allman, "Pressure ulcer prevalence, incidence, risk factors, and impact," *Clinics in Geriatric Medicine*, vol. 13, no. 3, pp. 421–436, 1997.

[7] E. F. Reilly, G. C. Karakousis, P. Sherwin et al., "Pressure ulcers in the intensive care unit: the forgotten enemy," *OPUS 12 Scientist*, vol. 1, no. 2, 2007.

[8] S. R. Eachempati, L. J. Hydo, and P. S. Barie, "Factors influencing the development of decubitus ulcers in critically ill surgical patients," *Critical Care Medicine*, vol. 29, no. 9, pp. 1678–1682, 2001.

[9] M. Edwards, "The rationale for the use of risk calculators in pressure sore prevention, and the evidence of the reliability and validity of published scales," *Journal of advanced nursing*, vol. 20, no. 2, pp. 288–296, 1994.

[10] L. E. Herman and K. F. Rothman, "Prevention, care, and treatment of pressure (decubitus) ulcers in intensive care unit patients," *Journal of Intensive Care Medicine*, vol. 4, no. 3, pp. 117–123, 1989.

[11] J. K. Stechmiller, L. Cowan, J. D. Whitney et al., "Guidelines for the prevention of pressure ulcers," *Wound Repair and Regeneration*, vol. 16, no. 2, pp. 151–168, 2008.

[12] Y. Xu, H. Hai, Z. Liang, S. Feng, and C. Wang, "Pedicled fasciocutaneous flap of multi-island design for large sacral defects," *Clinical Orthopaedics and Related Research*, vol. 467, no. 8, pp. 2135–2141, 2009.

[13] Y. Liu, X. Zhang, and C. Zhang, "Clinical typing and surgical principle of pressure sore," *Zhongguo xiu fu chong jian wai ke za zhi*, vol. 21, no. 9, pp. 932–936, 2007.

[14] H. Menke, "Infected decubitus ulcer in German," *Langenbecks Archiv für Chirurgie. Supplement. Kongressband*, vol. 114, pp. 517–520, 1997.

[15] J. L. Grolleau, J. F. Collin, J. P. Chavoin, and M. Costagliola, "Iliac transosseous transposition of a rectus abdominis flap to cover a sacral pressure sore," *Annales de Chirurgie Plastique et Esthetique*, vol. 39, no. 1, pp. 128–131, 1994 (French).

[16] V. Lemaire, K. Boulanger, and O. Heymans, "Free flaps for pressure sore coverage," *Annals of Plastic Surgery*, vol. 60, no. 6, pp. 631–634, 2008.

[17] J. Kottner, K. Raeder, R. Halfens, and T. Dassen, "A systematic review of interrater reliability of pressure ulcer classification systems," *Journal of Clinical Nursing*, vol. 18, no. 3, pp. 315–336, 2009.

[18] R. M. Allman, P. S. Goode, M. M. Patrick, N. Burst, and A. A. Bartolucci, "Pressure ulcer risk factors among hospitalized patients with activity limitation," *Journal of the American Medical Association*, vol. 273, no. 11, pp. 865–870, 1995.

[19] N. Graves, F. A. Birrell, and M. Whitby, "Modeling the economic losses from pressure ulcers among hospitalized patients in Australia," *Wound Repair and Regeneration*, vol. 13, no. 5, pp. 462–467, 2005.

[20] J. Schiffman, M. S. Golinko, A. Yan, A. Flattau, M. Tomic-Canic, and H. Brem, "Operative debridement of pressure ulcers," *World Journal of Surgery*, vol. 33, no. 7, pp. 1396–1402, 2009.

[21] P. C. Nogueira, M. H. L. Caliri, and V. J. Haas, "Profile of patients with spinal cord injuries and occurrence of pressure ulcer at a university hospital," *Revista Latino-Americana de Enfermagem*, vol. 14, no. 3, pp. 372–377, 2006.

[22] J. Alderden, J. D. Whitney, S. M. Taylor et al., "Risk profile characteristics associated with outcomes of hospital-acquired pressure ulcers: a retrospective review," *Critical Care Nurse*, vol. 31, pp. 30–43, 2011.

2

Clinical Features of Primary Vein Grafts in Free Tissue Transfers

**Mitsuru Nemoto, Kenichi Kumazawa, Eiju Uchinuma,
Natsuko Kounoike, and Akira Takeda**

*Department of Plastic and Reconstructive Surgery, Kitasato University Hospital, 1-15-1 Kitasato, Minami-ku,
Sagamihara, Kanagawa 252-0374, Japan*

Correspondence should be addressed to Mitsuru Nemoto; mnemoto@med.kitasato-u.ac.jp

Academic Editor: Lee L. Q. Pu

The outcomes of free tissue transfers combined with vein grafts have been inconsistent, and discussions continue regarding their appropriate use. Of the 142 free tissue transfers that we performed from January 2004 to December 2011, we retrospectively analyzed 15 consecutive patients who underwent free tissue transfers in combination with vein grafts. Etiologies included trauma (8 patients), infection (4), and tumor (3). Types of free tissue transfers were fibula (4), anterolateral thigh (3), groin (3), jejunum (3), latissimus dorsi (1), and dorsal pedis (1). Vein grafts were used for the artery (6), vein (2), or both (7). The donor veins were the saphenous vein (12) and the external jugular vein (3). The mean length of the grafted veins was 10.8 cm (range: 4–18 cm). Even though complications of congestion occurred in 2 patients, these flaps survived by reexploration. The flap success rate was 15 of 15 (100%) of vein grafted free flaps versus 124 of 127 (97.6%) of free flaps not requiring vein grafts. To improve the success rate of free tissue transfers combined with vein grafts, securing healthy recipient vessels, meticulous surgical handling, a reliable vascular anastomosis technique, and strict postoperative monitoring are crucial.

1. Introduction

Vein grafts used in combination with free tissue transfers are known to increase the risk of postoperative complications [1, 2]. Oliva [3] reported a failure rate of approximately 20% with this particular combined procedure. Miller et al. [4] stated that free tissue transfers to recipient sites that have been preoperatively exposed to radiation were unsuccessful in approximately 30% of the cases. Conversely, Germann and Steinau [5] reported that the success rate of free flaps combined with vein grafts was 96.7% and the success rate of free flaps without vein grafts was 96.2%, indicating a lack of significant difference between these two methods. Bayramiçli et al. [6] also reported that there were no significant differences in the success rates between free tissue transfers with or without vein grafts. The present study retrospectively analyzed the clinical features of 15 consecutive patients who underwent free tissue transfers with vein grafts to improve the flap success rate.

2. Patients and Methods

Using the medical records of all 142 patients who underwent free tissue transfers from January 2004 to December 2011 at our institution, we retrospectively analyzed 15 consecutive patients who underwent free tissue transfers combined with vein grafts. The analyzed items included etiology, timing, anatomic site, type of free tissue, grafted donor vein, length of grafted vein, recipient artery, recipient vein, and postoperative complications. The flap success rate of these 15 patients was compared with that of patients who underwent free tissue transfers without vein grafts using Fisher's exact test.

3. Results

The 15 patients were comprised of 13 males and 2 females, with a mean age of 45.8 years (range: 18–84 years) and the mean duration of follow-up was 62 months (range: 26–108 months). The etiologies were open fracture of the lower

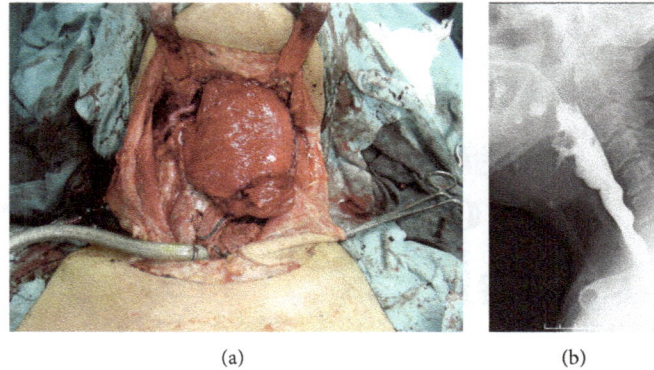

(a)   (b)

FIGURE 1: (a) The second jejunal vessels were anastomosed to lingual artery and internal jugular vein with vein grafts. (b) The postoperative X-ray finding of swallowing. There were no leakage and stenosis.

extremity in 6 patients, lower extremity osteomyelitis in 4 patients, hypopharyngeal carcinoma in 3 patients, and degloving injury in 2 patients. The timing of grafting was immediate in 3 patients, within 7 days in 8 patients, at 6–12 months after injury in 2 patients, and at 12–24 months after injury in 2 patients. Anatomic sites of free tissue transfers were the lower extremity in 10 patients, neck in 3 patients, forearm in 1 patient, and hand in 1 patient. Free tissue was obtained from the fibula in 4 patients, the anterolateral thigh in 3 patients, the groin in 3 patients, the jejunum in 3 patients, the latissimus dorsi in 1 patient, and the dorsal pedis in 1 patient. Grafted donor veins were the saphenous vein in 12 patients and the external jugular vein in 3 patients. The mean length of the grafted veins was 10.8 cm (range: 4–18 cm). Recipient arteries were the posterior tibial artery in 5 patients, the anterior tibial artery in 3 patients, the lingual artery in 3 patients, the popliteal artery in 1 patient, and the radial artery in 1 patient. The recipient veins were the posterior tibial vein in 4 patients, the anterior tibial vein in 2 patients, the saphenous vein in 1 patient, the internal jugular vein in 1 patient, and the cephalic vein in 1 patient. For vein graft-associated complications, congestion developed in 2 patients (1 patient with a degloving injury who underwent a free groin flap and 1 patient with osteomyelitis who underwent a free vascularized fibular flap), for whom additional vein grafts were performed. Though these 2 patients developed partial epidermal necrosis, these flaps survived. In the other 13 patients who received vein grafts, no postoperative complications were encountered, and all flaps survived (Table 1). During the study period, postoperative complications developed in 6 of the 127 patients who underwent a free tissue transfer without vein grafts, and necrosis was found in 3 of these 6 patients. Free flap survival was confirmed in 124 of the 127 patients who did not receive vein grafts. No significant differences in success rates were seen between patients who underwent free tissue transfers with or without vein grafts.

4. Case Reports

4.1. Case 6. A 71-year-old man with hypopharyngeal carcinoma (staging: T4N2M0) underwent esophageal reconstruction with a free jejunal transfer after undergoing a total pharyngolaryngoesophagectomy and selective neck dissection. With a free jejunal transfer, a second jejunal artery anastomosis to the lingual artery was performed, but thrombosis formation recurred at the anastomotic site. As a result, the free jejunum became a short pedicle, and a vein graft was therefore used to compensate for the insufficient vessel length. An 8 cm long vein harvested from the ipsilateral external jugular vein was interposed between the second jejunal artery and the lingual artery. In addition, a 5 cm external jugular vein was interposed between the second jejunal vein and the internal jugular vein, and the kinking of the vein at the anastomotic site was resolved. After vein graft, thrombosis did not develop, and the free jejunum survived. Neither postoperative leakage nor stenosis occurred at the anastomotic site of the intestinal tract (Figure 1).

4.2. Case 11. A 70-year-old man suffered from an open fracture of the left lower extremity in a traffic accident and underwent plate fixation. Because the fracture site became infected and osteomyelitis developed, the plate was removed, and the site of the bone defect was filled with antibiotic-impregnated cement after debridement. We decided to reconstruct the tibia with a free vascularized fibular flap from the opposite side. Due to the influence of scarring, the appropriate vessels for anastomosis could not be found at the recipient site. The recipient vessel was dissected on the proximal side, away from the zone of injury, and posterior tibial vessels were selected. The saphenous vein on the opposite thigh was harvested for vein grafting and was interposed in the approximately 7 cm length between the fibular vessels and the posterior tibial vessels. Thrombosis did not develop in the free vascularized fibular flap postoperatively and the flap survived. Union of the grafted fibula was obtained 8 months postoperatively. Tibial osteomyelitis has not recurred as of 50 months postoperatively (Figure 2).

4.3. Case 14. A 52-year-old man with diabetes mellitus sustained a deep burn injury to the left foot. The wound progressed to osteomyelitis of the 1st metatarsal bone. The bone defect was filled with antibiotic-impregnated cement after debridement. Six months later, we reconstruct the 1st

TABLE 1: Patients summary.

Patient number	Age, year	Sex	Etiology	Anatomic site	Type of free tissue	Recipient a.	Recipient v.	Vein graft	Complication	Result	Comments
1	39	M	Open fracture	Lower extremity	Groin	Ant. tibial a.	Ant. tibial v.	Interarterial and intervenous		Successful	
2	27	M	Degloving injury	Hand	Dorsal pedis	Radial a.		Interarterial		Successful	
3	18	M	Degloving injury	Forearm	Groin		Cephalic v.	Intervenous	Congestion	Reexploration	Survival
4	38	M	Open fracture	Lower extremity	Groin		Saphenous v.	Intervenous		Successful	
5	34	F	Open fracture	Lower extremity	ALT	Ant. tibial a.	Ant. tibial v.	Interarterial and intervenous		Successful	
6	71	M	Hypopharyngeal ca.	Neck	Jejunum	Lingual a.	Internal jugular v.	Interarterial and intervenous		Successful	
7	22	M	Open fracture	Lower extremity	ALT	Post. tibial a.		Interarterial		Successful	
8	21	M	Open fracture	Lower extremity	ALT	Ant. tibial a.		Interarterial		Successful	
9	65	M	Osteomyelitis	Lower extremity	Fibula	Post. tibial a.	Post. tibial v.	Interarterial and intervenous		Successful	
10	59	M	Hypopharyngeal ca.	Neck	Jejunum	Lingual a.		Interarterial		Successful	
11	70	M	Osteomyelitis	Lower extremity	Fibula	Post. tibial a.	Post. tibial v.	Interarterial and intervenous		Successful	
12	57	M	Osteomyelitis	Lower extremity	Fibula	Post. tibial a.	Post. tibial v.	Interarterial and intervenous		Successful	
13	30	F	Open fracture	Lower extremity	Latissimus dorsi	Popliteal a.		Interarterial		Successful	
14	52	M	Osteomyelitis	Lower extremity	Fibula	Post. tibial a.	Post. tibial v.	Interarterial and intervenous	Congestion	Reexploration	Survival
15	84	M	Hypopharyngeal ca.	Neck	Jejunum	Lingual a.		Interarterial		Successful	

ALT: anterolateral thigh.

(a)

(b)

(c)

(d)

(e)

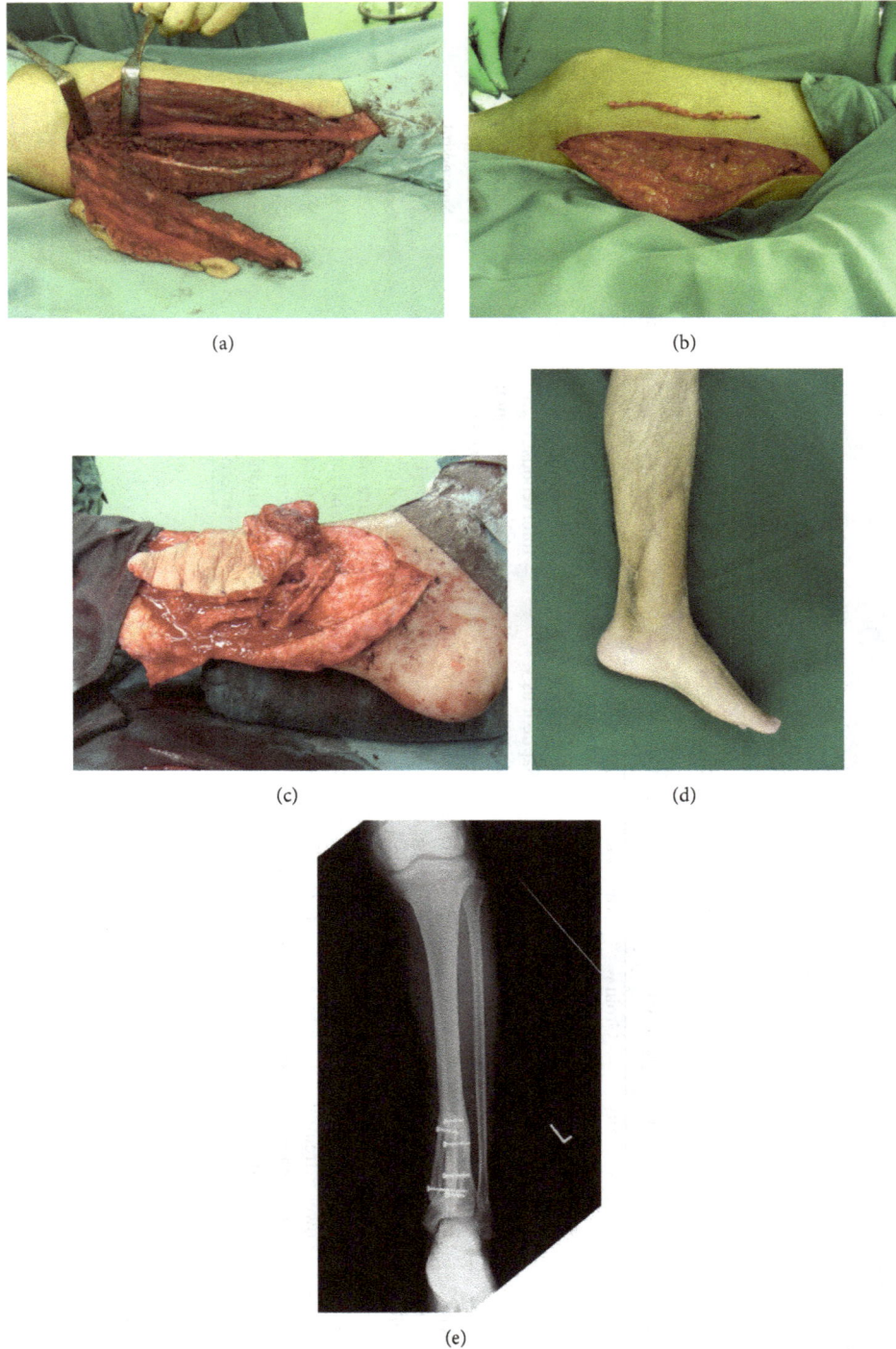

FIGURE 2: (a) The vascularized fibular flap. (b) The saphenous vein was harvested from right thigh. (c) The saphenous veins were interposed between fibular vessels and posterior tibial vessels. (d) The postoperative view of 50 months after surgery. (e) The osteomyelitis did not recur during the 50 months follow-up period.

metatarsal bone with a free vascularized ipsilateral fibular flap. Due to the avoidance of scarring around the 1st metatarsal bone, vein grafts were required to anastomose fibular vessels of the flap and the healthy recipient vessels. The vein grafts were the interposed fibular artery to the dorsal pedis artery and 2 comitant veins to 2 cutaneous veins. The vascularized fibular flap progressed to congestion the next day. We explored the anastomotic site and detected thrombosis in the interposed vein between the comitant vein and the cutaneous vein. The primary grafted vein with thrombosis

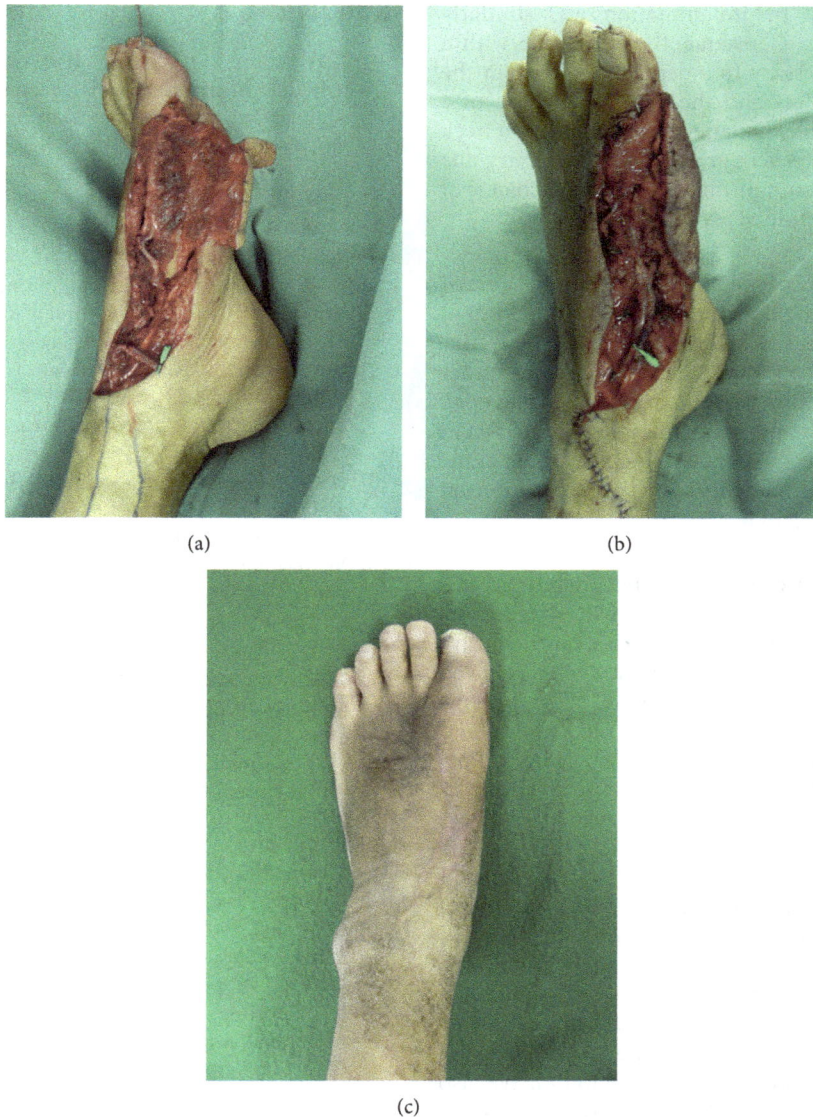

FIGURE 3: (a) Primary vein grafts were performed for an interarterial and 2 intervenous grafts. (b) Thrombosis was found in the primary vein graft between the comitant vein and the cutaneous vein. (c) Postoperative view 12 months after flap transfer with vein grafts.

was resected, and the contralateral small saphenous vein interposed the venous defect between the comitant vein and the healthy cutaneous vein. The congestion of the flap was ameliorated and survived. The osteomyelitis did not recur up to 12 months postoperatively (Figure 3).

5. Discussion

Vein grafting is an important technique in reconstructive microsurgery [7–13]. The combined usage of vein grafts with a free tissue transfer is applicable for trauma and neck dissection or when problems exist with the condition of recipient vessels due to radiation, pedicle length, or differences in the caliber of vessels for anastomosis. In animal studies [14, 15], the patency rate of vein grafts is similar to that for normal vascular anastomosis. Despite this, the success rate for a free

tissue transfer combined with vein grafts varies between 70% and 95%, depending on the report, and postoperative outcomes have not been consistent, leading to continual discussions on the appropriate use of vein grafting [3–6, 16]. Cheng et al. [17] stated that the failure rate of free tissue transfers combined with vein grafts is approximately 5 times greater than that of free tissue transfers without vein grafts and that the combined usage of vein grafts should be avoided if possible. However, we believe that this combined procedure cannot be avoided and that its usefulness will increase if the reliability of vein grafting can be improved.

In the free tissue transfer combined with vein graft that we performed, 8 patients underwent this operation due to trauma, 4 patients due to infection, and 3 patients due to malignant neck tumor. The soft tissue injury was extensive in degloving injury and open fracture of the lower extremity, and the scarring caused by inflammation was similarly extensive in osteomyelitis. Consequently, free tissue with a long pedicle became necessary to a degree greater than the amount of soft tissue defect and the combined usage of a vein graft became inevitable. In patients with malignant neck tumor, combined usage of a vein graft became necessary due to the extent of malignant tumor infiltration, aging change of recipient vessels, and the influence of radiation.

Bayramiçli et al. [6] succeeded in lower extremity reconstruction using a free tissue transfer with vein grafts in 21 of 22 patients and recommended having a detailed preoperative surgical plan and selecting appropriate recipient vessels under a magnifier when performing vein grafts. Schusterman et al. [13] also reported satisfactory outcomes in planned vein grafts. Planning free tissue transfer combined with vein grafts in advance is important in patients with poor conditions at the recipient sites.

Miller et al. [4] stated coagulation abnormality as well as scarring due to prior operation and radiation as factors affecting outcomes for vein grafts. In our series, postoperative congestion developed in 2 of the 15 patients who received free tissue transfer with vein grafts. One of these patients received a free vascularized fibular flap for osteomyelitis and the other received a groin flap for a degloving injury. Postosteomyelitis scarring and the influence on recipient veins due to the degloving injury were thought to be the causes of congestion. In both patients, we were able to achieve flap survival with early reexploration by dissecting the recipient vessel toward the healthy portion on the proximal side of the initial vessel anastomotic site. Germann and Steinau [5] stated that, although free tissue transfer combined with vein grafts carries a greater complication rate, no significant differences in the ultimate flap survival rate were seen when conducting strict postoperative monitoring and performing early revision when abnormal findings were found. We also salvaged free flaps where congestion occurred with strict monitoring and prompt reexploration, indicating that strict postoperative monitoring is essential for the success of free tissue transfers with vein grafts.

6. Conclusion

We obtained comparable clinical outcomes with both free tissue transfer combined with vein grafts and free tissue transfer without vein grafts. To improve the success rate of free tissue transfer combined with vein grafts, securing healthy recipient vessels, meticulous surgical handling, reliable vascular anastomosis techniques, and postoperative monitoring are crucial.

Acknowledgment

The authors thank Robert E. Brandt, Founder, CEO, and CME, of MedEd, Japan, for editing and preparing the paper.

References

[1] T. M. Whitney, H. J. Buncke, W. C. Lineaweaver, and B. S. Alpert, "Multiple microvascular transplants: a preliminary report of simultaneous versus sequential reconstruction," Annals of Plastic Surgery, vol. 22, no. 5, pp. 391–404, 1989.

[2] R. K. Khouri and W. W. Shaw, "Reconstruction of the lower extremity with microvascular free flaps: a 10-year experience with 304 consecutive cases," Journal of Trauma, vol. 29, no. 8, pp. 1086–1094, 1989.

[3] A. Oliva, "Interposition vein grafting in head and neck reconstructive microsurgery," Journal of Reconstructive Microsurgery, vol. 9, no. 4, pp. 319–320, 1993.

[4] M. J. Miller, M. A. Schusterman, G. P. Reece, and S. S. Kroll, "Interposition vein grafting in head and neck reconstructive microsurgery," Journal of Reconstructive Microsurgery, vol. 9, no. 3, pp. 245–251, 1993.

[5] G. Germann and H.-U. Steinau, "The clinical reliability of vein grafts in free-flap transfer," Journal of Reconstructive Microsurgery, vol. 12, no. 1, pp. 11–17, 1996.

[6] M. Bayramiçli, C. Tetik, A. Sönmez, R. Gürünlüoğlu, and F. Baltaci, "Reliability of primary vein grafts in lower extremity free tissue transfers," Annals of Plastic Surgery, vol. 48, no. 1, pp. 21–29, 2002.

[7] H. J. Buncke, B. Alpert, and K. G. Shah, "Microvascular grafting," Clinics in Plastic Surgery, vol. 5, no. 2, pp. 185–194, 1978.

[8] M. S. Moneim and N. E. Chacon, "Salvage of replanted parts of the upper extremity," The Journal of Bone and Joint Surgery Series A, vol. 67, no. 6, pp. 880–883, 1985.

[9] F. Nahai and R. Hagerty, "One-stage microvascular transfer of a latissimus flap to the sacrum using vein grafts," Plastic and Reconstructive Surgery, vol. 77, no. 2, pp. 312–315, 1986.

[10] G. G. Hallock, "The interposition arteriovenous loop revisited," Journal of Reconstructive Microsurgery, vol. 4, no. 2, pp. 155–159, 1988.

[11] J. C. Grotting, "Prevention of complications and correction of postoperative problems in microsurgery of the lower extremity," Clinics in Plastic Surgery, vol. 18, no. 3, pp. 485–489, 1991.

[12] S.-Y. Horng and M.-T. Chen, "Reversed cephalic vein: a lifeboat in head and neck free-flap reconstruction," Plastic and Reconstructive Surgery, vol. 92, no. 4, pp. 752–753, 1993.

[13] M. A. Schusterman, M. J. Miller, G. P. Reece et al., "A single center's experience with 308 free flaps for repair of head and neck cancer defects," Plastic and Reconstructive Surgery, vol. 93, no. 3, pp. 472–480, 1994.

[14] F. Zhang, A. Oliva, S. D. Kao, L. Newlin, H. J. Buncke, and A. Daniller, "Microvascular vein-graft patency in the rat model," Journal of Reconstructive Microsurgery, vol. 10, no. 4, pp. 223–227, 1994.

[15] F. Zhang, A. Oliva, S. D. Kao, L. Newlin, and H. J. Buncke, "Microvascular vein grafts in the rat cutaneous free-flap model," Journal of Reconstructive Microsurgery, vol. 10, no. 4, pp. 229–233, 1994.

[16] A. L. D. Kruse, H. T. Luebbers, K. W. Grätz, and J. A. Obwegeser, "Factors influencing survival of free-flap in reconstruction for cancer of the head and neck: a literature review," Microsurgery, vol. 30, no. 3, pp. 242–248, 2010.

[17] H. T. Cheng, F. Y. Lin, and S. C. N. Chang, "Evidence-based analysis of vein graft interposition in head and neck free flap reconstruction," Plastic and Reconstructive Surgery, vol. 129, no. 5, pp. 853e–854e, 2012.

3

Analysis of Complications in Postbariatric Abdominoplasty: Our Experience

Michele Grieco, Eugenio Grignaffini, Francesco Simonacci, and Edoardo Raposio

Department of Surgical Sciences, Plastic Surgery Division, University of Parma and Cutaneous, Regenerative,

Mininvasive and Plastic Surgery Unit, Azienda Ospedaliero-Universitaria di Parma, Via Gramsci 14, 43126 Parma, Italy

Correspondence should be addressed to Michele Grieco; dr.mgrieco@yahoo.it

Academic Editor: Selahattin Özmen

Abdominoplasty is one of the most popular body-contouring procedures. It is associated with a significant number of complications: the most common ones are seroma, hematoma, infection, wound-healing problems, and skin flap necrosis. From January 2012 to December 2014, 25 patients (18 women and 7 men) (mean age: 51 years) underwent abdominoplastic surgery at the Plastic Surgery Section, Department of Surgical Sciences, University of Parma, Italy. All patients reported a weight loss between 15 kg and 47 kg. All of the of 25 patients were included in the study; minor and major complications were seen in 17 (68%) and 8 (32%) patients, respectively. The percentage of complications in our patients was as follows: 9 patients with seroma (36%); 4 patients with wound dehiscence with delayed wound healing (16%); 3 cases with hematoma (12%); 2 patients with postoperative bleeding (8%); 1 patient (4%) with an umbilical necrosis; 1 patient (4%) with a deep vein thrombosis; 3 patients with infected seroma (12%); and 2 patients with wound infection (8%). There were no cases of postoperative mortality. The aim of this study is to analyze our complications in postbariatric abdominoplasty.

1. Introduction

Abdominoplasty is one of the most popular body-contouring procedures: it is a surgical technique reliable and safe. It is among the top five procedures in aesthetic surgery in the Unites States [1]. However, it is associated with a significant number of complications (32–37.4%) [2, 3]: the most common ones are seroma, hematoma, infection, wound-healing problems, and skin flap necrosis [4, 5]. The aim of postbariatric abdominoplasty was to remove the excess of skin and redundant fat in order to recreate a slim profile [6]. The bariatric population generally presents with a persistently elevated BMI despite having achieved massive weight loss [7]. Obesity is a known risk factor for complications after abdominoplasty [8], but nevertheless an increasing number of abdominoplasties are performed after the boom of bariatric procedures and consequently there are an increasing number of complications [9]. According to Hensel et al., we can define early or minor complications as those occurring in the immediate postoperative period and that were not life-threatening, did not extend hospital stay, and could be managed easily as an outpatient. All the other complications were defined as major ones [2].

2. Materials and Methods

From January 2012 to December 2014, 25 patients (18 women and 7 men) aged between 24 years and 79 years (mean age: 51 years) underwent abdominoplastic surgery at the Plastic Surgery Section, Department of Surgical Sciences, University of Parma, Italy. All patients reported a weight loss between 15 kg and 47 kg (average weight lost: 29 kg), obtained by previous bariatric surgery (14 Pt; 11 F and 3 M) or following a specific diet regimen (11 Pt; 7 F and 4 M). Six months after bariatric surgery, the patients were eligible for functional abdominoplasty. The patients were also advised to stop smoking and female patients were recommended to avoid oral contraception 1 month before surgery. All the procedures were performed with the patient under general anesthesia. The patient is marked in a standing position preoperatively. The skin incision was designed before the intervention as "transverse incision" designed at the superior level of the

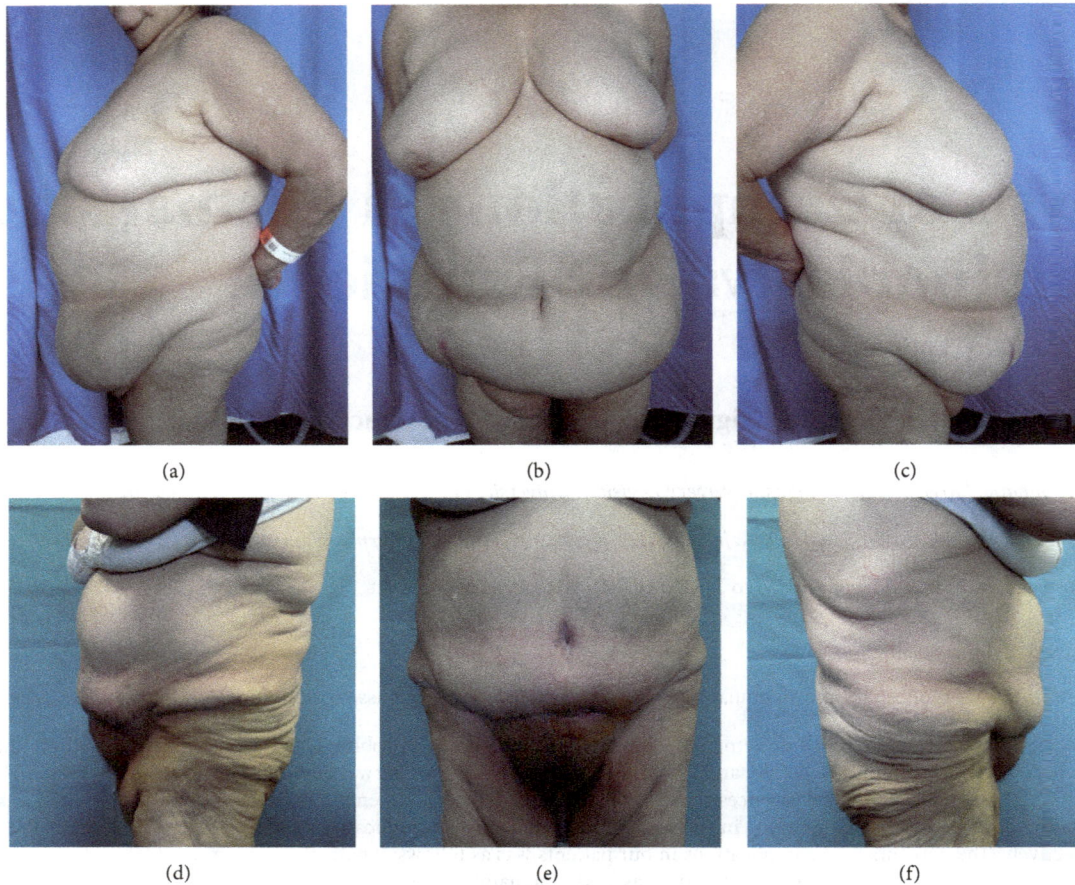

(a)   (b)   (c)

(d)   (e)   (f)

FIGURE 1: Patient with seroma: (a) + (b) + (c) preoperative case; (d) + (e) + (f) postoperative case.

symphysis pubis and continued laterally to the iliac spines or was designed as inverted "T." Intraoperatively, the patient was placed in a supine position with the arms abducted 90°. A single-shot second-generation cephalosporin was administered routinely. After the surgical incision of the skin, suprafascial dissection was carried out up to the xiphoid, with a lateral extension depending on the desired magnitude of medial skin shift. At this point, the stage is set to perform myofascial plication, to correct the rectus muscles diastasis. If there were important diastase, incisional hernias, and/or hernias, we prefer to place a polypropylene mesh that had been applied in collaboration with the general surgeons. Following skin resection and reinsertion of the umbilicus, skin closure was performed with absorbable monofilament (Vicryl 2/0 and 3/0 Monosyn). Routinely, two or four suction drains were placed. Postoperatively the drains were removed when fluid collection was <30 mL/24 h, and an abdominal binder was used for 4 weeks postoperatively. For all patients, antibiotic therapy was also administered immediately preoperatively and it was continued for 10 days. Postoperative care included 10 days of treatment with low molecular weight heparin to prevent major complications such as deep vein thrombosis and pulmonary embolism. Social activity was limited for 4 weeks after the discharge.

3. Results

Average weight of the 25 patients before surgery was 83,5 kg (range: 58 to 163 kg); average BMI was 31 kg/m^2 (range 24,77 to 57). All of the 25 patients were included in the study (18 females and 7 males), with a mean age of 51 years at the time of surgery; minor and major complications were seen in 17 (68%) and 8 (32%) patients, respectively. The percentage of complications in our patients was as follows: seroma in 9 patients (36%) (6 F and 3 M) (Figure 1); microbiological swab with antibiogram of the aspirated liquid for the evaluation of any superinfection was performed on all the 9 patients: the replacement of the specific home antibiotic therapy was necessary only for 3 among the 9 patients because of superinfection, in the absence of dehiscence of the wound. In 4 patients, we observed wound dehiscence whit delayed wound healing (16%) (3 F and 1 M) (Figure 2); in all these 4 patients, a punch biopsy from the diastasic wound was done to perform a microbiological analysis of the tissue and the related antibiogram: the home antibiotic therapy was necessarily replaced with a specific postbuffer therapy only in 2 patients (2 F). We observed hematoma in 3 cases (12%) (1 F and 2 M) and postoperative bleeding in 2 patients (8%) (1 F and 1 M) for whom it was necessary to reoperate within 24 hours from

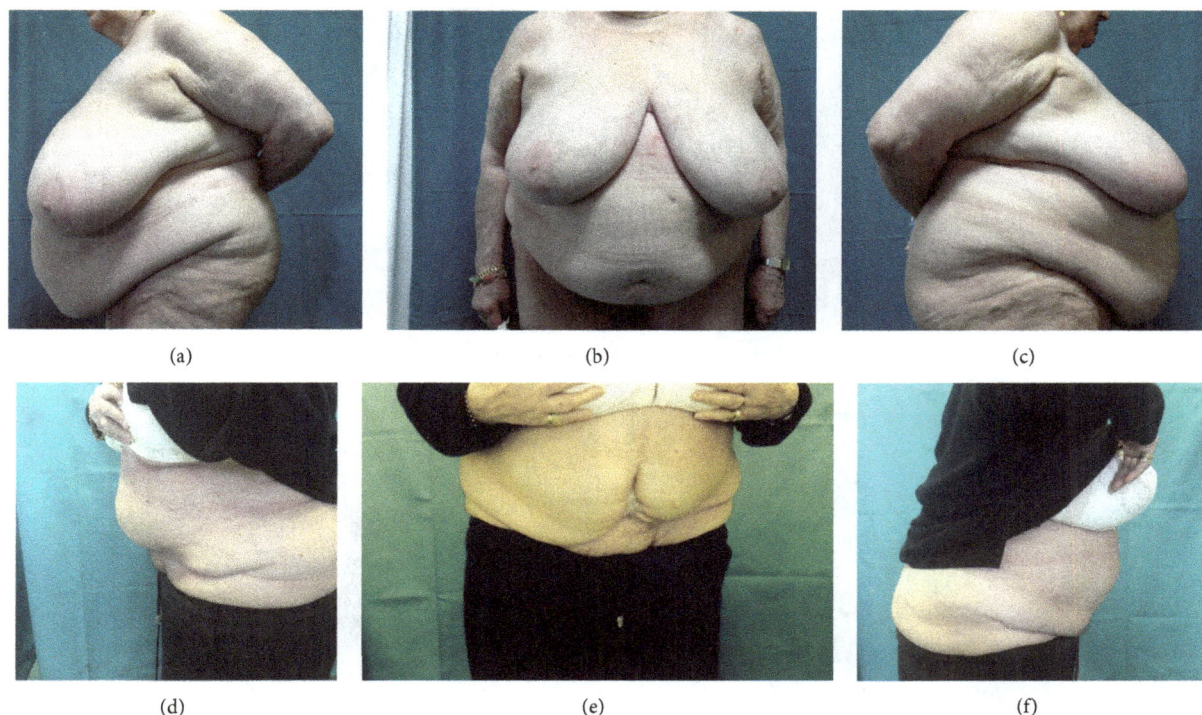

FIGURE 2: Patient with wound dehiscence: (a) + (b) + (c) preoperative case; (d) + (e) + (f) postoperative case.

TABLE 1: Minor complications after abdominoplasty in 25 patients.

Total minor complications	17 (68%)
Hematoma	3 (12%)
Seroma	9 (36%)
Skin necrosis	0
Umbilical necrosis	1 (4%)
Wound dehiscence/delayed wound healing	4 (16%)

TABLE 2: Major complications after abdominoplasty in 25 patients.

Total major complications	8 (32%)
Abscess	0
Bleeding	2 (8%)
Deep vein thrombosis and pulmonary embolism	1 (4%)
Infected seroma	3 (12%)
Wound infection	2 (8%)

the first surgery. Only in 1 female patient have we seen an umbilical necrosis (Figure 3), which was followed by a cycle of dressings until complete healing in a scar well accepted by the patient. Only in 1 male patient have we seen a deep vein thrombosis for which a therapy with low molecular weight heparin for 1 month was necessary (Tables 1-2).

4. Discussion

Abdominoplasty or abdominal dermolipectomy is a well-established procedure for improving body contour in aesthetic plastic surgery, with over a 100-year experience since its first publication by Kelly in 1899 [10]. Subsequently, the technique was perfected by Thorek [11] and Pitanguy [12], which, respectively, describe a procedure for preserving the navel and suturing the fascia of the rectus muscles. Considering the increasing popularity of abdominoplasty, there is renewed focus on technical refinements, not only to improve postoperative appearance but also to reduce postoperative complications. A multitude of risk factors has been proposed in the plastic surgery literature, which increased the rate of complications, including smoking [13], obesity [8], hypertension [14], and previous abdominal surgery (gynecologic versus weight-loss procedure) [15]. Obese patients (BMI > $30 \, \text{kg/m}^2$) had an increased total, major, and minor complication rate as compared with nonobese patients (BMI < $30 \, \text{kg/m}^2$) [7, 16]. These obese patients are bariatric patients who remain obese despite prior weight-reduction surgery [7]. Patients' expectations are sometimes underestimated, resulting in dissatisfaction and an increased frequency of follow-up. Our major and minor complication rate were 60% and 11,5%, respectively, which is seemingly consistent with the current literature. Seroma was our most frequent complication [4] according to the literature. It mainly occurs in overweight patients, in those who present a massive weight loss and in patients who present a dead space between the fascia and the abdominal flap after surgery [17], sequential aspirations may be necessary to treat this complication. Seroma is considered a minor complication and therefore is underreported by patients. This complication occurs in 38 to 42% of cases [4, 17, 18]. During abdominoplasty, the use of quilting suture technique described by Baroudi and Ferreira [19] or

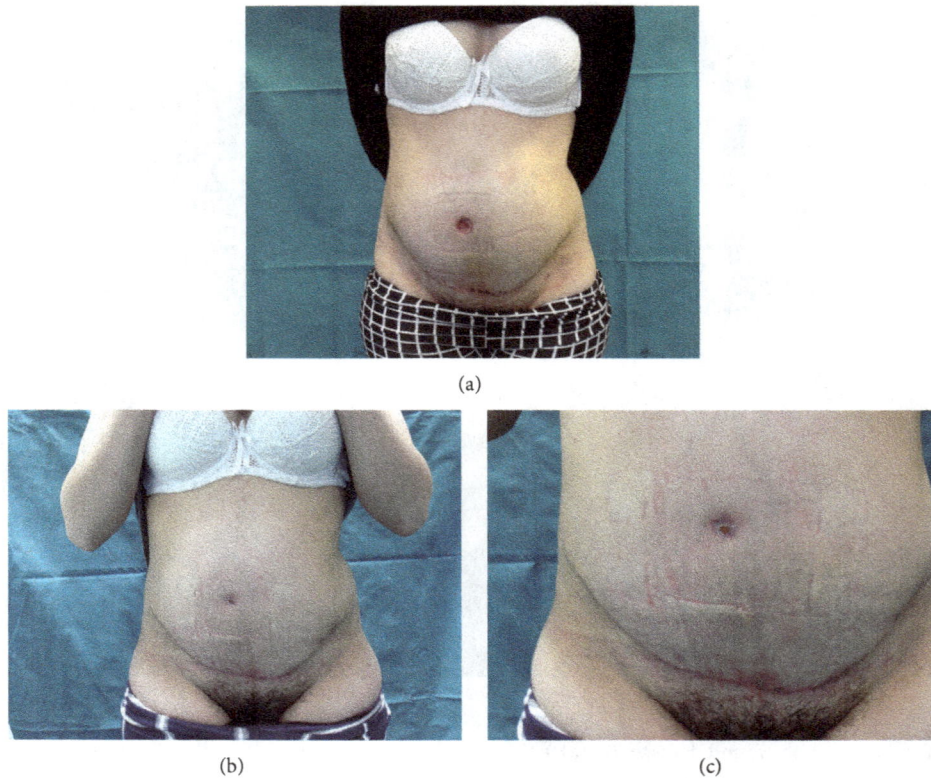

FIGURE 3: Patient with umbilical necrosis: (a) necrosis of the umbilicus; (b) + (c) navel closed.

the use of progressive tension sutures as described by H. Pollock and T. Pollock [20], between the abdominal flap and the rectus abdominis, might help in preventing seroma formation. Similarly, prophylactic drains placement in abdominoplasty has been described as an attempt to reduce seroma formation [21–23]. Hematomas are potential complications of any surgery including abdominoplasty. The frequency of hematoma was less than that of seroma; it occurs in 0.8% to 3% [24] of patients who have undergone abdominoplasty; however, the outcomes were more severe. Hematoma formation was detected by clinical examination, by abdominal ultrasound, and then by aspiration [25]. Abdominal wound-healing problems may occur more readily in previously obese patients [24]. It can arise due to inadequate deep closure or inadvertent straightening-up during the early postoperative period. Different factors can cause the rise of this complication: the presurgery BMI > 25 Kg/m^2, the concomitant mellitus diabetes, and the tabagism [13, 26]; also the tissue manipulation, associated with surgery, alters the healing process of the wound because of the release of a massive amount of mediators that influence both the coagulation and the complement activity and may therefore compromise the immune system [27, 28]. According to Araco [24, 26] in postbariatric patients, we performed a dissection with diathermocoagulation to reduce the occurrence of postoperative hematomas and wound infections with delayed healing compared with the cold knife. Generally, as long as they are small, conservative wound management and avoiding further stretch on the wound will allow these areas to heal by secondary

intention with no significant long-term effect on the overall quality of the scar. This complication is often associated with wound infection [8–13]. In our experience, the most common organisms isolated were *Staphylococcus epidermidis, Staphylococcus aureus,* and *Escherichia coli.* The treatment is appropriate antibiotics, evacuation and drainage of an abscess if present, and debridement and dressing changes. There were no cases of postoperative mortality.

5. Conclusion

Postoperative complications were frequent. Patients with complications had a significantly higher reoperation rate, longer hospital stay, and more dissatisfaction. Previous bariatric surgery procedure may play a role similar to so many other widely investigated risk factors such as smoking and BMI, and some categories of patients should require even more attention in the preoperative, intraoperative, and postoperative management. In our experience, often we find patients with great expectations prior to abdominoplasty. For this reason, we believe it is extremely important to inform these patients in the preoperative period about the increased risk of complications that may be incurred with respect to a patient who performs this surgery for aesthetic.

References

[1] American Society of Plastic Surgeons, http://www.plasticsurgery.org/.

[2] J. M. Hensel, J. A. Lehman Jr., M. P. Tantri, M. G. Parker, D. S. Wagner, and N. S. Topham, "An outcomes analysis and satisfaction survey of 199 consecutive abdominoplasties," *Annals of Plastic Surgery*, vol. 46, no. 4, pp. 357–363, 2001.

[3] C. Floros and P. K. B. Davis, "Complications and long-term results following abdominoplasty: a retrospective study," *British Journal of Plastic Surgery*, vol. 44, no. 3, pp. 190–194, 1991.

[4] F. Hafezi and A. H. Nouhi, "Abdominoplasty and seroma," *Annals of Plastic Surgery*, vol. 48, no. 1, pp. 109–110, 2002.

[5] J. H. Van Uchelen, P. M. N. Werker, and M. Kon, "Complications of abdominoplasty in 86 patients," *Plastic and Reconstructive Surgery*, vol. 107, no. 7, pp. 1869–1873, 2001.

[6] M. Fraccalvieri, G. Datta, P. Bogetti et al., "Abdominoplasty after weight loss in morbidly obese patients: a 4-year clinical experience," *Obesity Surgery*, vol. 17, no. 10, pp. 1319–1324, 2007.

[7] K. C. Neaman and J. E. Hansen, "Analysis of complications from abdominoplasty: a review of 206 cases at a university hospital," *Annals of Plastic Surgery*, vol. 58, no. 3, pp. 292–298, 2007.

[8] V. L. Vastine, R. F. Morgan, G. S. Williams et al., "Wound complications of abdominoplasty in obese patients," *Annals of Plastic Surgery*, vol. 42, no. 1, pp. 34–39, 1999.

[9] American Society of Plastic Surgeons, *2004 National Plastic Surgery Statistics*, American Society of Plastic Surgeons, 2005, http://www.plasticsurgery.org/public_education/2005Statistics.cfm.

[10] H. A. Kelly, "Report of gynecological cases (excessive growth of fat)," *The Johns Hopkins Medical Journal*, vol. 10, article 197, 1899.

[11] M. Thorek, "Plastic reconstruction of the female breasts and abdomen," *The American Journal of Surgery*, vol. 43, no. 2, pp. 268–278, 1939.

[12] I. Pitanguy, "Abdominal lipectomy: an approach to it trhough an analysis of 300 consecutive cases," *Plastic and Reconstructive Surgery*, vol. 40, pp. 384–391, 1967.

[13] E. H. Manassa, C. H. Hertl, and R.-R. Olbrisch, "Wound healing problems in smokers and nonsmokers after 132 abdominoplasties," *Plastic and Reconstructive Surgery*, vol. 111, no. 6, pp. 2082–2087, 2003.

[14] A. Momeni, M. Heier, H. Bannasch, and G. B. Stark, "Complications in abdominoplasty: a risk factor analysis," *Journal of Plastic, Reconstructive & Aesthetic Surgery*, vol. 62, no. 10, pp. 1250–1254, 2009.

[15] H. A. El-Khatib and A. Bener, "Abdominal dermolipectomy in an abdomen with pre-existing scars: a different concept," *Plastic and Reconstructive Surgery*, vol. 114, no. 4, pp. 992–997, 2004.

[16] M. Rogliani, E. Silvi, L. Labardi, F. Maggiulli, and V. Cervelli, "Obese and nonobese patients: complications of abdominoplasty," *Annals of Plastic Surgery*, vol. 57, no. 3, pp. 336–338, 2006.

[17] F. X. Nahas, L. M. Ferreira, and C. Ghelfond, "Does quilting suture prevent seroma in abdominoplasty?" *Plastic and Reconstructive Surgery*, vol. 119, no. 3, pp. 1060–1064, 2007.

[18] M. E. Bercial, M. S. Neto, J. A. Calil, L. A. Rossetto, and L. M. Ferreira, "Suction drains, quilting sutures, and fibrin sealant in the prevention of seroma formation in abdominoplasty: which is the best strategy?" *Aesthetic Plastic Surgery*, vol. 36, no. 2, pp. 370–373, 2012.

[19] R. Baroudi and C. A. A. Ferreira, "Seroma: how to avoid it and how to treat it," *Aesthetic Surgery Journal*, vol. 18, no. 6, pp. 439–441, 1998.

[20] H. Pollock and T. Pollock, "Progressive tension sutures: a technique to reduce local complications in abdominoplasty," *Plastic and Reconstructive Surgery*, vol. 105, no. 7, pp. 2583–2586, 2000.

[21] R. M. Najera, W. Asheld, S. M. Sayeed, and L. T. Glickman, "Comparison of seroma formation following abdominoplasty with or without liposuction," *Plastic and Reconstructive Surgery*, vol. 127, no. 1, pp. 417–422, 2011.

[22] R. C. Fang, S. J. Lin, and T. A. Mustoe, "Abdominoplasty flap elevation in a more superficial plane: decreasing the need for drains," *Plastic and Reconstructive Surgery*, vol. 125, no. 2, pp. 677–682, 2010.

[23] B. Teimourian, "Management of seroma in abdominoplasty," *Aesthetic Surgery Journal*, vol. 25, no. 5, pp. 510–511, 2005.

[24] A. Araco, R. Sorge, J. Overton, F. Araco, and G. Gravante, "Postbariatric patients undergoing body-contouring abdominoplasty: two techniques to raise the flap and their influence on postoperative complications," *Annals of Plastic Surgery*, vol. 62, no. 6, pp. 613–617, 2009.

[25] I. N. Stocchero, "Ultrasound and seromas," *Plastic and Reconstructive Surgery*, vol. 91, no. 1, p. 198, 1993.

[26] A. Araco, G. Gravante, R. Sorge et al., "Wound infections in aesthetic abdominoplasties: the role of smoking," *Plastic and Reconstructive Surgery*, vol. 121, no. 5, pp. 305e–310e, 2008.

[27] H. Sorg, T. Schulz, C. Krueger, and B. Vollmar, "Consequences of surgical stress on the kinetics of skin wound healing: partial hepatectomy delays and functionally alters dermal repair," *Wound Repair and Regeneration*, vol. 17, no. 3, pp. 367–377, 2009.

[28] A. Menderes, C. Baytekin, M. Haciyanli, and M. Yilmaz, "Dermalipectomy for body contouring after bariatric surgery in Aegean region of Turkey," *Obesity Surgery*, vol. 13, no. 4, pp. 637–641, 2003.

4

Complements C3 and C5 Individually and in Combination Increase Early Wound Strength in a Rat Model of Experimental Wound Healing

Hani Sinno,[1,2] Meenakshi Malhotra,[2] Justyn Lutfy,[2] Barbara Jardin,[2] Sebastian Winocour,[1] Fadi Brimo,[3] Lorne Beckman,[4] Kevin Watters,[4] Anie Philip,[1] Bruce Williams,[1] and Satya Prakash[2]

[1] Division of Plastic and Reconstructive Surgery, Department of Surgery, McGill University, Montreal, QC, Canada H3G 1A4
[2] Biomedical Technology and Cell Therapy Research Laboratory, Department of Biomedical Engineering, Faculty of Medicine, McGill University, 3775 Rue University, Room 311, Lyman Duff Medical Building, Montreal, QC, Canada H3A 2B4
[3] Department of Pathology, McGill University, Montreal, QC, Canada H3G 1A4
[4] Orthopedic Research Laboratory, McGill University, Montreal, QC, Canada H3A 1A1

Correspondence should be addressed to Satya Prakash; satya.prakash@mcgill.ca

Academic Editor: Adriaan O. Grobbelaar

Background. Complements C3 and C5 have independently been shown to augment and increase wound healing and strength. Our goal was to investigate the combinatorial effect of complements C3 and C5 on wound healing. *Methods.* Each rat served as its own control where topical collagen was applied to one incision and 100 nM of C3 and C5 in collagen vehicle was applied to the other incision ($n = 6$). To compare between systemic effects, a sham group of rats ($n = 6$) was treated with collagen alone on one wound and saline on the other. At day 3, the tissue was examined for maximal breaking strength (MBS) and sectioned for histological examination. *Results.* There was a statistically significant 88% increase in MBS with the topical application of C3C5 when compared to sham wounds ($n < 0.05$). This was correlated with increased fibroblast and collagen deposition in the treated wounds. Furthermore, there appeared to be an additive hemostatic effect with the C3C5 combination. *Conclusions.* The combination of complements C3 and C5 as a topical application drug to skin wounds significantly increased wound healing maximum breaking strength as early as 3 days.

1. Introduction

Wound healing can be problematic in several clinical settings. The current available surgical and medical options are not always ideal for all patients. The development of a novel therapeutic agent that may help augment the healing process is urgent. An understanding of the intricate cascade of events and cellular interactions is essential in the development of such therapeutic agents.

The complement cascade involves the interaction and cleavage of eleven proteins to form complexes responsible for hemostasis, chemotaxis, and bacterial lysis [1]. Complements

C3 and C5 have independently been shown to play a role in wound healing, augmenting wound strength, and increasing cellular infiltration and collagen deposition [2, 3]. Furthermore, C5 has been shown to accelerate healing by at least four days in the first week of wounding [3]. The synergistic effect of combining C3 and C5 to augment wound healing is not yet known.

We aim to decipher the potential synergistic effects that C3 and C5 may have on wound healing strength. Our objective is to combine C3 and C5 as a topical therapeutic agent to assess changes in wound strength and cellular infiltration. The potential synergistic effect on wound healing can be potentially a great advancement in the understanding of the complex processes of wound healing and translation to a novel therapeutic agent for the use and benefit for patients.

2. Materials and Methods

2.1. In Vivo Experimental Study. All procedures performed were in accordance with the guidelines of the McGill University Committee on Use and Care of Animals and have been approved by the McGill Animal Ethics Committee and Veterinary Care Services. Adult male Sprague-Dawley rats, 300 to 350 g (Charles River; Saint Constant, QC, Canada), were housed one week prior to surgery for acclimatization in clean separate cages and fed ad libitum water and standard rat chow. This study included two groups of experiments.

2.1.1. Group I: Sham Rats. This group ($n = 6$) was used as a control group. Type I collagen was purchased from PureCol (Inamed BioMaterials; Fremont, CA, USA) at concentrations of 6 mg/mL. The pH was adjusted to 4–4.5 by addition of 0.1 M NaOH. Collagen was chosen as a vehicle medium because of its relative inert nature and viscous properties that allows for a theoretical slow-release system [4]. The experimental wounds in the sham rats received collagen and the control side received normal saline (0.9% NaCl, 300 mOsm/L). 1 cc volume of solution was added to each incision.

2.1.2. Group II: C3C5 Rats. In the second group ($n = 6$), the synergistic effect of a combination of C3 and C5 in collagen solution was tested. C3 and C5 were purchased from VWR International (Montreal, Canada) as a stock solution of 250 μg/mL and were added to the collagen solution at concentrations of 100 nM each and were topically applied to the experimental wound and collagen alone on the control wound. 1 cc volume of solution was added to each incision.

2.1.3. Rational for Group Design. Group I rats were used as controls to compare with Group II experimental rats. Each group had two separate incisions. Each incision was treated with a different formulation. In Group I rats, one incision was treated with saline and the other was treated with collagen. Group I rats were not treated with any complement formulation. In Group II rats, one incision was treated with the C3C5 Collagen formulation and the other incision in only collagen formulation (no C3C5 was present). Any changes to wound strength, scar formation, histology, and protein content in Group II rats would be likely secondary to the presence of the C3 and C5 complements as Group I did not have any C3 or C5 treatment. In Group II, If only the C3C5 incisions showed increases in wound strength and not the collagen-treated incisions, then C3C5 does not have a systemic effect and only a local effect. The synergistic wound healing effects of C3 and C5 (Group II) were compared to the individual treatments of C3 (Sinno et al. [2]) and C5 (Sinno et al. [3]). All incision treatments were blinded and randomized to help eliminate any bias.

2.2. Surgical Protocol. Isoflurane gas (4-5% for induction, 1-2% for maintenance) and subcutaneous injection of Carbofen (5 mg/kg) were used to anesthetize the rats. The dorsum was shaved with an electric hair clipper and disinfected with 70% alcohol. Two full-thickness 6 cm linear skin incisions were made in the median plane (2 cm on either side of the midline), beginning 1 cm below the inferior edge of the scapula using sterile no. 10 surgical scalpels [5]. One wound received a single topical application of control solution and the other wound received the same volume of the experimental solution. This allowed each rat to serve as its own control. The incisions were reapproximated with five equidistant surgical clips, and the rats were monitored under heat lamp for an hour postoperatively. Animals were sacrificed on Day 3 using inhaled carbon dioxide gas followed by cervical dislocation. The central 3 cm of the wounds were harvested for tensometry measurements and the outer 3 cm strips were prepared for histological analysis.

2.3. Blood Analysis. To determine any measurable systemic effects on complement serum levels and inflammatory markers, blood tests were conducted during the recovery period at the day of surgery and on the day of sacrifice. A complete blood count and differential were measured looking at the cell count at day 3 as compared to that of the wounding day. Inflammatory markers in the serum such as CRP, C3, and C4 were examined to determine any measurable systemic changes at the different time points. Blood samples were retrieved from the right saphenous vein during the recovery period on the day of wounding and just before sacrifice.

2.4. Tensometry. The maximum wound breaking strength (MWBS) was calculated from three 10 mm strips from each wound ($n = 18$) with a tensometer (Tensometer 10; Monsanto Co., St. Louis, MO, USA). The 10 mm strips were precisely cut using a preformed instrument with two microtome blades separated by a 10 mm thick steel beam. The skin strips were placed vertically between the clamps of the tensometer with the wound at the center (2 cm from each jaw). A force was applied with a constant speed of 10 mm/s until rupture. The forces were plotted on computer software, and the MWBS was measured as the greatest force before rupture of the wounds. Tensile strength is the forces per unit of cross-sectional area. Since the cross-sectional area was made constant in all skin strips (10 mm wide, 40 mm jaw space, and similar adjacent skin width), the MWBS is directly proportional to tensile strength and is used interchangeably in this discussion.

2.5. Histopathology. At the time of sacrifice, the edges of the wounds and any open wounds not utilized for tensometry were excised for histological preparation. Three 5 mm perpendicular sections were placed in a tissue cassette between biopsy sponges. The specimens were then fixed in 10% Formalin, processed, and embedded in paraffin. The skin surface was identified and the specimens were cut at 5 μm intervals perpendicular to the long axis of the wound surface using an Olympus microtome. Hematoxylin and eosin staining was utilized to visualize the gross microscopic

TABLE 1: Effect of the topical application of collagen formulation and the combination of complements C3 and C5.

		Side	Maximal wound breaking strength (g)
Group I	Sham	Collagen	490 ± 57
		Saline	478 ± 86
Group II	C3C5	Collagen	787 ± 93*
		C3C5 in collagen	923 ± 191*

*$P < 0.05$, calculated using the unpaired t-test comparing the MWBS means of experimental wounds (Group II) to those of the Sham wounds (Group I).

cellular architecture. A blinded pathologist examined the slides for assessment of healing and cellular infiltration. A grading scheme was utilized to quantify differences between the specimens: Grade I, few fibroblast infiltrates; Grade II, moderate fibroblast infiltration; and Grade III, maximal fibroblast infiltration. The same grading scheme was used to assess the extent of inflammation and fibrosis in the wounds.

2.6. Statistical Analysis. A paired Student's t-test was utilized to compare means of experimental data between the same rats. The unpaired t-test was utilized to compare mean values of experimental data of different rats. A P value of <0.05 was considered statistically significant. The data is expressed as means ± SE.

3. Results

3.1. Tensometry Analysis. The blinded subjective assessment of the cosmetic appearance of the scars (raised borders, color, width, and general appearance) demonstrated no differences between the collagen-treated wounds as compared to the C3C5-treated wounds at all time points. Furthermore, there were no differences in the cosmetic appearance when Group I wounds were compared to Group II wounds at Day 3.

Mechanical analysis was then performed on the wounded skin. Values for maximal wound breaking strength (MWBS) are presented in Table 1. Values are presented in grams and are proportionally representative of wound tensile strength. *Group II.* C3C5 Rats: the synergistic effect of C3 and C5 was measured on MWBS in rat wounds. There was no difference in MWBS between the C3C5-treated wounds (923 ± 191 g) as compared to the contralateral collagen-treated wounds (787 ± 93 g) at Day 3 in the same rat. However, a significant increase in the MWBS of C3C5-treated wounds was measured when compared to the collagen treated wounds in sham rats ($P <$ 0.05) Figure 1. This translated into an 88% increase in wound tensile strength. Furthermore, the MWBS of the collagen-treated wounds in Group II rats (787 ± 93 g) was significantly higher than that in the collagen-treated wounds in Group I rats (490 ± 57 g), translating to a 61% increase in tensile strength ($P < 0.05$).

3.2. Comparison of C3, C5, and C3C5. C3 and C5 have previously shown to increase MWBS as compared to sham

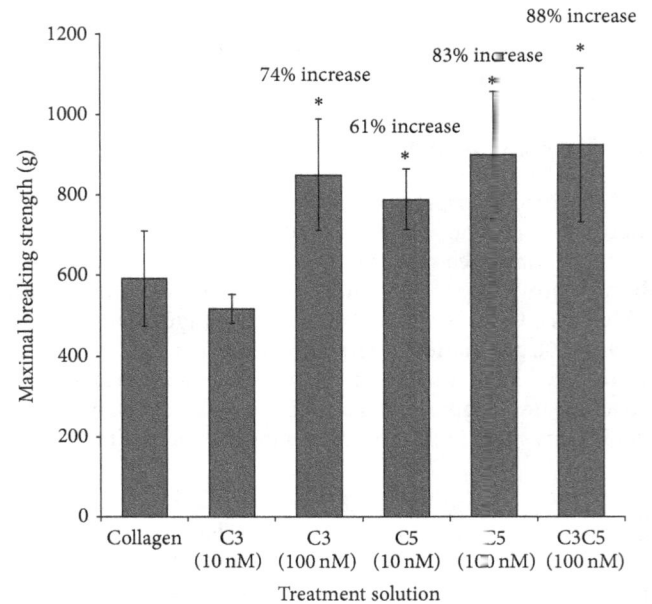

FIGURE 1: Maximal wound breaking strength of treated wounds as compared to control wounds at Day 3. In the horizontal axis, "collagen" represents the tensometry of the collagen treated wounds in the sham rats. The C3 (100 nM) [2], C5 (10 nM) [3], and C5 (100 nM) represent the tensometry of the complement (concentration) in collagen solution on experimental wounds. The C3C5 (100 nM) represents the combination of complements C3 and C5 in collagen formulation at concentrations of 100 nM on experimental wounds. Treatment of wounds with C3 (100 nM), and C5 (10 nM), C5 (100 nM) has been shown previously to increase MWBS as compared to sham wounds. The increase of MWBS attained with the application of C3C5 in combination does not seem to significantly differ than with the administration of C3 and C5 alone. A significant increase of 88% in maximal wound breaking strength can be seen with topical formulation of C3C5 at concentrations of 100 nM at Day 3. *$P < 0.05$.

wounds [2, 3]. Figure 1 illustrates that treatment of wounds with C3 100 nM [2], C5 10 and 100 nM [3], and C3C5 100 nM significantly increases MWBS as compared to the collagen-treated wounds in the sham rats at Day 3. No statistical difference is seen when a comparison between Day 3 MWBS of C3 100 nM, C5 10 nM, C5 100 nM, and C3C5 100 nM treated wounds was performed.

To determine any systemic hematologic or inflammatory effects from the topical application of complement, CBC, CRP, C3, and C4 blood levels were analyzed after the surgery and the day of sacrifice. Blood counts of neutrophils, lymphocytes, monocytes, and eosinophils were not different when compared between Day 0 and Day 3. Platelet count increased from day 0 (626 ± 193) to day 3 (1137 ± 80) in the C3C5-treated rats ($P < 0.05$) as was seen in the sham group. No differences were found in all the inflammatory markers (CRP, C3, and C4) and CBC when C3C5- (Group II) treated rats were compared with sham rats (Group I) except for haemoglobin levels on day 3. The C3C5-treated rats showed

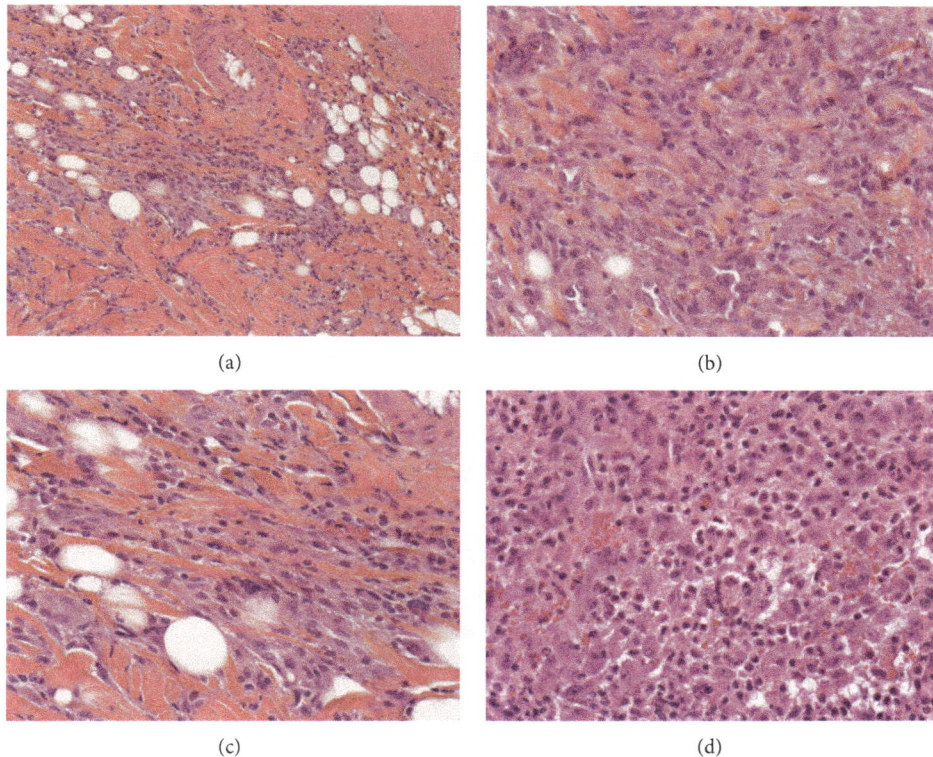

(a)

(b)

(c)

(d)

FIGURE 2: Histological imaging of control and experimental wounds stained with H&E. Blue represents nuclear staining. (a) 20x magnification of a representative control wound at Day 3; (b) 20x magnification of a representative C3C5-treated wound at Day 3; (c) 40x magnification of a representative control wound at Day 3; (d) 40x magnification of a representative C3C5-treated wound at Day 3. There is an increased cellular infiltration in the experimental wounds ((b) and (d)) as compared to control wounds ((a) and (c)) as represented by an increased inflammatory cell nuclear staining. It is evident that an increased extent of inflammation in the C3C5-treated wound beds exists as seen in the lower-power images. There is also an obvious increased collagen deposition and organization in the experimental wounds as seen in higher power images.

a higher haemoglobin content than sham rats at Day 3 after wounding (160 ± 3.3 versus 146 ± 2.2, resp., $P < 0.05$).

The histological analysis was utilized to determine any cellular effects that the C3C5 treatments may have had on wound healing. There was a trend toward a greater number of cellular infiltration and fibroblast deposition and collagen content in the C3C5-treated wounds as compared to the control rats (Figure 2).

4. Discussion

We have previously shown the role of complements C3 and C5 on wound healing [2, 3]. The topical application of either complement on wounds was associated with an increase in wound strength, fibroblasts infiltration, fibronectin, and collagen deposition [2, 3]. In the current study, we attempted to decipher a synergistic role of the application of both C3 and C5 on wounds.

The combination of C3 and C5 at doses of 100 nM showed significant increases in wound strength of up to 88% as compared to control rats. When C3C5-treated wounds were compared to C3-treated wounds and C5-treated wounds, there seemed to be no statistical differences in MWBS. The

combination of C3 and C5 did not show a significant additive effect although there was a trend toward such a difference. The combination of C3 and C5 to wound treatment did not show any significant hematologic or inflammatory changes as compared to sham rats except for an increase in haemoglobin level at Day 3. This increase in haemoglobin is a desirable postoperative feature. One explanation can be related to the haemostatic effect that the complement system has. It seems that combining C3 and C5 may lead to an increase in haemostasis at the time of wounding leading to reduction in intraoperative blood loss, which was visually appreciated but difficult to quantify. Clinically, this may translate to decreases in operative related bleeding and subsequent transfusions.

The application of C3C5 on one wound appeared to increase the wound strength of all wounds within the same rat. There appears to be a systemic effect of the topical application of C3 and C5 to increase wound strength, but this effect does not seem to be additive. This is a desirable feature in the development of a wound healing drug, as all wounds in the body seem to heal faster and stronger. As inflammatory levels including serum C3 levels do not seem to be different between the experimental groups, the cleaved products of C3 and C5 may be diffusing towards the adjacent wounds or even entering the blood stream resulting in the observed systemic wound healing effects. This whole-body healing effect of C3 and C5 seems to be primarily during the first phases of wound healing. It is known that C3 and C5 are spontaneously activated and help form a haemostatic plug in the first seconds of wound formation. Soon after, C3 and C5 become cleaved into smaller proteins that mobilize to form the membrane attach complex and are directly responsible for the opsonisation and death of foreign microorganisms. In addition, early in the inflammatory and proliferative phases of wound healing, C3 and C5 are active in inflammatory cellular chemotaxis. Their primary role in increasing vascular permeability may further accelerate healing by promoting cellular infiltration.

5. Conclusion

Our novel approach to the treatment of wounds with the topical application of complements C3 and C5 is based on the original idea that complements have a normal physiologic reaction in wound healing responsible for haemostasis, microorganism lysis, and inflammatory cell recruitment. We found a trend towards an additive effect on wound strength with the C3C5 combination topical formulation. Furthermore, there appeared to be an additive haemostatic effect leading to a significant decrease in the reduction of postoperative hemoglobin. The increase in wound healing and additive haemostatic effects further support the use of the combination of complements C3 and C5 as a therapeutic agent for incisional wounds.

Funding

The authors would like to acknowledge financial support from Bruce Williams, Division of Plastic Surgery Research Funds and the Canadian Institute of Health Research (CIHR) to Satya Prakash. They also acknowledge the National Sciences and Engineering Research Council of Canada (NSERC) and the McGill University Surgeon Scientist Fast Family Research Fund, and the Division of Plastic Surgery Research Fund to Hani Sinno.

Acknowledgments

The authors would also like to thank Pina Sorrini for her excellent secretarial help. They thank Genevieve Berube, Karen Zwiker, and the McGill University Animal Research Center Staff for their professional help with animal handling. They would also like to acknowledge the technical support of the McGill University Orthopedic Research Laboratory and the Small Animal Imaging Laboratory staff for their excellent technical support.

References

[1] W. K. Stadelmann, A. G. Digenis, and G. R. Totin, "Physiology and healing dynamics of chronic cutaneous wounds," *The American Journal of Surgery*, vol. 176, no. 2, supplement, pp. 26S–38S, 1998.

[2] H. Sinno, M. Malholtra, J. Lutfy et al., "Topical application of complement C3 in collagen formulation increases early wound healing," *Journal of Dermatological Treatment*, vol. 24, no. 2, pp. 141–147, 2011.

[3] H. Sinno, M. Malhotra, J. Lutfy et al., "Accelerated wound healing with topical application with of complement C5," *Plastic and Reconstructive Surgery*, vol. 130, no. 3, pp. 523–529, 2012.

[4] H. N. Fernandez, P. M. Henson, A. Otani, and T. E. Hugli, "Chemotactic response to human C3a and C5a anaphylatoxins. I. Evaluation of C3a and C5a leukotaxis in vitro and under simulated in vivo conditions," *Journal of Immunology*, vol. 120, no. 1, pp. 109–115, 1978.

[5] T. A. Mustoe, G. F. Pierce, A. Thomason, E. Gramates, M. B. Sporn, and T. F. Deuel, "Accelerated healing of incisional wounds in rats induced by transforming growth factor-β," *Science*, vol. 237, no. 4820, pp. 1333–1336, 1987.

5

FAMM Flap in Reconstructing Postsurgical Nasopharyngeal Airway Stenosis

Ferdinand Wanjala Nangole and Stanley Ominde Khainga

Department of Surgery (Plastic), University of Nairobi, Nairobi 00200, Kenya

Correspondence should be addressed to Ferdinand Wanjala Nangole; nangole2212@yahoo.com

Academic Editor: Georg M. Huemer

Introduction. Postsurgical nasopharyngeal airway stenosis can be a challenge to manage. The stenosis could be as a result of any surgical procedure in the nasopharyngeal region that heals extensive scarring and fibrosis. *Objective.* To evaluate patients with nasopharyngeal stenosis managed with FAMM flap. *Study Design.* Prospective study of patients with nasopharyngeal stenosis at the Kenyatta National Hospital between 2010 and 2013 managed with FAMM flap. *Materials and Methods.* Patients with severe nasopharyngeal airway stenosis were reviewed and managed with FAMM flaps at the Kenyatta National Hospital. Postoperatively they were assessed for symptomatic improvement in respiratory distress, patency of the nasopharyngeal airway, and donor site morbidity. *Results.* A total of 8 patients were managed by the authors in a duration of 4 years with nasopharyngeal stenosis. Five patients were managed with unilateral FAMM flaps in a two-staged surgical procedure. Four patients had complete relieve of the airway obstruction with a patent airway created. One patient had a patent airway created though with only mild improvement in airway obstruction. *Conclusion.* FAMM flap provides an alternative in the management of postsurgical severe nasopharyngeal stenosis. It is a reliable flap that is easy to raise and could provide adequate epithelium for the stenosed pharynx.

1. Introduction

Postsurgical nasopharyngeal airway obstruction is a relatively uncommon condition. The condition however when present can result in severe airway obstruction leading to both physical and psychosocial stress to the patients and the guardians. Patients with this condition are forced to breathe through the mouth and thus experience severe sleep apnea. Delayed management of this condition could result in failure to thrive, poor performance in school, and right-sided heart failure.

Management of this condition has traditionally involved relieving the obstruction by surgical or laser excision of scarred tissue [1–4]. The epithelial lining is then provided by either skin grafts, local flaps, or free flaps such as radial forearm flap [5, 6]. In some cases excision of scarred tissues followed by insertion of a stent for a duration of two to three weeks has proven sufficient [7]. Adequate excision of scarred tissue or inadequate epithelial lining after excision of scar

tissue would almost always result in the recurrence of the stenosis.

In this presentation we share our experience with the use of the facial artery muscular mucosa flap in the management of the nasopharyngeal stenosis (FAMM) at the Kenyatta National Hospital, a tertiary facility in Kenya.

2. Pertinent Literature

Nasopharyngeal stenosis is a relatively rare condition with an incident of about 3 in 100,000 cases after tonsillectomy surgery [8]. Infective causes such as syphilis and other granulomatous disease were a contributory to many cases before the Second World War. With the advent of better antibiotics, infection is not a big contributor to this condition.

Most cases of nasopharyngeal stenosis are due to either surgical procedures in the nasopharyngeal region or postradiation for nasopharyngeal tumours [9, 10]. The common surgical procedures attributed to the causation of nasopharyngeal stenosis are adenoidectomy and uvulopalatoplasties [9, 10]. Laser therapy for adenoids in the nasopharyngeal region has also been attributed to the causation of this disease [11].

Diagnosis of nasopharyngeal stenosis relies mainly on history and physical examination. History of surgery in the nasopharyngeal airway either for adenotonsillectomy, uvulopalatoplasty, and uvulectomy followed by difficulties in nasal breathing is highly suggestive. Other symptoms may be snoring, anosmia, rhinorrhea, otalgia, and dysphagia.

Physical examination will reveal absence or reduction of the nasopharyngeal orifice with scarring of the soft palate and the pharyngeal wall. Nasal endoscopy or postnasal mirror where they are available could assist in confirming the diagnosis.

Management of nasopharyngeal stenosis could be challenging. The condition is prone to high incidence of recurrence in spite of adequate planning and proper techniques.

The main modality in the management of nasopharyngeal stenosis is surgery. The principles entail the following:

(1) removal or excision of the scar tissues: this could either be through surgical excision or through the use of carbon dioxide laser,

(2) maintaining patency of the orifice until epithelialisation of the orifice tract (by use of stents or obturators),

(3) provision of epithelial lining: this could be provided by either skin grafts, local flaps, or regional or free flaps.

Due to the high recurrence rates noted in the management of this condition, many treatment modalities are now available in attempting to prevent the recurrences. The surgical options reported in literature include the use of either soft palate or pharyngeal wall flaps [12–14]. With this the scarred tissue is excised and the mucosal flaps either from the soft palate or the posterior pharyngeal wall mobilized to cover the defect. Other flaps reported in literature include the sternocleidomastoid myocutaneous flap [15]. Skin grafts and free flaps have also been used in the management of this condition with varying degrees of success [6].

Carbon dioxide laser has increasingly been utilized in the management of this condition. Krespi and Kacker probably report the largest series in the use of laser in the management of nasopharyngeal stenosis with good outcome [5]. Postexcision of an obturator is utilized by the patient for 2 to 6 months to prevent recurrence. Igwe et al. have utilized carbon dioxide laser to make radial cuts in the stenosed nasopharynx and then utilize controlled balloon dilatation to continuously expand the orifice [16]. Mitomycin c is then topically applied over the scar area to prevent fibroblast activities.

Plasma hook with mitomycin c as a modality for treatment of nasopharyngeal stenosis has also been reported with Madgy et al., though being only in a series of three patients [17].

Other nonsurgical techniques in the management of nasopharyngeal stenosis include the use of radiofrequency waves with or without mitomycin c. Hussein et al. with the use of radiofrequency and mitomycin c still advocated for the use of stents two weeks after surgery [18]. Wang et al. on the other hand found that this technique was best suited for patients with at least three months after the development of the stenosis [19].

3. Materials and Method

Patients with nasopharyngeal stenosis managed in the multidisciplinary clinic at the Kenyatta National Hospital were followed up during the study duration of four years between Jan 2010 and December 2013. Information gathered included the patients' demography, etiological cause of the nasopharyngeal airway obstructions, and any previous surgical interventions. A detailed history and clinical evaluation were then done to determine the severity of the airway obstructions. The severity of the obstruction was graded as follows.

Grade 1. Mild airway obstruction: these were patients who reported a good night sleep with only occasional episodes of dyspnoea. They predominantly breathe through the nose.

Grade 2. Moderately airway obstruction: these were patients who predominantly breathe through the nose during the day but had several episodes of nocturnal dyspnoea that disrupted their sleep pattern.

Grade 3. Severe airway obstruction: these were patients who could only breathe through the mouth. They persistently had sleep apnea and had other manifestations such as failure to thrive, poor school performance, and difficulties in feeding. Patients with previous surgical who attempt to relieve the stenosis with no success were also considered in this grade.

Patients who were classified in grade 3 were managed by the FAMM flap. The other patients in grades 1 and 2 were managed by the local flaps.

Operatively all the patients had oral intubation. Nasoendoscopy was done to confirm the presence of the stenosis. Tongue retractor was utilized to retract the tongue and keep the mouth wide open. Throat pack was inserted into the oral pharynx. After infiltration of lignocaine with adrenaline solution, the scarred tissue was excised until complete patency of the nasopharyngeal orifice was achieved. The facial artery was identified in the oral mucosa with the aid of hand held Doppler. Inferiorly based pedicle FAMM flap was then raised with the width of the flap corresponding to the extent of the defect to be covered (Figures 1 and 2). The dissection was carried out in the plane deep to the buccinators muscle. The parotid duct was identified and necessary precautions were taken not to injure it. The dissected flap was then advanced into the raw area over the soft palate ensuring complete separation of the soft palate from the nasopharyngeal wall (Figure 3). Suturing of the flap commenced between the flap and the soft palate nasal mucosa with interrupted Vicryl 2/0. This was followed by suturing the flap with soft palate oral mucosa. Upon completion nasogastric tube was passed through either of nostrils to confirm patency of the nasal airway. The donor site was closed primarily. Postoperatively

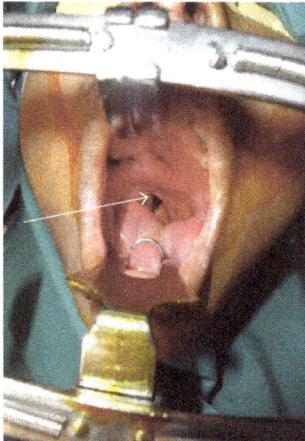

FIGURE 1: Patients with severe nasopharyngeal stenosis with extensive scarring of the soft palate.

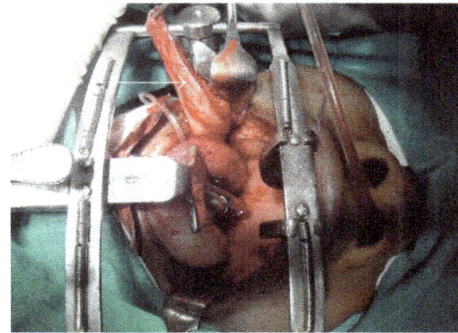

FIGURE 2: Patients with severe nasopharyngeal stenosis with extensive scarring of the soft palate.

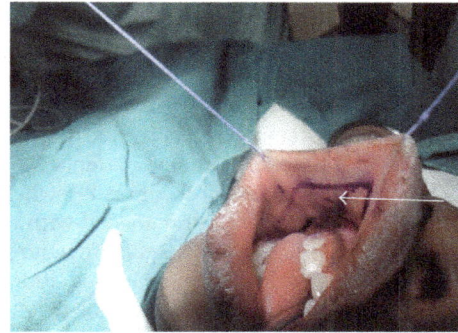

FIGURE 3: Markings for the FAMM FLAP.

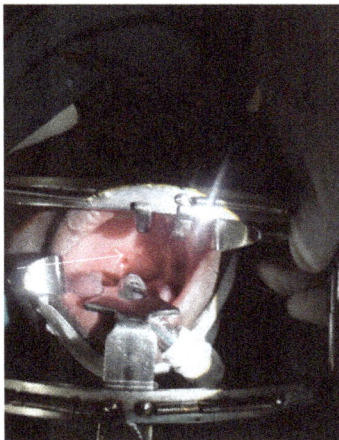

FIGURE 4: FAMM flap is raised.

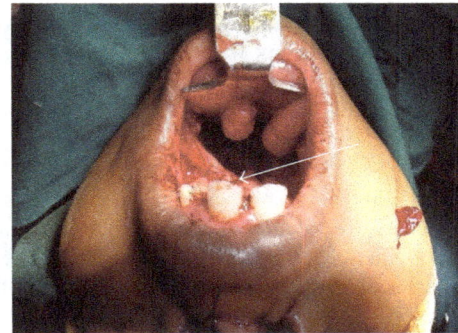

FIGURE 5: Flap inserted into the defect over the soft palate and pharyngeal wall.

the patient was intubated overnight in the intensive care unit to ensure patency of the airway.

The second stage procedure was done at about three weeks after the first surgery (Figure 4). Upon intubation patency of the nasal airway was checked by passing a nasogastric tube through either of the nostrils. The flap was detached from the buccal region and the facial artery ligated. Any redundant flap tissues were excised and proper positioning of the flap done (Figure 5).

After surgery, clinical evaluation of the patients was done by assessing improvement in airway obstruction, patency of the nasal airway, and healing of the donor site. Improvement in airway obstruction was graded as

(1) mild improvement: only slight improvement in airway obstruction with the patient still having predominantly oral breathing and sleep apnoea,

(2) moderate improvement: patient predominantly breathes through the nose but still has some episodes of sleep apnoea at night,

(3) great improvement: patient does not experience any more sleep apnoea and breathes through the nose.

The patients were followed up for at least one year in the clinic to check for any evidence of recurrence.

4. Results

A total of 8 patients with nasopharyngeal stenosis were reviewed in the multidisciplinary clinic at the Kenyatta National Hospital during the study duration of four years. Six patients had developed stenosis after traditional uvulectomy with 2 patients after adenoidectomy. The age range for the patients was 4 years to 12 years of age. Five were female patients with 3 male patients. Of the 8 patients seen 5 patients were classified as grade 3, with severe nasopharyngeal stenosis. The other 3 patients were classified as follows: grade 1, one patient, and grade 2, 2 patients. Patients with grades 1 and 2 (n = 3) were managed by excision of scar tissues and local pharyngeal flaps. All grade 3 patients (n = 5) had had an average of two surgical procedures elsewhere before referral to our clinic. They were all managed with unilateral inferiorly based FAMM flap in two staged procedures. Of the five patients managed with the FAMM flaps, four patients had complete relieve of the nasal airway obstruction with no sleep apnoea at one year of follow-up. One patient had mild improvement in the airway obstruction. All patients had patent nasal airway at one year of follow-up. The donor sites in all patients were closed primarily and healed with no complications. No facial nerve palsy nor injury to the parotid duct was noted in any patient. There was no flap loss or necrosis in any of the patients either.

5. Discussion

Traditional uvulectomy contributes to a big proportion of patients with nasopharyngeal stenosis in our setup. The belief in many African communities is that the uvula is responsible for recurrent respiratory tract infections especially in the pediatric age groups. The uvula should thus be excised to save the child from persistent throat or airway infections. Uvulectomy unfortunately in many communities is done in unhygienic conditions resulting in infections with resultant scarring of the nasopharynx with severe stenosis as seen in the majority of the patients in this study. There is thus a strong need for community education on the possible complications of this practice.

Nasopharyngeal stenosis in the literature could be managed by carbon dioxide laser for excision of scarred tissues [2–4]. After excision the patency of the airway is maintained by either a stent or an obturator for up to 6 months while waiting for epithelialisation of the orifice. Laser despite the fact that it is now widely used in the medical field is however not readily available in many countries like ours where resources are constrained. Our unit thus has no experience whatsoever on the management of nasopharyngeal stenosis with this modalities. It should however be noted that even in centers where it is widely practiced the patient still has to use a stent or an obturator for up to 6 months to prevent any recurrence. Mitomycin c may also have to be applied on the scar tissue after laser so as to suppress fibroblast activities. FAMM flap on the other hand provides adequate epithelial lining that allows tissues to heal by primary intention and hence there is no risk of recurrence due to healing by secondary intention. There is thus no need to use a stent or an obturator after surgical excision.

Surgical management of nasopharyngeal stenosis basically entails excision of the scar tissue with provision of an epithelial lining. A stent or an obturator may be utilized depending on the practice in the center. After excision of the scarred tissues, the epithelial ling could be provided by either skin grafts, local flaps, regional flaps, or even free flaps [12, 13]. The choice of which option to use could be influenced by many factors including severity of stenosis, quality of the surrounding mucosa, operating surgeons experience, and possible complications associated with the method chosen.

Skin graft is probably an easy option in the provision of epithelial lining anywhere on the body. It is easy to harvest with minimal donor site morbidity. Its biggest disadvantage however in the management of patient with nasopharyngeal stenosis is that the graft tends to contract and hence is prone to recurrence of the stenosis. It is also technically difficult to successfully secure the graft at the recipient site with pressure dressings and thus one is likely to experience poor graft take. Local pharyngeal and soft palatal flaps are probably the most quoted flaps in literature utilized in the management of nasopharyngeal stenosis [12–14]. These flaps have an advantage that they are proximal to the defect being reconstructed and thus are easier and faster to rise with minimal donor site morbidity.

Our experience however is such that they are probably only useful in patients with mild or moderate nasopharyngeal stenosis. Patients with severe stenosis usually have extensive scarring involving the mucosa and underlying tissues. It is thus technically difficult to raise such flaps and reconstruct defects appropriately. The flaps are also limited as to how much epithelial surface they could provide.

Regional flaps quoted in literature in the management of nasopharyngeal stenosis include the sternocleidomastoid musculocutaneous flap [15]. A possible shortcoming with this flap is an external skin incision that may not be cosmetically acceptable especially to our patients who have a tendency to form hypertrophic scars and keloids. Being a muscle flap it is also likely to be bulky and thus obliterate the nasopharyngeal orifice.

Facial artery musculomucosal flap (FAMM) is a pedicle flap that could be proximally or distally raised based on the facial artery. The facial artery is identified by a hand held Doppler and it is location mapped in the flap. The flap is able to provide mucosa lining of up to 3 cm in dimension while allowing for the closure of the donor site primarily [20]. This flap is well established in the reconstruction of multiple defects including palatal, nostril, nasal septal, and upper lip [20, 21].

Due to its wide arc of rotation the flap once fully mobilized is able to reach most parts of the soft palate and the nasopharynx. It is thus able to cover most of the raw area in patients with severe nasopharyngeal stenosis once the scar tissues are excised, providing adequate epithelial Lning and hence preventing recurrence of the stenosis. The flap is also thin and pliable, unlike most muscle or free flaps. It only provides mucosa with minimal muscle bulk to the scarred area. Due to its rich blood supply, flap necrosis is uncommon. The donor site in the majority of the patients heals without any complications.

In our patients a two-staged procedure was done. The first stage encompassed raising the flap and advancing it into the defect with the second stage detaching the flap from its donor site and excising any redundant tissues. This allows for proper insertion of the flap and removal of any unnecessary tissues in the oral cavity (see Figures 6 and 7). Neither stents

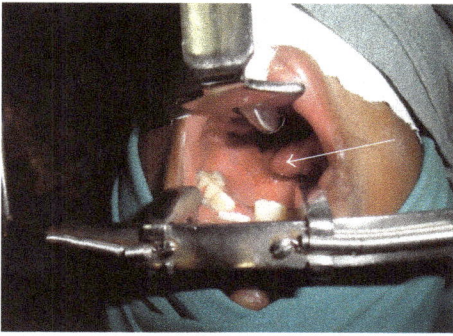

FIGURE 6: Patient with FAMM flap for the second staged procedure arrow indicating the redundant flap tissue around the pedicle to be excised

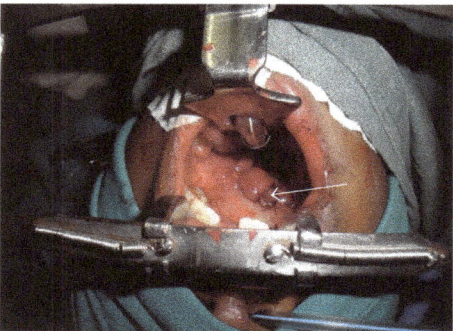

FIGURE 7: Patient after detaching the flap and excision of redundant tissues. Note patent airway as demonstrated by the nasogastric tube.

nor obturators were utilized since the epithelial surface was already established with the flap.

All our patients at one year of follow-up had a patent nasal passage with no recurrence of stenosis. However one patient had only mild improvement in his airway obstruction symptoms. This patient was however a syndromic patient with midface hypoplasia.

In conclusion FAMM flap provides an alternative in the management of nasopharyngeal stenosis. It is a relatively easy flap to raise and has less donor site morbidity. The flap is able to provide adequate epithelial lining of the scarred raw soft palatal region and thus reduce chances of healing by scarring. It should thus be considered in the management of patient with severe nasopharyngeal stenosis with extensive scarring of the pharynx and the soft palate.

References

[1] D. W. Stepnick, "Management of total nasopharyngeal stenosis following UPPP," *Ear, Nose and Throat Journal*, vol. 72, no. 1, pp. 86–90, 1993.

[2] J. Van Duyne and J. A. Coleman Jr., "Treatment of nasopharyngeal inlet stenosis following uvulopalatopharyngoplasty with the CO_2 laser," *Laryngoscope*, vol. 105, no. 9, article 1, pp. 914–918, 1995.

[3] D. Sidell and D. K. Chhetri, "CO_2 laser ablation and balloon dilation for acquired nasopharyngeal stenosis: a novel technique," *Laryngoscope*, vol. 121, no. 7, pp. 1486–1489, 2011.

[4] L. M. Jones, V. L. Guillory, and E. A. Mair, "Total nasopharyngeal stenosis: treatment with laser excision, nasopharyngeal obturators, and topical mitomycin-c," *Otolaryngology—Head and Neck Surgery*, vol. 133, no. 5, pp. 795–798, 2005.

[5] Y. P. Krespi and A. Kacker, "Management of nasopharyngeal stenosis after uvulopalatoplasty," *Otolaryngology—Head and Neck Surgery*, vol. 123, no. 6, pp. 692–695, 2000.

[6] K. E. McLaughlin, I. N. Jacobs, N. W. Todd, G. S. Gussack, and G. Carlson, "Management of nasopharyngeal and oropharyngeal stenosis in children," *Laryngoscope*, vol. 107, no. 10, pp. 1322–1331, 1997.

[7] B. L. Eppley, A. M. Sadove, D. Hennon, and J. A. Van Aalst, "Treatment of nasopharyngeal stenosis by prosthetic hollow stents: clinical experience in eight patients," *Cleft Palate-Craniofacial Journal*, vol. 43, no. 3, pp. 374–378, 2006.

[8] C. J. Imperatori, "Atresia of the pharynx operated upon by the MacKenty method," *Annals of Otology, Rhinology & Laryngology*, vol. 53, pp. 329–334, 1944.

[9] P. Bonfils, N. de Preobrajenski, A. Florent, and J.-L. Bensimon, "Choanal stenosis: a rare complication of radiotherapy for nasopharyngeal carcinoma," *Cancer/Radiotherapie*, vol. 11, no. 3, pp. 143–145, 2007.

[10] L. B. Johnson, R. G. Elluru, and C. M. Myer III, "Complications of adenotonsillectomy," *Laryngoscope*, vol. 112, no. 8, pp. 35–36, 2002.

[11] C. Giannoni, M. Sulek, E. M. Friedman, and N. O. Duncan III, "Acquired nasopharyngeal stenosis: a warning and review," *Archives of Otolaryngology—Head and Neck Surgery*, vol. 124, no. 2, pp. 163–167, 1998.

[12] E. Toh, A. W. Pearl, E. M. Genden, W. Lawson, and M. L. Urken, "Bivalved palatal transposition flaps for the correction of acquired nasopharyngeal stenosis," *The American Journal of Rhinology*, vol. 14, no. 3, pp. 199–204, 2000.

[13] G. Abdel-Fattah, "Palatal eversion: a new technique in treatment of nasopharyngeal stenosis," *International Journal of Pediatric Otorhinolaryngology*, vol. 76, no. 6, pp. 879–882, 2012.

[14] R. T. Cotton, "Nasopharyngeal stenosis," *Archives of Otolaryngology*, vol. 111, no. 3, pp. 146–148, 1985.

[15] M. E. Smith, "Prevention and treatment of nasopharyngeal stenosis," *Operative Techniques in Otolaryngology—Head and Neck Surgery*, vol. 16, no. 4, pp. 242–247, 2005.

[16] C.-N. Igwe, R. Sharma, D. Roberts, and C. Hopkins, "Use of balloon dilatation as an adjunctive treatment for complete nasopharyngeal stenosis: a technical innovation," *Clinical Otolaryngology*, vol. 37, no. 1, pp. 88–89, 2012.

[17] D. N. Madgy, W. Belenky, B. Dunkley, and S. Shinhar, "A simple surgical technique using the plasma hook for correcting acquired nasopharyngeal stenosis," *Laryngoscope*, vol. 115, no. 2, pp. 370–372, 2005.

[18] J. Hussein, T. S. Tan, A. W. Chong, P. Narayanan, and R. Omar, "Velopharyngeal and choanal stenosis after radiotherapy for nasopharyngeal carcinoma," *Auris Nasus Larynx*, vol. 40, no. 3, pp. 323–326, 2013.

[19] Q. Y. Wang, L. Chai, S. Q. Wang, S. H. Zhou, and Y. Y. Lu, "Repair of acquired posterior choanal stenosis and atresia by temperature-controlled radio frequency with the aid of an endoscope," *Archives of Otolaryngology: Head & Neck Surgery*, vol. 135, no. 5, pp. 462–466, 2009.

[20] J. Pribaz, W. Stephens, L. Crespo, and G. Gifford, "A new intraoral flap: facial artery musculomucosal (FAMM) flap," *Plastic and Reconstructive Surgery*, vol. 90, no. 3, pp. 421–429, 1992.

[21] A. Joshi, J. S. Rajendraprasad, and K. Shetty, "Reconstruction of intraoral defects using facial artery musculomucosal flap," *British Journal of Plastic Surgery*, vol. 58, no. 8, pp. 1061–1066, 2005.

6

Sociodemographic Predictors of Breast Reconstruction Procedure Choice: Analysis of the Mastectomy Reconstruction Outcomes Consortium Study Cohort

Tiffany N. S. Ballard,[1] Yeonil Kim,[2] Wess A. Cohen,[3] Jennifer B. Hamill,[1] Adeyiza O. Momoh,[1] Andrea L. Pusic,[3] H. Myra Kim,[2,4] and Edwin G. Wilkins[1]

[1]Section of Plastic Surgery, University of Michigan, Ann Arbor, MI 48109, USA
[2]Center for Statistical Consultation and Research, University of Michigan, Ann Arbor, MI 48109, USA
[3]Division of Plastic and Reconstructive Surgery, Memorial Sloan-Kettering Cancer Center, New York, NY 10065, USA
[4]Department of Biostatistics, University of Michigan, Ann Arbor, MI 48109, USA

Correspondence should be addressed to Tiffany N. S. Ballard; tballard@med.umich.edu

Academic Editor: Hiroshi Mizuno

Background. To promote patient-centered care, it is important to understand the impact of sociodemographic factors on procedure choice for women undergoing postmastectomy breast reconstruction. In this context, we analyzed the effects of these variables on the reconstructive method chosen. *Methods.* Women undergoing postmastectomy breast reconstruction were recruited for the prospective Mastectomy Reconstruction Outcomes Consortium Study. Procedure types were divided into tissue expander-implant/direct-to-implant and abdominally based flap reconstructions. Adjusted odds ratios were calculated from logistic regression. *Results.* The analysis included 2,203 women with current or previous breast cancer and 202 women undergoing prophylactic mastectomy. Compared with women <40 years old with current or previous breast cancer, those 40 to 59 were significantly more likely to undergo an abdominally based flap. Women working or attending school full-time were more likely to receive an autologous procedure than those working part-time or volunteering. Women undergoing prophylactic mastectomy who were ≥50 years were more likely to undergo an abdominal flap compared to those <40. *Conclusions.* Our results indicate that sociodemographic factors affect the reconstructive procedure received. As we move forward into a new era of patient-centered care, providing tailored treatment options to reconstruction patients will likely lead to higher satisfaction and better outcomes for those we serve.

1. Introduction

Breast cancer, with an estimated 296,980 cases of invasive or in situ breast cancer diagnosed in 2013, is the most common non-skin cancer neoplasm of women in the US [1]. It is a diagnosis that is not limited by race, income, education, or geographic location. While many women still choose breast conservation for the primary treatment of breast cancer, the rates of mastectomy among women eligible for breast conserving surgery have increased over the past decade [2, 3]. Today most women undergo a skin-sparing mastectomy, during which the skin of the nipple, areola, and biopsy scar is removed with the breast tissue and the rest of the skin remains intact, or nipple-sparing mastectomy, in which the skin of the nipple and areola is also preserved. For women undergoing mastectomy, the benefits of breast reconstruction in preserving body image, self-esteem, sexuality, and quality of life are widely recognized [4–8]. With the growing availability of implant-based and autogenous tissue options in recent years, patients now have a wide range of procedures from which to choose. However, little is known about how and why procedure choices are made by patients and their surgeons. In fact, the decision-making process for mastectomy reconstruction remains poorly understood.

Previous studies have focused on clinical factors, such as body mass index (BMI), disease stage, and cancer treatment, as the primary determinants of procedure choice [9, 10]. However, the reconstruction decision may also be impacted by other, less obvious influences. A growing body of research suggests that sociodemographic factors have significant effects on health care treatment choices: that is, a patient's age, ethnicity, education, and income may play important roles in determining the treatment she receives [11–13]. Although the impact of these variables on the utilization of breast reconstruction has been studied in large database analyses with a focus on clinical factors [14, 15], little is known about the effects of sociodemographic variables on procedure choice in this population.

Surgeons accustomed to basing their reconstructive recommendations on purely clinical considerations may question the importance of these less "tangible" variables. However, patients' ethnic, social, educational, and financial backgrounds may significantly affect decision-making, processes of care, and outcomes [11, 16]. Growing awareness among providers and policy-makers of the importance of these factors has given rise to a "patient-centered care" movement in US health care. The concept of patient-centered care as outlined in the Institute of Medicine's (IOM) 2001 report, *Crossing the Quality Chasm*, is rooted in the recognition of patients as unique individuals [17]. The IOM calls for physicians to provide "care that is respectful and responsive to individual patient preferences, needs, and values." Patient-centered care means tailoring treatment interventions based on patients' backgrounds and preferences. This approach rejects the traditional "one size fits all" model of health care in favor of providing individualized care, including educating patients on treatment choices and helping patients choose options which best fit their values and lifestyles.

One of the first steps in designing individualized care for breast reconstruction patients is to better understand how social and demographic factors are related to the selection of reconstructive options. In this context, we sought to assess the impact of these variables on procedure type for postmastectomy reconstruction in a large, multicenter, prospective study.

2. Methods

2.1. Study Population. Patients were recruited as part of the Mastectomy Reconstruction Outcomes Consortium (MROC) Study, a prospective, multicenter cohort study funded by the National Cancer Institute. Women 18 years or older undergoing first-time, immediate, or delayed breast reconstruction following skin-sparing or nipple-sparing mastectomy for cancer treatment or prophylaxis were eligible for participation. Immediate reconstruction was performed at the time of mastectomy, and delayed reconstruction was performed at a subsequent date. Women undergoing a secondary attempt at reconstruction or revisions were excluded. Women receiving expander/implant or abdominally based autologous tissue reconstruction were included in this analysis. Autogenous tissue reconstructions included pedicle transverse

rectus abdominis musculocutaneous (pTRAM), free transverse rectus abdominis musculocutaneous (fTRAM), deep inferior epigastric perforator (DIEP), and superficial inferior epigastric artery (SIEA) flaps. Both unilateral and bilateral procedures were evaluated. Choices of reconstructive options were based on patient and surgeon preferences. Over 60 plastic surgeons from 10 centers in Michigan, New York, Illinois, Ohio, Massachusetts, Washington, DC, Georgia, Texas, and Manitoba have contributed patients to the study. The MROC Study follows patients from immediately prior to reconstruction to two years postoperatively. Appropriate approval from all participating site Institutional Review Boards (IRBs) was obtained. The electronic medical record for each patient was reviewed to obtain clinical data. All data were collected via Velos (Velos Inc., Fremont CA), a web-based clinical trial management system.

2.2. Dependent Variable. In this analysis, the dependent variable of interest was reconstructive procedure choice, categorized as tissue expander/implant or abdominally based flap reconstructions. Implant procedures included tissue expander (TE) and direct-to-implant (DTI) techniques, while abdominally based flaps included pTRAM, fTRAM, DIEP, and SIEA flaps. Due to their small numbers, patients undergoing latissimus dorsi flaps (with or without implants), superior gluteal artery perforator (SGAP) flaps, and inferior gluteal artery perforator (IGAP) flaps or patients undergoing a combination of implant and autologous procedures in bilateral reconstructions were excluded.

2.3. Independent Variables. Demographic variables were self-reported and included age, race, ethnicity (Hispanic/non-Hispanic), marital status, employment status, smoking status, highest level of education, and household income. Categories for racial group were "white," "black," and "other" (American Indians, Asians, Hawaiians, and Pacific Islanders). Employment was described as full-time (including students); part-time (including those seeking employment, homemaker, or other); unable to work or disabled; or retired. The educational categories were defined as high school diploma or less; some college or college/trade degree; and some graduate school or graduate degree. Household income (dollars per year) categories included low income (<$50,000), mid income ($50,000 to $100,000), and high income (≥$100,000).

To control for potential confounding, a group of clinical variables were also incorporated into the analysis. These included body mass index (BMI), medical comorbidities, procedure laterality (unilateral versus bilateral), and cancer status. In accordance with Centers for Disease Control guidelines, BMI (kg/m^2) was categorized as normal (less than 25), overweight (25 to less than 30), moderately obese/obesity class I (30 to less than 35), and severely obese/obesity class II (35 or above). Medical comorbidities were scored by the Charlson Index [18] and categorized as none, one, or two or more. Patients were categorized into three groups based on the indication for mastectomy and timing of the procedure: (1) patients with active cancer undergoing immediate reconstruction, (2) a history of breast cancer undergoing immediate reconstruction, or (3) a history of breast cancer undergoing delayed reconstruction. Patients with active cancer in one breast undergoing bilateral mastectomies (with a contralateral prophylactic mastectomy) and reconstruction were classified in the group of patients with active cancer undergoing immediate reconstruction. Women undergoing prophylactic mastectomies were analyzed as a separate cohort and were classified as unilateral or bilateral immediate reconstructions.

2.4. Statistical Analysis. As the determinants for procedural choices were expected to differ between women undergoing reconstruction following mastectomies for breast cancer and those choosing prophylactic mastectomies with reconstruction, all analyses were conducted separately for the cohorts of patients with cancer and those without cancer. Determinants for the two procedure types (abdominally based autologous flap procedures versus TE/DTI) were evaluated. Initially, chi-square tests were performed to determine significant differences in the demographic and clinical variables between procedure types. To further evaluate the effects of the sociodemographic and clinical factors on the choice of procedure, a mixed-effects logistic regression was used, with procedure type as the dependent variable and patient factors as the independent variables. The model included study site as random intercepts to adjust for between-site differences. Both unadjusted (crude) and adjusted odds ratios (OR) of choosing an abdominally based flap versus TE/DTI, along with the corresponding 95% confidence intervals, were calculated from the mixed-effects logistic regression model parameter estimates. Because the main objective of the analysis was to show the adjusted relationship between each carefully defined factor level and the choice of procedure type, even when no significant effects were seen for a factor or a subset of factor levels, all predictors were included in the model for the cohort of women undergoing reconstruction following mastectomies for breast cancer. Factors were dropped from the model for women undergoing prophylactic mastectomies if they caused quasi- or complete-separation from the small sample size. Statistical analysis was performed using Stata 13.1 (StataCorp LP, College Station, TX), and statistical significance was set at 0.05.

3. Results

A total of 2,405 women were included in this analysis: 2,203 women with current or previous breast cancer and 202 women undergoing prophylactic mastectomy. Demographic and clinical variables with their associated bivariate analyses are summarized in Table 1 for each cohort. Among the 2,203 women with breast cancer, 70.7% underwent TE/DTI and 29.3% received abdominally based flap reconstructions. Over 90% (n = 2027) underwent immediate reconstruction, while 8% (n = 176) underwent delayed reconstruction. For the 202 women undergoing prophylactic mastectomy and reconstruction, 77.7% received TE/DTI, while 22.3% underwent abdominally based flap reconstructions. All women undergoing prophylactic mastectomy underwent immediate

reconstruction. The majority of women were white and non-Hispanic. Among all women reporting their smoking status (n = 2,381), 59 (2.5%) were current smokers.

3.1. Women with Current or Previous Breast Cancer. Bivariate analyses showed no significant differences in race, ethnicity, or marital status between women receiving TE/DTI and abdominal flaps. Reconstruction with an abdominally based flap was significantly associated with older age ($p < 0.001$); being retired or unable to work ($p < 0.001$); having a high school diploma or less ($p < 0.001$); and an annual income of less than \$50,000 ($p < 0.001$). Clinical variables, including BMI, number of comorbidities, procedure laterality, cancer status, and timing of the reconstruction, were also significantly different between the two procedure types.

Table 2 summarizes the crude and the adjusted odds ratios for each factor based on the logistic regression models. Controlling for other variables in the model, age had a statistically significant effect on procedure choice: compared with women under 40 years old, those 40 to 49 and 50 to 59 years old were significantly more likely to undergo an abdominal flap than a TE/DTI reconstruction (OR 1.88, p = 0.009; OR 1.98, p = 0.006, resp.). Employment status also had a significant effect on procedure type: women working or attending school full-time were more likely to receive autologous procedures than those in part-time or volunteer occupations (OR 1.56, p = 0.006).

After adjusting for other variables, significant procedure choice differences were no longer observed for the education and income variables. Although not significant, statistical trends were noted for the effects of race and ethnicity on procedure choice: compared to white women, black women were less likely to undergo abdominally based flaps than TE/DTI procedures (OR 0.74, p = 0.25). Hispanic women were more likely to receive abdominal flaps than non-Hispanic women (OR 1.41, p = 0.23).

Clinical factors including BMI, laterality, and timing of reconstruction had statistically significant effects on procedure choice among women with breast cancer. Compared to women with BMIs less than 25, women with higher BMIs were more likely to undergo abdominally based flaps. Women undergoing bilateral procedures were half as likely to receive abdominal flaps compared with those undergoing unilateral reconstructions (OR 0.55, $p < 0.001$). Patients undergoing delayed reconstruction were more likely to undergo autologous procedures than their counterparts receiving immediate reconstructions (OR 11.40, $p < 0.001$).

3.2. Women with No Previous History of Breast Cancer. Bivariate analyses showed no significant differences in procedure choice by race, ethnicity, marital status, or employment status (Table 1). A significantly higher proportion of women undergoing prophylactic mastectomy and abdominally based flap reconstruction attended some college or had a college degree (p = 0.01), had an income between \$50,000 and \$99,999, and had BMIs over 25 ($p < 0.001$) than patients receiving TE/DTI procedures.

After adjusting for other variables, age remained significantly associated with procedure type: women with no cancer

TABLE 1: Patient characteristics by cancer status and procedure type.

Variable	Number of women (%) with current or previous cancer by reconstructive procedure type N = 2203			Number of women (%) undergoing prophylactic mastectomy by reconstructive procedure type N = 202		
	TE/DTI	Abdominal flap[†]	p	TE/DTI	Abdominal flap[†]	p
	1557 (70.7)	646 (29.3)		157 (77.7)	45 (22.3)	
Age (years)	1557	646	<0.001	157	45	0.01
<40	282 (84.7)	51 (15.3)		71 (85.5)	12 (14.5)	
40–49	577 (72.9)	215 (27.1)		52 (78.8)	14 (21.2)	
50–59	439 (63.8)	249 (36.2)		34 (64.2)	19 (35.8)	
≥60	259 (66.4)	131 (33.6)				
Race	1538	635	0.49	157	45	0.30
White	1346 (70.4)	565 (29.6)		147 (77.8)	42 (22.2)	
Black	114 (75.0)	38 (25.0)		8 (88.9)	1 (11.1)	
Other*	78 (70.9)	32 (29.1)		2 (50.0)	2 (50.0)	
Ethnicity	1524	634	0.34	156	43	0.93
Non-Hispanic	1423 (70.4)	599 (29.6)		152 (78.4)	42 (21.7)	
Hispanic	101 (74.3)	35 (25.7)		4 (80.0)	1 (20.0)	
Marital status	1542	644	0.13	157	45	0.32
Not married	402 (68.1)	188 (31.9)		43 (82.7)	9 (17.3)	
Married	1140 (71.4)	456 (28.6)		114 (76.0)	36 (24.0)	
Employment status	1538	638	<0.001	155	45	0.40
Full-time/student	866 (69.3)	383 (30.7)		96 (77.4)	28 (22.6)	
Part-time/volunteer[‡]	512 (76.2)	160 (23.8)		50 (74.6)	17 (25.4)	
Unable to work/disabled	41 (61.2)	26 (38.8)		5 (100)	0 (0.0)	
Retired	119 (63.3)	69 (36.7)		4 (100)	0 (0.0)	
Smoking status	1539	643	<0.001	154	45	0.25
Never smoker	1019 (73.6)	366 (26.4)		116 (79.5)	30 (20.5)	
Previous smoker	483 (65.2)	258 (34.8)		35 (70.0)	15 (30.0)	
Current smoker	37 (66.1)	19 (33.9)		3 (100)	0 (0.0)	
Education	1549	643	<0.001	157	45	0.01
High school diploma or less	115 (51.1)	110 (48.9)		8 (88.9)	1 (11.1)	
Some college or college degree	837 (68.6)	383 (31.4)		78 (70.3)	33 (29.7)	
Some graduate or graduate degree	597 (79.9)	150 (20.1)		71 (86.6)	11 (13.4)	
Income	1505	627	<0.001	153	45	0.04
<$50,000	238 (58.5)	169 (41.5)		18 (78.3)	5 (21.7)	
$50,000–$99,999	439 (64.2)	245 (35.8)		47 (67.1)	23 (32.9)	
≥$100,000	828 (79.5)	213 (20.5)		88 (83.8)	17 (16.2)	
BMI	1557	646	<0.001	157	45	<0.001
<25	788 (84.4)	146 (15.6)		101 (93.5)	7 (6.5)	
25–29.9	458 (66.4)	232 (33.6)		35 (72.9)	13 (27.1)	
30–34.9	192 (53.3)	168 (46.7)		13 (43.3)	17 (56.7)	
≥35	119 (54.3)	100 (45.7)		8 (50.0)	8 (50.0)	
Medical comorbidities	1557	646	0.001	157	45	0.75
None	32 (64.0)	18 (36.0)		126 (78.8)	34 (21.2)	
One	1393 (72.1)	540 (27.9)		29 (74.4)	10 (25.6)	
More than two	132 (60.0)	88 (40.0)		2 (66.7)	1 (33.3)	

TABLE 1: Continued.

Variable	Number of women (%) with current or previous cancer by reconstructive procedure type N = 2203			Number of women (%) undergoing prophylactic mastectomy by reconstructive procedure type N = 202		
	TE/DTI	Abdominal flap[†]	p	TE/DTI	Abdominal flap[†]	p
Procedure laterality	1557	646	<0.001	157	45	0.34
Unilateral	652 (62.9)	384 (37.1)		9 (90.0)	1 (10.0)	
Bilateral[¥]	905 (77.5)	262 (22.5)		148 (77.1)	44 (22.9)	
Cancer status, timing of reconstruction	1557	646	<0.001			
Active cancer, immediate	1492 (75.2)	492 (24.8)				
Cancer history, immediate	27 (62.8)	16 (37.2)				
Cancer history, delayed	38 (21.6)	138 (78.4)				

[†]Pedicled transverse rectus abdominis myocutaneous, free transverse rectus abdominis myocutaneous, deep inferior epigastric perforator, and superficial inferior epigastric artery flaps.
[*]American Indians, Asians, Hawaiians, and Pacific Islanders.
[‡]Includes homemakers and women seeking employment.
[¥]Includes contralateral prophylactic mastectomy and reconstruction.
TE/DTI, tissue expander/direct-to-implant; BMI, body mass index.

history, aged 50 years or older, were more likely to undergo an abdominal flap compared to those under 40 years old (OR 4.44, p = 0.02, Table 3). Race and ethnicity did not have significant effects on procedure choice for these women. Among the clinical variables, BMI had a significant effect: women with BMIs of 25 to 29.9, 30 to 34.9, and 35 and above were more likely to undergo flaps than women with BMIs less than 25 (OR 10.35, p = 0.001; OR 27.29, p < 0.001; OR 26.48, p < 0.001, resp.).

4. Discussion

Women undergoing postmastectomy reconstruction have a wide variety of reconstructive options, including tissue expander/implant-based techniques and autogenous tissue procedures utilizing a variety of donor sites. Providing patient-centered care requires awareness of patients' backgrounds and preferences in order to tailor treatment and determine the best option for each woman. Our analysis found that a number of sociodemographic variables, including age, race, ethnicity, and employment status, impact the type of reconstructive procedure received. Additional research is needed to determine whether the procedure differences observed reflect patient preferences or other more concerning factors, such as disparities either in access to care or in the quality of information received during the surgical decision-making process.

This study has multiple strengths. First, the multicenter design enables the study team to enroll patients from 10 different sites across the US and Canada, which allows us to control for site differences and increases the potential generalizability of results, compared with single-center designs. A previous study by Katz et al. demonstrated the impact that treatment site and surgeon can have on the receipt of reconstruction [19], with much wider variation in treatment rates across surgeons noted for reconstructive

procedures compared to mastectomy. Therefore, controlling for site variation is a critical step in the analysis of procedure choice. The second strength is that the study is prospective, which enables us to control for multiple variables which may not be available in retrospective study designs or databases. Over 2,400 women are currently enrolled in the MROC Study and will be followed for two years postoperatively as we track longitudinal outcomes.

We found that reconstructive procedure choice varied across several demographic variables. Age plays a key role in determining which reconstructive procedure a woman chooses. Women 40 to 60 years old with current or previous cancer and women aged 50 to 60 undergoing prophylactic mastectomy were more likely to undergo an abdominally based flap compared to women less than 40 years old, a finding that has been previously demonstrated [20, 21]. A number of factors may contribute to this difference, including pregnancy, breast shape, and lifestyle. Younger women have a greater likelihood for being nulliparous with insufficient soft tissue for autologous reconstruction. Additionally, the shape of implants more closely resembles that of a nonptotic, youthful breast. Lifestyle and personal preference may also lead to younger patients' increased reluctance to undergo autologous reconstruction due to concerns over the longer recovery time and the possible impact on an active lifestyle.

Although we noted race and ethnicity effects on procedure choice, these differences were not statistically significant. In the current study, black women were less likely to undergo an abdominally based flap than white women, and Hispanic women were more likely to undergo an abdominal flap compared to non-Hispanic women. This lack of statistical significance is likely attributable to the relatively small number of minority patients in the analysis. Although the MROC Study includes 10 sites serving demographically diverse patient populations, our study cohorts are limited to evaluating the women treated at these centers. When

TABLE 2: Factors associated with undergoing abdominal flap versus TE/DTI among women undergoing mastectomy for current or previous breast cancer[†].

Variable	Unadjusted OR (95% CI)	Adjusted OR (95% CI)	p[††]
Age			
<40	1.0	1.0	
40–49	2.06 (1.51–2.80)	1.88 (1.17–3.02)	0.009
50–59	3.26 (2.40–4.43)	1.98 (1.22–3.22)	0.006
≥60	2.89 (2.06–4.05)	1.63 (0.92–2.90)	0.10
Race			
White	1.0	1.0	
Black	0.77 (0.53–1.12)	0.74 (0.44–1.24)	0.25
Other[*]	1.05 (0.70–1.58)	1.27 (0.65–2.50)	0.49
Ethnicity			
Non-Hispanic	1.0	1.0	
Hispanic	0.83 (0.56–1.22)	1.41 (0.81–2.48)	0.23
Marital status			
Not married	1.0	1.0	
Married	0.88 (0.72–1.07)	1.05 (0.75–1.47)	0.77
Employment status			
Part-time/volunteer[‡]	1.0	1.0	
Full-time/student	1.32 (1.08–1.62)	1.56 (1.14–2.15)	0.006
Unable to work/disabled	1.75 (1.05–2.91)	0.68 (0.31–1.46)	0.32
Retired	1.77 (1.27–2.48)	1.04 (0.58–1.87)	0.89
Smoking status			
Never smoker	1.0	1.0	
Previous smoker	1.35 (0.78–2.37)	0.54 (0.24–1.24)	0.15
Current smoker			
Education			
High school diploma or less	1.0	1.0	
Some college or college degree		1.11 (0.70–1.77)	0.66
Some graduate or graduate degree		1.19 (0.71–2.01)	0.51
Income			
<$50,000	1.0	1.0	
$50,000–$99,999	0.81 (0.63–1.03)	0.94 (0.63–1.39)	0.75
≥$100,000	0.37 (0.29–0.47)	0.76 (0.50–1.18)	0.22
BMI			
<25	1.0	1.0	
25–29.9	2.94 (2.33–3.69)	3.02 (2.15–4.25)	<0.001
30–34.9	5.25 (4.04–6.82)	5.58 (3.74–8.32)	<0.001
≥35	4.99 (3.67–6.79)	4.99 (3.12–8.00)	<0.001
Medical comorbidities			
None	1.0	1.0	
One	1.13 (0.82–1.56)	1.50 (0.62–3.62)	0.37
≥Two	1.94 (1.29–2.91)	1.63 (0.61–4.33)	0.33
Procedure laterality			
Unilateral	1.0	1.0	
Bilateral[¥]	0.51 (0.43–0.61)	0.55 (0.42–0.73)	<0.001
Cancer status, timing of reconstruction			
Active cancer, immediate	1.0	1.0	
Cancer history, immediate	1.80 (0.96–3.36)	2.09 (0.88–4.99)	0.10
Cancer history, delayed	11.01 (7.58–16.00)	11.40 (7.22–18.02)	<0.001

[†]Reference group is women undergoing tissue expander- (TE-) implant or direct-to-implant (DTI).

[††]p value corresponds to the adjusted odds ratios.

[*]American Indians, Asians, Hawaiians, and Pacific Islanders.

[‡]Includes homemakers and women seeking employment.

[¥]Includes contralateral prophylactic mastectomy and reconstruction.

TE/DTI, tissue expander/direct-to-implant; OR, odds ratios; BMI, body mass index.

TABLE 3: Factors associated with undergoing TE/DTI versus abdominal flap among women undergoing prophylactic mastectomy and immediate reconstruction[†].

Variable	Unadjusted OR (95% CI)	Adjusted OR (95% CI)	$p^{††}$
Age			
<40	1.0	1.0	
40–49	2.06 (1.51–2.80)	2.03 (0.62–6.64)	0.24
50–59	3.12 (2.33–4.19)	4.44 (1.30–15.22)	0.02
Race			
White	1.0	1.0	
Black	0.77 (0.53–1.12)	0.34 (0.02–5.76)	0.46
Other[*]	1.05 (0.70–1.58)	10.03 (0.51–195.93)	0.13
Marital status			
Not married	1.0	1.0	
Married	0.88 (0.72–1.07)	0.70 (0.19–2.54)	0.58
Education			
High school diploma or less	1.0	1.0	
Some college or college degree	0.48 (0.36–0.64)	6.60 (0.49–89.04)	0.16
Some graduate or graduate degree	0.26 (0.19–0.35)	4.16 (0.27–62.97)	0.30
Income			
<$50,000	1.0	1.0	
$50,000–$99,999	0.81 (0.63–1.03)	1.83 (0.34–9.93)	0.49
≥$100,000	0.37 (0.29–0.47)	1.41 (0.23–8.45)	0.71
BMI			
<25	1.0	1.0	
25–29.9	2.94 (2.33–3.69)	10.35 (2.70–39.72)	0.001
30–34.9	5.25 (4.04–6.82)	27.29 (6.45–115.49)	<0.001
≥35	4.99 (3.67–6.79)	26.48 (4.92–142.49)	<0.001
Medical comorbidities			
None	1.0	1.0	
One	1.13 (0.82–1.56)	0.84 (0.24–2.90)	0.78
≥Two	1.94 (1.29–2.91)	0.61 (0.02–15.34)	0.77
Procedure laterality, timing			
Unilateral, immediate	1.0	1.0	
Bilateral, immediate	2.68 (0.33–21.70)	6.37 (0.39–104.01)	0.19

[†]Reference group is women undergoing tissue expander- (TE-) implant or direct-to-implant (DTI).
[††]p value corresponds to the adjusted odds ratios.
[*]American Indians, Asians, Hawaiians, and Pacific Islanders.
TE/DTI, tissue expander/direct-to-implant; OR, odds ratios; BMI, body mass index.

choosing sites for MROC, particular emphasis was placed on recruiting centers from urban areas with large minority populations. However, attracting sufficient numbers of minorities for study participation remains challenging. This issue is not unique to MROC and has been described in previous prospective cohort studies and clinical trials [22, 23].

Previous large studies of databases, such as the American College of Surgeons National Surgical Quality Improvement Program (ACS-NSQIP) and the Surveillance, Epidemiology, and End Results (SEER) program, have suggested that black women are more likely to undergo autologous reconstruction compared to TE/DTI procedures [15, 21]. This observation has been attributed to minority patients' concerns over implant-related health risks and fears that reconstruction may negatively impact their cancer treatment [24, 25]. By contrast, black women in our study were less likely to undergo abdominally based flaps compared with white women. There are several possible explanations for this finding. First, the increasing use of implants nationally [26] in recent years may reflect diminishing public concerns about possible implant-related connective-tissue diseases and breast cancer. These issues prompted a Federal moratorium in April 1992, limiting implant use to reconstructive cases [27]. The moratorium was lifted in 2006 after multiple studies failed to find a link between silicone implants and systemic disease [28].

In our study, employment and education status were significant determinants of procedure choice. Women with current or previous cancer who were full-time students or employees were more likely to undergo flap-based reconstruction than TE/DTI. Even for a woman who would be a good candidate for DTI reconstruction, her surgeon cannot guarantee that an implant can be placed until examination of the mastectomy flaps intraoperatively. Therefore, women opting for implant-based reconstruction must be prepared for the possibility of requiring multiple follow-up visits for tissue expansion and a second surgery for implant exchange. These follow-up visits and subsequent surgeries requiring additional time off may negatively impact women's ability to resume working full-time. Thus, although the immediate postoperative physical recovery and restrictions are greater, autologous reconstructions may be preferred for some women as their expected return to work will be more predictable barring any major complications.

This study has several notable limitations. As with any prospective cohort design, there is potential for confounding by additional known or unknown variables. Although use of a randomized, controlled design would limit confounding, randomization would defeat the objective of this analysis, since its purpose was to examine procedure choice. Also, the feasibility of a RCT design in breast reconstruction studies is problematic, given patients' and surgeons' strong preferences for procedure types. In this study, chemotherapy and radiation were not included in the regression; these variables will be the focus of future studies assessing one- and two-year outcomes. Radiation is known to impact the reconstructive options available to a woman and has been associated with increased complications [29–32]. As mentioned above, our analyses were also limited by relatively small numbers of minority patients, despite inclusion of study sites for MROC with relatively large minority populations. While the MROC Study is a multicenter project, the majority of sites are based within large academic medical centers. Thus, our findings may not be generalizable to all patients, particularly those in smaller practice settings. Finally, we did not evaluate the mechanics of the patient decision-making process, evaluating how patients learn about their choices and subsequently choose their procedure; this is a fertile area for future research.

5. Conclusions

In summary, our analysis suggests that sociodemographic variables impact procedure choice in women undergoing postmastectomy breast reconstruction. Given the changing trends in mastectomy and reconstruction over the last 15 years, it is important to better understand the patient factors that impact surgical decision-making in socially, ethnically, and economically diverse populations. As we move forward into a new era of patient-centered care, providing tailored treatment options to reconstruction patients will likely lead to higher satisfaction and better outcomes for those we serve.

Acknowledgments

The study was supported by grants from the National Cancer Institute (1RO1CA152192) and a Research Fellowship grant from the Plastic Surgery Foundation. The authors gratefully acknowledge the contributions of their colleagues at the following centers who contributed their expertise to this multicenter trial: University of Michigan Health System, Ann Arbor, MI; Memorial Sloan-Kettering Cancer Center, New York City, NY; St. Joseph Mercy Hospital, Ypsilanti, MI; Northwestern Memorial Hospital, Chicago, IL; Ohio State Medical Center, Columbus, OH; Brigham and Women's Hospital, Boston, MA; Georgetown University Medical Center, Washington, DC; Georgia Institute of Plastic Surgery, Savannah, GA; M.D. Anderson Cancer Center, Houston, TX; and University of Manitoba, Winnipeg, MB.

References

[1] American Cancer Society, *Breast Cancer Facts and Figures 2013-2014*, 2014, http://www.cancer.org/acs/groups/content/@research/documents/document/acspc-042725.pdf.

[2] K. L. Kummerow, L. Du, D. F. Penson, Y. Shyr, and M. A. Hooks, "Nationwide trends in mastectomy for early-stage breast cancer," *JAMA Surgery*, vol. 150, no. 1, pp. 9–16, 2015.

[3] A. E. Dragun, J. Pan, E. C. Riley et al., "Increasing use of elective mastectomy and contralateral prophylactic surgery among breast conservation candidates: a 14-year report from a comprehensive cancer center," *American Journal of Clinical Oncology*, vol. 36, no. 4, pp. 375–380, 2013.

[4] L. A. Stevens, M. H. McGrath, R. G. Druss, S. J. Kister, F. E. Gump, and K. A. Forde, "The psychological impact of immediate breast reconstruction for women with early breast cancer," *Plastic and Reconstructive Surgery*, vol. 73, no. 4, pp. 619–628, 1984.

[5] J. H. Rowland, J. C. Holland, T. Chaglassian, and D. Kinne, "Psychological response to breast reconstruction. Expectations for and impact on postmastectomy functioning," *Psychosomatics*, vol. 34, no. 3, pp. 241–250, 1993.

[6] W. S. Schain, "Breast reconstruction. Update of psychosocial and pragmatic concerns," *Cancer*, vol. 68, no. 5, supplement, pp. 1170–1175, 1991.

[7] E. G. Wilkins, P. S. Cederna, J. C. Lowery et al., "Prospective analysis of psychosocial outcomes in breast reconstruction: one-year postoperative results from the Michigan Breast Reconstruction Outcome Study," *Plastic and Reconstructive Surgery*, vol. 106, no. 5, pp. 1014–1027, 2000.

[8] D. Atisha, A. K. Alderman, J. C. Lowery, L. F. Kuhn, J. Davis, and E. G. Wilkins, "Prospective analysis of long-term psychosocial outcomes in breast reconstruction: two-year postoperative results from the Michigan breast reconstruction outcomes study," *Annals of Surgery*, vol. 247, no. 6, pp. 1019–1028, 2008.

[9] J. E. Lang, D. E. Summers, H. Cui et al., "Trends in postmastectomy reconstruction: a SEER database analysis," *Journal of Surgical Oncology*, vol. 108, no. 3, pp. 163–168, 2013.

[10] S. Agarwal, L. Pappas, L. Neumayer, and J. Agarwal, "An analysis of immediate postmastectomy breast reconstruction frequency using the surveillance, epidemiology, and end results database," *Breast Journal*, vol. 17, no. 4, pp. 352–358, 2011.

[11] G. D. Rosson, N. K. Singh, N. Ahuja, L. K. Jacobs, and D. C. Chang, "Multilevel analysis of the impact of community vs

patient factors on access to immediate breast reconstruction following mastectomy in Maryland," *Archives of Surgery*, vol. 143, no. 11, pp. 1076–1081, 2008.

[12] L. Kruper, A. Holt, X. X. Xu et al., "Disparities in reconstruction rates after mastectomy: patterns of care and factors associated with the use of breast reconstruction in Southern California," *Annals of Surgical Oncology*, vol. 18, no. 8, pp. 2158–2165, 2011.

[13] B. C. Reuben, J. Manwaring, and L. A. Neumayer, "Recent trends and predictors in immediate breast reconstruction after mastectomy in the United States," *The American Journal of Surgery*, vol. 198, no. 2, pp. 237–243, 2009.

[14] A. K. Alderman, S. T. Hawley, N. K. Janz et al., "Racial and ethnic disparities in the use of postmastectomy breast reconstruction: results from a population- based study," *Journal of Clinical Oncology*, vol. 27, no. 32, pp. 5325–5330, 2009.

[15] A. C. Offodile II, T. C. Tsai, J. B. Wenger, and L. Guo, "Racial disparities in the type of postmastectomy reconstruction chosen," *Journal of Surgical Research*, vol. 195, no. 1, pp. 368–376, 2015.

[16] R. Jagsi, J. Jiang, A. O. Momoh et al., "Trends and variation in use of breast reconstruction in patients with breast cancer undergoing mastectomy in the United States," *Journal of Clinical Oncology*, vol. 32, no. 9, pp. 919–926, 2014.

[17] Committee on Quality of Health Care in America and Institute of Medicine, *Crossing the Quality Chasm: A New Health System for the 21st Century*, National Academy Press, Washington, DC, USA, 2001.

[18] W. H. Hall, R. Ramachandran, S. Narayan, A. B. Jani, and S. Vijayakumar, "An electronic application for rapidly calculating Charlson comorbidity score," *BMC Cancer*, vol. 4, article 94, 2004.

[19] S. J. Katz, S. T. Hawley, P. Abrahamse et al., "Does it matter where you go for breast surgery?: attending surgeon's influence on variation in receipt of mastectomy for breast cancer," *Medical Care*, vol. 48, no. 10, pp. 892–899, 2010.

[20] C. R. Albornoz, P. B. Bach, A. L. Pusic et al., "The influence of sociodemographic factors and hospital characteristics on the method of breast reconstruction, including microsurgery: a U.S. population-based study," *Plastic and Reconstructive Surgery*, vol. 129, pp. 1071–1079, 2012.

[21] A. K. Alderman, L. McMahon Jr., and E. G. Wilkins, "The national utilization of immediate and early delayed breast reconstruction and the effect of sociodemographic factors," *Plastic and Reconstructive Surgery*, vol. 111, no. 2, pp. 695–705, 2003.

[22] P. F. Pinsky, M. Ford, E. Gamito et al., "Enrollment of racial and ethnic minorities in the prostate, lung, colorectal and ovarian cancer screening trial," *Journal of the National Medical Association*, vol. 100, no. 3, pp. 291–298, 2008.

[23] E. T. Hawk, E. B. Habermann, J. G. Ford et al., "Five National Cancer Institute-designated cancer centers' data collection on racial/ethnic minority participation in therapeutic trials: a current view and opportunities for improvement," *Cancer*, vol. 120, supplement 7, pp. 1113–1121, 2014.

[24] L. R. Rubin, J. Chavez, A. Alderman, and A. L. Pusic, "'Use what God has given me': difference and disparity in breast reconstruction," *Psychology and Health*, vol. 28, no. 10, pp. 1099–1120, 2013.

[25] M. Morrow, Y. Li, A. K. Alderman et al., "Access to breast reconstruction after mastectomy and patient perspectives on reconstruction decision making," *JAMA Surgery*, vol. 149, no. 10, pp. 1015–1021, 2014.

[26] C. R. Albornoz, P. B. Bach, B. J. Mehrara et al., "A paradigm shift in U.S. Breast reconstruction: increasing implant rates," *Plastic and Reconstructive Surgery*, vol. 131, no. 1, pp. 15–23, 2013.

[27] S. L. Spear, P. M. Parikh, and J. A. Goldstein, "History of breast implants and the food and drug administration," *Clinics in Plastic Surgery*, vol. 36, no. 1, pp. 15–21, 2009.

[28] F. A. Medeiros, L. M. Alencar, P. A. Sample, L. M. Zangwill, R. Susanna Jr., and R. N. Weinreb, "The relationship between intraocular pressure reduction and rates of progressive visual field loss in eyes with optic disc hemorrhage," *Ophthalmology*, vol. 117, no. 11, pp. 2061–2066, 2010.

[29] O. O. Afolabi, D. H. Lalonde, and J. G. Williams, "Breast reconstruction and radiation therapy: a Canadian perspective," *Canadian Journal of Plastic Surgery*, vol. 20, no. 1, pp. 43–46, 2012.

[30] R. Gurunluoglu, A. Gurunluoglu, S. A. Williams, and S. Tebockhorst, "Current trends in breast reconstruction: survey of american society of plastic surgeons 2010," *Annals of Plastic Surgery*, vol. 70, no. 1, pp. 103–110, 2013.

[31] A. Alderman, K. Gutowski, A. Ahuja, and D. Gray, "ASPS clinical practice guideline summary on breast reconstruction with expanders and implants," *Plastic and Reconstructive Surgery*, vol. 134, no. 4, pp. 648e–655e, 2014.

[32] E. M. Hirsch, A. K. Seth, J. Y. Kim et al., "Analysis of risk factors for complications in expander/implant breast reconstruction by stage of reconstruction," *Plastic and Reconstructive Surgery*, vol. 134, no. 5, pp. 692e–699e, 2014.

7

Aesthetic and Functional Outcomes of the Innervated and Thinned Anterolateral Thigh Flap in Reconstruction of Upper Limb Defects

Carlos Alberto Torres-Ortíz Zermeño[1] and Javier López Mendoza[2]

[1] Plastic and Reconstructive Surgery, General Hospital Dr. Manuel Gea González, Calzada de Tlalpan No. 4800, 14080 Mexico City, DF, Mexico
[2] Hand and Microsurgery Clinic, General Hospital Dr. Manuel Gea González, Calzada de Tlalpan No. 4800, 14080 Mexico City, DF, Mexico

Correspondence should be addressed to Carlos Alberto Torres-Ortíz Zermeño; torresortiz_plastica@hotmail.com

Academic Editor: Georg M. Huemer

Background. The anterolateral thigh (ALT) flap has been widely described in reconstruction of the upper extremity. However, some details require refinement to improve both functional and aesthetic results. *Methods*. After reconstruction of upper extremity defects using thinned and innervated ALT flaps, functional and aesthetic outcomes were evaluated with the QuickDASH scale and a Likert scale for aesthetic assessment of free flaps, respectively. *Results*. Seven patients with a mean follow-up of 11.57 months and average flap thickness of 5 mm underwent innervation by an end-to-end neurorrhaphy. The average percentage of disability (QuickDASH) was 21.88% with tenderness, pain, temperature, and two-point discrimination present in 100% of cases, and the aesthetic result gave an overall result of 15.40 (good) with the best scores in color and texture. *Conclusions*. Simultaneous thinning and innervation of the ALT flap lead to a good cosmetic result and functional outcome with a low percentage of disability, which could result in minor surgical procedures and better recovery of motor and sensory function. *Level of Evidence*. IV.

1. Introduction

The most appropriate procedure to correct a defect is currently chosen according to the best possible functional and aesthetic outcome. This represents a change in the reconstructive ladder, improving the functional and aesthetic results that can be achieved with currently free flaps.

The anterolateral thigh (ALT) flap was described in 1984 by Song et al. as a fasciocutaneous flap based on perforators of the descending branch of the lateral femoral circumflex artery. This artery runs caudally in the intermuscular septum between the rectus femoris and vastus lateralis, giving off multiple septocutaneous and musculocutaneous perforators. The flap dimensions vary according to whether it is based on a perforator vessel (up to 20 × 12 cm) or musculocutaneous vessels (up to 34 × 14 cm) [1–3].

Thinning and innervation of the ALT flap have been partially studied by several centers worldwide, but there are still discussions about the limit of thinning of the ALT flap and the prognosis when it is innervated [4], even when there are some studies about the vascular supply and the limits that its perforator vessel can irrigate [5].

In the field of the reconstruction of the upper extremity and, even more, in the hand, the ideal selected flap should meet certain requirements like tissue for replacing like area, thin and pliable flap for molding the hand contour, minimal donor-site morbidity, and sizable pedicle for microsurgical anastomosis; also, change of position intraoperatively should not be necessary [6].

Thinning of the ALT flap has become a popular choice in the reconstruction of soft tissues because it obtains a high-quality and less bulky tissue. The results of reconstruction are more functional and aesthetic and, in some cases, do not require additional debulking procedures [7].

Successful thinning of the ALT flap has been described in both Asian and Western patients. In 2003, Alkureishi et al.

TABLE 1: Demographic data, showing age, gender, anatomic region where the flap was inset, and the etiology.

Patient	Age	Gender	Upper limb defect	Etiology
1	3	Male	Dorsal side of the left hand	Burn sequelae
2	6	Male	Volar side of the distal right forearm and hand	Trauma sequelae
3	2	Male	Dorsal and lateral side of the distal left forearm	Acute trauma
4	27	Male	Dorsal side of the right hand	Burn sequelae
5	28	Male	Dorsal side of the distal right forearm	Acute trauma
6	18	Male	Volar side of the left 4th finger	Acute trauma
7	3	Female	Volar side of the right hand	Burn sequelae

analyzed a series of 10 ALT flaps in Western patients using arterial markers and flap measures. Partial loss of subdermal plexus blood, enough to produce skin necrosis at the distal areas of the flap, was observed [8].

Reconstruction with the ALT flap is a commonly performed surgery, at least in our center. However, we believe that simultaneous thinning and innervation of the ALT flap improve the aesthetic result, promote early rehabilitation, improve the functionality of the limb, and recreate as much as possible the healthy tissue characteristics of the recipient zone. In addition, it preserves motor activity and the perceptions of touch, pain, and temperature in the reconstructed area.

Most published studies refer to the thinning or innervation of free flaps, but not the combination of these techniques. The purpose of this study was to evaluate the functional and aesthetic results of the ultrathin ALT flap and its innervation in soft tissue reconstruction in the upper extremity.

2. Material and Methods

We analyzed seven patients from June 2010 to May 2011 who were considered to be reconstructed by the herein-described method according to the criteria here exposed. Inclusion criteria were sequelae of previous trauma or acute trauma, by a sequential presentation of cases, whose defect was not a candidate for local or regional flap reconstruction, with exposure of deep structures, abundant scar tissue that generates the joint limitation to the flexion or extension, or the joint distortion. And our last inclusion criteria was the reconstruction of the limb with the recovery of the sensibility.

In this series, the indication for reconstruction was acute trauma in three patients, sequelae of crushing trauma in one patient, and burn sequelae in the remaining three patients (Table 1).

2.1. Surgical Technique.
The ALT flap was marked in the habitual manner, and the perforators vessels were identified preoperatively by Doppler US. The rise begins with blunt undermining from medial to lateral, until the localization of the major perforator vessel, preserving the superficial fascia, and a ratio around the perforator vessel of 2 cm to ensure flap survival. The dominant nerve (lateral femoral cutaneous nerve) was identified and preserved. The vascular pedicle was followed in a retrograde fashion to its origin to obtain a

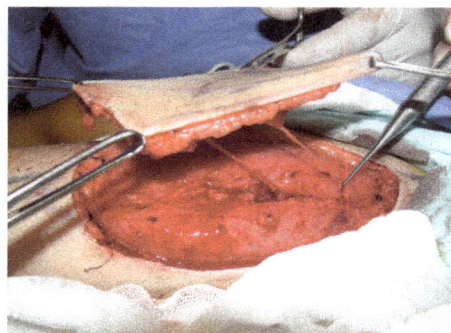

FIGURE 1: Thinned anterolateral thigh flap, with its vascular pedicle and the nerve.

length of at least 7 to 10 cm for comfortable anastomoses. The thinning of the flap was performed with curved iris scissors, leaving a homogenous thickness in most of the flap, outside the security perforator ratio (Figure 1). The thickness of the flap was measured in all the flaps with a centimeters rule, 2 cm outside the security ratio. Vessel and nerve anastomoses were performed with 9-0 nylon, and the extremity was immobilized by a splint. All patients underwent thinning and innervation of the flap by neurorrhaphy to a sensory nerve adjacent to the reconstructed area, usually to one of the sensory branches of the radial nerve.

2.2. Evaluation.
The aesthetic outcome was assessed using the Likert scale for evaluation of aesthetic results in free flaps, in which four main factors are evaluated on a numerical scale: general appearance, shape, color, and texture [9] (Figure 2).

The combined numerical score of the Likert scale (min, 4; max, 20) was classified as follows: 4 to 6, poor; 7 to 9, bad; 10 to 13, regular; 14 to 16, good; and 17 to 20, very good. This evaluation was performed for each patient by three plastic and reconstructive surgeons not involved in the research, an associated researcher (second-year resident), and a close relative. We averaged the scores and obtained a total that was used for classification within the ranges mentioned above.

In addition to evaluation of the overall aesthetic result, we analyzed each one of the four evaluated aesthetic aspects: general appearance, contour, color, and texture. These factors were compared with the features of a normal extremity on a scale of 1 to 5 in which 1 was the worst rating and 5 the best

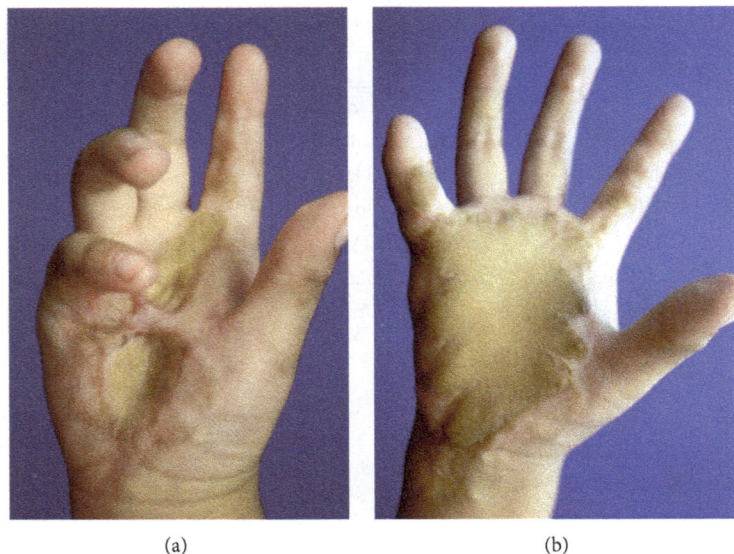

(a)   (b)

FIGURE 2: Before and after images of a 4-year-old child with burn sequelae on her dominant hand.

(1, strongly disagree; 2, disagree; 3, neither agree nor disagree; 4, agree; 5, strongly agree).

Functionality was evaluated by the Spanish validated version of the QuickDASH scale [10, 11], which assesses motor functions of the upper extremity using a simple questionnaire of 11 items. This value was then converted to a score of 0 to 100 using the formula described within the scale. This questionnaire was answered by the patient or, in the case of infants, a parent or guardian.

The data were validated using descriptive statistics (means, confidence intervals, and percentages) with SPSS version 19.0 statistical software. The study was approved by the Research Ethics Committee of our center, the Hospital General Dr. Manuel Gea Gonzalez. All procedures were in accordance with the Regulations of the General Health Law in the Field of Health Research.

TABLE 2: Anterolateral thigh flap characteristics among patients.

Px	Thickness flap (mm)	Length (cm)	Width (cm)
1	6	6	5
2	6	12	8
3	5	11	6
4	4	14	10
5	5	26	15
6	4	12	6
7	5	10	8
Mean: 5 mm		Min: 6 cm Max: 26 cm Mean: 13	Min: 5 cm Max: 15 cm Mean: 8.2

Abbreviations: Px: patient, mm: millimeters, and cm: centimeters.

3. Results

According to the patients analyzed, 6 were male (85.7%) and 1 was female (14.3%), with a mean age of 12.43 years (min: 2 and max: 28, confidence interval 95% (95% CI) 1.66–23.20), with a mean follow-up evaluation of 11.5 months (min: 7 and max: 18, 95% CI 7.62–15.53).

The mean flap thickness was 5 mm, and the mean size was 13 × 8.2 cm (min: 6 × 5 cm, max 26 × 15 cm), taking care to maintain a safe ratio around the perforating vessels to ensure survival of the flap (1 cm) (Table 2). It is important to mention that the different areas of the defects to be reconstructed had the same dimensions of the designed flaps for each one.

The aesthetic outcome was assessed using the Likert scale for evaluation of aesthetic results in free flaps, and each patient was evaluated in the manner previously mentioned (Table 3).

The differences between the overall score of the evaluators means and their associated procedures were measured with the ANOVA (analysis of variance). Concordance among the first three evaluators was good (>0.61) and without statistically significant difference in the overall scores (ANOVA) of the rest of the evaluators (Table 4).

The global analysis results for each characteristic of the aesthetic evaluation scale are shown in Table 3.

Evaluation of general aesthetics revealed a mean of 15.4 (good), CI (95%): 1.50–2.20, with the value of each characteristic evaluated as follows: appearance mean, 3.60 (CI (95%): 3.11–4.1); contour: mean, 3.85 (CI (95%): 3.28–4.42); color: mean, 3.91 (CI (95%): 3.47–4.35); and texture: mean, 3.97 (CI (95%): 3.62–4.31).

The best rated features were color and texture, with a mean score of 3.9; the worst rated feature was overall appearance, with a score of 3.6 (Figure 3, Table 5).

Functional aspects showed a mean of 21.88% (CI (95%): 6.37–37.39) as evaluated by the QuickDASH scale (Table 6, Figure 4). This percentage represents a low disability that

TABLE 3: Aesthetic evaluation.

Px	ESP 1	ESP 2	ESP 3	Relative	2nd Y.R.	Min/max	Mean	Qualification
1	19	20	20	20	15	15/20	**18.8**	**Very good**
2	17	14	19	13	11	11/19	**14.8**	**Good**
3	17	19	19	10	13	10/19	**15.6**	**Good**
4	14	16	16	14	13	13/16	**14.6**	**Good**
5	13	19	18	16	12	12/19	**15.6**	**Good**
6	14	16	18	13	11	11/18	**14.4**	**Good**
7	18	19	13	8	12	8/19	**14**	**Good**

Abbreviations: Px: patient; ESP: evaluating specialist; 2nd Y.R: second-year resident.

TABLE 4: ANOVA for evaluators.

Analysis by the evaluators (ANOVA)	
Evaluator 1 (specialist 1):	0.747
Evaluator 2 (specialist 2):	0.327
Evaluator 3 (specialist 3):	0.205
Evaluator 4 (2nd year resident):	0.681
Evaluator 5 (relative):	0.343
	(>0.5)

Abbreviations: Evaluator 1: specialist 1; evaluator 2: specialist 2; evaluator 3: specialist 3; evaluator 4: second-year resident; evaluator 5: relative.

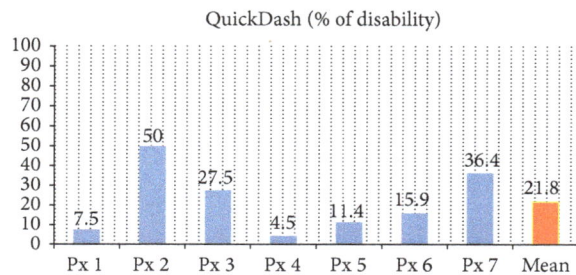

FIGURE 4: Rating of QuickDASH scale.

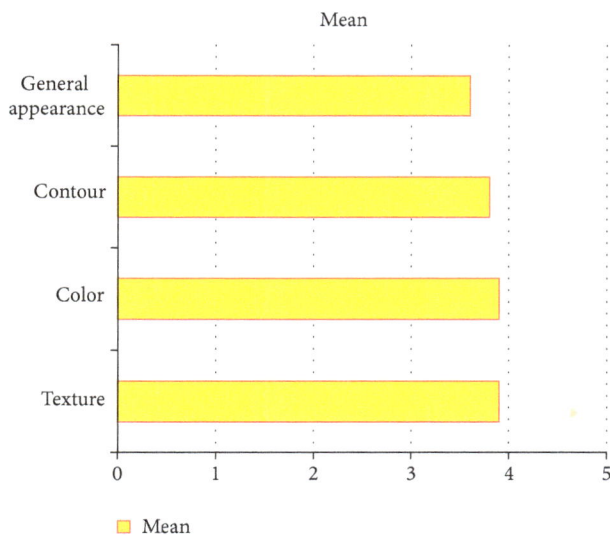

FIGURE 3: Aesthetic evaluation characteristics.

means that most of the common uses of the upper limb, as grabbing or taking a pen or a glass of water, could be done.

Perception of pain and touch was present in 100% of patients. The temperatures (cold and heat) were positive in 85% of patients on the entire flap. Just in one patient (15%) the perception of both cold and heat was absent in the distal half of the flap.

Two-point discrimination showed a mean of 8.57 mm (CI (95%): 3.05–14.09) in the proximal half of the flap and a mean of 9.71 mm (CI (95%): 4.33–15.10) in the distal half. Note that the youngest patient (Px 3) failed to perform this evaluation because of the patient's difficulty in interpretation (Table 6).

4. Discussion

Thinning of the ALT free flap was described by Kimura et al. in 2011. They defined an ultrathin flap as a flap with a 6 mm thickness [12]. Our series is in line with this definition in which we achieved minimum and maximum thickness of 4 and 6 mm, respectively.

A clear understanding of the vascular anatomy of a perforator flap is mandatory, and the *perforasome* concept helps to achieve this understanding. Each perforator possesses a unique tridimensional vascular territory and can be linked by direct or indirect linking vessels to other perforators, increasing the potential size of a flap.

These linking vessels, as described by Taylor and Saint-Cyr, can be established by two mechanisms: (1) the direct linking vessels located in the suprafascial plexus and adipose layer and (2) the indirect linking vessels that depend on a low-pressure reflux phenomenon in the subdermal plexus. These systems also have communications between them to maintain the perfusion pressure. Their distribution is tridimensional and allows for differences in pressure, inversion of flow, and bidirectional flow to recruit adjacent perforasomes, first in the axial plane and later in the transverse plane [13, 14]. The significance of these concepts of perforator flow between perforators directly impacts flap design and survival. We believe that this helped us to achieve a 100% survival rate.

The innervation of the ALT flap has been widely studied. Innervation is heavily reliant on the femoral cutaneous nerve as the dominant nerve. There are two other well-identified

TABLE 5: Aesthetic evaluation by characteristics.

Px	General appearance	Contour	Color	Texture	Mean patients
1	4.8	4.8	4.6	4.6	**4.7**
2	3.4	3.4	4	4	**3.7**
3	4	3.4	4.4	3.8	**3.9**
4	3.4	3.8	3.4	4	**3.6**
5	3.6	4.6	3.6	3.8	**3.9**
6	3	3.2	4	4.2	**3.6**
7	3.4	3.8	3.4	3.4	**3.5**
Mean characters	**3.6**	**3.8**	**3.9**	**3.9**	**3.8**

Abbreviations: Px: patient.

TABLE 6: Functional evaluation.

Px	QuickDASH (% of disability)	Touch	Pain	temp hot	temp cold	2-point disc. proximal (mm)	2-point disc. distal (mm)
1	7.5	+	+	+	+	8	10
2	50	+	+	+	+	10	10
3	27.5	+	+	+	+	Unable	
4	4.5	+	+	+	+	6	10
5	11.4	+	+	+	+	8	10
6	15.9	+	+	+ (1/2 prox)	+ (1/2 prox)	20	20
7	36.4	+	+	+	+	8	8
	Mean: 21.8					Mean: 8.57 mm	Mean: 9.71 mm

Abbreviations: Px: patient; temp: temperature; prox: proximal.

but inconsistent branches: the superior and medial perforator nerves. They share territory with the lateral femorocutaneous nerve because of anastomoses between them [15].

An important factor in the neurorrhaphy is the axonal charge of the receptor nerve because it has a direct impact on the velocity of nerve regeneration. In a terminolateral neurorrhaphy, the axonal charge provided to the nerve is smaller, and the regeneration time is thus longer. This knowledge prompted us to perform terminoterminal neurorrhaphies, decreasing the reinnervation time.

The largest report of an ultrathin ALT flap was reported by Kimura et al. [12]. Their study involved 31 patients during a 6-year period. There were variations in width and length, but the average was 7.7 × 14.7 cm to preserve flap vascularity and survival. Our series had an average size of 13 × 8.2 cm, and every flap was designed to cover a specific defect. Thinning of the flap is a challenge for the surgeon, but it could be made easier by following general principles such as blunt dissection of the vascular pedicle, maintaining a minimum thickness of 3 to 4 mm, and designing the skin paddle with a minimum of 4.5 cm safe ratio around the vascular pedicle, for a total diameter of 9 cm. Following these principles will ensure the safety of the procedure, with the advantage of a one-stage reconstruction that allows a wide and early range of movement, especially in the hand and fingers.

Our series did not have a control group with which to compare our flap because of the presence of different types of defects, making it impossible to create an identical flap in every patient. However, based on the aesthetic scale for free flaps (Likert scale), we provided a good general contour and avoided numerous debulking procedures or liposuction to achieve a good appearance [15].

There is not enough evidence to conclude that flap thinning will compromise the vascularity of the flap. In addition, thinning will not affect the degree of reinnervation of the flap or the velocity of sensibility restoration in the reconstructed area, primarily when the dominant nerve of the flap is well identified. There are currently no reports on this relationship, and more specific studies are necessary to define the timing of nerve regeneration.

Postsurgical sensory evaluation is limited in pediatric patients because of difficulties related to the children's cooperation and interpretation of the two-point discrimination test, as in one of our cases. An excellent option in this circumstance is the neurophysiologic test known as somatosensorial evoked potentials [16]. However, the increased cost and requirement for human resources should be taken into account. These factors justified the absence of this test in our series. Otherwise, performance of this test should be considered when a sensory evaluation cannot be accurately performed for any reason (age, psychiatric illness, etc.). As previously mentioned and observed in our series, the optimal age for this reconstruction, with the exception of emergency cases, is >3 years; at this age, the patient is usually psychologically and physically able to cooperate with the evaluation.

Previous reports on the aesthetic evaluation of free flaps have been published. Parret et al. used the Likert scale to evaluate different types of free flaps for reconstruction of the dorsum of the hand. In their report, venous flaps provided the best cosmetic appearance among fascial, muscular, and fasciocutaneous flaps [9]. Our series included the entire hand, wrist, and forearm, unlike Parret's report, which focused only on dorsum defects. Another critical point is the size of our defects; unlike Parret, we did not use venous flaps. Previous reports mentioned the small size of the venous flap and that its vascularity depends on neovascularization from the arteriovenous shunt created within the flap; trying to increase its size could jeopardize the vascularity, producing venous congestion and necrosis [9, 17].

Making a comparison of our results with the publication of Parret, which makes a similar aesthetic assessment, we can say that our results are better in general appearance and contour than his fasciocutaneous flaps (3.6 versus 2.24 and 3.8 versus 1.95, resp.), better in color than his fascial, muscle, and fasciocutaneous flaps (3.9 versus 3.62, 3.76, and 2.52, resp.), and better in texture, also compared with his fascial, muscle, and fasciocutaneous flaps (3.9 versus 3.29, 3.48, and 3.1, resp.).

From the functional point of view, our assessment was made by the validated scale QuickDASH, which is a shortened version of the DASH scale to measure the degree of disability of the upper extremity (for its acronym in English, Disability of the Arm and Shoulder). This scale does not measure the degree of disability as mild, moderate, or severe. Instead, the result is expressed as a percentage of disability. According to the article published by Kovacs et al. [18], which is the largest series so far studied, with 118 patients, he performs a comparative analysis of the injured reconstructed limb with the healthy contralateral limb. According to these reports, we observed that the scale measured a diminishing result as the patient adapted to the conditions of his injured limb and was still able to perform more tasks as time passed, even without rehabilitation exercises. According to the average result in our study in the QuickDASH scale of 21.88%, with a mean follow-up of 11.57 months, we find a very low disability percentage in our patients, compared with those described in the international literature, and it is even better than those assessed by Kovacs, who concluded that the average rating of the DASH scale before 3 years after the injury is of 28.7% and is of 20.2% after 3 years.

An important difference in our report is the heterogeneous group of evaluators (three certified plastic surgeons, one second-year plastic surgery resident, and a first-degree relative of the patient), which provides a more objective result. In this study, we ruled out the patients' opinions because of the young age of many of the patients; otherwise, this may be studied in the future as a new line of investigation. The concordance among the three first evaluators was good (>0.61), and that between evaluators 4 and 5 was regular (0.54). Otherwise, after statistically analyzing the results of all of the evaluators (one-way ANOVA), no significant statistical differences were found (>0.5).

5. Conclusions

Simultaneous thinning and innervation of the ALT flap lead to a good cosmetic result and functional outcome with a low percentage of disability according to the rating scales in the present study. This technique may result in fewer surgeries, better recovery of motor and sensory function, and significant improvement in color and texture on the reconstructed tissue.

Disclosure

This paper was presented in "Dr. Fernando Ortiz Monasterio residents free papers contest" at the XLII Mexican Congress of Plastic and Reconstructive Surgery and it was the winner of the 1st place in the residents free papers contest.

References

[1] Y.-G. Song, G.-Z. Chen, and Y.-L. Song, "The free thigh flap: a new free flap concept based on the septocutaneous artery," *British Journal of Plastic Surgery*, vol. 37, no. 2, pp. 149–159, 1984.

[2] Y. Kimata, K. Uchiyama, S. Ebihara, T. Nakatsuka, and K. Harii, "Anatomic variations and technical problems of the anterolateral thigh flap: a report of 74 cases," *Plastic and Reconstructive Surgery*, vol. 102, no. 5, pp. 1517–1523, 1998.

[3] F. Demirkan, H.-C. Chen, F.-C. Wei et al., "The versatile anterolateral thigh flap: a musculocutaneous flap in disguise in head and neck reconstruction," *British Journal of Plastic Surgery*, vol. 53, no. 1, pp. 30–36, 2000.

[4] D. Ribuffo, E. Cigna, F. Gargano, C. Spalvieri, and N. Scuderi, "The innervated anterolateral thigh flap: anatomical study and clinical implications," *Plastic and Reconstructive Surgery*, vol. 115, no. 2, pp. 464–470, 2005.

[5] K. Nojima, S. A. Brown, C. Acikel et al., "Defining vascular supply and territory of thinned perforator flaps: part I. Anterolateral thigh perforator flap," *Plastic and Reconstructive Surgery*, vol. 116, no. 1, pp. 182–193, 2005.

[6] R. Adani, L. Tarallo, I. Marcoccio, R. Cipriani, C. Gelati, and M. Innocenti, "Hand reconstruction using the thin anterolateral thigh flap," *Plastic & Reconstructive Surgery*, vol. 116, no. 2, pp. 467–473, 2005.

[7] B.-J. Jeon, S.-Y. Lim, J.-K. Pyon, S.-I. Bang, K. S. Oh, and G.-H. Mun, "Secondary extremity reconstruction with free perforator flaps for aesthetic purposes," *Journal of Plastic, Reconstructive & Aesthetic Surgery*, vol. 64, no. 11, pp. 1483–1489, 2011.

[8] L. W. T. Alkureishi, J. Shaw-Dunn, and G. L. Ross, "Effects of thinning the anterolateral thigh flap on the blood supply to the skin," *British Journal of Plastic Surgery*, vol. 56, no. 4, pp. 401–408, 2003.

[9] B. M. Parrett, J. S. Bou-Merhi, R. F. Buntic, B. Safa, G. M. Buncke, and D. Brooks, "Refining outcomes in dorsal hand coverage: consideration of aesthetics and fonor-Site morbidity," *Plastic and Reconstructive Surgery*, vol. 126, no. 5, pp. 1630–1638, 2010.

[10] Institute for Work & Health, "QuickDASH scale. Versión Española (España)," Spanish (Spain) translation courtesy of Dr. R.S. Rosales, Institute for Research in Hand Surgery, GECOT, Unidad de Cirugía de La Mano y Microcirugía, Tenerife, Spain, 2006.

[11] http://www.dash.iwh.on.ca/assets/images/pdfs/quickdash_info _2010.pdf.

[12] N. Kimura, K. Satoh, T. Hasumi, and T. Ostuka, "Clinical application of the free thin anterolateral thigh flap in 31 consecutive patients," *Plastic and Reconstructive Surgery*, vol. 108, no. 5, pp. 1197–1208, 2001.

[13] G. I. Taylor, "The angiosomes of the body and their supply to perforator flaps," *Clinics in Plastic Surgery*, vol. 30, no. 3, pp. 331–342, 2003.

[14] M. Saint-Cyr, C. Wong, M. Schaverien, A. Mojallal, and R. J. Rohrich, "The perforasome theory: vascular anatomy and clinical implications," *Plastic and Reconstructive Surgery*, vol. 124, no. 5, pp. 1529–1544, 2009.

[15] E. P. Askouni, A. Topping, S. Ball, S. Hettiaratchy, J. Nanchahal, and A. Jain, "Outcomes of anterolateral thigh free flap thinning using liposuction following lower limb trauma," *Journal of Plastic, Reconstructive and Aesthetic Surgery*, vol. 65, no. 4, pp. 474–481, 2012.

[16] O. Papazian, I. Alfonso, and V. F. García, "Evaluación neurofisiológica de los niños con neuropatías periféricas," *Revista de Neurologia*, vol. 35, no. 3, pp. 254–268, 2002.

[17] Y.-T. Lin, S. L. Henry, C.-H. Lin, H.-Y. Lee, W.-N. Lin, and F.-C. Wei, "The shunt-restricted arterialized venous flap for hand/ digit reconstruction: enhanced perfusion, decreased congestion, and improved reliability," *Journal of Trauma: Injury Infection & Critical Care*, vol. 69, no. 2, pp. 399–404, 2010.

[18] L. Kovacs, M. Grob, A. Zimmermann et al., "Quality of life after severe hand injury," *Journal of Plastic, Reconstructive and Aesthetic Surgery*, vol. 64, no. 11, pp. 1495–1502, 2011.

8

Evaluation of the Use of Auricular Composite Graft for Secondary Unilateral Cleft Lip Nasal Alar Deformity Repair

Percy Rossell-Perry[1,2] **and Carolina Romero-Narvaez**[2,3]

[1] *Faculty of Medicine, San Martin de Porres University, Lima, Peru*
[2] *Outreach Surgical Center Program Lima Peru, ReSurge International, 120 Schell Street Apartment 1503 Miraflores, Lima 18, Peru*
[3] *San Bartolome Children Hospital, Lima, Peru*

Correspondence should be addressed to Percy Rossell-Perry; prossellperry@gmail.com

Academic Editor: Stephen M. Warren

The purpose of this study is to evaluate the surgical outcome after using composite grafts for secondary cleft lip nasal deformities. A retrospective cohort study of one surgeon's outcome of 35 consecutive performed secondary cleft lip nasal deformity repair. Thirty-five patients with secondary nose deformity related to unsatisfactory cleft lip repair were operated using the proposed surgical technique since 2008. All these patients met the study criterion of having anthropometric measurements performed at least one year postoperatively. Measurement of nostril size was performed at the right and left side of the nose, preoperatively and at least one year postoperatively. The study found statistically significant differences between the preoperatory and postoperatory nose measurements. In addition, we have not found statistically significant differences between the cleft and noncleft nostril sizes measured at least one year postoperatively. The findings suggest that the proposed technique is a good alternative to address secondary nose deformity related to cleft lip primary repair.

1. Introduction

Secondary alar deficiencies are a common undesirable outcome after primary unilateral cleft lip nose repair.

Even when this technique has been published previously by many authors, it was not well studied and most of the articles are cases series including a few number of patients.

This problem may be in relation to congenital hypoplasia or surgical technique deficiencies (commonly observed using Millard's subnasal incision).

Proper location of this incision would be difficult to be established in some cases.

If the incision is done in a higher position, the alar nose is shortened with the consequent nose asymmetry (Figure 1).

Different techniques have been described for alar reconstruction like local flaps and grafts.

Auricular composite graft is one of the most advantageous methods because it is possible to reconstruct the structural cartilage and skin in one stage.

The use of auricular composite grafts was first described by Koenig in 1902 and the use of two surfaces of skin and cartilage as composite graft was first described by Brown and Cannon in 1946 [1, 2].

Rettinger and O'Connell in 2002 and Ayhan et al. in 2006 described the use of composite grafts for nasal base correction in patients with cleft lip nose in a case series study observing symmetrical and functional results in a small number of patients [3, 4].

Another case series study developed by Cho et al. in 2002 [5] in patients with secondary cleft lip nasal deformity observed an absorption rate of 10% of the graft.

The purpose of this study is to evaluate the symmetry of the nose after using auricular composite grafts for secondary unilateral cleft lip nasal deformities.

2. Methods

This is a prospective cohort study of one surgeon's (corresponding author) outcome of 35 consecutive secondary

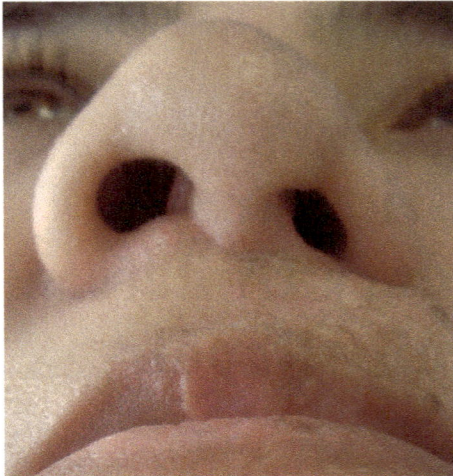

FIGURE 1: Patient with secondary unilateral cleft lip nose deformity and nose asymmetry related to the use of Millard's subnasal incision.

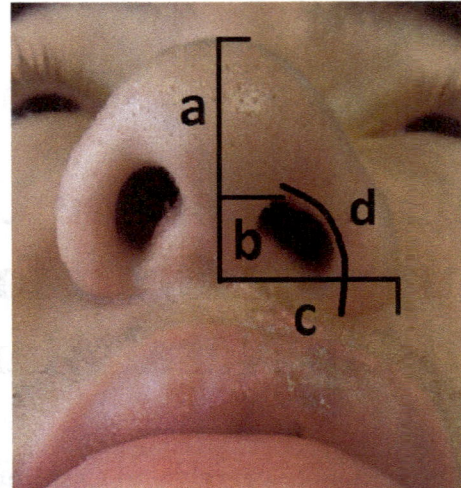

FIGURE 2: Standard anthropometric measurements. (a) Nostril dome height, (b) nostril apex height, (c) alar width, and (d) alar length.

unilateral cleft lip nasal deformity repair from the Outreach Surgical Center Program Lima Peru.

These patients had an open rhinoplasty and the following associated procedures based on Millard Jr. principles [6]:

(a) previously alveolar bone graft during mixed dentition period,

(b) vestibular nose lengthening (composite V-Y method) [7],

(c) medial mobilization of the lateral alar crus (composite V-Y method),

(d) shortening of the nasal base width (when necessary),

(e) septoplasty.

All these patients met the study criterion of having anthropometric measurements performed preoperatively and at least one year postoperatively.

These were the standard anthropometric measurements (Figure 2):

(a) nostril dome height, which was measured from the midway point at the base of the columella to the highest point on the nasal dome;

(b) nostril apex height, which was measured from the midway point at the base of the columella to the highest point of the nostril;

(c) alar width, which was measured from the midway point at the base of the columella to the most lateral point of the nostril in a line perpendicular to the axis of the columella;

(d) alar length, measured from the alar columellar junction to the alar base.

Measurements were performed at the right and left side of the nose, preoperatively and at least one year postoperatively.

These measurements were compared in order to determine pre- and postoperatively nose symmetry.

Outcomes were additionally determined by a parent questionnaire assessment.

Differences in alar length were identified in these patients in order to evaluate the amount of tissue necessary for alar reconstruction.

The tissue's requirement is estimated using the length of the alar nose measured from the alar-columellar junction to the alar base.

Based on our experience, the graft is designed 50% larger than the estimated defect due to the scar contracture of the graft observed during the healing process.

In order to maximize graft survival, careful preoperative design, preparation of the recipient site, meticulous surgical technique, and diligent postoperatory care are mandatory.

The recipient bed of the graft located at the deficient alar base must be in good condition for proper development of the process of plasmatic imbibition, vascular inosculation, and neovascularization.

All the scar tissue should be excised from the recipient site leaving a healthy raw surface to receive the auricular composite graft. The use of electrocautery should be avoided as possible.

2.1. Surgical Technique. After design with marking pen of the required auricular tissue in the ear, local anesthetic without epinephrine is injected around the designed composite graft avoiding any hydrodissection of the skin off the cartilage (Figure 3).

The skin and cartilage are incised in one block with 15C blade following the skin markings.

The size of the cartilage component should be a few millimeters bigger than the skin component in order to guarantee their integrity as composite graft (Figure 4).

The graft should be harvested carefully and manipulated gently grabbing the cartilage and skin with the forceps

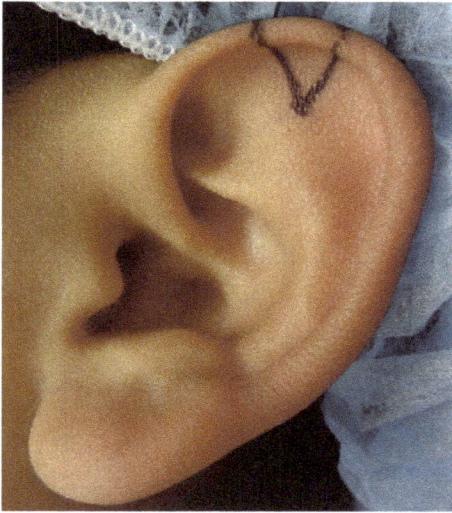

FIGURE 3: Designed area of the required auricular tissue from the helix.

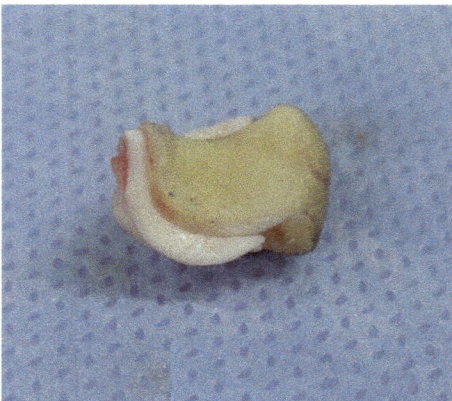

FIGURE 4: Auricular composite graft. The size of the cartilage component should be a few millimeters bigger than the skin component. This is a 15 × 18 mm composite graft.

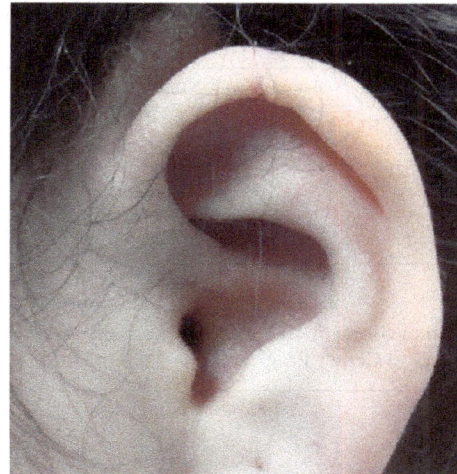

FIGURE 5: Long term appearance of the donor site after 18 months.

simultaneously. Any skin traction alone may separate it from the cartilage losing the tissue connection between them.

After this, carefully edge to edge closure is performed at the donor site using skin stitches.

Up to 1.5 centimeter defect can be closed primarily without problems. Larger grafts are rarely required for secondary alar nose repair in these patients.

Long term appearance of the donor site is acceptable (Figure 5).

The affected alar nose is incised at the level of the scar and this scar tissue should be removed carefully leaving healthy tissue at the borders to receive the composite graft and guarantee its survival. Use of cautery should be avoided as possible.

The skin edges of the auricular composite graft are directly closed to the defect's skin edges with simple resorbable sutures.

The composite graft is located between the alar nose and upper lip suturing the skin component only using resorbable simple stitches.

Stitches are placed first at the corners (internal and external) and between the graft and alar nose and upper lip, making easier the application of the following sutures. These stitches should not include the cartilage component and must be placed superficially in order to avoid any bad alignment between the borders.

Special attention must be taken with the sutures located around the medial surface of the graft where the skin is firmly attached to the cartilage. At this level the stitches should include only the skin avoiding any disruption between the component's graft.

Antibiotic ointment is applied to the surgical surfaces.

Moisturizing ointment is recommended to be applied over the graft during one week in order to avoid graft desiccation (greatest risk for graft failure).

Appearance of the grafts is not good during the first days becoming first blue and then pink after epidermolysis. Complete survival was confirmed after 7 days.

We did not use any drug to improve graft survival in the studied group.

2.2. Statistical Analysis. A two-sample test of proportions was performed to assess the statistical significance between the two methods. $P < 0.05$ yielded a confidence level of 95%.

The data were analyzed using Stata 11.0 software.

3. Results

Thirty-five patients with secondary alar nose deformity related to unsatisfactory unilateral cleft lip repair were operated using the proposed surgical technique since 2008.

The mean age at the time of the surgery was 11.57 years (range 8 to 14 years).

Gender: men 24 (68.57%) and women 14 (31.43%).

Side: left 23 (65.71%) and right 12 (34.29%)

TABLE 1: Comparisons of cleft side and noncleft side using auricular composite graft technique preoperatively by the Outreach Surgical Center Program Lima 2008 to 2013.

Nose segment	Noncleft n: 35 Mean	Cleft n: 35 Mean	P	CL
Nostril apex height	13 ± 1.22	8.82 ± 1.78	0.0003	−4.18 (−6.08; −2.29)
Alar width	17.33 ± 2.66	21.92 ± 1.61	0.0002	4.59 (2.53; 6.65)
Alar length	20 ± 2.57	14.94 ± 1.06	0.00001	−5.06 (−5.45; −2.66)

TABLE 2: Comparisons of cleft side and noncleft side using auricular composite graft technique at 1 year or more postoperatively by the Outreach Surgical Center Program Lima 2008 to 2013.

Nose segment	Noncleft n: 35 Mean	Cleft n: 35 Mean	P	CL
Nostril apex height	13 ± 1.22	11 ± 0.58	0.05	2 (0.02; 3.99)
Alar width	17.33 ± 2.66	18.11 ± 2.86	0.21	0.78 (−0.54; 2.09)
Alar length	20 ± 2.57	20.21 ± 1.76	0.41	−0.21 (−2.74; 1.17)

TABLE 3: Comparisons of cleft side pre- and postoperative nose measurements after 1 year using the proposed technique in patients with secondary unilateral cleft lip nose deformity by the Outreach Surgical Center Program Lima 2008 to 2013.

Nose segment	Preoperatory n: 35 Mean	Postoperatory n: 35 Mean	P
Nostril apex height	8.82 ± 1.78	11 ± 0.58	0.004
Alar width	21.92 ± 1.61	18.11 ± 2.86	0.001
Alar length	14.94 ± 1.06	20.21 ± 1.76	0.00001
Nostril dome height	19.31 ± 1.65	20.67 ± 2.07	0.14

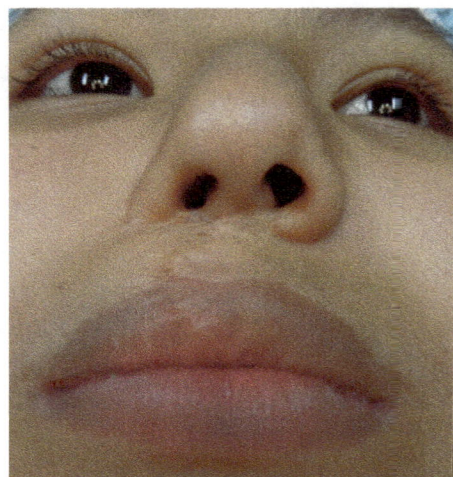

FIGURE 6: Case 1: A 9-year-old female patient with a right unilateral cleft lip initially treated using conventional Millard technique. At this time the nose is asymmetric with deficiency of the right alar nose.

The preoperatively mean height and width of auricular composite tissue were 16.21 mm (range: 18 to 13 mm) and 10.35 mm (range: 13 to 8 mm), respectively.

We observed statistically significant preoperatory differences between the cleft and noncleft sides and between the preoperatory and postoperatory nose measurements (Tables 1 to 3).

In addition, we have not found statistically significant differences between the cleft and noncleft sides measured at least one year postoperatively (Table 2).

Observed rate of graft survival was 100% with 2 partial necroses.

90.35% of the patients were very satisfied with the surgical outcomes.

Three patients (8.5%) showed fair results with some recurrence of the asymmetry of both nostrils.

Surgical outcomes are presented in Tables 1 to 3 and Figures 6, 7, 8, 9, 10, 11, 12, and 13.

4. Discussion

Surgical repair of the nasal deformity caused by trauma, tumor extirpation, burns, and cleft lip nose is challenging because it requires reconstruction of the outer and inner skin and supporting cartilage [3–5, 8–12].

The auricular composite graft let us reconstruct the three-layered structure of the alar and has a similar shape, curve, color, and texture. In addition, the graft is similar to the recipient site because the ear has components with various shapes and curves.

Primary closure of the donor site can be achieved for a defect less than 15 mm as described by Singh and Bartlett in 2007 [13] (Figures 4 and 5).

In case of secondary cleft lip nasal deformity with severe tissue deficiency, auricular composite graft can be useful for columellar lengthening or for creating symmetrical nostrils [10–12].

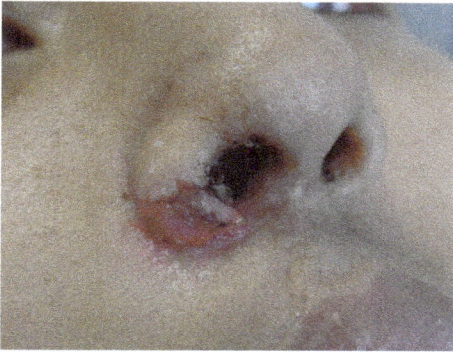

FIGURE 7: The patient is shown one week after secondary rhinoplasty using auricular composite graft. The graft is having some epidermolysis.

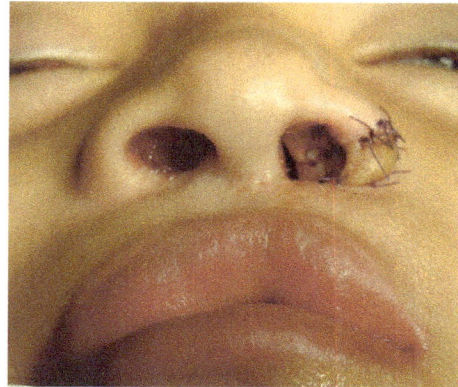

FIGURE 10: Intraoperative image shows nose asymmetry using the auricular composite graft for nose repair.

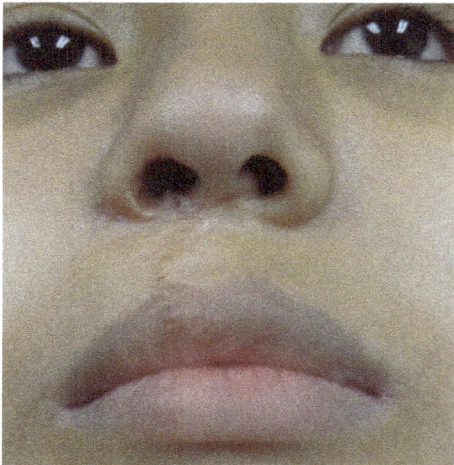

FIGURE 8: Postoperative view of the patient two years after surgery.

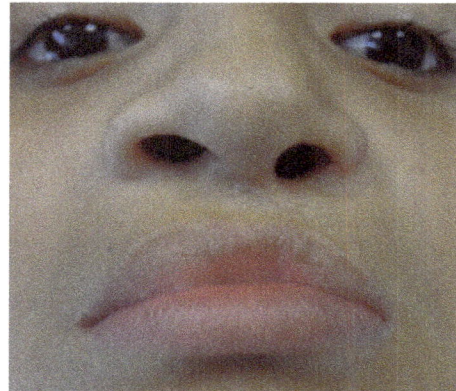

FIGURE 11: Postoperative view of the patient three years after surgery illustrating cosmetic and functional improvement of the nose with small contracture of the graft after the healing process.

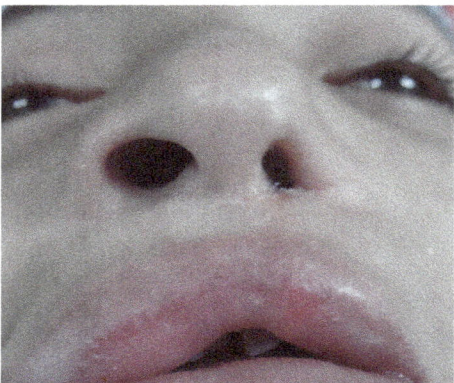

FIGURE 9: Case 2: A 12-year-old female patient with a left unilateral cleft lip initially treated using conventional Millard technique. At this time the nose has a severe deformity with functional impairment and nose asymmetry.

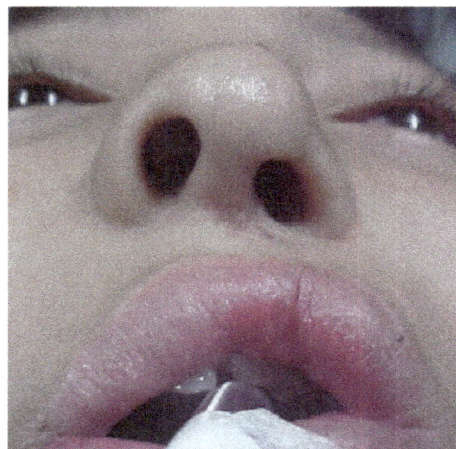

FIGURE 12: Case 3: A 10-year-old female patient with a left unilateral cleft lip initially treated using conventional Millard technique. The nose has a severe deformity with nose asymmetry.

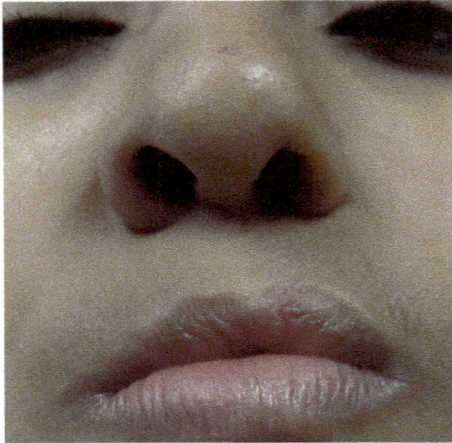

FIGURE 13: Postoperative view of the patient four years after surgery.

The main disadvantage of this method is the contracture of the graft after the healing process which has been observed in all cases.

Difference between pre- and postoperative width of the graft was 5.27 mm and represents 50.91% of the initial width of the graft (10.35 mm).

This percentage represents the contracture of the graft and supports our preoperatory design considering a composite graft 50% larger than the estimated defect.

This outcome is similar to the initial report made by Rees [14] with 53% of reabsorption.

Grafted tissues frequently shrink their width and thickness. In order to improve this situation, we design the composite grafts larger than the estimated defect preoperatively.

Cosmetic appearance of the graft is difficult to be improved and this is the main limitation of this technique.

In relation with the size of the graft, initial studies concluded that a graft larger than 10 mm results in subsequent necrosis of the graft [2, 15].

However, we use larger grafts (mean 20 × 12 mm) with high rate of survival (85.71%).

Parkhouse and Evans [16] reported similar results with a successful graft of 10 × 18 mm for alar reconstruction.

Previous anthropometric studies described by Farkas et al. [17] did not conclude major differences in relation to the age (range: 6 to 13 years old) and gender.

This is the reason why these variables are not affecting our results and any stratification was not necessary in the studied group.

Many papers have been published about the use of auricular composite graft in aesthetic and reconstructive surgery.

Most of them are case series studies including a small number of patients.

This is the first analytic research to evaluate objectively differences between the cleft and noncleft side of the nose pre- and postoperatively.

Objective evaluation of the cleft nose deformity after using conventional Millard's technique for primary repair

has been done and nostril apex height, alar length, and width asymmetry have been determined in all the cases preoperatively (Table 1).

Effectiveness of the proposed technique for secondary nose deformity repair has been confirmed with this comparative study observing nonstatistical significant differences between the cleft and noncleft side and statistical significant differences between pre- and postoperatively anthropometric nose measurements (Tables 2 and 3) (Figures 6 to 13).

We observe some small differences between the cleft and noncleft side in the presented cases; however, they are small and nonstatistically significant. These differences are mainly related to the recurrence of the septal deviation.

An adequate and symmetrical nasal tip projection was obtained by repositioning the cleft lower lateral cartilage; however, these were not statistically significant (P: 0.14) (Table 3).

Nasal retainers are commonly used in cleft nose deformity repair; however, we did not use any molding device in this study due to the observed complications related to their use, like skin reaction, infection, ulceration, recurrence, pain, and others.

This problem requires additional studies to evaluate cosmetic appearance of the graft.

5. Conclusions

The proposed technique of open rhinoplasty in combination with auricular composite grafts has been useful for gaining additional alar length in patients who otherwise have a satisfactory relationship between the anatomic subunits.

The findings suggest that the proposed technique is a good alternative to address secondary nose deformity related to unilateral cleft lip primary repair.

Acknowledgment

The authors would like to thank Dr. Paul Rottler for his assistance with native English speaker paper revision.

References

[1] F. Koenig, "Zur deckung von defekten der nasenflügel," Berl Klein Wochenschr, vol. 39, p. 137, 1902.

[2] J. B. Brown and B. Cannon, "Composite free grafts of two surfaces of skin and cartilage from the ear," Annals of Surgery, vol. 124, no. 6, pp. 1101–1107, 1946.

[3] G. Rettinger and M. O'Connell, "The nasal base in cleft lip rhinoplasty," Facial Plastic Surgery, vol. 18, no. 3, pp. 165–178, 2002.

[4] M. Ayhan, M. Gorgu, B. Erdogan et al., "Various applications of chondrocutaneous composite grafts in secondary cleft lip nose patients," Journal of Craniofacial Surgery, vol. 17, no. 6, pp. 1065–1071, 2006.

[5] B. C. Cho, J. W. Park, and B. S. Baik, "Correction of severe secondary cleft lip nasal deformity using a composite graft: current approach and review," *Annals of Plastic Surgery*, vol. 48, no. 2, pp. 131–137, 2002.

[6] D. R. Millard Jr., "Earlier correction of the unilateral cleft lip nose," *Plastic and Reconstructive Surgery*, vol. 70, no. 1, pp. 64–73, 1982.

[7] J. Potter, "Some nasal tip deformities due to alar cartilage abnormalities," *Plastic and Reconstructive Surgery*, vol. 13, no. 5, pp. 358–366, 1954.

[8] R. Gurunluoglu, M. Shafighi, A. Gardetto, and H. Piza-Katzer, "Composite skin grafts for basal cell carcinoma defects of the nose," *Aesthetic Plastic Surgery*, vol. 27, no. 4, pp. 286–292, 2003.

[9] D. Son, M. Kwak, S. Yun, H. Yeo, J. Kim, and K. Han, "Large auricular chondrocutaneous composite graft for nasal alar and columellar reconstruction," *Archives of Plastic Surgery*, vol. 39, no. 4, pp. 323–328, 2012.

[10] Y. W. Cheon and B. Y. Park, "Long-term evaluation of elongating columella using conchal composite graft in bilateral secondary cleft lip and nose deformity," *Plastic and Reconstructive Surgery*, vol. 126, no. 2, pp. 543–553, 2010.

[11] S. Saha, V. Kumar, R. Kashanchi, and A. Agrawal, "Correction of the nose in patients with unilateral cleft lip with composite grafts," *Scandinavian Journal of Plastic and Reconstructive Surgery and Hand Surgery*, vol. 39, no. 6, pp. 344–348, 2005.

[12] K. Matsuo and T. Hirose, "Secondary correction of the unilateral cleft lip nose using a conchal composite graft," *Plastic and Reconstructive Surgery*, vol. 86, no. 5, pp. 991–995, 1990.

[13] D. J. Singh and S. P. Bartlett, "Aesthetic management of the ear as a donor site," *Plastic and Reconstructive Surgery*, vol. 120, no. 4, pp. 899–908, 2007.

[14] T. D. Rees, "The transfer of free composite grafts of skin and fat: a clinical study," *Plastic and Reconstructive Surgery*, vol. 25, pp. 556–564, 1960.

[15] J. A. Lehman Jr., W. S. Garrett Jr., and R. H. Musgrave, "Earlobe composite grafts for the correction of nasal defects.," *Plastic and Reconstructive Surgery*, vol. 47, no. 1, pp. 12–16, 1971.

[16] N. Parkhouse and D. Evans, "Reconstruction of the ala of the nose using a composite free flap from the pinna," *British Journal of Plastic Surgery*, vol. 38, no. 3, pp. 306–313, 1985.

[17] L. G. Farkas, C. R. Forrest, and J. H. Phillips, "Comparison of the morphology of the "cleft face" and the normal face: defining the anthropometric differences," *Journal of Craniofacial Surgery*, vol. 11, no. 2, pp. 76–82, 2000.

9

Effect of Extracorporeal Shock Wave Treatment on Deep Partial-Thickness Burn Injury in Rats

Gabriel Djedovic,[1] Florian Stefan Kamelger,[1,2] Johannes Jeschke,[1] and Hildegunde Piza-Katzer[1]

[1] *Department of Plastic, Reconstructive and Aesthetic Surgery, Innsbruck Medical University, Anichstraße 35, 6020 Innsbruck, Austria*
[2] *Department of Traumatology and Sports Medicine, Innsbruck Medical University, Anichstraße 35, 6020 Innsbruck, Austria*

Correspondence should be addressed to Florian Stefan Kamelger; floriankamelger@yahoo.de

Academic Editor: Marcus Lehnhardt

Extracorporeal shock wave therapy (ESWT) enhances tissue vascularization and neoangiogenesis. Recent animal studies showed improved soft tissue regeneration using ESWT. In most cases, deep partial-thickness burns require skin grafting the outcome is often unsatisfactory in function and aesthetic appearance. The aim of this study was to demonstrate the effect of ESWT on skin regeneration after deep partial-thickness burns. Under general anesthesia, two standardized deep partial-thickness burns were induced on the back of 30 male Wistar rats. Immediately after the burn, ESWT was given to rats of group 1 ($N = 15$), but not to group 2 ($N = 15$). On days 5, 10, and 15, five rats of each group were analyzed. Reepithelialization rate was defined, perfusion units were measured, and histological analysis was performed. Digital photography was used for visual documentation. A wound score system was used. ESWT enhanced the percentage of wound closure in group 1 as compared to group 2 ($P < 0.05$). The reepithelialization rate was improved significantly on day 15 ($P < 0.05$). The wound score showed a significant increase in the ESWT group. ESWT improves skin regeneration of deep partial-thickness burns in rats. It may be a suitable and cost effective treatment alternative in this type of burn wounds in the future.

1. Introduction

Burn wounds are a response to thermic, chemical, or electric forces and, depending on the depth of the burn, acute surgical debridement of the burned skin layers may be necessary. Wounds that affect the superficial skin layers including the reticular stratum characterize deep partial-thickness burns. Thus, destruction of structures that play an important role in skin regeneration leads to scar formation as well as to decreased functional and aesthetical outcome. However, in contrast to full-thickness burn wounds, blood supply to the affected area is still intact.

Extracorporeal shock wave therapy (ESWT) has been used for over 30 years in lithotripsy. Besides its mechanical effects, its biological effects were first described nearly 15 years ago by orthopedic surgeons. Still, the exact mechanisms are not perfectly known yet; however, experimental studies could reveal the potential of shock waves to increase growth factors, which are known to be crucial for wound healing and angiogenesis [1]. Angiogenesis is an essential component of wound healing and, thus, of healing of burn wounds. Other studies showed an increase in skin flap survival in rats or described effects improving the clinical outcome in patients with plantar fasciitis, tennis elbow, or nonunions [2–6].

The purpose of this study was to investigate the effect of ESWT on wound healing in deep partial-thickness burns and to develop a standardized protocol for an animal model that allows further investigations of burns of this kind.

Thereto, we modified the burn animal model originally described by Kaufman et al. and modified by Kuroda et al. [7, 8]. Macroscopical and histological examinations were carried out for measuring wound surface and courting epithelial layers. Additionally, a score system was used that combines epithelialization, granulation, cell density, and vascularization [9, 10] to measure the improvement in wound healing with and without ESWT.

We hypothesize that ESWT of deep partial thickness burns leads to an increase of perfusion in the wound and thus to a better healing in terms of a faster reepithelialization as well as of a lack of scar formation.

2. Material and Methods

2.1. Animals. The animals (300–380 grams) used in the present study were maintained and used in conformity with Austrian national regulations and international guidelines of the Council of Europe on animal welfare. All 30 Wistar rats (Charles River Laboratories, Sulzfeld, Germany) were kept in separate cages with a 12-hour light/12-hour night circle and free access to pellets and water. Rats were sedated with sevoflurane and anesthetized with ketamine hydrochloride. Postoperatively, the animals were treated with 0.1 mg/kg BW/12 h buprenorphine for adequate analgesia.

2.2. Burn Stamp. After anesthesia, the dorsal fur of the rats was trimmed and the skin depilated with Veet, a commercially available depilation cream. Anatomical structures that defined the burn areas were the iliac crest, the 12th rip, and the spinous process. In accordance with the protocol of Kaufman et al. [7], modified by Kuroda et al. [8], two standardized deep partial-thickness burns were inflicted on the dorsal skin of each animal with a specially constructed burn stamp made of steel with a tare weight of exactly 500 grams and a diameter of 2 cm. The burn stamp was preoperatively heated in a 70°C water bath for two hours. Induction of a burn wound with the heated stamp was for 9 seconds and no additional pressure was applied in order to keep standardized conditions. Preliminary histological investigation established the presence of a deep partial-thickness burn wound using the described protocol (data not shown).

2.3. Extracorporeal Shock Wave Therapy. After standardized infliction of two burn wounds in all animals, rats were randomly divided into two groups of 15 animals each. Group 1 was treated with ESWT, whereas group 2 served as control. In group 1, immediately after infliction of the burn wound, the shock wave applicator (Evotron, High Medical Technologies, Lengwil, Switzerland) was held perpendicularly to the wound and 500 shocks were applied with an energy flux density of 0.11 mJ/mm^2 and a frequency of 240/min. A commercially available ultrasonic gel served as contact medium. The burn wounds of group 2 were covered with ultrasound gel, which was then removed after two minutes. To authors' knowledge, commercially available ultrasonic gel does not influence water loss and wound healing.

The wound was not subjected to any further manipulation.

2.4. Analysis. Two investigators performed analysis in a blinded fashion. All wounds were photo-documented daily, pictures were transferred to hard disk, and wound surfaces were quantified with standard analysis software. Each group was divided into three subgroups. Five animals of each group were killed on day five, day ten, and day fifteen, respectively, with an overdose of pentobarbital. Before the animals were sacrificed, wounds were investigated with a Laser Doppler Imager (LDI, Moor Inc., Sussex, England) and the data were transferred to hard disk. We attached great importance to a sufficient sedation status of the animals to avoid artifacts and corruptions because of movement during LDI-measurement. Nevertheless, measurements were repeated if artifacts occurred.

Percentage of open wound surface on day$_x$ was calculated:

$$\frac{\varnothing \text{ of wound surface of day}_x}{\varnothing \text{ of wound surface of day}_1} \times 100 \tag{1}$$

$$= \text{percentage (\%) of surface on day}_x.$$

Additionally, on day 1 and on day$_x$, the burn wounds were measured with the LDI. Regions of interest (ROI) were defined 2 × 2 cm. Percentage of perfusion units (PU) of day$_x$ was calculated as follows:

$$\frac{\text{mean of PU of day}_x}{\text{mean of PU of day}_1} \times 100 \tag{2}$$

$$= \text{percentage (\%) of PU on day}_x.$$

Wound areas were harvested, fixed in 4% formaldehyde and embedded in paraffin wax, and prepared for histological analysis. H&E staining was performed. The number of epithelial cell layers on days 5, 10, and 15 was counted. Furthermore, wound healing was assessed histologically within the wound center with the score system of Yu et al. [9] as modified by Schlager et al. [10]; this system combines the parameters of the degree of reepithelialization, cell number, granulation tissue, and vascularization for classifying burn wounds (Table 1). The determined scores for each parameter were summed up and presented for days 5, 10, and 15.

2.5. Statistical Analysis. The Mann-Whitney U test was used. Results are expressed as mean ± standard deviation (SD) and considered significant when $P < 0.05$ and highly significant when $P < 0.01$. All statistical analyses were performed using SPSS 12.0 software (SPSS, Chicago, Illinois).

3. Results

3.1. Macroscopical Analysis. None of the animals showed any signs of infection. Animals lost 10 to 20 grams of body weight from day 0 to day 1. Body weight normalized during the study period.

Wound measurements on day 5 showed a remaining surface of 48.5% ± 10.0 in the ESWT group (group 1) and of 43.6% ± 8.6 in animals of the control group (group 2) in comparison to the measured wound area on day 1. No significance could be calculated. Day 10 showed 6.8% ± 6.6 of remaining wound surface in the ESWT group and 7.9% ± 8.8 in the control group. On day 15, a statistically significant difference between the ESWT group (0.1% ± 0.1) and the control group (3.8% ± 5.5) could be seen (Figure 1; $P < 0.05$).

TABLE 1: Histologic scoring of burn wounds according to Schlager et al. [10].

1	EP	None to very minimal epithelialization
	CC	None to very minimal (mainly inflammatory cells)
	GT	None
	V	None
2	EP	Minimal epithelialization
	CC	Predominately inflammatory cells, few fibroblasts
	GT	None to a thin layer of granulation tissue
	V	Few capillaries
3	EP	Completely thin layer
	CC	More fibroblasts, still with inflammatory cells
	GT	Thicker layer of granulation tissue
	V	Well-defined capillary system
4	EP	Completely thick layer
	CC	Fewer numbers of fibroblasts in dermis
	GT	Uniformly thick layer of granulation tissue
	V	Extensive neovascularization

EP: epithelialization; CC: cellular content; GT: granulation tissue; V: vascularity.

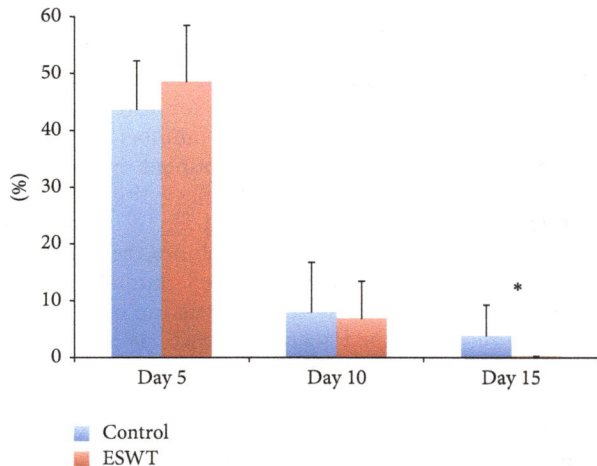

FIGURE 2: Percentage of perfusion units of the control compared to the ESWT-treated group in correlation to the measurements taken on day one. Day 5 showed statistically higher perfusion of the wound ($^{**}P < 0{,}01$).

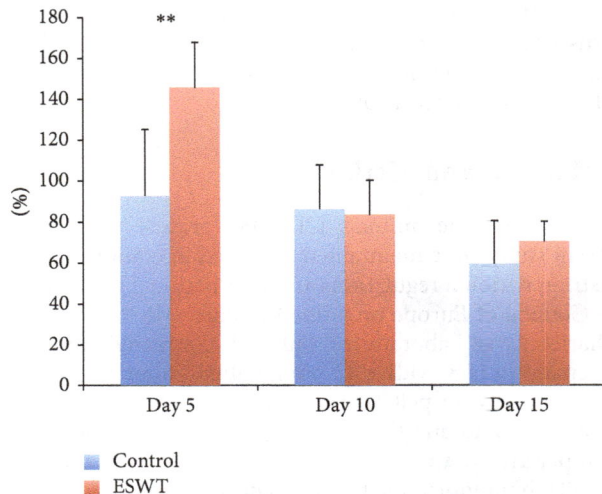

FIGURE 1: Percentage of remaining wound areas of the control group compared to the ESWT-treated group in correlation to the measurements taken on day one. Day 15 showed statistically different wound surfaces ($^{*}P = 0.028$).

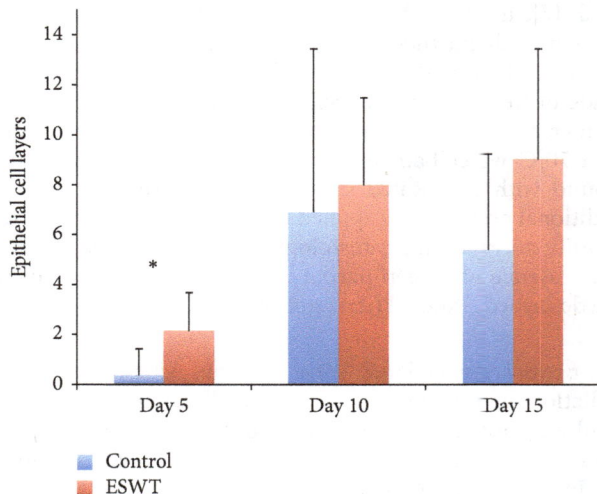

FIGURE 3: Number of epidermal cell layers at the centre of the burn wound of the control group compared to the ESWT-treated group. Day 5 shows statistical significance with a P-value of 0.038.

Perfusion measurements using the Laser Doppler Imager showed no statistically significant difference between the two groups on day 10 (group 1: 83.3% ± 16.9, group 2: 86.0% ± 21.7) and day 15 (group 1: 70.3% ± 9.8, group 2: 59.5% ± 20.9) in comparison to the measured perfusion units on day 1. Only the measurements on day 5 showed a high statistical significance (group 1: 145.2% ± 22.7, group 2: 92.7% ± 32.6; Figure 2; $P < 0.01$).

3.2. Microscopical Analysis. Prior to the main study, three rats (number of burn wounds = 6) were sacrificed after the application of the burn stamp and wounds were excised and applied to histological assessment. All wounds revealed affection of the epidermal as well as the reticular dermal layer, which classified them as deep partial-thickness burns.

Histological analysis revealed no signs of infection.

Counting of epithelial cell layers showed significant differences between the ESWT group (2.1 ± 1.6 layers) and the control group (0.4 ± 1.1 layers) on day 5 (Figure 3; $P < 0.05$). On day 10 (group 1: 8 ± 3.6 layers, group 2: 6.9 ± 6.6 layers) and day 15 (group 1: 9 ± 4.4 layers, group 2: 5.4 ± 3.5 layers), the ESWT group showed a greater number of cell layers than animals of the control group. However, this difference did not reach statistical significance.

TABLE 2: Summary of macroscopical and histological findings of the ESWT group compared to the control group.

Day	Group	Wound surface		Perfusion index		Epithelial cell layers		Score system	
		Mean	SD	Mean	SD	Mean	SD	Mean	SD
5	Control	43.6	8.6	92.7	32.6	0.4	1.1	5.8	0.7
	ESWT	48.5	10.0	145.2**	22.7	2.1*	1.6	7.4**	0.5
10	Control	7.9	8.8	86.0	21.7	6.9	6.6	10.0	1.7
	ESWT	6.8	6.6	83.3	16.9	8.0	3.6 *	11.9*	1.6
15	Control	3.8	5.5	59.5	20.9	5.4	3.9	11.6	1.5
	ESWT	0.07*	0.1	70.3	9.8	9.0	4.4	14.3**	0.5

*$P < 0.05$; **$P < 0.01$.

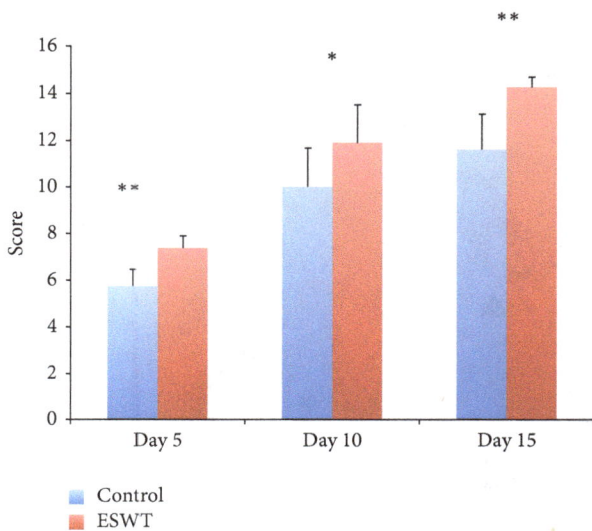

FIGURE 4: Calculated score after Schlager et al. [10] of burn wound healing in the control compared to the ESWT-treated group on days 5, 10, and 15 (*$P < 0,05$, **$P < 0,01$).

The wound score system showed a highly significant improvement of the healing process on day 5 (group 1: 7.4 ± 0.5; group 2: 5.8 ± 0.7) and day 15 (group 1: 14.3 ± 0.5; group 2: 11.6 ± 1.5) and a significant improvement of the healing process on day 10 (group 1: 11.9 ± 1.6; group 2: 10.0 ± 1.7) (Figure 4).

Macroscopical and histological findings are summarized in Table 2. Wound surface decreased in both groups over time; however, just one animal of the ESWT group showed a minimally open wound ground on day 15. Moreover, the perfusion index showed a highly significant difference in perfusion on day 5. According to these findings, the ingrowth of new epithelial tissue into the wounds was faster and differed significantly on day 5 in the ESWT group. The wound score, which summarizes histological parameters like epithelialization, cellular content, granulation, and vascularity, differed significantly on all days of measurement and thus indicated the formation of a well vascularized and reepithelialized tissue. During the entire investigation period group 1 showed a higher reepithelialization rate in the wound center, more vessels in the reticular layer, and a faster-developing granulation, accompanied by a faster appearance of fibroblasts, compared to the untreated group. Figure 6 shows the wound areas of the ESWT group and Figure 5 the control group, respectively. The wounds in the ESWT group already showed a thin but continuous epithelial covering. Vessels in the reticular stratum were common.

4. Discussion

Shock waves are high-amplitude sound waves that extend in a three-dimensional manner. They are characterized by a fast and intense pressure boost, in which a positive pressure phase is followed by a negative one [11].

ESWT has shown its effectiveness in urology, in orthopedics, and recently in plastic and reconstructive surgery [1–6, 12–16].

In the current study we found that the treatment with this noninvasive technique resulted in a clinical tendency towards better wound healing, shown by a significantly smaller and well-epithelialized wound area in the treatment group on day 15. Interestingly, on day 5 the measured wound area of the ESWT-treated group was still larger than the respective one of the untreated group. One possible explanation of this phenomenon is that this initially delayed wound closure could be due to an additional tissue injury caused by the highly energetic shock waves, as observed in bones [17] and endothelial cells [18, 19]. Petechial bleeding observed immediately after the shock-wave treatment lends some support to this assumption. However, in previous investigations performed by our group, no such bleeding was observed [3–5]. A possible explanation for this observation might be that in those studies shock waves were applied to uninjured skin whereas in the current study to skin that had undergone burn injury. It is fair to assume that injured skin is liable to be more sensitive to additional forces.

Already on day 5 a significantly higher number of epithelial cell layers could be counted in the burn injury center, although the macroscopically observed wound area was yet larger. This trend could be seen during the entire investigation period. Histological examination and the wound score evaluated important factors of wound healing (granulation, vascularization, epithelialization, and cellular content) [10]. During the entire investigation period, the ESWT group showed a higher reepithelialization rate in the wound center and more vessels in the reticular layer compared to the untreated

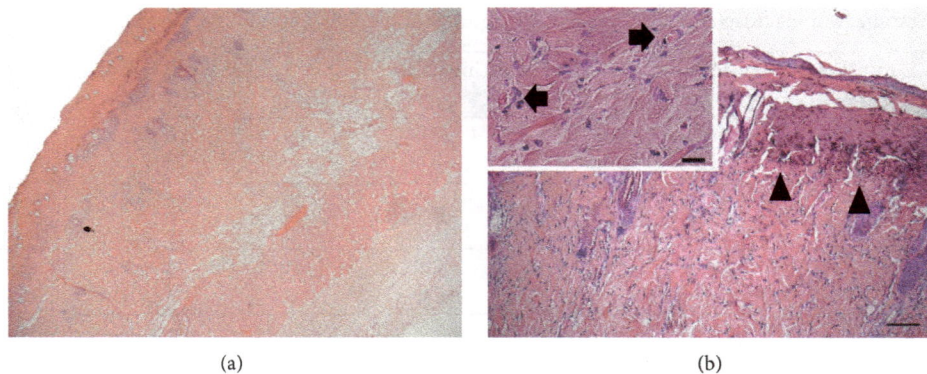

(a)

(b)

FIGURE 5: (a) This haematoxylin-eosin- (H.E.-) stained histological section shows the centre of the burn wound of the control group on day 5. (b) The burn wound has not yet reepithelialized (arrowheads); vessels in the reticular stratum are rare (scale bar = 100 μm). The inset shows the distribution of vessels (arrows) in the reticular stratum in a higher magnification (scale bar = 20 μm).

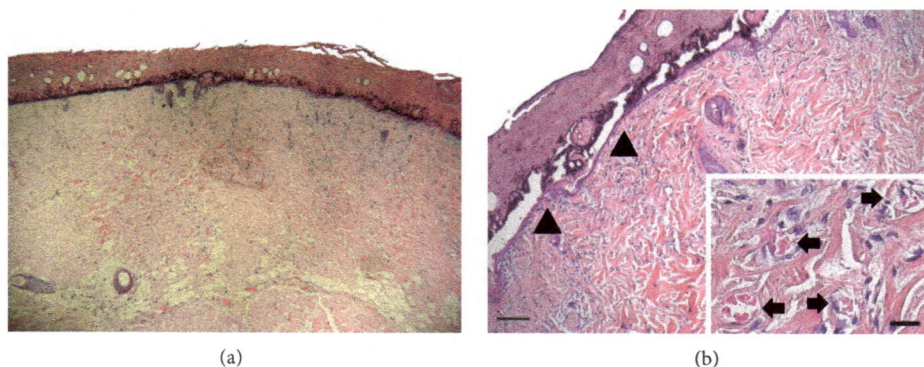

(a)

(b)

FIGURE 6: (a) The H.E.-stained histological section shows the centre of the burn wound of the ESWT-treated group on day 5. (b) The burn wound is closed by a thin continuous layer of epithelial cells (arrowheads). The reticular layer shows a higher number of vessels, compared to the control group (scale bar = 100 μm). The inset shows the distribution of vessels (arrows) in the reticular stratum in a higher magnification (scale bar = 20 μm).

group. Moreover, a lower number of inflammatory cells, less fibroblasts, and a uniform layer of granulation could be seen. Thus, a significantly better healing on days 5, 10, and 15 could be shown. These effects may be mediated by growth factors, which are known to be upregulated after ESWT and moreover within the first days after trauma and damage to the skin [14, 15, 20–23]. However, this assumption is highly speculative, due to the fact that staining of these factors was not performed in our study. With the establishment of a day 1 group of killed rats, the wound score system might have shown proper time comparison between the control and the treatment group. Nevertheless, we abstained from a further group to decrease the number of sacrificed rats needed for this study.

Inflammatory response and formation of granulation tissue, however, play a major role in burn wound healing. It is a well-known fact that rats heal mostly by contraction. Therefore, the histological findings of reepithelialization and the reduction of the number of fibroblasts and inflammatory cells in the ESWT group stay even more for an improvement in the healing of the burn wound after ESWT.

Wound perfusion was measured with the Laser Doppler Imager. The Laser Doppler perfusion image index (LDPII) is a standard tool in the determination of perfusion and microcirculation in the investigation of different diseases correlating to tissue ischemia [24, 25]. It directly correlates with arteriogenesis [26]. Blood flow in ESWT-treated rats significantly increased over the first five days. ESWT is known to contribute to the release of growth and angiogenic factors [4]. Therefore, together with the physiological response after trauma, ESWT may lead to an immediate increase of capillary perfusion and thus to a better blood supply and perfusion as well as to prevention of ischemia, a major problem in the zone of stasis of an acute burn wound. The increased number of vessels in the reticular layer of wounds of the ESWT group through all specimens supports these theories. Huemer et al. showed similar results after shock wave treatment of abdominal skin flaps [5]. An alternative working mechanism of ESWT could be vasodilatation and thus increased perfusion of the damaged tissue, as already shown in the literature [27].

5. Conclusion

The present study demonstrates significant benefits of ESWT in regeneration of skin and wound closure after deep partial-thickness burns. These findings might be confirmed by the fact that in first clinical reports deep partial-thickness burns show the tendency to heal without any surgical intervention when they are treated with ESWT [28]. We believe that ESWT represents a simple, noninvasive, and cost-effective treatment approach to deep partial-thickness burns, which may help avoid skin grafting or flap surgery by exploiting the vascular supply that is left intact after burn injuries and by accelerating the wound healing process. Nevertheless, further investigations, for example, a multiarm study with multiple ESWT treatments over a set treatment period instead of one treatment immediate status after injury, have to be performed to fully understand the mechanisms and benefits of ESWT treatment on burns.

Disclosure

Florian Stefan Kamelger, M. D., has to disclose a consulting agreement with Sanuwave, Inc., Alpharetta, Georgia.

Acknowledgments

The authors are indebted to Ing. Gaston Glock for generously providing them with the Laser Doppler Imager, to Professor Hanno Ulmer for statistical support, and to Professor Dagmar Födinger and Professor Hartmut Glossmann for laboratory facilities.

References

[1] C. J. Wang, F. S. Wang, K. D. Yang et al., "Shock wave therapy induces neovascularization at the tendon-bone junction. A study in rabbits," *Journal of Orthopaedic Research*, vol. 21, no. 6, pp. 984–989, 2003.

[2] C.-J. Wang, "An overview of shock wave therapy in musculoskeletal disorders," *Chang Gung Medical Journal*, vol. 26, no. 4, pp. 220–232, 2003.

[3] R. Meirer, F. S. Kamelger, G. M. Huemer, S. Wanner, and H. Piza-Katzer, "Extracorporal shock wave may enhance skin flap survival in an animal model," *British Journal of Plastic Surgery*, vol. 58, no. 1, pp. 53–57, 2005.

[4] R. Meirer, A. Brunner, M. Deibl, M. Oehlbauer, H. Piza-Katzer, and F. S. Kamelger, "Shock wave therapy reduces necrotic flap zones and induces VEGF expression in animal epigastric skin flap model," *Journal of Reconstructive Microsurgery*, vol. 23, no. 4, pp. 231–235, 2007.

[5] G. M. Huemer, R. Meirer, R. Gurunluoglu et al., "Comparison of the effectiveness of gene therapy with transforming growth factor-β or extracorporal shock wave therapy to reduce ischemic necrosis in an epigastric skin flap model in rats," *Wound Repair and Regeneration*, vol. 13, no. 3, pp. 262–268, 2005.

[6] R. Meirer, G. M. Huemer, M. Oehlbauer, S. Wanner, H. Piza-Katzer, and F. S. Kamelger, "Comparison of the effectiveness of gene therapy with vascular endothelial growth factor or shock wave therapy to reduce ischaemic necrosis in an epigastric skin flap model in rats," *Journal of Plastic, Reconstructive & Aesthetic Surgery*, vol. 60, no. 3, pp. 266–271, 2007.

[7] T. Kaufman, S. N. Lusthaus, U. Sagher, and M. R. Wexler, "Deep partial skin thickness burns: a reproducible animal model to study burn wound healing," *Burns*, vol. 16, no. 1, pp. 13–16, 1990.

[8] T. Kuroda, T. Harada, H. Tsutsumi, and M. Kobayashi, "Hypernatremia deepens the demarcating borderline of leukocytic infiltration in the burn wound," *Burns*, vol. 23, no. 5, pp. 432–437, 1997.

[9] W. Yu, J. O. Naim, and R. J. Lanzafame, "Effects of photostimulation on wound healing in diabetic mice," *Lasers in Surgery and Medicine*, vol. 20, no. 1, pp. 56–63, 1997.

[10] A. Schlager, K. Oehler, K.-U. Huebner, M. Schmuth, and L. Spoetl, "Healing of burns after treatment with 670-nanometer low-power laser light," *Plastic and Reconstructive Surgery*, vol. 105, no. 5, pp. 1635–1639, 2000.

[11] W. Folberth, G. Köhler, A. Rohwedder, and E. Matura, "Pressure distribution and energy flow in the focal region of two different electromagnetic shock wave sources," *The Journal of stone disease*, vol. 4, no. 1, pp. 1–7, 1992.

[12] F.-S. Wang, C.-J. Wang, H.-J. Huang, H. Chung, R.-F. Chen, and K. D. Yang, "Physical shock wave mediates membrane hyperpolarization and Ras activation for osteogenesis in human bone marrow stromal cells," *Biochemical and Biophysical Research Communications*, vol. 287, no. 3, pp. 648–655, 2001.

[13] F.-S. Wang, C.-J. Wang, Y.-J. Chen et al., "Ras induction of superoxide activates ERK-dependent angiogenic transcription factor HIF-1alpha and VEGF-A expression in shock wave-stimulated osteoblasts," *Journal of Biological Chemistry*, vol. 279, no. 11, pp. 10331–10337, 2004.

[14] Y.-J. Chen, T. Wurtz, C.-J. Wang et al., "Recruitment of mesenchymal stem cells and expression of TGF-β1 and VEGF in the early stage of shock wave-promoted bone regeneration of segmental defect in rats," *Journal of Orthopaedic Research*, vol. 22, no. 3, pp. 526–534, 2004.

[15] Y. J. Chen, C. J. Wang, K. D. Yang et al., "Extracorporeal shock waves promote healing of collagenase-induced Achilles tendinitis and increase TGF-β1 and IGF-I expression," *Journal of Orthopaedic Research*, vol. 22, no. 4, pp. 854–861, 2004.

[16] W. Schaden, R. Thiele, C. Kölpl et al., "Shock wave therapy for acute and chronic soft tissue wounds: a feasibility study," *Journal of Surgical Research*, vol. 143, no. 1, pp. 1–12, 2007.

[17] D. M. K. S. K. Sukul, E. J. Johannes, E. G. J. M. Pierik, G. J. W. M. Van Eijck, and M. J. E. Kristelijn, "The effect of high energy shock waves focused on cortical bone: an in vitro study," *Journal of Surgical Research*, vol. 54, no. 1, pp. 46–51, 1993.

[18] A. Sondén, A.-S. M. Johansson, J. Palmblad, and B. T. Kjellström, "Proinflammatory reaction and cytoskeletal alterations in endothelial cells after shock wave exposure," *Journal of Investigative Medicine*, vol. 54, no. 5, pp. 262–271, 2006.

[19] A. Sondén, B. Svensson, N. Roman, B. Brismar, J. Palmblad, and B. T. Kjellström, "Mechanisms of shock wave induced endothelial cell injury," *Lasers in Surgery and Medicine*, vol. 31, no. 4, pp. 233–241, 2002.

[20] P. Martin, "Wound healing—aiming for perfect skin regeneration," *Science*, vol. 276, no. 5309, pp. 75–81, 1997.

[21] L. F. Brown, K.-T. Yeo, B. Berse et al., "Expression of vascular permeability factor (Vascular endothelial growth factor) by epidermal keratinocytes during wound healing," *The Journal of Experimental Medicine*, vol. 176, no. 5, pp. 1375–1379, 1992.

[22] N. N. Nissen, P. J. Polverini, A. E. Koch, M. V. Volin, R. L. Gamelli, and L. A. DiPietro, "Vascular endothelial growth factor mediates angiogenic activity during the proliferative phase of wound healing," *The American Journal of Pathology*, vol. 152, no. 6, pp. 1445–1452, 1998.

[23] P. Fritsch, *Dermatologie und Venerologie: Lehrbuch und Atlas (German Edition)*, Springer, 1st edition, 1999.

[24] C. K. Enestvedt, L. Hosack, S. R. Winn et al., "VEGF gene therapy augments localized angiogenesis and promotes anastomotic wound healing: a pilot study in a clinically relevant animal model," *Journal of Gastrointestinal Surgery*, vol. 12, no. 10, pp. 1762–1770, 2008.

[25] S. C. Bir, M. Fujita, A. Marui et al., "New therapeutic approach for impaired arteriogenesis in diabetic mouse hindlimb ischemia," *Circulation Journal*, vol. 72, no. 4, pp. 633–640, 2008.

[26] S. Clark, F. Campbell, T. Moore, M. I. V. Jayson, T. A. King, and A. L. Herrick, "Laser doppler imaging—a new technique for quantifying microcirculatory flow in patients with primary Raynaud's phenomenon and systemic sclerosis," *Microvascular Research*, vol. 57, no. 3, pp. 284–291, 1999.

[27] A. Schwentker and T. R. Billiar, "Nitric oxide and wound repair," *Surgical Clinics of North America*, vol. 83, no. 3, pp. 521–530, 2003.

[28] R. Meirer, F. S. Kamelger, and H. Piza-Katzer, "Shock wave therapy: an innovative treatment method for partial thickness burns," *Burns*, vol. 31, no. 7, pp. 921–922, 2005.

10

Use of Lateral Calcaneal Flap for Coverage of Hindfoot Defects: An Anatomical Appraisal

Panagiotis Zygouris, Adamantios Michalinos, Vassilis Protogerou, Evangelos Kotsiomitis, Antonios Mazarakis, Ioannis Dimovelis, and Theodore Troupis

Department of Anatomy, National and Kapodistrian University of Athens, Mikras Asias 75 Street, Goudi, 11527 Athens, Greece

Correspondence should be addressed to Theodore Troupis; ttroupis@gmail.com

Academic Editor: Malcolm W. Marks

Lateral calcaneal flap is an established surgical option for coverage of lateral calcaneum and posterior heel defects. Lateral calcaneal flap vascularization and innervations are based on lateral calcaneal artery neurovascular bundle, that is, lateral calcaneal artery, small saphenous vein, and sural nerve. Anatomical research has allowed exploration of its many advantages but can also lead to its various modifications, permitting a wide variety of clinical applications. In this paper the authors report an anatomical and clinical study on lateral calcaneal artery course and lateral calcaneal flap clinical applications. Anatomic part of our study focused on lateral calcaneal artery course and optimization of surgical technique for flap harvesting. Data were used for design of lateral calcaneal flap in 5 patients. Our results were satisfactory in terms of coverage adequacy, perioperative morbidity, and functional and aesthetical outcome.

1. Introduction

Posterior heel and lateral calcaneum defects are often difficult in their restoration because of their osseous or tendinous bed, poor area vascularization, continuous movement, and high functional demands. Conservative treatment usually fails; use of split of full-thickness skin grafts often leads to unacceptable results while free flaps transfer is technically demanding and presents significant perioperative morbidity [1, 2].

Lateral calcaneal flap is based on lateral calcaneal artery (LCA) neurovascular bundle consisting of LCA, small saphenous vein, and sural nerve. Lateral calcaneal flap is an important surgical option for coverage of hindfoot defects. Its advantages include adequate coverage of posterior heel and lateral calcaneum [3], high success rate, low perioperative morbidity [4], and good functional results [5]. Investigation of LCA anatomy has led to various modifications of lateral calcaneal flap, including its island form [6], its adipofascial form [7], its reverse form [8], and its V-Y advancement form [9].

While being widely used, anatomical details on lateral calcaneal flap vascularization are still lacking, yet their impact is important for final result. The aim of this study is to investigate LCA anatomy and lateral calcaneal flap clinical results.

2. Materials and Methods

Twelve cadaveric legs were dissected for creation of lateral calcaneal flap at the Laboratory of Forensic Medicine and Toxicology, National and Kapodistrian University of Athens, Greece. Flap was dissected at its short straight form at 6 legs and at its long curved at 6 legs. We based the design of the flap on the estimated course of the LCA, as described in morphometric studies [4, 10], using 3 anatomical landmarks. First landmark was origin of LCA from peroneal artery, approximately 6 cm above the middle of the line connecting lateral malleolus and insertion of Achilles tendon. Second landmark was the middle of the line connecting between lateral malleolus and insertion of the Achilles tendon. Third landmark was 1 cm proximal to the tuberosity of the fifth metatarsal. Based on those 3 landmarks, curved course of LCA was designed and flap, in its short straight or long curved form, was designed. Dissection of the flap began from distal to proximal. As soon as LCA was identified, it was ligated and injected with methylene blue. Then dissection continued

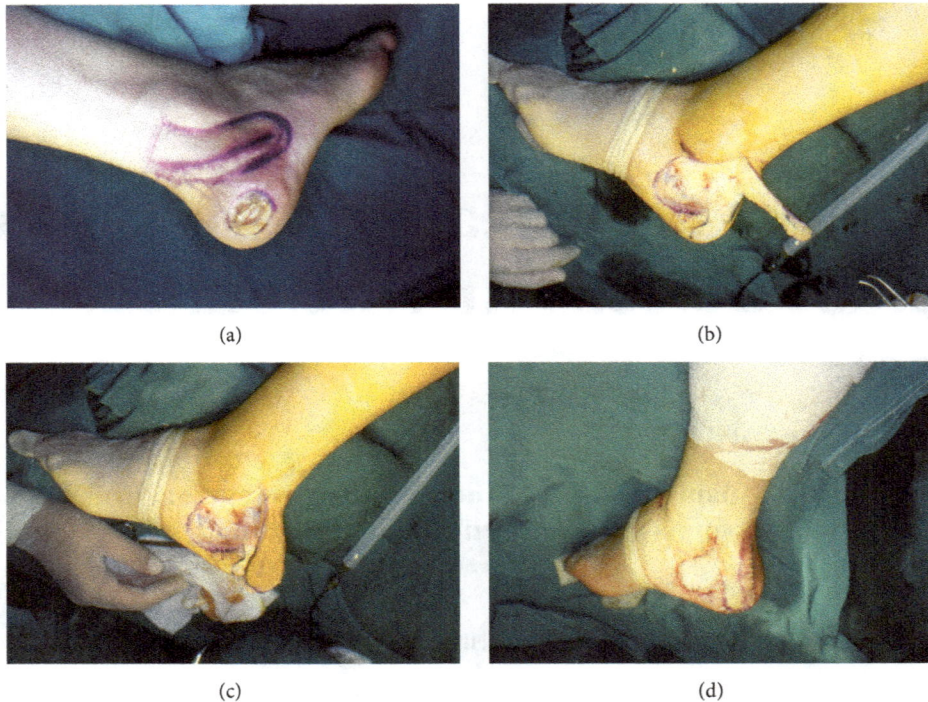

FIGURE 1: Lateral calcaneum defect covered by lateral calcaneal flap, straight form. (a) Preoperative design of lateral calcaneal flap. (b) Harvesting of the flap. (c) Alignment of the flap. (d) Immediate postoperative result.

along the course of LCA from distal to proximal so as to identify its area of vascularization. Distance between lateral malleolus and LCA was measured, as was flap's ideal pivot point.

Clinical part of the study included use of lateral calcaneal flap for rerepair of defects of posterior heel in 5 patients between 2005 and 2010. Mean age of the patients was 33 years old (20–62). All defects were consequence of motorcycle injury. In all patients defect had been covered in the past with split thickness skin grafts. Result was unacceptable in terms of functionality and appearance because of hyperkeratosis (3 patients) and ulceration (2 patients). One of our patients suffered from moderate atherosclerosis. Apart from that, no other health issues were encountered (Figures 1 and 2).

Preoperatively course of LCA was outlined with Doppler ultrasound. Surgical procedure was performed under a tourniquet and surgical loupes of 4.3 magnification.

The defect was measured at its two maximal dimensions and then the flap was marked on the skin (as a transposition or island flap). The damaged skin graft was totally removed; the defect was measured and the required size of the flap was marked on the skin as a skin transposition or island flap. When a skin transposition flap was used an incision was made to the skin until under the fascia. The incision at the posterior edge of the flap was carried down to the periosteum close to the Achilles tendon and near the calcaneum under the inferior border of the line connecting lateral malleolus and Achilles tendon. Undermining of the fascia was straightforward when the dissection was done immediately over the periosteum. The flap was raised proximally to the pivot point and was rotated to cover the defect.

When an island flap was used the surgical procedure to elevate the fascial side of the flap was similar to its long version. The differences were the carrying skin, the pedicle preparation, and the tunnel we created so that the flap could approach the defect. For the pedicle construction an incision was made posterior to the lateral malleolus and extended proximally along the fibula and the peroneus longus and the pedicle was separated from the overlying skin. The sural nerve and the accompanying vessels in the suprafascial layer were identified and kept into the pedicle of the flap and a tunnel was created to approach the defect.

Middle size of the defects was 4 × 4.5 cm. Donor site was covered with full-thickness skin graft.

3. Results

LCA was found 1.1 cm behind lateral malleolus, on the line connecting lateral malleolus with insertion of Achilles tendon, above deep fascia. Small saphenous vein coursed subcutaneously, parallel with sural nerve and above LCA. Based on visualized branches of LCA, ideal size of the flap was measured at 7-8 cm length for its straight form and 12-13 cm length for its curved form. Width was measured at 4 cm and pivot point at 3 cm above the inferior border of lateral malleolus. Size and dimensions of lateral calcaneal flap are adequate for coverage of deficits of posterior heel (Figure 3).

Good correspondence was always found between estimated course of LCA and its course radiographically and surgically identified. Based on that, dissection should always start outside the triangle bounded by inferior border of lateral calcaneus, Achilles tendon, and a point about 6 cm above the

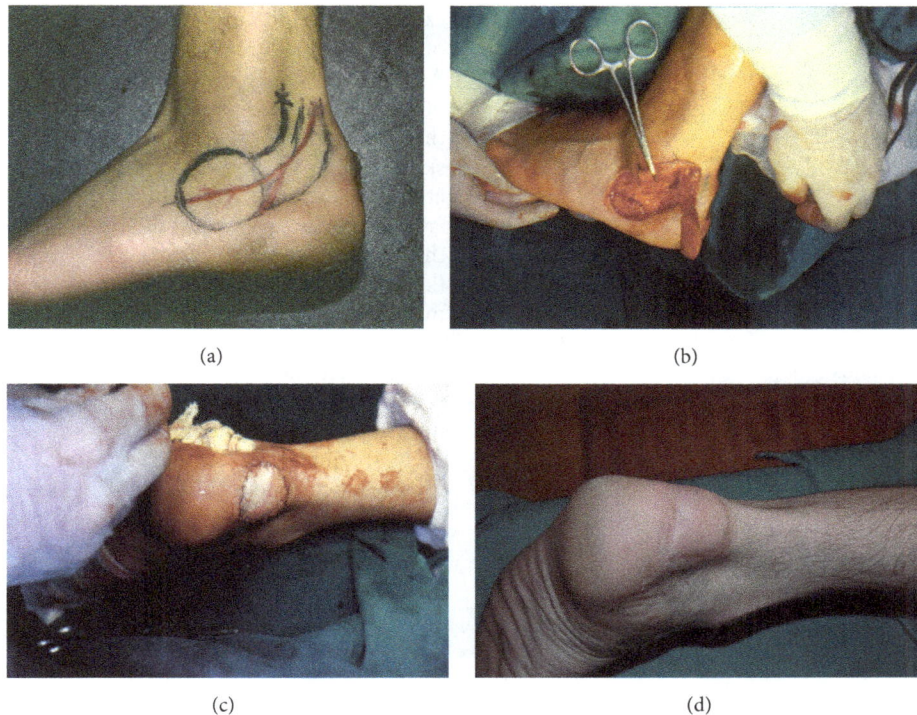

FIGURE 2: Posterior heel defect covered by lateral calcaneal flap, island form. (a) Preoperative design of the flap. (b) Harvesting of the flap. (c) Immediate postoperative result. (d) Long-term result.

TABLE 1

Number	Sex, age	Defect	Previous operation	Comorbidities	Flap form	Follow-up (y)	Complications
1	M, 20	Posterior heel, Achilles tendon—ulceration	Split thickness graft	No	Island	1	None
2	M, 30	Achilles tendon—hyperkeratosis	Split thickness graft	No	Short straight	0.5	None
3	M, 27	Posterior heel, Achilles tendon—hyperkeratosis	Split thickness graft	No	Long straight	1	None
4	M, 26	Posterior heel, Achilles tendon—ulceration	Split thickness graft	No	Island	10	None
5	M, 62	Posterior heel defect—ulceration, hyperkeratosis	Split thickness graft	Atherosclerosis	Long straight	3	Venous oedema—superficial necrosis

line connecting those two points. Dissection should proceed to the level of the deep fascia early since depth of LCA course and its branches is not stable. A generous lateral margin should be left since the donor area can usually be covered satisfactorily and the flap can be trimmed before its final positioning.

Concerning surgical results, only the atherosclerotic patients presented venous edema and a small area of superficial necrosis, treated conservatively. Apart from that, no morbidity concerning the flap and the donor region appeared. All operated patients were ambulatory at 8th postoperative day. Sensitivity of the flap was conserved intact except for 2 points discrimination in the lateral part of the dorsum of the foot. All

patients are able to wear shoes and no restriction concerning leg movement has been observed. Follow-up of the patients ranges between 5 months and 10 years (Table 1).

4. Discussion

Reconstruction of soft tissue defects of calcaneal region and posterior heel is demanding because of their osseous or tendinous bed, poor vascularization, and constant area movement. Their restoration necessitates tissues with reliable blood supply, adequate elasticity, and sensitivity. Furthermore they are often of traumatic origin and endorse young persons, causing significant morbidity if suboptimally treated.

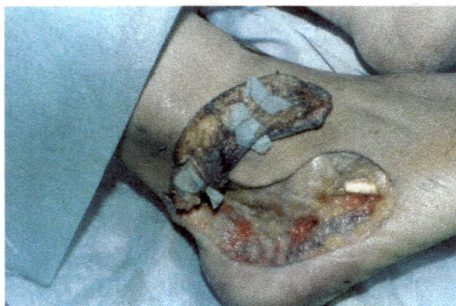

FIGURE 3: Cadaveric dissection of lateral calcaneal flap, showing LCA (left) and small saphenous vein (SSV) (right).

Lateral calcaneal flap was introduced by Grabb and Argenta in 1981 [11]. Based on course and distribution of LCA they described two possible forms, short straight and long curved. While being widely used, relative few anatomical details are known over flap's vascularization.

Peroneal artery divides approximately 6 cm above the tip of the lateral malleolus into LCA and its anterior perforating branch [5]. LCA courses downward and penetrates deep fascia at a distance of 3.8 cm (range: 3–4.5 cm) above the tip of lateral malleolus [3]. It acquires a deeper yet almost parallel course to small saphenous vein and sural nerve, forming the neurovascular bundle of lateral calcaneal flap. Small saphenous vein and sural nerve course at the level of the superficial fascia [3]. At the level of the ankle, LCA follows a curve lying approximately in the middle of the distance between tip of lateral malleolus and insertion of Achilles tendon. Through this part various branches follow a downward and posterior course and form a superficial course around calcaneus. LCA continues distally until the tip of the fifth metatarsal and there it divides into its dorsal branch that anastomoses with lateral tarsal artery and its plantar branch that anastomoses with lateral plantar artery [2, 8]. In 12% of the cases LCA is a branch of posterior tibial artery [4].

From a surgical point of view, most important morphometric characteristics of LCA are its depth from skin level, its adequacy as arterial network, and its distance from surgically important landmarks like the tip of the lateral malleolus. Distance between LCA and tip of lateral malleolus was calculated at 1 cm by Demirseren et al. [2]. The same distance was measured at 3 cm according to Freeman et al. [4] and at 2.6 cm according to Elsaidy and El-Shafey [3]. Distance of LCA from Achilles tendon was measured at 1.35 cm from Borrelli and Lashgari [10] and at 5–8 mm from Demirseren et al. [2]. Diameter of LCA is measured at 1.75 ± 0.12 mm and its depth at 7.5–8 cm [3]. Distance between LCA and sural nerve has been measured at approximately 1 cm [8, 12]. Based on the above measurements, Elsaidy and El-Shafey described a "danger triangle" during dissection of LCA between Achilles tendon, lateral malleolus, and penetration point of deep fascia from LCA [3].

Based on the anatomic characteristics of the LCA, various modifications of the lateral calcaneal flap have been invented. In 1984 Holmes and Rayner [6] utilizing the length and stable caliper of LCA introduced the island form of lateral

calcaneal flap. Its longer pedicle allows coverage of defects of anterior malleolus, posterior aspect of calcaneum, and Achilles tendon. Island form prevents problems like kinking of the pedicle, dog-ear deformity, and the need for sacrificing the normal skin bridge for flap insetting. Undermining of the skin during flap creation might lead to necrosis [2]. Ishikawa et al. [8] studied the rich anastomotic network of LCA with lateral plantar artery and lateral tarsal artery and invented the reverse lateral calcaneal flap. Reverse lateral calcaneal flap's pivot point is positioned about 20 mm proximal to fifth metatarsal and its proximal edge one or two fingers proximal to inferior portion of lateral malleolus. Its vascularization does not depend on peroneal artery and thus should be meticulously tested for adequacy both preoperatively with Doppler ultrasound and intraoperatively with vascular clamping of LCA. Its diminished vascularization makes it inappropriate for atherosclerotic patients. Furthermore mandatory division of sural nerve compromises flap's sensitivity. Lin et al. in 1996 [7] designed the adipose lateral calcaneal flap utilizing the deep position of LCA. Adipose lateral calcaneal flap's softness and pliability provides a beneficial filling for defects after debridement and minimizes donor size morbidity. Its small pedicle and size make it improper for coverage of large defects [13].

5. Conclusions

Lateral calcaneal flap presents good functional and aesthetical results for coverage of posterior heel and lateral calcaneum defects. Its advantages are its good functional results, its small perioperative morbidity, and its relative easiness for its design and creation. It is also a flap resistant to atherosclerosis, a common problem in patients with posterior heel defects.

Good knowledge of LCA anatomy ensures optimal design of the flap and maximum utilization of its length, protects from operative accidents including accidental devascularization or denervation of the flap, and allows optimum usage of lateral calcaneal flap various form, in respect to defect's particular characteristics.

Parallel anatomical and surgical research allows surgeon to benefit from classical anatomical knowledge, put it in use, and ensure the best for their patients' interests.

References

[1] A. Yanai, S. Park, T. Iwao, and N. Nakamura, "Reconstruction of a skin defect of the posterior heel by a lateral calcaneal flap," *Plastic and Reconstructive Surgery*, vol. 75, no. 5, pp. 642–647, 1985.

[2] M. E. Demirseren, K. Efendioglu, C. O. Demiralp, K. Kilicarslan, and H. Akkaya, "Clinical experience with a reverse-flow anterolateral thigh perforator flap for the reconstruction of soft-tissue defects of the knee and proximal lower leg," *Journal of*

Plastic, Reconstructive and Aesthetic Surgery, vol. 64, no. 12, pp. 1613–1620, 2011.

[3] M. A. Elsaidy and K. El-Shafey, "The lateral calcaneal artery: anatomic basis for planning safe surgical approaches," *Clinical Anatomy*, vol. 22, no. 7, pp. 834–839, 2009.

[4] B. J. C. Freeman, S. Duff, P. E. Allen, H. D. Nicholson, and R. M. Atkins, "The extended lateral approach to the hindfoot. Anatomical basis and surgical implications," *The Journal of Bone & Joint Surgery—British Volume*, vol. 80, no. 1, pp. 139–142, 1998.

[5] S.-J. Wang, Y.-D. Kim, H. Huang et al., "Lateral calcaneal artery perforator-based skin flaps for coverage of lower-posterior heel defects," *Journal of Plastic, Reconstructive & Aesthetic Surgery*, vol. 68, no. 4, pp. 571–579, 2015.

[6] J. Holmes and C. R. W. Rayner, "Lateral calcaneal artery island flaps," *British Journal of Plastic Surgery*, vol. 37, no. 3, pp. 402–405, 1984.

[7] S.-D. Lin, C.-S. Lai, Y.-T. Chiu, and T.-M. Lin, "The lateral calcaneal artery adipofascial flap," *British Journal of Plastic Surgery*, vol. 49, no. 1, pp. 52–57, 1996.

[8] K. Ishikawa, N. Isshiki, K. Hoshino, and C. Mori, "Distally based lateral calcaneal flap," *Annals of Plastic Surgery*, vol. 24, no. 1, pp. 10–16, 1990.

[9] A. Hayashi and Y. Maruyama, "Lateral calcaneal V-Y advancement flap for repair of posterior heel defects," *Plastic and Reconstructive Surgery*, vol. 103, no. 2, pp. 577–580, 1999.

[10] J. Borrelli and C. Lashgari, "Vascularity of the lateral calcaneal flap: a cadaveric injection study," *Journal of Orthopaedic Trauma*, vol. 13, no. 2, pp. 73–77, 1998.

[11] W. C. Grabb and L. C. Argenta, "The lateral calcaneal artery skin flap (the lateral calcaneal artery, lesser saphenous vein, and sural nerve skin flap)," *Plastic and Reconstructive Surgery*, vol. 68, no. 5, pp. 723–730, 1981.

[12] A. Freeman, N. Geddes, P. Munson et al., "Anaplastic lymphoma kinase (ALK 1) staining and molecular analysis in inflammatory myofibroblastic tumours of the bladder: a preliminary clinico-pathological study of nine cases and review of the literature," *Modern Pathology*, vol. 17, no. 7, pp. 765–771, 2004.

[13] M. S. Chung, G. H. Baek, H. S. Gong et al., "Lateral calcaneal artery adipofascial flap for reconstruction of the posterior heel of the foot," *Clinics in Orthopedic Surgery*, vol. 1, no. 1, pp. 1–5, 2009.

11

Complements and the Wound Healing Cascade: An Updated Review

Hani Sinno and Satya Prakash

Division of Plastic and Reconstructive Surgery, Department of Surgery, McGill University, Montreal, QC, Canada H3A 2B4

Correspondence should be addressed to Satya Prakash; satya.prakash@mcgill.ca

Academic Editor: Georg M. Huemer

Wound healing is a complex pathway of regulated reactions and cellular infiltrates. The mechanisms at play have been thoroughly studied but there is much still to learn. The health care system in the USA alone spends on average 9 billion dollars annually on treating of wounds. To help reduce patient morbidity and mortality related to abnormal or prolonged skin healing, an updated review and understanding of wound healing is essential. Recent works have helped shape the multistep process in wound healing and introduced various growth factors that can augment this process. The complement cascade has been shown to have a role in inflammation and has only recently been shown to augment wound healing. In this review, we have outlined the biology of wound healing and discussed the use of growth factors and the role of complements in this intricate pathway.

1. Introduction

From birth to old age, skin has the vital role of regulating fluid balance, infection control, and thermogenesis. Disruption of this regenerating protective layer can be devastating to the patient and society. More than 2 million burn cases [1] and 7 million chronic skin ulcers caused by pressure, arterial or venous insufficiency, and diabetes mellitus each year in the United States alone are affected by abnormal wound healing [2]. This translates to annual costs of $9 billion in attempt to reduce the major disability and consequent death of such severe skin injury [3].

To help reduce patient morbidity and mortality related to abnormal or prolonged skin healing, an understanding of wound healing is essential. Recent works have helped shape the multistep process in wound healing and introduced various growth factors that can augment this process. The complement cascade has been shown to have a role in inflammation and has only recently been shown to augment wound healing (Figure 3). In this work, we will review the biology of wound healing and discuss the use of growth factors and the role of complements in this intricate pathway.

2. Wound Healing

Normal wound healing is a dynamic series of events involving the coordinated interaction of blood cells, proteins, proteases, growth factors, and extracellular matrix components. The wound healing process can be divided into three phases: (1) inflammatory phase; (2) proliferative phase; and (3) maturational phase. Although different predominant cells characterize these phases at differing times, a considerable amount of overlap can occur (Figure 1).

2.1. Inflammatory Phase. The inflammatory phase is the first phase of wound healing and is characterized by hemostasis and inflammation. Hemostasis is initiated during the exposure of collagen during wound formation that activates the intrinsic and extrinsic clotting cascade. In addition, the injury to tissue causes a release of thromboxane A2 and prostaglandin 2-alpha to the wound bed causing a potent vasoconstrictor response. Furthermore, the extravasation of blood constituents provides the formation of the blood clot reinforcing the hemostatic plug. This initial response helps to limit hemorrhage and provides an initial extracellular matrix for cell migration.

Prostaglandin-2α

Time	Phase	Growth factor	Source	Target/effect	Vascular response	Cellular response	Event
Injury	Inflammatory	Clotting cascade	Tissue injury	Platelet, hemostatic plug, vasoconstriction	Vasoconstriction	Platelet	Clot formation
		Thromboxane A2	Tissue injury	Vasoconstriction			
		Prostaglandin F2α	Tissue injury	Vasoconstriction			
		Complement C3	Spontaneous, foreign tissue	Vasoactive and spasmogenic, activation of complement cascade, mast cell degranulation			
3 days		Complement C5	C3, platelet	Mast cell degranulation, chemotaxis of monocytes and neutrophil, vasoactive and spasmogenic, bacterial lysis		Neutrophil	Growth factor elaboration
		EGF	Platelet	Reepithelialization, pleiotropic cell proliferation			
	Proliferative	TGF-β1 and β2	Platelet, macrophage, and keratinocyte	Chemotaxis of macrophages and fibroblasts, matrix formation and remodeling		Macrophage	
		PDGF	Platelet, macrophage, and epidermal cell	Platelet, macrophages, epidermal cells, fibroblast			
		IL-i and IL-6	Neutrophil, macrophage	Inflammation, reepithelialization			
		TNF	Neutrophil, macrophage	Inflammation, reepithelialization			
7 days		VEGF	Platelet, neutrophil, macrophage, epidermal cells, and fibroblast	Angiogenesis, granulation tissue formation, increased vascular permeability			Collagen deposition
		FGF	Macrophage, endothelial cell	Granulation tissue formation, angiogenesis, fibroblast		Fibroblast	
		IGF	Epidermal cell, fibroblast	Reepithelialization, granulation tissue formation			
Weeks	Remodeling						Collagen cross-linking

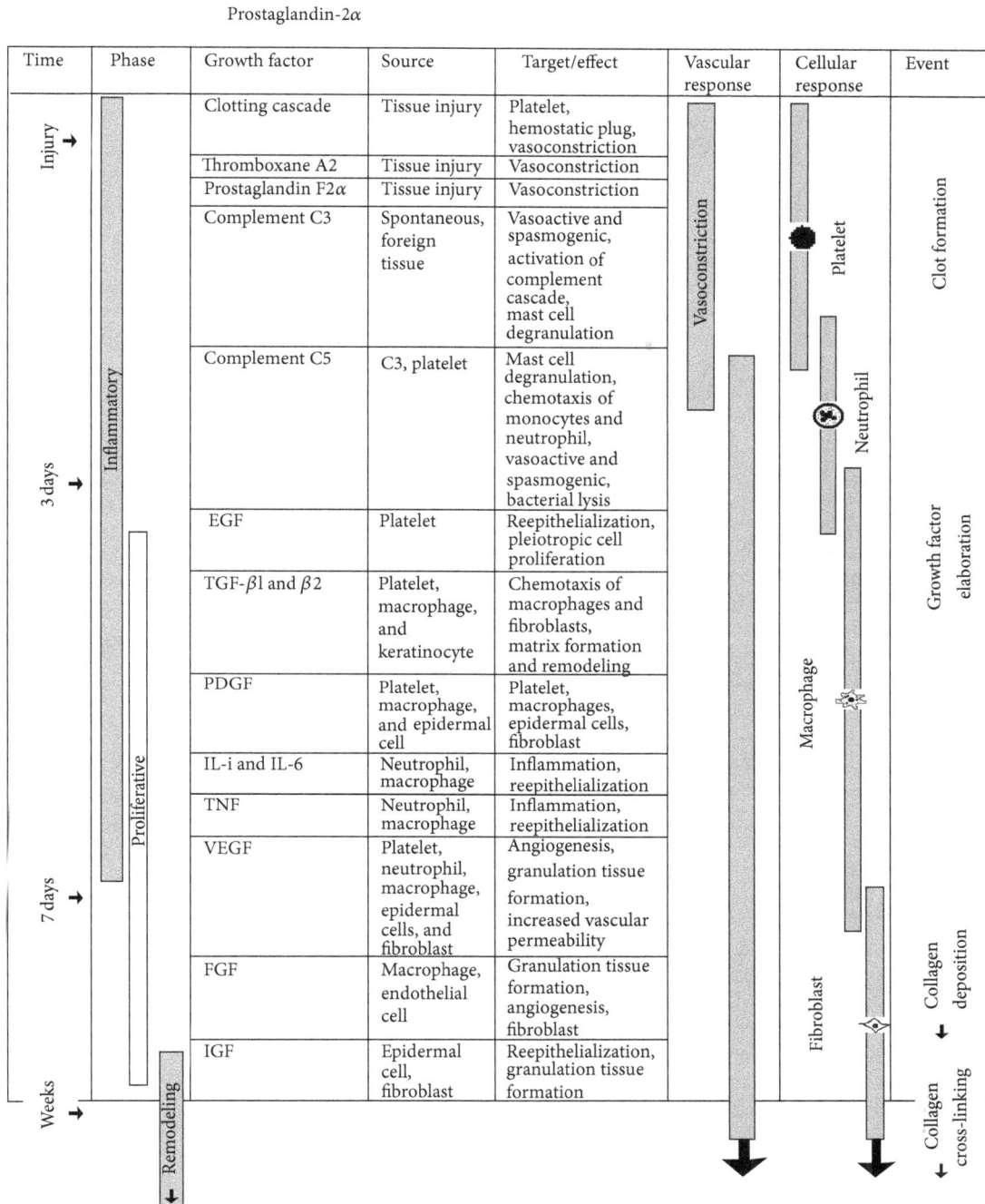

FIGURE 1: Cytokines and complements involved in inflammation. The three phases of wound healing are associated with different growth factors and subsequent cellular infiltration. Although the complement system is involved in inflammation, its role in wound healing has never been proposed. Complements C3 and C5, epidermal growth factor (EGF), transforming growth factor (TGF), platelet-derived growth factor (PDGF), tumor necrosis factor (TNF), vascular endothelial growth factor (VEGF), and insulin-like growth factor (IGF).

Platelets are among the first response cells that play a key role in the formation of the hemostatic plug. They secrete several chemokines such as epidermal growth factor (EGF), fibronectin, fibrinogen, histamine, platelet-derived growth factor (PDGF), serotonin, and von Willebrand factor. These factors help stabilize the wound through clot formation and also attract and activate macrophages and fibroblasts [4].

They also act to control bleeding and limit the extent of injury. Platelet degranulation activates the complement cascade, specifically C5, a potent neutrophils chemotactic protein [5]. Vasoactive mediators and chemokines are released by the activated coagulation cascade, complement pathways, and parenchymal cells which play a key role in the recruitment of inflammatory leukocytes to injured skin [6].

After hemostasis is achieved, capillary vasodilatation and leakage result secondary to local histamine release by the activated complement cascade. The increased blood flow and altered vascular permeability allow for the migration of inflammatory cells to the wound bed. The presence of foreign organisms further stimulates the activation of the alternate complement pathway. Complement C3 activation results in a cascade of nonenzymatic protein cleavage and interactions that eventually stimulate inflammatory cells and the lysis of bacteria.

The second response cell to migrate to the wound after complement activation and platelet recruitment is the neutrophil. It is responsible for debris scavenging, complement-mediated opsonization and lysis of foreign organisms, and bacterial destruction via oxidative burst mechanisms (i.e., superoxide and hydrogen peroxide formation). Neutrophils kill bacteria and decontaminate the wound from foreign debris. These wastes are later extruded with the eschar or phagocytosed by macrophages.

Macrophages are important phagocytic cells that play a key role in wound healing. They are formed from monocytes stimulated by fragments of the extracellular matrix protein, transforming growth factor β, and monocyte chemoattractant protein 1 [7]. In addition to direct phagocytosis of bacteria and foreign materials, macrophages secrete numerous enzymes and cytokines; collagenases, which debride the wound; interleukins and tumor necrosis factor (TNF), which stimulate fibroblasts and promote angiogenesis; and transforming growth factor (TGF), which stimulates keratinocytes [8]. Macrophages also secrete platelet-derived growth factor and vascular endothelial growth factor which initiate the formation of granulation tissue and thus initiate the transition into the proliferative phase and tissue regeneration [6].

2.2. Proliferative Phase.
The proliferative phase is marked by epithelialization, angiogenesis, granulation tissue formation, and collagen deposition. Epithelialization occurs within hours after injury in wound repair. With an intact basement membrane, the epithelial cells migrate upwards in the normal pattern as occurs in a first-degree skin burn whereby the epithelial progenitor cells remain intact below the wound and the normal layers of epidermis are restored in 2-3 days. If the basement membrane has been damaged, similar to a deeper burn, then the normal epidermal cells from skin appendages (e.g., hair follicles, sweat glands) and the wound periphery reepithelialize the wound.

Neovascularization is necessary to deliver nutrients to the wound and help maintain the granulation tissue bed. Angiogenesis has been attributed to many molecules including fibroblast growth factor, vascular endothelial growth factor, transforming growth factor β, angiogenin, angiotropin, angiopoietin 1, tumor necrosis factor alpha, and thrombospondin [9–11]. In different clinical scenarios such as diabetes and vascular disease, this critical nutrient supply by capillaries is insufficient to sustain the tissue deposition in the granulation phase and thus results in a chronically unhealed wound.

The proliferative phase ends with granulation tissue formation. This new stroma begins to invade the wound space close to four days after injury. The new blood vessels at this time have provided a facilitated entry point into the wound to cells such as macrophages and fibroblasts. Macrophages continue to supply growth factors stimulating further angiogenesis and fibroplasia. The secreted platelet-derived growth factor [4] and transforming growth factor β [12] along with the extracellular matrix molecules [13] stimulate fibroblasts differentiation to produce ground substance and then collagen. Fibroblasts are the key players in the synthesis, deposition, and remodeling of the extracellular matrix providing strength and substance to the wound.

2.3. Maturational Phase.
The third and final phase of wound healing is the maturational phase. This is characterized by the transition from granulation tissue to scar formation. Close to two weeks after injury, the wound undergoes contraction, ultimately resulting in a smaller amount of apparent scar tissue. Collagen deposition by fibroblasts continues for a prolonged period with a net increase in collagen deposition reached after three weeks from tissue injury. The entire process is a dynamic continuum dictated by numerous growth factors and cells with an overlap of each of the three phases of wound healing to provide continued remodeling. The human wound is estimated to reach its maximal strength at one year, with a maximal tensile strength that is 70% of normal skin [14].

2.4. Healing of Tendons, Ligaments, Bones, and Muscles.
Wound healing of tendons, ligaments, bones, and muscles is generally similar to that of skin and other tissues which include the three different phases of inflammation, proliferation, and maturation. Certainly, many of the same growth factors are also involved in these intricate processes.

2.4.1. Tendons and Ligaments.
Heal through "extrinsic" and "intrinsic" processes. The former healing process is based on immobilization whereby fibroblast-dependent ingrowth and neovascularization from the tendon sheath take place. This creates fibrosis and adhesion formation incorporating into the site of tendon injury. The growth factors which stimulate fibroblast are similar to those found in the skin wound healing process described above. Intrinsic healing involved inflammation, proliferation, and remodeling which occur from within the tendon itself. Blood clot and granulation tissue fill the tendon and ligament gaps, Epitenon cells proliferate and transform into fibroblasts, and the wound healing cascade continues to form a stable scar bridging the injured gaps.

2.4.2. Muscles.
Skeletal muscles cells do not regenerate once torn. A similar scar formation can occur to bridge injured gaps.

2.4.3. Bone.
Has the unique property of "Creeping Substitution" in which a process in a fracture site or necrotic bone is resorbed and replaced by new tissue moving along channels created by invading host blood vessels found within the periosteum and Volkmann's canals. This process is governed

by osteoblasts, osteoclasts and the arcade of cytokines, and growth factors including bone morphogeneic proteins (BMPs), TGF-β, fibroblast growth factors (BFGFs), PDGF, and interleukins.

3. Complements

The complement system is known to have a profound inflammatory response. It is composed of bactericidal and haemolytic proteins. These eleven molecules interact in two different enzymatic cascades: the classical and the alternative pathways (Figure 2). The resulting membrane attack complex (MAC) is directly responsible for the lysis of foreign organisms. Furthermore, the complement cascade plays an important role in many acute inflammatory processes and host defences.

The *classical pathway* is activated by an antibody bound to a foreign particle. The first component is complement 1 (C1), which can also be activated by IgM and IgG immunoglobulins. C4 then C2 are cleaved to activate C3 and C5 [15]. Through the *lectin pathway*, the mannan-binding protein (MBP) can activate the classical pathway independent of antibody by substituting for C1 [16].

The *alternate pathway* functions in an antibody-independent route and thus does not require prior exposure to a particle for activation. It allows for rapid complement activation and amplification on foreign microorganisms and surfaces. Factors B and D are key proteins that promote the activation of C3 and C5. Damaged tissue may contain proteases capable of proteolytic cleavage of C3 and C5 [17]. C3 is cleaved to form C3a and C3b. C5 also becomes C5a and C5b when activated. The "a" component is generally the chemotactic protein, while the "b" component further stimulates the proliferation of the complement cascade.

The final enzymatic step in the complement pathway allows for cleavage of C5 and the initiation of MAC formation. The membrane attack complex is composed of C5,6,7,8, and 9 [18]. Complements C5 to C9 are noncovalently bound to form MAC which causes pore development in membranes of microorganisms and consequent lysis and death [18].

Other activators of the complement pathway exist. C-reactive protein (CRP) has been shown to bind damaged host tissue and microorganisms, consequently activating C1 [16]. This activation of the classical pathway of complement enhances phagocyte recruitment. Serum protein amyloid P component also binds damaged cells and activates complement [19].

The most common complement protein in human serum is C3. C3a, originally identified as an anaphylatoxin, was shown to act as a mediator of inflammatory reactions with effects on polymorphonuclear leukocytes (PMNLs), vascular tone, and leakage. C3a has spasmogenic activities [20] and increases microvascular permeability [5]. Its effects on wound strength and healing have not yet been shown.

C3a and C5a are released through the proteolytic cleavage in the activation pathways. They have a chemotactic response to neutrophils [21]. C3a and C5a bind to specific receptors on mast cells and basophils and trigger degranulation, releasing inflammatory agents into the tissues. This anaphylactic response is controlled by carboxypeptidase N which cleaves the carboxy-terminal arginine residue from both C3a and C5a [22]. This cleavage prevents the activated complements from binding receptors on mast cells. Cleaved C5a, however, retains its chemotactic activity to recruit neutrophils and activate basophils.

C5a has been shown to be chemotactically active for monocytes and PMNL and also promotes the release of free radicals and tissue-digesting enzymes from these cells [23]. C5a promotes neutrophil migration during acute inflammation [24]. The oxidative burst power of neutrophils is further strengthened by C5a binding allowing for augmented bacterial phagocytosis. C5a also has spasmogenic activities [20] and increases microvascular permeability [5].

4. Complements and Wound Healing

Both complements C3 and C5 have been recently shown to augment wound healing [25–27]. Sinno et al. demonstrated that the topical application of C3 in a collagen vehicle can successfully increase wound healing. There was a measured increase in maximal breaking strength by 74% [25]. The authors also found a correlation of increased inflammatory cellular recruitment and increased collagen deposition and organization along with this increase in wound strength. Furthermore, Sinno et al. further demonstrated that the topical application of C5 in collagen vehicle also accelerated wound healing [26]. In fact, C5-treated wounds maximal breaking strength increased by 83 percent at day 3 and by 64 percent at day 7 when compared to sham wounds. They also found an increase in the inflammatory cellular recruitment, which they attributed to the likely mechanism of action of complement wound healing effects. They also found an objective increase in fibroblast infiltration and collagen deposition. Moreover, complements C3 and C5 have both independently and in combination been shown to accelerate and increase wound healing [27].

5. Current Trends and Growth Factors

With an understanding of the phases of wound healing and the associated inflammatory cytokines such as complements and other growth factors, therapeutic modalities can be investigated for the management of problematic wounds. It is vital to understand that inflammation and wound healing are governed by an array of growth factors and cytokines and the inflammatory cells that produce them (Figure 1). Platelet-activating factor (PAF), transforming growth factor-beta (TGF-β), and platelet-derived growth factor (PDGF), for example, have been shown to affect inflammation and repair by their chemotactic activity for monocytes, neutrophils, smooth muscle cells, and fibroblasts [28–30].

Current pharmacologic cytokines and growth factors have a limited role in clinical practice. In one clinical study led by Crovetti and colleagues, a platelet gel was used on cutaneous chronic ulcers in twenty-four patients [31]. They hypothesized that the effects of their topically applied hemoproduct would provide a supplemental load of PDGF, TGF-β,

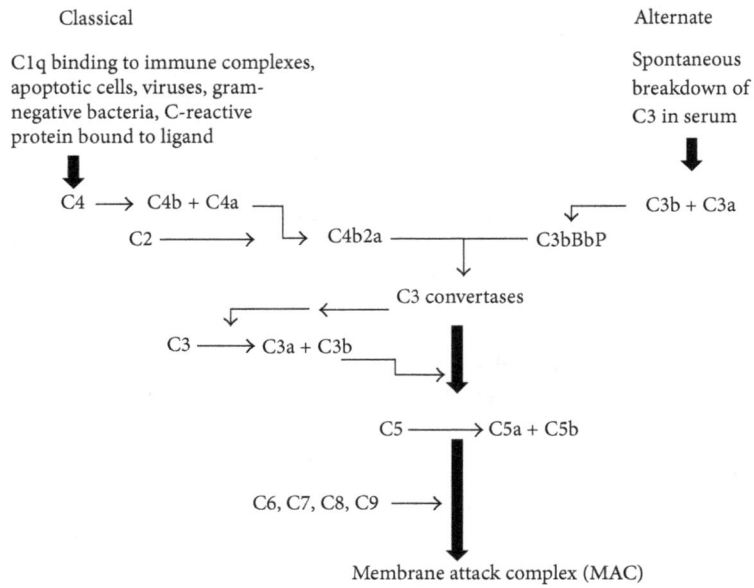

FIGURE 2: Complement cascade. The complement system converges with the activation of complements C3 and C5 with the subsequent formation of the membrane attack complex. The C3a and C5a proteins are responsible for chemotaxis. The C3b and C5b are responsible for the continued proliferation of the complement cascade.

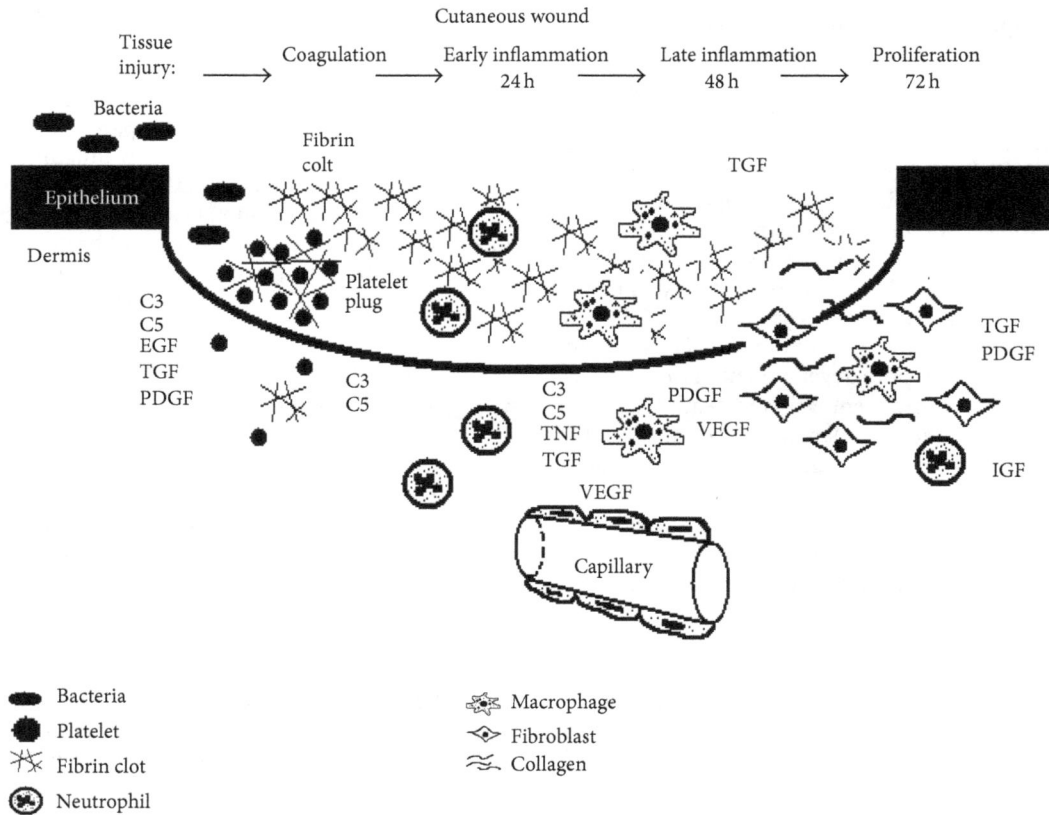

FIGURE 3: Cutaneous wound healing in time. A schematic representation of cutaneous wound healing and the growth factors and cellular participants in the first 72 hours of injury. The complement cascade appears to be involved in many stages of the wound healing. Platelets, macrophages, fibroblasts, and the formation of the fibrin clot are the major cellular players in early cutaneous, tendon, ligament muscle, and bone healing.

and vascular endothelial growth factor (VEGF). Although a complete response was only observed in less than half of the patients in the treatment group, in each case, granulation tissue formation increased after the first application of the product. This product still remains under investigation.

Tumor necrosis factor-alpha (TNF-α) has been associated with inhibition of normal wound healing when found in high levels. In chronic wounds, the levels of TNF-α have been found to be 100-fold higher when compared to levels in acute wounds [32]. Streit and colleagues demonstrated promising results with infliximab (acting as a TNF-α inhibitor) on chronic wounds in a small case series [33].

Diabetes is one metabolic disease that has been associated with problematic wounds. It is hypothesized that impaired wound healing in diabetic patients is a result of decreased angiogenesis that may be secondary to a diminished production of vascular endothelial growth factor (VEGF). Galiano and colleagues demonstrated the effects of topical VEGF to have a significant accelerated repair in experimental wounds in diabetic mice [34]. This study demonstrated a potential role for VEGF therapy in the treatment of diabetic complications characterized by impaired neovascularization. Furthermore, Zhang and colleagues revealed that exogenous application of VEGF can increase early angiogenesis and tensile strength in the ischemic wound in a rat model [35].

Platelet-activating factor (PAF) has been studied by Porras-Reyes and Mustoe as a chemotactic agent with no cell proliferative properties [36]. They found an increase in maximal breaking strength of wounds treated with PAF at five and seven days after injury compared to controls. Furthermore, with the PAF receptor antagonist introduction, the PAF response was blocked. This revealed that PAF can promote wound healing, but its endogenous supply is not essential for this purpose.

Transforming growth factor-beta (TGF-β) has been described as a potent growth factor involved in wound healing. It has been shown to influence the inflammatory response, angiogenesis, reepithelialization, extracellular matrix deposition, and remodeling [12, 37, 38]. Targeting of TGF-β has been shown to accelerate wound healing and reduce scarring [38, 39].

Another precursor for the development of problematic wounds is previous radiotherapy exposure. It has been clinically shown to impair wound healing [40]. These effects were attributed to the diminished hematopoiesis with whole body radiation and local tissue mesenchymal injury with surface irradiation. Mustoe and colleagues observed a fifty percent increase in the strength of radio-treated wounds with the topical application of platelet-derived growth factor-BB homodimers (PDGF-BB) [29]. They attributed this to the increase in macrophage recruitment during the early phases of wound healing.

Currently, only few cytokines and growth factors are used clinically. To date, one of the few available commercial products proven to be efficacious in randomized, double-blind-studies is PDGF [41–43]. In multiple studies, recombinant human PDGF-BB has been demonstrated to reduce healing time and improve the incidence of complete wound healing in stages III and IV ulcers. Within the realm of bone healing,

BMP have also had great promise. The delivery of these active peptides has also had great research and has been shown to influence the healing rates [44].

The limitations of current wound healing treatments call for an urgent development of a safe, effective, and economical formulation for use in wound healing that is associated with so many other diseases and a variety of the population. An effective therapy would ideally decrease the bacterial load, establish stringent inflammatory control, and concomitantly increase wound tensile strength. Furthermore, a rigorous search for optimal peptide-carrier combination along with timing of growth factor administration is warranted.

6. Conclusion

The wound healing cascade is a complex milieu of regulated pathways, secreted growth factors, cytokines, and inflammatory cells. Throughout the three phases of healing, different growth factors and cells have been shown to be essential during each step. Different cytokines have been clinically studied to help augment wound healing. Recently, complements have been shown to augment wound healing. These naturally secreted proteins have innate hemostatic, antibacterial, and inflammatory effects that have now been shown to also accelerate wound healing. We recommend further human phase I clinical trials to further understand the role of complements and other growth factors in wound healing.

References

[1] P. A. Brigham and E. McLoughlin, "Burn incidence and medical care use in the United States: estimates, trends, and data sources," *Journal of Burn Care and Rehabilitation*, vol. 17, no. 2, pp. 95–107, 1996.

[2] "U.S. markets for wound management products," Medical Data International, Irvine, Calif, USA, August 1997.

[3] G. S. Ashcroft, S. J. Mills, and J. J. Ashworth, "Ageing and wound healing," *Biogerontology*, vol. 3, no. 6, pp. 337–345, 2002.

[4] C.-H. Heldin and B. Westermark, *Role of Platelet-Derived Growth Factor in Vivo*, Plenum Press, New York, NY, USA, 2nd edition, 1996.

[5] J. Bjork, T. E. Hugli, and G. Smedegard, "Microvascular effects of anaphylatoxins C3a and C5a," *Journal of Immunology*, vol. 134, no. 2, pp. 1115–1119, 1985.

[6] R. A. F. Clark and P. M. Henson, *The Molecular and Cellular Biology of Wound Repair*, Plenum Press, New York, NY, USA, 2nd edition, 1996.

[7] S. J. Leibovich and R. Ross, "The role of the macrophage in wound repair. A study with hydrocortisone and antimacrophage serum," *American Journal of Pathology*, vol. 78, no. 1, pp. 71–100, 1975.

[8] E. J. Brown, "Phagocytosis," *BioEssays*, vol. 17, no. 2, pp. 109–117, 1995.

[9] J. Folkman and P. A. D'Amore, "Blood vessel formation: what is its molecular basis?" *Cell*, vol. 87, no. 7, pp. 1153–1155, 1996.

[10] M. L. Iruela-Arispe and H. F. Dvorak, "Angiogenesis: a dynamic balance of stimulators and inhibitors," *Thrombosis and Haemostasis*, vol. 78, no. 1, pp. 672–677, 1997.

[11] W. Risau, "Mechanisms of angiogenesis," *Nature*, vol. 386, no. 6626, pp. 671–674, 1997.

[12] A. B. Roberts, *Transforming Growth Factor-Beta*, Plenum Press, New York, NY, USA, 2nd edition, 1996.

[13] J. Xu and R. A. F. Clark, "Extracellular matrix alters PDGF regulation of fibroblast integrins," *Journal of Cell Biology*, vol. 132, no. 1-2, pp. 239–249, 1996.

[14] S. M. Levenson, E. F. Geever, L. V. Crowley, J. F. Oates III, C. W. Berard, and H. Rosen, "The healing of rat skin wounds," *Annals of surgery*, vol. 161, pp. 293–308, 1965.

[15] M. Loos, "Classical pathway of activation," in *The Complement System*, K. T. G. Rother, Ed., pp. 136–154, Springer, Berlin, Germany, 1985.

[16] U. Holmskov, R. Malhotra, R. B. Sim, and J. C. Jensenius, "Collectins: collagenous C-type lectins of the innate immune defense system," *Immunology Today*, vol. 15, no. 2, pp. 67–74, 1994.

[17] O. Gotze, "The alternate pathway of activation," in *The Complement System*, K. T. G. Rother, Ed., pp. 154–168, Springer, Berlin, 1985.

[18] D. K. Imagawa, N. E. Osifchin, and W. A. Paznekas, "Consequences of cell membrane attack by complement: release of arachidonate and formation of inflammatory derivatives," *Proceedings of the National Academy of Sciences of the United States of America*, vol. 80, no. 21 I, pp. 6647–6651, 1983.

[19] P. S. Hicks, L. Saunero-Nava, T. W. Du Clos, and C. Mold, "Serum amyloid P component binds to histones and activates the classical complement pathway," *Journal of Immunology*, vol. 149, no. 11, pp. 3689–3694, 1992.

[20] T. E. Hugli, F. Marceau, and C. Lundberg, "Effects of complement fragments on pulmonary and vascular smooth muscle," *American Review of Respiratory Disease*, vol. 135, no. 6, pp. S9–13, 1987.

[21] H. N. Fernandez, P. M. Henson, A. Otani, and T. E. Hugli, "Chemotactic response to human C3a and C5a anaphylatoxins. I. Evaluation of C3a and C5a leukotaxis in vitro and under simulated in vivo conditions," *Journal of Immunology*, vol. 120, no. 1, pp. 109–115, 1978.

[22] T. E. Hugli, "Biochemistry and biology of anaphylatoxins," *Complement*, vol. 3, no. 3, pp. 111–127, 1986.

[23] N. Schupf, C. A. Williams, A. Berkman, W. S. Cattell, and L. Kerper, "Binding specificity and presynaptic action of anaphylatoxin C5a in rat brain," *Brain Behavior and Immunity*, vol. 3, no. 1, pp. 28–38, 1989.

[24] K. E. Foreman, A. A. Vaporciyan, B. K. Bonish et al., "C5a-induced expression of P-selectin in endothelial cells," *Journal of Clinical Investigation*, vol. 94, no. 3, pp. 1147–1155, 1994.

[25] H. Sinno, M. Malholtra, J. Lutfy et al., "Topical application of complement C3 in collagen formulation increases early wound healing," *Journal of Dermatological Treatment*, vol. 24, no. 2, pp. 141–147, 2011.

[26] H. Sinno, M. Malhotra, J. Lutfy et al., "Accelerated wound healing with topical application of complement C5," *Plastic and Reconstructive Surgery*, vol. 130, no. 3, pp. 523–529.

[27] H. Sinno, M. Malhotra, J. Lutfy et al., "Complements c3 and c5 individually and in combination increase early wound strength in a rat model of experimental wound healing," *Plastic Surgery International*, vol. 2013, Article ID 243853, 5 pages, 2013.

[28] B. H. Porras-Reyes and T. A. Mustoe, "Platelet-activating factor: improvement in wound healing by a chemotactic factor," *Surgery*, vol. 111, pp. 416–423, 1992, Erratum in *Surgery*, vol. 112, no. 3, pp. 612, 1992.

[29] T. A. Mustoe, J. Purdy, P. Gramates, T. F. Deuel, A. Thomason, and G. F. Pierce, "Reversal of impaired wound healing in irradiated rats by platelet-derived growth factor-BB," *American Journal of Surgery*, vol. 158, no. 4, pp. 345–350, 1989.

[30] T. A. Mustoe, G. F. Pierce, and A. Thomason, "Accelerated healing of incisional wounds in rats induced by transforming growth factor-β," *Science*, vol. 237, no. 4820, pp. 1333–1336, 1987.

[31] G. Crovetti, G. Martinelli, M. Issi et al., "Platelet gel for healing cutaneous chronic wounds," *Transfusion and Apheresis Science*, vol. 30, no. 2, pp. 145–151, 2004.

[32] R. W. Tarnuzzer and G. S. Schultz, "Biochemical analysis of acute and chronic wound environments," *Wound Repair and Regeneration*, vol. 4, no. 3, pp. 321–325, 1996.

[33] M. Streit, Z. Beleznay, and L. R. Braathen, "Topical application of the tumour necrosis factor-α antibody infliximab improves healing of chronic wounds," *International Wound Journal*, vol. 3, no. 3, pp. 171–191, 2006.

[34] R. D. Galiano, O. M. Tepper, C. R. Pelo et al., "Topical vascular endothelial growth factor accelerates diabetic wound healing through increased angiogenesis and by mobilizing and recruiting bone marrow-derived cells," *American Journal of Pathology*, vol. 164, no. 6, pp. 1935–1947, 2004.

[35] F. Zhang, M. P. Lei, T. M. Oswald et al., "The effect of vascular endothelial growth factor on the healing of ischaemic skin wounds," *British Journal of Plastic Surgery*, vol. 56, no. 4, pp. 334–341, 2003.

[36] B. H. Porras-Reyes and T. A. Mustoe, "Platelet-activating factor: improvement in wound healing by a chemotactic factor," *Surgery*, vol. 111, no. 4, pp. 416–423, 1992.

[37] D. R. Edwards, G. Murphy, J. J. Reynolds et al., "Transforming growth factor beta modulates the expression of collagenase and metalloproteinase inhibitor," *EMBO Journal*, vol. 6, no. 7, pp. 1899–1904, 1987.

[38] M. F. Cordeiro, A. Mead, R. R. Ali et al., "Novel antisense oligonucleotides targeting TGF-β inhibit in vivo scarring and improve surgical outcome," *Gene Therapy*, vol. 10, no. 1, pp. 59–71, 2003.

[39] J. S. Huang, Y.-H. Wang, T.-Y. Ling, S.-S. Chuang, F. E. Johnson, and S. S. Huang, "Synthetic TGF-beta antagonist accelerates wound healing and reduces scarring," *The FASEB Journal*, vol. 16, no. 10, pp. 1269–1270, 2002.

[40] W. E. Powers, J. H. Ogura, and L. A. Palmer, "Radiation therapy and wound healing delay. Animals and man," *Radiology*, vol. 89, no. 1, pp. 112–115, 1967.

[41] M. C. Robson, L. G. Phillips, A. Thomason, L. E. Robson, and G. F. Pierce, "Platelet-derived growth factor BB for the treatment of chronic pressure ulcers," *Lancet*, vol. 339, no. 8784, pp. 23–25, 1992.

[42] T. A. Mustoe, N. R. Cutler, R. M. Allman et al., "A phase II study to evaluate recombinant platelet-derived growth factor-BB in the treatment of stage 3 and 4 pressure ulcers," *Archives of Surgery*, vol. 129, no. 2, pp. 213–219, 1994.

[43] M. C. Robson, L. G. Phillips, A. Thomason et al., "Recombinant human platelet-derived growth factor-BB for the treatment of chronic pressure ulcers," *Annals of Plastic Surgery*, vol. 29, no. 3, pp. 193–201, 1992.

[44] P. Yilgor Huri, G. Huri, U. Yasar et al., "A biomimetic growth factor delivery strategy for enhanced regeneration of iliac crest defects," *Biomedical Materials*, vol. 8, no. 4, Article ID 045009.

12

Assessing Improvement in Quality of Life and Patient Satisfaction following Body Contouring Surgery in Patients with Massive Weight Loss: A Critical Review of Outcome Measures Employed

Shehab Jabir

St. Andrews Centre for Plastic Surgery and Burns, Broomfield Hospital, Chelmsford, Essex CM1 7ET, UK

Correspondence should be addressed to Shehab Jabir; shihab.jabir@googlemail.com

Academic Editor: Marcus Lehnhardt

Body contouring following massive weight loss is a rapidly expanding field in plastic surgery. However, healthcare payers are reluctant to fund such procedures, viewing them as purely cosmetic. This has resulted in a flurry of studies assessing quality of life (QoL) and patient satisfaction following body contouring surgery in this cohort of patients to establish an evidence base to support the idea that body contouring is as much (or even more) a functional procedure as it is cosmetic. However, the methods employed in these studies are seldom ideal, and hence the conclusions are unreliable. The gold standard to assess QoL and patient satisfaction is to use patient specific psychometrically validated patient reported outcome (PRO) measures. Developing such measures consists of a three-step process which includes a review of the current literature, qualitative patient interviews to determine what patients consider the most important, and expert opinion. This study aims to appraise the currently available literature on assessment of QoL and patient satisfaction in body contouring surgery patients. This will hopefully provide an understanding of methodological weaknesses in current studies and inform future investigators of the design of ideal instruments for assessing QoL and patient satisfaction in body contouring patients.

1. Introduction

Body contouring surgery has undergone a rapid expansion in the last decade, becoming one of the fastest growing areas within plastic surgery. As the number of obese individuals continues to increase, bariatric surgery has come to the fore as the method of choice for rapidly losing excess weight with approximately one quarter of patients opting for bariatric surgery [1]. However, when a previously obese or morbidly obese individual loses a massive amount of weight, it results in cutaneous contour deformities on various parts of the body. These cutaneous deformities may then lead to psychological distress as well as functional problems, offsetting the positive benefits brought about by weight loss surgery [2–4]. Hence body contouring surgery would intuitively appear to be the next step in rehabilitating the obese patient with massive weight loss (MWL).

However, it has been a challenge to convince healthcare payers of the importance of body contouring procedures to the overall outcome of massive weight loss patients. Whereas funding for bariatric surgery has become easier to obtain due to mounting evidence of its benefits on the health of obese individuals and the economic implications of this benefit, it has yet to filter down to body contouring surgery. Most healthcare systems still consider body contouring to be a cosmetic procedure and are reluctant to fund such operations. This in turn has led to a number of studies addressing body contouring surgery following massive weight loss in patients who have already had bariatric surgery. The primary areas of focus of this research can be divided into two: (1) surgical outcomes in terms of procedure related complications and (2) the quality of life (QoL) and psychosocial outcome of body contouring in massive weight loss patients. In terms of procedure related complications, it has been shown that

TABLE 1: Search terms used with the Boolean operation AND to combine terms.

Body contouring		Body image		Massive weight loss/MWL
Abdominoplasty				
Panniculectomy				Postbariatric
Torsoplasty		Psychological function		
Thoracoplasty	AND		AND	
Brachioplasty/arm lift		Quality of life		Weight reduction
Thigh lift				
Reduction mammaplasty/breast reduction		QoL		
Facelift		Psychosocial function		

as operator experience increases, complication rates drop [5, 6]. However, the second category of research, that is, QoL and psychosocial outcome, is far more important from a funding perspective. If we are able to demonstrate that body contouring surgery results in a significant improvement of the patient's QoL and psychosocial state, then it seizes to be viewed as a purely cosmetic procedure and may make it even obligatory for healthcare payers to fund body contouring surgery as the completion step to rehabilitating the obese patient.

The gold standard for measuring the impact of body contouring surgery on massive weight loss individuals is to use patient-specific, well-constructed psychometrically validated patient reported outcome (PRO) measures (also known as instruments). PRO instruments are any report of the status of a patient's condition that comes directly from the patient without interpretation by a surgeon or other healthcare professional [7]. These measures usually consist of a number of sections which are designed to include key aspects of a conceptual framework. The conceptual framework explicitly defines the concepts measured by the instrument in a diagram that presents a description of the relationships between items, domain (subconcepts), and concepts measured and the scores produced by a PRO instrument [7].

A systematic review of PRO instruments to measure quality of life and patient satisfaction following body contouring surgery was undertaken by Reavey et al. They identified five PRO measures with varying psychometric validity: one general plastic surgery (DAS 59), three breast reduction (BRASSQ, BRS, Breast-Q), and one liposuction instrument (FQAD). Following this, Reavey et al. called for the development of new PRO measures specific to this population [8]. The development of PRO measures consists of a thorough review of currently available literature, qualitative patient interviews to determine what patients consider most important, and expert opinion [9]. A comprehensive understanding of issues that are critical to patients can be obtained from these three sources of information which may then help to inform development of scales and items for inclusion in a new PRO instrument. The aim of this study is to review the methods of assessing QoL and patient satisfaction in postbody contouring MWL patients. This would enable us to delineate what measures have already been employed to assess QoL and patient satisfaction in this domain and where improvements are necessary. It is hoped that by doing so, we would be fulfilling another step toward developing new specific PRO instruments for this fast growing population of patients.

2. Methods

An attempt was made to make the search for the literature as systematic as possible. Hence, the PRISMA statement for systematic reviews was adhered to [10]. Items 12–16 of the PRISMA statement were not applicable to this study as it was not possible to undertake quantitative data synthesis due to wide heterogeneity in the reported outcome measures.

The predetermined inclusion and exclusion criteria for this review were used to determine eligibility of a study to be included in the review.

Inclusion criteria include the following:

(i) the study population was restricted to massive weight loss patients;

(ii) patients included in the study had either one or more of what is considered a body contouring procedure (e.g., abdominoplasty, panniculectomy, thoracoplasty, brachioplasty, mastopexy/plasty, thigh lif, etc.);

(iii) a clearly defined method of measuring improvement in quality of life and/or psychosocial function;

(iv) english language publication.

Exclusion criteria include the following:

(i) Studies measuring only overall "satisfaction" with body contouring procedures.

(ii) Studies measuring the desire for body contouring in postmassive weight loss patients who believed they may attain some functional/psychosocial benefits from body.

The literature search was then carried out on Medline, Embase, CINAHL, PsycINFO, Google Scholar, and the Cochrane databases from inception till March 2013 for studies on the topic of improvement in quality of life and psychosocial function following body contouring surgery in massive weight loss patients. The keywords used are shown in Table 1. The terms in each column were combined with the Boolean operator "OR" while terms between columns were combined with "AND." The output was limited to citations in the English language. Reference lists of identified studies were then hand searched for additional reports.

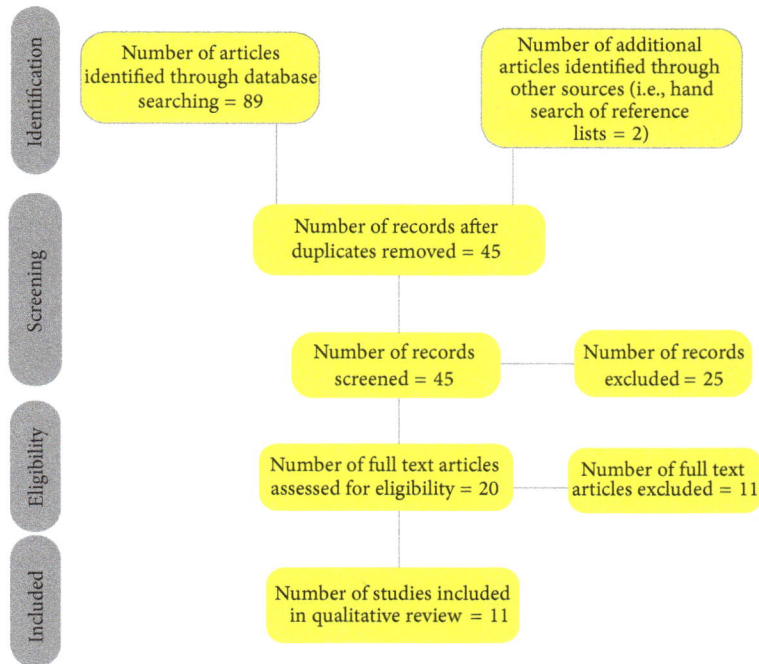

FIGURE 1: Systematic review flow diagram.

The title and abstract of all identified studies were examined. In cases where suitability of a study for inclusion in the review was unclear, the entire paper was obtained and assessed for suitability. Data was extracted onto a Performa which included the data categories listed.

Demographics include the following:

(i) mean age of study subjects;

(ii) number of subjects;

(iii) gender distribution, male: female;

(iv) BMI postbariatric surgery/postmassive weight loss.

Preoperative characteristics (i.e., prior to body contouring surgery but post-bariatric/massive weight loss):

(i) time period between bariatric surgery and body contouring surgery;

(ii) instrument for measurement of quality of life (QoL) and QoL as per that particular instrument of prebody contouring;

(iii) instrument for measurement of psychosocial function and psychosocial function prebody contouring;

(iv) body contouring procedures performed.

Postoperative characteristics (i.e., following body contouring surgery):

(i) QoL following body contouring surgery;

(ii) psychosocial function following body contouring surgery;

(iii) length of follow-up postbody contouring surgery.

Other considerations:

(i) psychometric assessment of tools employed;

(ii) validity and test-retest reliability.

3. Results

The search retrieved a total of 89 studies. Following removal of duplicates, 45 studies remained. 25 studies were excluded following screening of the title and abstract. The entire papers of the remaining 20 articles were reviewed to establish suitability for inclusion. 11 studies were excluded as they did not meet the eligibility criteria leaving 9 studies for inclusion. The reference lists of these 9 studies were then hand searched to identify any further studies. Two studies were identified in this manner, resulting in a total of 11 studies for inclusion in the review. A flow diagram of the search strategy is provided in Figure 1.

A summary of the characteristics of each study is provided in Table 2. Due to the wide heterogeneity in study design and instruments employed to measure psychosocial function and quality of life in body contouring patients, a narrative review of all studies included was undertaken.

3.1. Lazer et al. [11]. Two questionnaires that had been designed specifically for the study yet had not been validated were administered to 41 patients. The first tool was a three-item subjective questionnaire that assessed:

(1) the patient's most problematic body areas after weight loss: abdomen, breasts, thigh, and/or arms;

TABLE 2: Summary of characteristics of studies cited for this review.

Study	Number of patients	Procedure(s)	Control group	Psychosocial function assessed	Quality of life assessed	Average weight loss following bariatric surgery	Study design: prospective (P)/ retrospective (R)	Mean age
Lazar et al. [11]	41 (32 females, 9 males)	Abdominoplasty	No	Yes	Yes	40.2 kg	R	Median age 38 years
Song et al. [12]	18 (16 females, 2 males)	Panniculectomy or abdominoplasty. Eleven patients underwent lower body lift or breast reduction or brachioplasty	No	Yes	Yes	138 ± 76 lbs	P	46 ± 10 years
Cintra Jr. et al. [13]	16 (all females)	Abdominoplasty	No	Yes	Yes	23.8 kg/m^2	R	40.1 ± 8 years
Stuerz et al. [14]	34 (30 females, 4 males)	Abdominoplasty	Yes	Yes	Yes	16 kg/m^2	P	37.1 ± 9.3 years
Pecori et al. [15]	10 (all females)	Abdominoplasty (7), leg and/or arm lifts (8), torsoplasty (2)	Yes	Yes	No	49 kg	R	Range 28–56 years
Lanier [16]	50 (28 females, 22 males)	Abdominoplasty (24), facelift (18), Reduction mammaplasty (10)	No	Yes	No	126 lbs	R	Not stated
Menderes et al. [17]	11 (7 females, 4 males)	Blepharoplasty (8), mastopexy (8), thigh reduction (5), arm reduction (2), Abdominoplasty (11), reduction mammaplasty (3), lateral thigh lift (2), gynaecomastia (3), medial thigh lift (1), liposuction (3)	No	Yes	No	57.6 kg	R	37.4 years
Van Der Beek et al. [18]	43 (41 females, 2 males)	Primarily abdominoplasty and breast reduction/augmentation	No	No	Yes	51.3 kg	R	41.5 years
Singh et al. [19]	104 (85 females, 19 males)	Unspecified	Yes	Yes	Yes	N/A	R	42
Coriddi et al. [20]	49 (40 females, 9 males)	Panniculectomy and abdominoplasty	No	Yes	Yes	21.5 k/m^2	P	45.8
Klassen et al. [21]	43 (40 females, 3 males)	Abdominoplasty (31), liposuction (18), Upper arm lift (14), breast lift (10), lift (9), buttock lift (6)	No	Yes	Yes	N/A	R	47

TABLE 3: Psychological evaluation questionnaire and patient answers.

Questions	Yes (%)	Good (%)	No (%)	Bad (%)	Intermediate opinion (%)
How do you feel today?		65.4		15.4	19.2
What is your opinion about abdominoplasty?		50		23.1	26.9
Are the results in accordance with your expectations?	61.5				38.5
Are the scars a problem for you?	61.5		11.6		26.9
Do you like your new body?	53.9		11.5		34.6
Do other people regard you differently now?	61.5		38.5		
Has your daily life improved?	84.6		7.7		7.7
What if abdominoplasty had been contraindicated?		38.5		61.5	
Would you agree to redo abdominoplasty?	96.1		3.9		

TABLE 4: Instruments used by Song et al. [12].

Area of assessment	Outcome measures	General or specifically developed for study
Body perception and ideals	Pictorial body image assessment (PBIA)	Modified version of the Stunkard Silhouette tool developed specifically for this study
Body image satisfaction and areas of distress	(i) Body image and satisfaction assessment (BISA) (ii) Current body image assessment (CBIA)	(i) Specifically developed for this study (ii) Specifically developed for this study
General and condition specific quality of life	(i) Health related quality of life (HR-QoL) (ii) The postbariatric surgery quality of life (PBSQoL) survey	(i) A general instrument to measure QoL (ii) Specifically developed for this study
Mood	Beck's inventory	General instrument to assess mood

(2) consequences on QoL of abdominal skin overhanging: current life, dressing, aesthetics, psychological status, and/or sexual relations;

(3) ranking the effects of abdominoplasty on each of the previously mentioned QoL areas as: very good, good, average quite bad, or bad.

The second tool was a nine-item questionnaire designed by a trained psychologist to assess psychological status. The questions in this tool were as follows:

(1) How do you feel today?

(2) What is your opinion of your abdominoplasty?

(3) Are the results in accordance with your expectations?

(4) Are the scars a problem for you?

(5) Do you like your new body?

(6) Do other people regard you differently now?

(7) Has your daily life improved?

(8) What if abdominoplasty had been contraindicated?

(9) If you had to do it over again, would you undergo abdominoplasty?

The first questionnaire was administered once to assess preabdominoplasty body perception and QoL and for a second time to assess postbody contouring perception of improvement. The second tool was administered once to assess psychological status with all data being collected after an average follow-up period of 57.7 months (range 41 to 80 months).

In terms of the 5 areas of QoL assessed, aesthetics was the primary area of concern with 38 patients stating that they considered the abdomen an area of concern affecting their QoL prior to abdominoplasty. The next most concerning areas in terms of QoL were psychological status (36), dressing (33), sexual relations (27), and current life (15). After abdominoplasty, patients evaluated their QoL as good or very good in all of the above domains.

The second tool to assess psychological status following abdominoplasty again seemed to suggest that abdominoplasty did have a positive impact on their psychological status with 84.6% saying their daily life improved following the procedure. The results of the psychological questionnaire are presented in Table 3.

3.2. Song et al. [12]. Assessed body image, quality of life, and other measures in a prospective manner using a number of different instruments as shown in Table 4. A description of each of these instruments is provided in Table 5. Outcomes were assessed immediately prior to body contouring surgery, 3 months, and then 6 months after body contouring surgery. We will restrict ourselves here to the outcomes of body image and QoL. The study included a total of 18 patients, 16 females, and 2 males.

At 3 months, body image and satisfaction as measured by the BISA tool improved significantly ($P < 0.01$). The improvement remained stable at 6 months.

In terms of QoL measured by the HR-QoL, the mean score prebody contouring at 3 months postbody contouring and at 6 months postbody contouring remained around

TABLE 5: Description of each of the outcome tools employed by Song et al. [12].

Outcome measure	Description
PBIA	A pictorial representation from underweight to severely obese on a 13-point scale on which the patient indicates which one they believe they were before bariatric surgery, their appearance before body contouring surgery, and their personal ideal silhouette
BISA	Divides the body into 10 areas (e.g., thighs, abdomen) with a visual analogue scale from 0, signifying extreme dissatisfaction, to 10, signifying perfect satisfaction. A possible maximum score of 100 and minimum of 0
CBIA	Assesses areas of greatest dissatisfaction. The patient is handed a blank canvass of human outlines representing the front and back views on which they circle up to three areas of distress. These areas are anatomically coded in order to detect changes in areas of distress as patients underwent body contouring
HR-QoL	A modification of the SF-36 questionnaire which is used to assess physical function, self-esteem, sexual function, physical distress, and work function
PBSQoL	A quality of life measure that was specifically designed for the postbariatric weight loss patient population. It assessed areas such as feelings of attractiveness, skin rash and infection, ease of exercise, public embarrassment about loose skin, ease of shopping, and clothing fit
Beck's inventory	A highly sensitive and validated measure of depression symptoms used to assess mood

the same mark and there was not a statistically significant improvement. On the other hand, the PBSQoL scores which were collated from 13 patients however revealed a statistically significant improvement in the quality of life.

3.3. Cintra et al. [13]. Assessed quality of life in 16 female patients following abdominoplasty after massive weight loss. A validated tool known as the Adaptive Operationalized Diagnostic Scale (AODS)—as described below—was used to assess QoL.

Description of AODS Used by Cintra et al. to Assess QoL

> AODS: A 31-item instrument consisting of 4 domains: affectivity/personal relations, productivity, social/cultural performance, and organic/somatic health. Together they evaluate physical and mental health, social adjustment, body image, self-concept, self-esteem, and mood and feelings. Results are summarized in five levels of adaptation from good (level 1) to very severe maladaptation (level 5) for each domain and as a final score for a complete test.

The patients were questioned by a trained psychologist using this tool after an interval of approximately 1–3 years following abdominoplasty. The best overall response corresponded to the social and cultural domain, where 81.3% of patients had good adaptation (level 1). For the other three domains, results were remarkably similar with 62.5% of the tests displaying the highest value of adaptation (level 1) and few complete failures. Final scoring for the complete test is demonstrated in Table 6.

In terms of specific subtopics in the domains sited in Table 5, points of note include the fact that 87.5% had a very good self-image, 87.5% displayed adequate self-esteem, and around 68.8% noticed a better sex life after abdominoplasty.

3.4. Stuerz et al. [14]. Carried out a prospective study including 31 postbody contouring patients with a control group of 26 patients who had undergone gastric banding and who

TABLE 6: Final results of the quality of life questionnaire.

Category	Level	Result (%)
Good adaptation	1	43.8
Mild adaptation	2	37.5
Moderate maladaptation	3	6.3
Severe maladaptation	4	6.3
Very severe maladaptation	5	6.3

had lost weight but who had not undergone body contouring surgery for comparison. The instruments used in this study are listed in Table 7 and were administered to the body contouring group 1 day before body contouring surgery and then at 3 and 12 months after the procedure.

In terms of body image which was assessed via the Strauss and Appelt's Questionnaire, there were improvements in all four areas listed in Table 7 with a statistically significant improvement ($P < 0.001$) in the attractiveness/self-esteem subscale in the surgery group compared with the control group. However, no significant difference was detected on the "Emphasis on attractiveness" subscale of the Body Perception Questionnaire by Paulus between the two groups. Furthermore, no change was detected in terms of life satisfaction (assessed via the Life Satisfaction Questionnaire) or anxiety and depression between the two groups (assessed via the Hospital Anxiety and Depression Scale).

The author's General Questionnaire after surgery revealed that abdominoplasty resulted in a change in leisure activities in 21 patients, reduced inhibitions in 20 patients, and improved sexual relationships in 27 patients.

3.5. Pecori et al. [15]. Studied body image issues in four groups of patients who are described in Table 8

The two groups particularly relevant to our purposes are the POST-A group and POST-B group. Body image in each of the groups was evaluated by means of the Body Uneasiness Test (BUT), a self-administered questionnaire which had displayed satisfactory test-retest reliability and internal consistency in previous studies. A description of the domains

TABLE 7: Description of outcome tools used by Stuerz et al. [14].

Outcome measure	Description
Strauss and Appelt's Questionnaire for assessing one's own body	This questionnaire consists of 52 items which are answered with "true" or "not true" and consists of four subscales: (1) Attractiveness/self-confidence (2) Accentuation of external appearance (3) Worry about possible physical defects (4) Problems regarding sexuality
Subscale "Emphasis on attractiveness" of the Body Perception Questionnaire by Paulus	This is a 22-item scale which assesses the extent to which appearance is adjusted to meet social norms
The Life Satisfaction Questionnaire	Covers ten areas of life, is, an index of general life satisfaction, and includes, healthiness, work life, financial status, leisure, partnership, relationship to own children, own person, sexuality, friends/relatives, and residence
The Hospital Anxiety and Depression Scale	A self-rating scale which consists of two separate subscales for anxiety and depression (each with 7 items) and is used to detect states of depression and anxiety
Author's general questionnaire	Developed by the authors of the study and inquires about factors such as financing, expectations, reasons, desire for any other plastic surgery, dealing with the scar, satisfaction, effects on leisure activities, sexuality, inhibitions, and preoperative surgical information

TABLE 8: Description of patient groups in the study carried out by Pecori et al. [15].

Group	Number of patients	Description
OB group	20	Morbidly obese women prior to biliopancreatic diversion (BPD)
POST group	20	>2 years following BPD
POST-A group	10	Postobese women following BPD who required cosmetic procedures
POST-B group	10	Postobese women after BPD and subsequent cosmetic surgery
Control	20	Lean and healthy individuals

assessed by the BUT questionnaire is provided in the description of the two parts of the body uneasiness test used by Pecori et al. below.

Body Uneasiness Test (Divided into Two Parts)

Part 1: explores body-related and shape-related psychopathology. Results are expressed in both a combined Global Severity Index and in scores of 5 subscales:

(1) weight phobia (fear of being or becoming fat);

(2) body image concerns (overconcerned with physical appearance);

(3) avoidance;

(4) compulsive self-monitoring (rituals involving checking physical appearance);

(5) depersonalization (feelings of detachment or estrangement from one's body).

Part 2: indicates dissatisfaction with the overall body shape and with the different parts of one's body. Results are expressed in two domains: Positive Symptom Total and Positive Index Distress Symptom.

Table 9 demonstrates the mean scores with the standard deviation for the POST-A and POST-B groups for parts 1 and 2 of the BUT questionnaire. There is a clear improvement in all domains in the POST-B group (i.e., postobese women at

TABLE 9: BUT score data in subjects of POST-A and POST-B groups (mean ± SD).

	POST-A	POST-B
Global severity index	1.68 ± 1.13	1.04 ± 0.63
Weight phobia	2.31 ± 1.41	1.80 ± 0.88
Body image concern	2.23 ± 1.54	1.28 ± 0.72
Avoidance	1.07 ± 1.1	0.35 ± 0.55
Compulsive self-monitoring	1.02 ± 0.64	1.09 ± 0.79
Depersonalization	1.09 ± 0.91	0.46 ± 0.56
Positive symptoms total	10.7 ± 7.01	10.1 ± 9.30
Positive index distress	4.10 ± 0.81	4.07 ± 1.37

>2 years after BPD who have undergone cosmetic surgery) compared to the POST-A group (i.e., postobese women at 2 years after BPD requiring cosmetic surgery). No statistical significance testing was carried out by the authors.

3.6. Lanier et al. [16]. 50 patients (28 women and 22 men) underwent a variety of body contouring procedures. Following these procedures, a questionnaire was administered to the patients asking the following questions:

(1) Did the surgical procedure enable you to feel better about yourself in regard to the way you look and feel?

(2) Did the operative procedure provide you an incentive to maintain your weight reduction goal?

TABLE 10: Modification of the Derriford Appearance Scale by Menderes et al. [17] leads to fewer questions in each section of the scale.

Derriford appearance scale (DAS-59)	Original no. of questions	No. of questions in modified questionnaire
GSC	17	12
SSC	20	9
SBSC	9	5

Forty-eight of the 50 patients returned the questionnaire (96% response rate). Thirty-nine patients (82%) answered "Yes" when asked whether plastic surgery after weight reduction had improved their self-esteem. Thirty-four patients (72%) stated that the body contouring surgery did not provide an incentive to maintain their weight reduction goal. Thus this study showed that self-esteem in massive weight loss patients could be improved by body contouring surgery but did not affect long-term weight maintenance which may require behaviour modification through the team efforts of a weight reduction counselor, therapist, and surgeon.

3.7. Menderes et al. [17]. 11 patients (7 women and 4 men) who underwent body contouring surgery following vertical banded gastroplasty (VBG) had their self-consciousness assessed by the Derriford Appearance Scale. The questionnaire administered was modified from its original structure, taking into account local norms. The modified questionnaire consisted of 3 subscales:

(1) general self-consciousness (GSC) of appearance;

(2) social self-consciousness (SSC) of appearance; and

(3) sexual and bodily self-consciousness of appearance (SBSC).

The difference between the original questionnaire and the final modified version is given in Table 10.

Each of the patients were asked to answer each of the questions in each subscale with one of five possible statements (from almost never to almost always), and the level of distress was measured with statements (from not at all distressed to extremely distressed) in a Likert type format.

The results are shown in Table 11. As can be seen, there is a significant improvement in GSC and SBSC after bariatric surgery and then after body contouring surgery. SSC also improved to a substantial degree after bariatric surgery and then after body contouring surgery. No statistical analysis was carried out.

3.8. Van Der Beek et al. [18]. Assessed quality of life and satisfaction with body contouring surgery in 43 patients who had undergone bariatric surgery. Quality of life was assessed by the Obesity Psychosocial State Questionnaire (OPSQ) (Table 12) which measures seven domains with items in each domain having a five-point rating from 1 (almost never) to 5 (almost always). The questionnaire was administered twice retrospectively following body contouring surgery, the first time to record their prebody contouring quality of life and a second time to record their postbody contouring quality of life. Satisfaction was measured simply by asking the patient about their overall satisfaction with the procedure.

There were improvements in almost all domains with the greatest improvements being in the physical functioning and physical appearance domains ($P < 0.001$). They felt less depressed, more satisfied with their appearance, and felt that they had more control over their eating behaviours following reconstructive surgery ($P < 0.001$). In terms of overall satisfaction with the procedure, sixty-seven percent of patients felt satisfied with the overall result of the operation.

3.9. Singh et al. [19]. Applied the SF-36 questionnaire to a total of 104 individuals belonging to four groups of patients including a control group (27 patients), an obese group (31 patients), a postbariatric surgery group (30 patients), and a postbody contouring surgery group (16 patients). The SF-36 questionnaire consists of 8 scales that assess both physical and mental components of health as shown in Table 13.

Comparison of the outcomes for the social functioning and role-emotional components of the SF-36 questionnaire between the postbariatric surgery and postbody contouring groups found a statistically significant reduction in QoL in the postbody contouring group compared to the postbariatric surgery group. However, physical functioning was considerably improved in the postbody contouring group compared to the postbariatric surgery group, although not to a statistically significant degree.

3.10. Coriddi et al. [20]. Conducted a prospective telephone survey assessing several functional outcomes and satisfaction before and after body contouring surgery (Table 14). 52 patients who had abdominal contouring procedures (41 had panniculectomies and 11 had abdominoplasties) were recruited with 49 responding to the survey (94% response rate).

Apart from shoulder pain, there were statistically significant improvements in all functional outcomes between the pre- and postbody contouring groups. In terms of satisfaction, 91.8 percent of patients said that they would have their body contouring procedure again or would recommend it to a friend.

3.11. Klassen et al. [21]. Used qualitative patient interviews to obtain information regarding quality of life and satisfaction issues in body contouring surgery. Forty-three massive weight loss postbody contouring surgery patients were interviewed. The interviews took the form of patients describing their weight loss journey with probes to explore the impact of obesity, weight loss, and body contouring surgery on their quality of life. Analysis of the interviews revealed a number of important health and aesthetic concerns which were explained in terms of 5 core themes.

(1) Appearance-related concerns.

(2) Physical health concerns.

(3) Sexual health concerns.

TABLE 11: Evaluation of self-consciousness.

	Preoperative perception of SC	Perception of SC between bariatric and plastic surgical interventions	Perception of SC after bariatric and plastic surgery interventions
General self-consciousness	34.3 (3.1)	27.6 (2.5)	21.2 (1.9)
Social self-consciousness	25.1 (2.8)	19.4 (2.1)	16.6 (1.8)
Self-consciousness of appearance	17.7 (3.5)	11.8 (2.3)	8.2 (1.6)

TABLE 12: The Obesity Psychosocial State Questionnaire (OPSQ).

Scales	Example item
Physical function	To kneel or duck easily
Mental well-being	To feel depressed (reversed score)
Physical appearance	To feel fat when someone takes a picture (reverse score)
Social acceptance	To be discriminated because of my weight (reverse score)
Self-efficacy	To feel helpless toward my eating behaviour (reversed score)
Intimacy	To have sexual problems because of my weight (reversed score)
Social network	To visit friends and acquaintances

TABLE 13: The eight scales of the SF-36 which assess physical and mental components of health.

Scale	Measures
Physical component	
Physical functioning	Limitations in physical activities due to health problems
Role-physical	Limitations in usual daily activities due to health problems
Bodily pain	Pain experienced due to health problems
General health	General health perceptions
Vitality	Self-perceived energy and fatigue
Mental component	
Social functioning	Limitations in social activities due to physical or emotional problems
Role-emotional	Limitations in usual daily activities due to emotional problems
Mental health	Perceived well-being and the presence of any psychological distress

(4) Psychological health concerns.

(5) Social health concerns.

Although no quantitative methods were employed to assess the impact of body contouring surgery on massive weight loss patients, this qualitative study demonstrated that body contouring leads to an overall improvement in the 5 core themes cited above and was an important step in the completion of the entire weight loss process for patients. Furthermore, the issues cited above enable investigators to appreciate QOL issues from the patient's perspective and may

provide the conceptual framework necessary to help develop more specific PRO instruments.

4. Discussion

Table 15 provides a summary of the instruments used in each study, if the instruments were psychometrically validated, were patient reported, and if they were modified from their original format by the investigators.

Psychometric validity includes a number of concepts. Some of the essential concepts include:

(i) content validity—refers to the instrument incorporating relevant questions/sections of interest within it (i.e., how adequately the sampling of items reflects its aims). The questions included within an instrument are usually determined by experts within the field in which the instrument was designed for use;

(ii) construct validity—essentially involves a conceptual definition of the construct to be measured by the instrument and then assessing the internal structure of its components and the theoretical relationship of its item and subscale scores;

(iii) concurrent validity—compares the outcomes of the newly developed instrument with established "gold standard" instruments to determine how well the new instrument purports to measure what it measures in comparison to older, better established instruments;

(iv) predictive validity—this assesses an instrument's ability to predict future outcomes (e.g., resource use or treatment outcomes);

(v) test-retest reliability—this ascertains the extent of agreement when the same instrument is applied to the same cohort of patients by the same investigator at two different time points;

(vi) interrater reliability—refers to the degree of agreement between outcomes when the same instrument is applied to the same cohort of patients by two or more different investigators;

(vii) sensitivity to change—the extent to which the instrument demonstrates change over time in comparison to "gold standard" measures (e.g., change measured my more established measures);

(viii) acceptability/Feasibility/Utility—this is a measure of how useful and acceptable the instrument is to the investigator and or patient.

In an ideal setting, each PRO instrument would have been validated for every category mentioned above. This would

Table 14: Functional status survey before and after abdominal contouring surgery.

Question*	Before body contouring	After body contouring
Neck pain		
Back pain		
Shoulder pain		
Abdominal pain		
Pain during exercise		
Difficulties with walking		
Difficulties with standing		
Difficulties with posture		
Difficulties with sleeping		
Difficulties with travel		
Difficulties with work tasks		
Difficulties with personal hygiene		
Difficulties with toilet habits		
Difficulties finding clothes		
Lymphedema		
Skin irritation		
Lower extremity paresthesias (numbness/tingling)		
Lower extremity weakness		

Question†	Before body contouring	After body contouring
Ability to climb stairs		
Ability to descend stairs		
Ability to jog/run		
Ability to rise from a squatting position		
Ability to play with kids		
Ability to do household tasks		

Satisfaction‡		
Would you have this procedure again? yes/no		
Would you recommend this procedure to a friend? yes/no		

*Respondents reported on a 10-point Likert scale ranging from 1 (infrequent) to 10 (often).
†Respondents reported on a 10-point Likert scale ranging from 1 (completely able) to 10 (unable).
‡Respondents reported on a 10-point Likert.

ensure that the instrument measures what it was designed for with a high degree of accuracy. However, this is not always possible or necessary. As long as content validity, construct validity, and predictive validity are satisfactory, the instrument could potentially provide accurate measures of the concept of interest. Table 15 shows that most studies used psychometrically validated instruments while some used measures that were nonpsychometrically validated. A detailed discussion of the psychometric properties of each of the measures employed by the different studies is beyond the scope of this review. However, an important point of note is that all psychometric measures employed by the different studies were not developed to provide outcomes in postbody contouring surgery patients. In other words, none of the psychometrically validated instruments employed within the studies reviewed were developed specifically for the population of interest, that is, postmassive weight loss body contouring surgery patients. Hence, from the outset, content validity of the PRO instruments used is breached. This makes the QoL outcomes obtained from these instruments (in postmassive weight loss body contouring surgery patients) questionable. As a result, this review has identified the need for condition-specific outcome measures. Furthermore, certain studies modified the psychometrically validated measures used. It is hard to predict the impact of modification on each particular instrument, but taking into consideration the type and extent of modification mentioned in each study report, it would be reasonable to assume that the modification may have led to a slight improvement in the validity of the instrument. This is because they were modified to take into account the population of interest, that is, to improve construct validity. For example, the modifications made to the original Derriford appearance scale, a validated outcome instrument, used by Menderes et al. were modified taking into account local norms and patient participation. It is less likely, but not impossible, that the modification might have negatively impacted the validity.

Squires et al. present an advanced protocol for the psychometric assessment of instruments based on the Standards for Educational and Psychological Testing [22]. Validity, reliability, and acceptability are all assessed. A unitary approach to validity consisting of accumulating evidence based on instrument content, response processes, internal structure, and relations to other variables is taken while reliability is assessed with internal consistency coefficients and information functions. Acceptability of the instrument is assessed with missing data frequencies and the time required to complete the survey. Apart from this "traditional" method of assessing psychometric properties, other more modern methods of psychometric assessment have been developed, most useful of which is the Rasch model analysis which was developed by Rasch [23]. Rasch model analysis provides psychometric information that is not provided with the above mentioned more traditional analyses. Rasch model analysis is a probability model that converts the ordinal scores obtained by summing item scores into interval measures [24]. While the ordinal raw scores used in traditional analyses are typically used as if they were interval in nature, the measures produced by Rasch analysis are on an equal-interval scale that is common to both persons and items. *Rasch analysis uses these equal-interval measures to assess multiple psychometric characteristics specific to the population for which the PRO instrument is being developed. This enables the design of PRO instruments which are more accurate and sensitive to clinical changes.*

All measures used were patient reported as indicated in Table 15. The advantage of patient reported measures includes

TABLE 15: Summary of instruments employed in each study, psychometric validity, modification by investigators, and if they were patient reported outcome measures.

Study	Questionnaire/s employed	Psychometrically validated?	Modified for study?	Patient reported?
Lazar et al. [11]	(1) Three-item subjective questionnaire	(1) No	(1) N/A	(1) Yes
	(2) Nine-item psychological status questionnaire designed by trained psychologist	(2) No	(2) N/A	(2) Yes
Song et al. [12]	(1) Pictorial body image assessment	(1) No	(1) N/A	(1) Yes
	(2) Body image and satisfaction assessment	(2) No	(2) N/A	(2) Yes
	(3) Current body image assessment	(3) No	(3) N/A	(3) Yes
	(4) Health related quality of life	(4) Yes	(4) Yes	(4) Yes
	(5) The postbariatric surgery quality of life survey	(5) No	(5) N/A	(5) Yes
	(6) Becks inventory	(6) Yes	(6) No	(6) Yes
Stuerz et al. [14]	(1) Strauss and Appelt's questionnaire (for assessing body image)	(1) Yes	(1) No	(1) Yes
	(2) "Emphasis on attractiveness" subscale of the Body Perception Questionnaire by Paulus	(2) Yes	(2) Yes	(2) Yes
	(3) The life satisfaction questionnaire	(3) Yes	(3) No	(3) Yes
	(4) The hospital anxiety and depression scale	(4) Yes	(4) No	(4) Yes
	(5) Author's general questionnaire	(5) No	(5) N/A	(5) Yes
Cintra et al. [13]	Adaptive Operationalized Diagnostic Scale	Yes	No	Yes
Pecori et al. [15]	Body uneasiness test	Yes	No	Yes
Lanier [16]	2 questions devised by investigators	No	N/A	Yes
Menderes et al. [17]	Derriford appearance scale	Yes	Yes	Yes
Van Der Beek et al. [18]	The obesity psychosocial state questionnaire	Yes	No	Yes
Singh et al. [19]	SF-36	Yes	No	Yes
Coriddi et al. [20]	(1) Functional status survey (2) Two Question Satisfaction survey	No	N/A	Yes
Klassen et al. [21]	Qualitative interview	N/A	N/A	Yes

the fact that the individual who was subjected to the intervention who should theoretically have most insight into the impact of the intervention provides the outcome. In addition, in a more general sense, it enables healthcare payers to appreciate the views of patients on particular interventions and may provide a less biased perspective to a particular treatment option. Hence, patient reported outcomes may have more weight when healthcare payers decide to fund a particular procedure.

5. Conclusion

As mentioned above, a systematic review of PRO instruments to measure quality of life and patient satisfaction following body contouring surgery identified five PRO measures with varying psychometric validity. However, it must be pointed out that none of these measures have been specifically developed for body contouring surgery patients, and hence the title of the study is a misnomer to its content. Reavey et al. conclude that there is a need to develop specific PRO measures for this group of patients. This review has found a number of studies which have attempted to assess QoL and patient satisfaction in postbody contouring massive weight loss patients with less than ideal PRO measures.

Hence, the author agrees that there is an urgent need to develop specific and well constructed PRO instruments in order to obtain reliable information regarding QoL and patient satisfaction following body contouring surgery in MWL patients. Furthermore, future investigators should use newer techniques of assessing psychometric validity of newly developed instruments which are both more convenient and reliable compared to more traditional techniques.

Acknowledgment

The author would like to thank Ian Wilkes, Pauline Kewell, and the rest of the staff at the Warner Library for their assistance in obtaining papers for this review.

References

[1] D. B. Sarwer and A. N. Fabricatore, "Psychiatric considerations of the massive weight loss patient," *Clinics in Plastic Surgery*, vol. 35, no. 1, pp. 1–10, 2008.

[2] "Psychological considerations of the massive weight loss patient," *Plastic and Reconstructive Surgery*, vol. 117, supplement 1, pp. 17S–21S, 2006.

[3] R. Y. Chandawarkar, "Body contouring following massive weight loss resulting from bariatric surgery," *Advances in Psychosomatic Medicine*, vol. 27, pp. 61–72, 2006.

[4] R. J. Hafner, J. M. Watts, and J. Rogers, "Quality of life after gastric bypass for morbid obesity," *International Journal of Obesity*, vol. 15, no. 8, pp. 555–560, 1991.

[5] J. M. Hensel, J. A. Lehman Jr., M. P. Tantri, M. G. Parker, D. S. Wagner, and N. S. Topham, "An outcomes analysis and satisfaction survey of 199 consecutive abdominoplasties," *Annals of Plastic Surgery*, vol. 46, no. 4, pp. 357–363, 2001.

[6] M. A. Van Huizum, N. A. Roche, and S. O. P. Hofer, "Circular belt lipectomy: a retrospective follow-up study on perioperative complications and cosmetic outcome," *Annals of Plastic Surgery*, vol. 54, no. 5, pp. 459–464, 2005.

[7] U.S. Food and DrugAdministration. Patient reported outcome measures: use in medical product development to support labeling claims, 2009, http://www.fda.gov/downloads/Drugs/Guidances/UCM193282.pdf.

[8] P. L. Reavey, A. F. Klassen, S. J. Cano et al., "Measuring quality of life and patient satisfaction after body contouring: a systematic review of patient-reported outcome measures," *Aesthetic Surgery Journal*, vol. 31, no. 7, pp. 807–813, 2011.

[9] K. N. Lohr, "Assessing health status and quality-of-life instruments: attributes and review criteria," *Quality of Life Research*, vol. 11, no. 3, pp. 193–205, 2002.

[10] A. Liberati, D. G. Altman, J. Tetzlaff et al., "The PRISMA statement for reporting systematic reviews and meta-analyses of studies that evaluate health care interventions: explanation and elaboration," *Annals of Internal Medicine*, vol. 151, no. 4, pp. W-65–W-94, 2009.

[11] C. C. Lazar, I. Clerc, S. Deneuve, I. Auquit-Auckbur, and P. Y. Milliez, "Abdominoplasty after major weight loss: improvement of quality of life and psychological status," *Obesity Surgery*, vol. 19, no. 8, pp. 1170–1175, 2009.

[12] A. Y. Song, J. P. Rubin, V. Thomas, J. R. Dudas, K. G. Marra, and M. H. Fernstrom, "Body image and quality of life in post massive weight loss body contouring patients," *Obesity*, vol. 14, no. 9, pp. 1626–1636, 2006.

[13] W. Cintra Jr., M. L. A. Modolin, R. Gemperli, C. I. C. Gobbi, J. Faintuch, and M. C. Ferreira, "Quality of life after abdominoplasty in women after bariatric surgery," *Obesity Surgery*, vol. 18, no. 6, pp. 728–732, 2008.

[14] K. Stuerz, H. Piza, K. Niermann, and J. F. Kinzl, "Psychosocial impact of abdominoplasty," *Obesity Surgery*, vol. 18, no. 1, pp. 34–38, 2008.

[15] L. Pecori, G. G. Serra Cervetti, G. M. Marinari, F. Migliori, and G. F. Adami, "Attitudes of morbidly obese patients to weight loss and body image following bariatric surgery and body contouring," *Obesity Surgery*, vol. 17, no. 1, pp. 68–73, 2007.

[16] V. C. Lanier, "Body contouring surgery after weight reduction," *Southern Medical Journal*, vol. 80, no. 11, pp. 1375–1380, 1987.

[17] A. Menderes, C. Baytekin, M. Haciyanli, and M. Yilmaz, "Dermalipectomy for body contouring after bariatric surgery in Aegean region of Turkey," *Obesity Surgery*, vol. 13, no. 4, pp. 637–641, 2003.

[18] E. S. J. Van Der Beek, W. Te Riele, T. F. Specken, D. Boerma, and B. Van Ramshorst, "The impact of reconstructive procedures following bariatric surgery on patient well-being and quality of life," *Obesity Surgery*, vol. 20, no. 1, pp. 36–41, 2010.

[19] D. Singh, H. R. Zahiri, L. E. Janes et al., "Mental and physical impact of body contouring procedures on post-bariatric surgery patients," *Eplasty*, vol. 12, p. e47, 2012.

[20] M. R. Coriddi, P. F. Koltz, R. Chen, and J. A. Gusenoff, "Changes in quality of life and functional status following abdominal contouring in the massive weight loss population," *Plastic and Reconstructive Surgery*, vol. 128, no. 2, pp. 520–526, 2011.

[21] A. F. Klassen, S. J. Cano, A. Scott, J. Johnson, and A. L. Pusic, "Satisfaction and quality-of-life issues in body contouring surgery patients: a qualitative study," *Obesity Surgery*, vol. 22, no. 10, pp. 1527–1534, 2012.

[22] J. E. Squires, L. Hayduk, A. M. Hutchinson et al., "A protocol for advanced psychometric assessment of surveys," *Nursing Research and Practice*, vol. 2013, Article ID 156782, 8 pages, 2013.

[23] P. W. Duncan, R. K. Bode, S. M. Lai, and S. Perera, "Rasch analysis of a new stroke-specific outcome scale: the stroke impact scale," *Archives of Physical Medicine and Rehabilitation*, vol. 84, no. 7, pp. 950–963, 2003.

[24] B. D. Wright and J. M. Linacre, "Observations are always ordinal; measurements, however, must be interval," *Archives of Physical Medicine and Rehabilitation*, vol. 70, no. 12, pp. 857–860, 1989.

13

The Lateral Port Control Pharyngeal Flap: A Thirty-Year Evolution and Followup

Sean Boutros[1,2] and Court Cutting[3]

[1] Hermann Memorial Hospital and Hermann Children's Hospital, Houston, TX 77030, USA
[2] Houston Plastic and Craniofacial Surgery, 6400 Fannin Suite 2290, Houston, TX 77030, USA
[3] Institute for Reconstructive Plastic Surgery, New York University, New York, NY 10016, USA

Correspondence should be addressed to Sean Boutros; drseanboutros@drseanboutros.com

Academic Editor: Luis Bermudez

In 1971, Micheal Hogan introduced the Lateral Port Control Pharyngeal Flap (LPCPF) which obtained good results with elimination of VPI. However, there was a high incidence of hyponasality and OSA. We hypothesized that preoperative assessment with videofluoroscopy and nasal endoscopy would enable modification and customization of the LPCPF and result in improvement in the result in both hyponasality and obstructive apnea while still maintaining results in VPI. Thirty consecutive patients underwent customized LPCPF. All patients had preoperative diagnosis of VPI resulting from cleft palate. Patient underwent either videofluoroscopy or nasal endoscopy prior to the planning of surgery. Based on preoperative velar and pharyngeal movement, patients were assigned to wide, medium, or narrow port designs. Patients with significant lateral motion were given wide ports while patients with minimal movement were given narrow ports. There was a 96.66% success rate in the treatment of VPI with one patient with persistent VPI (3.33%). Six patients had mild hyponasality (20%). Two patients had initial OSA (6.67%), one of which had OSA which lasted longer than six months (3.33%). The modifications of the original flap description have allowed for success in treatment of VPI along with an acceptably low rate of hyponasality and OSA.

1. Introduction

In 1971, Micheal Hogan introduced the lateral port control pharyngeal flap [1–3]. This flap was conceived out of frustration over the inconsistent results obtained in the correction of velopharyngeal insufficiency with pharyngeal flaps. By noting important contributions to the understanding of physiology and dynamics of hypernasal speech by Warren, Isshiki, and Bjork [4–7], he devised a technique that could be universally applied to all patients with velopharyngeal insufficiency and obtain good result with consistent elimination of hypernasal speech [1–3, 8]. In his technique, the superiorly based flap, lined by the nasal side of the soft palate [9–12], was designed so that the lateral aperture size was controlled by the passage of a 4 mm diameter catheter. This effectively created an air passage that allowed the oropharyngeal pressure build up necessary to eliminate hypernasal speech.

After his initial description, the procedure evolved due to observation of the results. At the time Hogan described the LPC pharyngeal flap, sleep apnea had not yet been described as a clinical entity [13, 14]. In terms of speech intelligibility, hyponasality is preferred over hypernasality. The idea that many cleft palate patients with VPI often had good lateral wall movement allowing a "tailored width" pharyngeal flap [15] was also not yet widely known. For this reason, Hogan initially described a single-size flap that tended to produce very small lateral ports. Dr. Hogan intuitively began constructing larger ports in most patients and still maintained adequate results. In the past 30 years, the Hogan LPC flap became well known for the production of hyponasality and sleep apnea. The subsequent modifications of Hogan's original description, which takes these factors into account, are the subject of this paper.

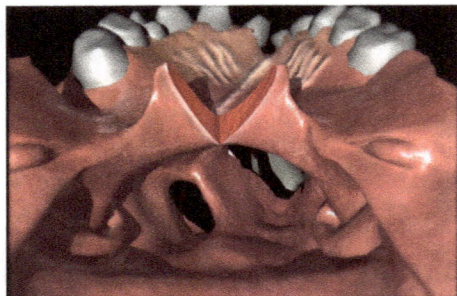

FIGURE 1: Division of soft palate.

2. Materials and Methods

Thirty consecutive patients undergoing pharyngeal flap procedures for velopharyngeal insufficiency (VPI) were identified. Twenty-seven of these patients had VPI as a result of cleft palate, and 23 of these patients had adequate followup (greater than one year) for inclusion in this study. Patients were treated at the Institute of Reconstructive Plastic Surgery and either operated on or supervised by the senior surgeon (CC). Patients were treated according to the cleft VPI protocol as outlined later on. All patients were followed by the senior surgeon, pediatric otolaryngologist, and speech therapist.

2.1. Preoperative Evaluation. Patients with velopharyngeal insufficiency underwent evaluation with videofluoroscopy or fiberoptic nasal endoscopy [16, 17]. The findings are reviewed in a multidisciplinary clinic with a plastic surgeon, a pediatric otolaryngologist, and a speech therapist. Together, a consensus was reached as to the amount of velar and pharyngeal movement.

In patients between 2.5 and 3 years of age who have not undergone intravelar veloplasty with the initial palate repair (palate closure performed at another institution), this procedure is the first-line treatment [18]. Many patients will attain adequate velar closure and have complete elimination of hypernasality with this procedure alone. These patients were excluded from this study.

In patients over four years, in whom the time course is more pressed due to the difficulty in elimination of compensatory articulations acquired after prolonged time with nasal escape, the pharyngeal flap is the procedure of choice if the nasal endoscopy shows lateral wall movement with poor central closure [8, 15–17, 19]. In a small minority of patients (none in our sample group), there may be good central movement with poor lateral closure. These rare patients are treated with a sphincter procedure. In addition, patients who have had previous intravelar veloplasty are also candidates for pharyngeal flaps. Based on the fiberoptic and videofluoroscopic findings, these patients are assigned to a small, medium-small, medium, medium-large, and large ports sizes. This corresponds with wide, medium-wide, medium, medium-narrow, and narrow pharyngeal flaps [13, 15, 17, 20, 21].

2.2. Operation. Prior to prep and drape, the posterior pharyngeal wall and the soft palate are infiltrated with approximately 10 cc of 0.5% lidocaine with 1 : 200,000 epinephrine. The posterior pharynx should always be palpated prior to infiltration, as patients with undiagnosed velo-cardio-facial syndrome are likely to have medialization of the carotid arteries, and care must be taken to avoid their injury. A Dingman's mouth gag is placed with the smallest tongue gag that will adequately hold the tongue on the floor of the mouth. Placement of a larger gag will limit the ability to reach the posterior pharyngeal wall. The handle of the gag is hung on the Mayo stand edge fully open and protrudes the mandible for optimal access.

The soft palate is split in the midline (Figure 1) and retraction sutures are placed. This split should stop just prior to the hard/soft palate junction (see supplementary video available online at doi:10.1155/2012/237308). The posterior pharyngeal wall is visualized, and the superiorly based pharyngeal flap of the appropriate width is outlined. As the flap is superiorly based, its mucosal surface will be reflected to the nasal side. It should be based as high as possible, approximately 15 mm caudal to the Eustachian tube orifices. The flap is incised to the parapharyngeal space. It is not necessary to incise to the prevertebral fascia as it does not contribute to the vascularity of the flap and results in a more painful donor site. The paired parapharyngeal spaces can be confirmed by the presence of the midline raphe. The flap is elevated with a peanut and the midline raphe cut with scissors. A suture is placed in the tip of the flap for retraction.

The donor site should be closed directly except for the most proximal area. Closure decreases the postoperative pain, infection rate, and decreases downward migration of the flap with time. It will also allow for reestablishment of the sphincteric action of the pharyngeal wall with approximation of the muscles. It is best to close the middle of the donor site first and use the long end of a suture for retraction to expose the most caudal aspect of the donor site. Attempting to close the most cranial or proximal area of the donor site will cause the flap to take a tube shape and make creation of the appropriate size port difficult. Care must be taken to cauterize the edges of the cut posterior pharynx prior to closure as this is the most likely site of postoperative bleeding. This bleeding will most likely be from a cut ascending pharyngeal artery or one of its branches. Bleeding in this area may cause loss of airway and preclude oral intubation. Hemostasis is best performed with a suction cautery device. Although commercial suction cauteries are available, passing a neuro-tip suction through a red rubber catheter can easily create a suction cautery.

Attention should be turned to the creation of the lining flaps. It is important to consider the width of the lateral port much more than the width of the lining flap. The lining flaps are elevated from the nasal side of the soft palate and will line the oral side of the pharyngeal flap (Figure 2). They are based on the posterior edge of the soft palate, and the tip of the flap is at the hard/soft palate junction. The split soft palate should be reflected laterally. The rhomboidal-shaped flap is elevated off the underlying velar musculature. Starting at the most anterior aspect of the soft palate split, an incision

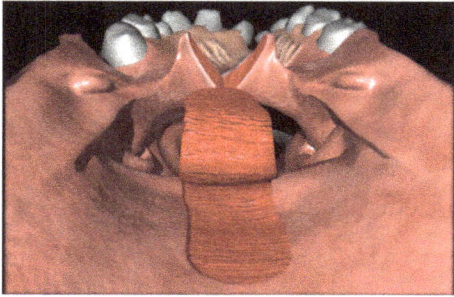

FIGURE 2: Elevation of superiorly based pharyngeal flap.

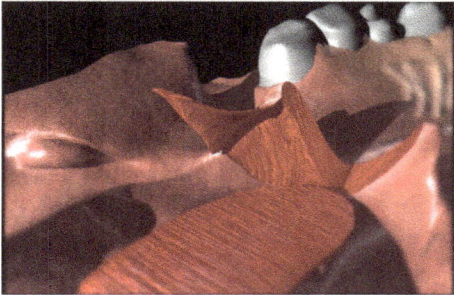

FIGURE 3: Elevation of the lining flap from the nasal side of the soft palate. Note that the lateral extent of the lining flap will help determine the size of the resulting lateral port.

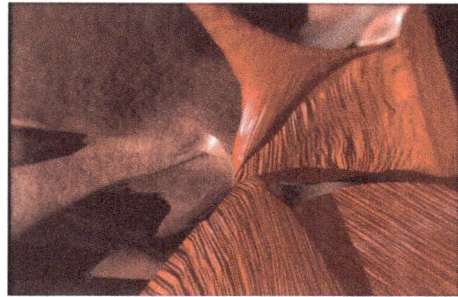

FIGURE 4: The key suture brings the lateral aspect of the lining flap to the superiorly based pharyngeal flap. This suture sets the size of the lateral port.

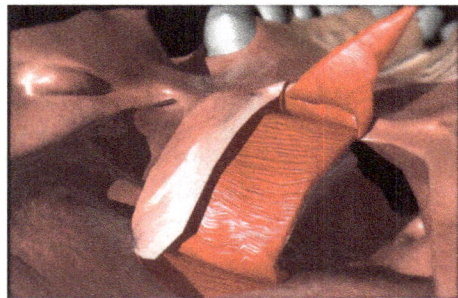

FIGURE 5: The lining flap is brought down to cover the raw side of the pharyngeal flap. This lining is crucial to prevention of contraction and tabularization of the pharyngeal flap.

is created toward the lateral/posterior edge of the soft palate. The lateral cut edge on the nasal surface of the soft palate will determine the size of the port.

The nasal lining flaps are then turned out to cover the raw surface of the pharyngeal flap. The port is created by suturing of the lateral cut edge to a point 5 mm from the base of the pharyngeal flap (Figures 3, 4, and 5). The lateral edge of the pharyngeal flap is sutured to the lateral cut edge from the elevation of the lining flaps, that is, the nasal side of the soft palate. The final suture is a horizontal mattress suture setting the tip of the flap well beyond the most anterior soft palate split in order to prevent formation of a fistula at this critical location. The suture is passed through and through (oral to nasal) the most anterior soft palate. It is passed through the tip of the pharyngeal flap in a mattress fashion and "through and through" (nasal to oral) the soft palate.

The lateral edge of the tip of the lining flaps, elevated from the nasal side of the soft palate, is sutured to the lateral defect of the posterior pharyngeal wall. The medial edges of both lining flaps are sutured to the midline raphe at the base of the pharyngeal flap and to each other. The medial edges of the lining flaps are sutured together with each suture catching the midline raphe of the pharyngeal flap. The uvula is reconstructed, and the oral side of the soft palate is repaired.

A tongue stitch is placed in lieu of an oral airway as passage of an oral or nasal airway may disrupt the flap. The air and fluid are evacuated from the stomach, and blood is suctioned from the nose and pharynx. The patient is only extubated when fully awake, and the surgeon must be present in the room. After extubation, the patient is placed in a tonsillar position and kept awake. Traction on the tongue suture will both open the airway and stimulate the patient as needed.

2.3. Postoperative Management. In the initial postoperative period, airway observation is critical. The patients are kept on continuous pulse oximetry in the initial postoperative period. The intensive care unit is usually not required. The tongue suture is usually removed the next morning. Patients are given pain control with per rectum acetaminophen and codeine and kept on IV antibiotics to decrease the risk of streptococcal infection until they are taking liquids by mouth at which time they can be converted to oral antibiotics. They are allowed fluids immediately but are unlikely to take anything by mouth for the first few days. At the time they are taking adequate liquids, they can be discharged. The time course for oral intake varies dramatically. It ranges from three to nine days, but most patients take adequate fluids by mouth between three and four days. After several days of liquids, the patient is slowly transitioned to a soft diet, which is maintained for two to three weeks.

3. Results

Based on the preoperative evaluation of lateral wall motion, the procedures were divided as such: 6 patients had large port design (small flaps), 3 patients had large/medium port design (small/medium flaps), 14 patients had medium port design (medium flaps), and 6 patients had small/medium port design (medium/wide flaps). The incidence of small ports (wide flaps) was zero.

There was one patient with persistent VPI (4.3%). Five patients had mild hyponasality (21.7%). Two patients had initial sleep apnea (8.7%). One of the two had sleep apnea which lasted longer than six months (4.3%). This patient's flap was taken down with resolution of the VPI and no hypernasality. There was no airway compromise most likely due to hemostasis obtained prior to back wall closure.

In all patients, there was some initial nocturnal obstruction due to swelling associated with the procedure. Overall, we have seen two patterns of sleep apnea in our patients. The first is obstruction at five to six weeks when wound contracture is at its highest. The obstruction resolves over several weeks as the contracture relaxes. There is a separate group in whom the contracture does not relax and there is resulting long-term obstruction. This may resolve over the next six to nine months, but if it does not resolve, the flap is taken down. Contraction of the pharyngeal flap may also lengthen the scarred soft palate [22].

4. Discussion

4.1. Preoperative Assessment. At the time of Hogan's original publication, there was no way to accurately assess the amount of velar or lateral pharyngeal movement preoperatively. The only measure of success was the postoperative result. As a result, in patients with some degree of pharyngeal movement, the results were typically good, and in patients with poor movement, the results were poor. There was no way to preoperatively stratify patients into the good or poor responder groups.

Videofluoroscopy and nasal endoscopy opened a new understanding of the movement of the velum and how surgical procedures could benefit patients [8, 16, 17, 23]. Videofluoroscopy allowed for direct visualization of the lateral pharyngeal wall movement, identifying the location and degree of the pathology and allowing formation of a reconstructive plan. This, along with the fundamentals of lateral port control technique of described by Hogan, allow for surgeons to customize the procedure to allow for appropriately sized flaps for each patient based on the amount of movement they have prior to surgery. This results in nasal competence, good speech, and limited hyponasality.

4.2. Port Diameter. Dr. Hogan was inspired to develop the lateral port control pharyngeal flap by the works of Drs. Warren and Isshiki. Both showed that the critical closing diameter allowing normal speech was 20 mm² (Dr. Isshiki's critical diameter was 19.6 mm²). Dr. Hogan observed these facts and made two ports that would have a sum total of 25 mm², ("...slightly larger than our threshold value of 20 mm². Because of the mesial movement of the lateral pharyngeal walls which occurs during speech") [19, 24]. In his design, Dr. Hogan focused on cross-sectional area of the ports not the airflow through the ports which is more

important. According to Poiseuille's law, airflow is directly proportional to the fourth power of the radius. Thus, small changes in diameter have a dramatic effect on airflow.

$$\text{Flow} = \frac{\Pi \, (\text{pressure difference}) \, \text{radius}^4}{8 \, (\text{viscosity}) \, (\text{length})}. \quad (1)$$

A 20 mm port has a radius of 2.526 mm,

$$\text{Flow} = \frac{\Pi \, (\text{pressure difference}) \, (2.526 \, \text{mm})^4}{8 \, (\text{viscosity}) \, (\text{length})}. \quad (2)$$

By this, half the flow or flow prime would be described by the following equation:

$$\text{Flow prime} = \frac{\text{Flow}}{2} = \frac{\Pi \, (\text{pressure difference}) \, (2.526 \, \text{mm})^4}{16 \, (\text{viscosity}) \, (\text{length})},$$

$$\text{Flow prime} = \frac{\Pi \, (\text{pressure difference}) \, (2.526 \, \text{mm})^4}{16 \, (\text{viscosity}) \, (\text{length})},$$

$$\frac{\Pi \, (\text{pressure difference}) \, (\text{radius prime})^4}{8 \, (\text{viscosity}) \, (\text{length})}$$

$$= \frac{\Pi \, (\text{pressure difference}) \, (2.526 \, \text{mm})^4}{16 \, (\text{viscosity}) \, (\text{length})},$$

$$\frac{(\text{radius prime})^4}{8} = \frac{(2.526)^4}{16},$$

$$(\text{radius prime})^4 = 20.36 \, \text{mm},$$

$$\text{radius prime} = 2.125 \, \text{mm}.$$

$$(3)$$

Therefore, two ports with a radius of 2.125 mm each (cross sectional area of 14.19 mm² each and a total cross sectional area of 28.38 mm²) would have the same airflow as one port with a radius of 2.5 mm (cross sectional area of 19.63 mm² each).

In essence, a 50% larger sum total cross sectional area of two ports would have the exact same air flow resistance as a single port of 20 mm². This of course assumes that there would be no pharyngeal movement. It can then be extrapolated that after pharyngeal flap, with the creation of ports, where with pharyngeal and velar movement the size of each of the two ports is reduced to an area of 14.19 mm², there would be no clinically apparent hypernasality.

In today's evaluation of the patient with velopharyngeal insufficiency, this becomes more significant as presurgical evaluation of the patient can give a much clearer picture of the pharyngeal movement. The procedure is no longer forced to address the least common denominator, that is, paralytic velum and pharyngeal wall, as it can be customized for each patient depending on the specific needs and level of dysfunction.

Presently, the goal is to have complete velar closure. However, with two ports, even if there is not complete closure, the resulting nasal air escape would be less than that found with one port.

4.3. Sleep Apnea. Not until recently did obstructive sleep apnea come into the attention of physicians treating velopharyngeal insufficiency [3]. Prior to this, nighttime obstruction and the resulting clinical symptoms after pharyngeal flap surgery were largely ignored, and the procedures touted as a success or failure solely on the effect on hypernasality. Nighttime snoring was even considered a measure of success as it indicated a low likelihood of nasal escape. However, more recent studies have shown that this important clinical entity is not only a source of significant morbidities including snoring, excessive daytime sleepiness, learning disabilities, irritability, perioperative aspiration pneumonia, growth retardation, heart disease, and hypertension, but also mortality with perioperative respiratory arrest and sudden death.

The incidence of obstructive sleep apnea is controversial. Some authors report that with objective testing in a series of patients, over 90% will have some degree of sleep apnea after pharyngeal flap, and only some of which are clinically significant [25]. Most generally, it is quoted that an approximately 10% incidence of clinically apparent obstructive apnea and that only a fraction of these cases will require intervention [26–28]. In any event, the risk of postsurgical sleep apnea should be taken into account when approaching patients. With preoperative assessment and procedure individualization as we have shown, the incidence of clinically important sleep apnea can be significantly decreased resulting in few patients with this complication.

5. Conclusions

With some modifications from the original description by incorporation of preoperative diagnostic testing, the lateral port control pharyngeal flap has stood the test of time and has proven to be a powerful procedure in treatment of velopharyngeal insufficiency. Like all pharyngeal flaps, it serves to limit airflow from the oropharynx to the nasopharynx by forming an obstruction in the dysfunctional central area. It does not add any scarring or injury to the area where there is normal anatomy and the muscle function is good, that is, laterally. It uses this lateral pharyngeal sphincteric motion, along with the motion of the levator veli palatini muscle, to create a functional, dynamic obstruction to air flow. The lateral port control method turns the attention of the procedure to what is necessary for cure as it forces the surgeon to design a flap where the goal is the creation of a port of appropriate size that will prevent hypernasality while still resulting in an acceptable incidence of hyponasality and obstructive sleep apnea.

Acknowledgment

This work was presented at the American Cleft Palate Association Meeting, Myrtle Beach, South Carolina in March 2005.

References

[1] V. M. Hogan, "A clarification of the surgical goals in cleft palate speech and the introduction of the Lateral Port Control (L.P.C.) pharyngeal flap," *Cleft Palate Journal*, vol. 10, no. 4, pp. 331–345, 1973.

[2] P. A. Levine and R. L. Goode, "The lateral port control pharyngeal flap: a versatile approach to velopharyngeal insufficiency," *Otolaryngology*, vol. 90, no. 3, Part 1, pp. 310–314, 1982.

[3] J. W. Canady, B. B. Cable, M. P. Karnell, and L. H. Karnell, "Pharyngeal flap surgery: protocols, complications, and outcomes at the University of Iowa," *Otolaryngology*, vol. 129, no. 4, pp. 321–326, 2003.

[4] D. W. Warren, "Velopharangeal orifice size and upper pharangeal pressure flow patterns in normal speech," *Plastic and Reconstructive Surgery*, vol. 33, pp. 148–154, 1964.

[5] D. W. Warren and J. L. Devereux, "An analog study of cleft palate speech," *Cleft Palate Journal*, vol. 3, pp. 103–114, 1966.

[6] N. Isshiki, I. Honjow, and M. Morimoto, "Effects of velopharyngeal incompetence upon speech," *Cleft Palate Journal*, vol. 5, pp. 297–310, 1968.

[7] L. Bjork, "Velopharangeal function in connected speech," *Acta Radiologica*. In press.

[8] B. B. Cable and J. W. Canady, "The endoscopically assisted pharyngeal flap," *Cleft Palate-Craniofacial Journal*, vol. 40, pp. 114–115, 2003.

[9] C. Stoll, M. Hochmuth, P. Meister, and F. Soost, "Refinement of velopharyngoplasty in patients with cleft palate by covering the pharyngeal flap with nasal mucosa from the velum," *Journal of Cranio-Maxillofacial Surgery*, vol. 28, no. 3, pp. 171–175, 2000.

[10] F. J. Newman and A. Messinger, "A method for lining the superiorly based pharyngeal flap," *Annals of Plastic Surgery*, vol. 14, no. 4, pp. 346–350, 1985.

[11] M. J. Vandevoort, N. S. Mercer, and E. H. Albery, "Superiorly based flap pharyngoplasty: the degree of postoperative 'tubing' and its effect on speech," *British Journal of Plastic Surgery*, vol. 54, no. 3, pp. 192–196, 2001.

[12] S. B. Hardy and M. Spira, "Lining the superiorly based pharyngeal flap," *Annals of Plastic Surgery*, vol. 11, no. 4, pp. 289–290, 1983.

[13] D. D. Daly and R. E. Yoss, "Pathologic sleep," *International Journal of Neurology*, vol. 5, no. 2, pp. 195–206, 1965.

[14] R. T. Brouillette, S. K. Fernbach, and C. E. Hunt, "Obstructive sleep apnea in infants and children," *Journal of Pediatrics*, vol. 100, no. 1, pp. 31–40, 1982.

[15] R. V. Argamaso, R. J. Shprintzen, and B. Strauch, "The role of lateral pharyngeal wall movement in pharyngeal flap surgery," *Plastic and Reconstructive Surgery*, vol. 66, no. 2, pp. 214–219, 1980.

[16] D. M. Crockett, R. M. Bumsted, and D. R. Van Demark, "Experience with surgical management of velopharyngeal incompetence," *Otolaryngology*, vol. 99, no. 1, pp. 1–9, 1988.

[17] B. C. Sommerlad, F. V. Mehendale, M. J. Birch, D. Sell, C. Hatte, and K. Harland, "Palate re-repair revisited," *Cleft Palate-Craniofacial Journal*, vol. 39, pp. 295–307, 2002.

[18] R. J. Shprintzen, M. L. Lewin, and C. B. Croft, "A comprehensive study of pharyngeal flap surgery: tailor made flaps," *Cleft Palate Journal*, vol. 16, no. 1, pp. 46–55, 1979.

[19] M. P. Karnell, K. Ibuki, H. L. Morris, and D. R. Van Demark, "Reliability of the nasopharyngeal fiberscope (NPF) for assessing velopharyngeal function: analysis by judgment," *Cleft Palate Journal*, vol. 20, no. 3, pp. 199–208, 1983.

[20] B. G. Peat, E. H. Albery, K. Jones, and R. W. Pigott, "Tailoring velopharyngeal surgery: the influence of etiology and type of

operation," *Plastic and Reconstructive Surgery*, vol. 93, no. 5, pp. 948–953, 1994.

[21] R. J. Shprintzen, G. N. McCall, and M. L. Skolnick, "The effect of pharyngeal flap surgery on the movements of the lateral pharyngeal walls," *Plastic and Reconstructive Surgery*, vol. 66, no. 4, pp. 570–573, 1980.

[22] T. Agarwal, G. M. Sloan, D. Zajac, K. S. Uhrich, W. Meadows, and J. A. Lewchalermwong, "Speech benefits of posterior pharyngeal flap are preserved after surgical flap division for obstructive sleep apnea: experience with division of 12 flaps," *The Journal of Craniofacial Surgery*, vol. 14, no. 5, pp. 630–636, 2003.

[23] A. Ysunza, M. C. Pamplona, E. Ramírez, S. Canún, M. C. Sierra, and A. Silva-Rojas, "Videonasopharyngoscopy in patients with 22q11.2 deletion syndrome (Shprintzen syndrome)," *International Journal of Pediatric Otorhinolaryngology*, vol. 67, no. 8, pp. 911–915, 2003.

[24] J. Karling, G. Henningsson, O. Larson, and A. Isberg, "Adaptation of pharyngeal wall adduction after pharyngeal flap surgery," *Cleft Palate-Craniofacial Journal*, vol. 36, pp. 166–172, 1999.

[25] Y. F. Lia, M. L. Chuang, P. K. Chen, N. H. Chen, C. Yun, and C. S. Huang, "Incidence and severity of obstructive sleep apnea following pharyngeal flap surgery in patients with cleft palate," *Cleft Palate-Craniofacial Journal*, vol. 39, pp. 312–316, 2002.

[26] M. D. Wells, T. A. Vu, and E. A. Luce, "Incidence and sequelae of nocturnal respiratory obstruction following posterior pharyngeal flap operation," *Annals of Plastic Surgery*, vol. 43, no. 3, pp. 252–257, 1999.

[27] M. Sirois, L. Caouette-Laberge, S. Spier, Y. Larocque, and E. P. Egerszegi, "Sleep apnea following a pharyngeal flap: a feared complication," *Plastic and Reconstructive Surgery*, vol. 93, no. 5, pp. 943–947, 1994.

[28] A. Ysunza, M. Garcia-Velasco, M. Garcia-Garcia, R. Haro, and M. Valencia, "Obstructive sleep apnea secondary to surgery for velopharyngeal insufficiency," *Cleft Palate-Craniofacial Journal*, vol. 30, no. 4, pp. 387–390, 1993.

14

Telemedicine and Plastic Surgery

Denis Souto Valente,[1] **Luciano Silveira Eifler,**[2] **Lauro Aita Carvalho,**[2]
Gustavo Azambuja Pereira Filho,[2] **Vinicius Weissheimer Ribeiro,**[2]
and Alexandre Vontobel Padoin[1]

[1]*Graduate Program in Medicine and Health Sciences, PUCRS School of Medicine (FAMED), Avenida Ipiranga 6681,
90619-900 Porto Alegre, RS, Brazil*
[2]*Mae de Deus Health System, Rua Soledade 569, 90470-340 Porto Alegre, RS, Brazil*

Correspondence should be addressed to Denis Souto Valente; denisvalentedr@gmail.com

Academic Editor: Lee L. Q. Pu

Background. Telemedicine can be defined as the use of electronic media for transmission of information and medical data from one site to another. The objective of this study is to demonstrate an experience of telemedicine in plastic surgery. *Methods.* 32 plastic surgeons received a link with password for real-time streaming of a surgery. At the end of the procedure, the surgeons attending the procedure by the Internet answered five questions. The results were analyzed with descriptive statistics. *Results.* 27 plastic surgeons attended the online procedure in real-time. 96.3% considered the access to the website as good or excellent and 3.7% considered it bad. 14.8% reported that the transmission was bad and 85.2% considered the quality of transmission as good or excellent. 96.3% classified the live broadcasting as a good or excellent learning experience and 3.7% considered it a bad experience. 92.6% reported feeling able to perform this surgery after watching the demo and 7.4% did not feel able. 100% of participants said they would like to participate in other surgical demonstrations over the Internet. *Conclusion.* We conclude that the use of telemedicine can provide more access to education and medical research, for plastic surgeons looking for medical education from distant regions.

1. Introduction

Telemedicine can be defined as the use of electronic media for transmission of information and medical data from one site to another. It is a vague term which cover a wide range of topics, all concerning the delivery of health care at a distance, encompassing diagnosis and treatment of patients, education of staff, patients, and the general public, and administrative activities, such as collecting public health data, as well as research. All of these may be assisted by judicious use of telemedicine. The exchange of medical information over distances by electronic means is an emerging area [1, 2].

The main advantage of telemedicine is that it can improve access to health care, often by reducing the need to travel or by increasing the speed with which a specialist opinion can be obtained. The classical telemedicine programs have mainly used store-and-forward methods, although there has been some limited use of real-time video. Its applications range from data collection for diagnostic purposes to telesurgery [3]. The objective of this study is to demonstrate the initial experience of the authors in the application of telemedicine in plastic surgery.

2. Materials and Methods

The demonstration of a malar fat pad removal surgery for aesthetic purposes is reported. After obtaining informed consent from the patient, and with the support of the Hospital Telemedicine Service, a demonstrative surgery was scheduled. 32 members of the Brazilian Society of Plastic Surgery who wanted to see how this surgery was done were warned by e-mail 12 days in advance and received a link with password for real-time streaming. This study is in accordance with the 2000 Edinburgh, Scotland Revision of

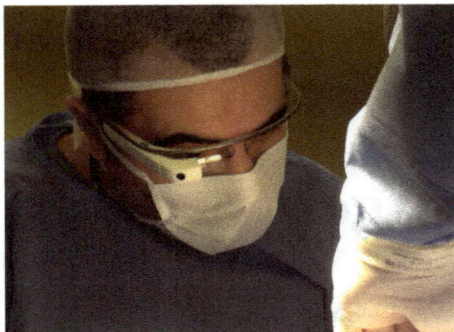

FIGURE 1: The plastic surgeon wearing the Glass.

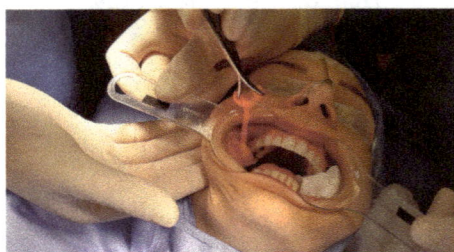

FIGURE 2: An image captured by the equipment.

the Declaration of Helsinki, applicable ICH guidelines, and Guidelines on Research Practice.

On the day of surgery, the plastic surgeon wore a Google Glass (Google Inc., California, USA) and performed the surgery with transmission via Internet in real time. The live broadcast was interactive and the observers were able to interact remotely with the operating surgeon. Figure 1 shows the plastic surgeon wearing the Glass, and Figure 2 shows an image captured by the equipment. At the end of the procedure, the surgeons who attended the procedure by the Internet answered five questions, two related to transmission and three related to the learning goals in this broadcast. At the end of data collection, the results were presented and analyzed with descriptive statistics.

3. Results

Among the 32 invited plastic surgeons, 27 attended the online procedure in real time. 96.3% considered the access to the website as good or excellent and 3.7% considered it bad. 14.8% reported that the transmission was bad and 85.2% considered the quality of transmission as good or excellent. 96.3% classified the live broadcasting as a good or excellent learning experience and 3.7% considered it a bad learning experience. 92.6% reported feeling able to perform this surgery after watching the demo and 7.4% did not feel able. 100% of participants said they would like to participate in other surgical demonstrations over the Internet.

4. Discussion

Telemedicine allows a reduction in consultation time, training, and mentoring among different geographic areas without the expensive mobilization of experts. Telemedicine modalities can range from elementary transmission of digital texts or images with medical context, through live interactive videoconference, to complex procedures as performing surgery in a remote location via robotic tools. E-health and telehealth refer to the delivery of remote clinical and nonclinical services using technology. The transmission of still images, patient consultations by videoconferencing, patient interactive portals, continuing medical education, patient-focused wireless applications, remote monitoring of vital signs, and nursing call centers, among other utilizations, are all considered as telemedicine. Technological advances in picture, audio, and video tools for Internet sharing, wireless broadband availability, and the evolution of handheld devices allowed patients to access medical services without the need to travel long distances shortening the gap among medical facilities and persons needing medical care. The first generation telemedicine systems were "point-to-point" models over landlines, confining health care providers to fixed workstations within hospitals. The involvement of the World Wide Web heralded the second generation of telemedicine, allowing consultations to be conducted from anywhere at any time [1, 4].

Plastic surgery can benefit from telemedicine more than other medical specialties because the clinical visual assessment is the basis of the diagnosis of traumatic injuries, burns, wounds, and the arrangement of transoperative care. Usually, plastic surgery does not depend on laboratorial or imaging tests. The advanced broadcasting technology has been convenient to plastic surgeons as a diagnostic gadget and can simplify the clinical assessment from a distance [5].

An important benefit of telemedicine is to provide skilled medical care. Complex wounds and severe traumatic injuries can be evaluated remotely to afford the appropriate venue for transfer and treatment. Persons with chronic wounds usually have several mobility limitations; telemedicine can be useful in these patients allowing plastic surgeon evaluation, as well as wound monitoring and care, generating logistic and financial benefits. Patients who do not have access to specialist care for geographical reasons can benefit from telemedicine consultations without the need to travel long distances, thus generating savings from work or school absence prevention, and the suffering of elongated waiting periods to achieve specialist evaluations. Telemedicine has been used in military facilities and also by humanitarian purposes to provide international multidisciplinary care to war victims living in remote areas who do not have access to specialty care [6, 7].

There is a debate about the ethical aspect of telemedicine. The Federal Council of Medicine in Brazil defines and regulates the provision of services through telemedicine as practice of medicine through the use of interactive methodologies, audiovisual communication, and data, for care, education, and research in health. The services provided through telemedicine should have the infrastructure and appropriate technology, to comply with the technical standards relevant to custody, handling, data transmission, confidentiality, privacy, and assurance of medical secrecy [8].

By analyzing the data obtained in our work, we see that the vast majority of study participants found the experience useful and all of which accompanied the surgical procedure wanted to participate in new dynamics using the same technology. This opens an important path for worldwide plastic surgery information exchange among plastic surgeons. The American Society of Plastic Surgeons believes that telemedicine is one of the future fields of research in this specialty [9]. In our paper, there is not a conflict of interests, because the only quoted equipment (Google Glass) is no longer manufactured worldwide. This study's main limitations include the small sample size, the short study duration, and the observational design.

This technology allows surgeons to track one procedure to their displacement distance decreasing costs and time and exposing the patient to lower risk of infection if there were more people in the operating room. In addition, the images may be stored in Cloud enabling better low-cost medical documentation. Data support Google Glass positive impact on health care delivery, clinical training, medical documentation, and patient safety. Concerns exist regarding patient confidentiality, technical issues, and limited software [10].

Telemedicine is now widely used in surgery from performing operations to teaching and can be divided into three main components: telesurgery, telementoring, and teleconsultation. Developments across these fields have led to remarkable achievements such as intercontinental telesurgery and telementoring [11]. In plastic surgery, it is now being performed for burn management, real-time video consultation, cleft care, microsurgery monitoring, hand surgery, and wound management [1, 2, 4–7, 12, 13].

Although telemedicine technologies are considered promising, most telemedicine applications have failed to survive beyond the funded research phase to be embedded as methods of routine health care delivery [14, 15]. An important issue in our study is the interaction possibility. If there was not an interactive component, there would not be an educational benefit of the live broadcast studied by just watching a recorded video through Google Glass. As the observers were permitted to interact with the surgeon, we found a use of telemedicine that has been a well-described tool for surgical education and the observers feedback was an interesting analysis. Currently, medical education has not taken advantage of the advances in telemedicine. Information about this mode of medical delivery remains absent from the medical school curriculum. The next generations of physicians, who will be the users of this new transformative system, have little foundation in telemedicine. This is something that needs to change.

5. Conclusion

The use of telemedicine can provide more access to education and medical research, for plastic surgeons looking for medical education from distant regions. This translational technology can positively impact health care delivery, medical documentation, surgical training, and patient safety.

Disclosure

Level V is descriptive studies.

References

[1] M. A. Costa, C. A. Yao, T. J. Gillenwater et al., "Telemedicine in cleft care: reliability and predictability in regional and international practice settings," *Journal of Craniofacial Surgery*, vol. 26, no. 4, pp. 1116–1120, 2015.

[2] N. Panse, "Telemedicine and plastic surgery in India," *World Journal of Plastic Surgery*, vol. 3, no. 1, pp. 70–71, 2014.

[3] J. A. M. Paro, R. Nazareli, A. Gurjala, A. Berger, and G. K. Lee, "Video-based self-review: comparing Google Glass and GoPro technologies," *Annals of Plastic Surgery*, vol. 74, supplement 1, pp. S71–S74, 2015.

[4] J. Niamtu III, "Google glass: dermatologic and cosmetic surgery applications," *Dermatologic Surgery*, vol. 40, no. 10, pp. 1150–1152, 2014.

[5] B. Atiyeh, S. A. Dibo, and H. H. Janom, "Telemedicine and burns: an overview," *Annals of Burns and Fire Disasters*, vol. 27, no. 2, pp. 87–93, 2014.

[6] N. H. Naam and S. Sanbar, "Advanced technology and confidentiality in hand surgery," *Journal of Hand Surgery*, vol. 40, no. 1, pp. 182–187, 2015.

[7] K. Kiranantawat, N. Sitpahul, P. Taeprasartsit et al., "The first Smartphone application for microsurgery monitoring: silpaRamanitor," *Plastic and Reconstructive Surgery*, vol. 134, no. 1, pp. 130–139, 2014.

[8] E. J. C. Rezende, E. C. Tavares, C. de Souza, and M. do Carmo Barros de Melo, "Telehealth: confidentiality and informed consent," *Revista Médica de Minas Gerais*, vol. 23, no. 3, pp. 367–373, 2013.

[9] American Society of Plastic Surgeons, Study: Google Glass Shows Promising Uses in Plastic Surgery, July 2015, http://www.plasticsurgery.org/news/2015/google-glass-shows-promising-uses-in-plastic-surgery.html.

[10] C. R. Davis and L. K. Rosenfield, "Looking at plastic surgery through Google Glass: part 1. Systematic review of Google Glass evidence and the first plastic surgical procedures," *Plastic and Reconstructive Surgery*, vol. 135, no. 3, pp. 918–928, 2015.

[11] N. Raison, M. S. Khan, and B. Challacombe, "Telemedicine in surgery: what are the opportunities and hurdles to realising the potential?" *Current Urology Reports*, vol. 16, no. 7, article 43, 2015.

[12] I. Westra and F. B. Niessen, "Implementing real-time video consultation in plastic surgery," *Aesthetic Plastic Surgery*, vol. 39, no. 5, pp. 783–790, 2015.

[13] R. K. Chittoria, "Telemedicine for wound management," *Indian Journal of Plastic Surgery*, vol. 45, no. 2, pp. 412–417, 2012.

[14] S. J. Cho, I. H. Kwon, and J. Jeong, "Application of telemedicine system to prehospital medical control," *Healthcare Informatics Research*, vol. 21, no. 3, pp. 196–200, 2015.

15

Surgical Implications of Asymmetric Distribution of Dermal Collagen and Elastic Fibres in Two Orientations of Skin Samples from Extremities

Naveen Kumar,[1] Pramod Kumar,[2] Satheesha Nayak Badagabettu,[1] Keerthana Prasad,[3] Ranjini Kudva,[4] and Raghuveer Coimbatore Vasudevarao[5]

[1]*Department of Anatomy, Melaka Manipal Medical College, Manipal Campus, Manipal University, Manipal 576104, India*
[2]*Department of Plastic Surgery, King Abdul Aziz Hospital, Sakaka, Al-Jouf 42421, Saudi Arabia*
[3]*Department of Information Science, Manipal School of Information Science, Manipal University, Manipal 576104, India*
[4]*Department of Pathology, Kasturba Medical College, Manipal University, Manipal 576104, India*
[5]*Department of Pathology, Yenepoya University, Deralakatte, Mangalore 575018, India*

Correspondence should be addressed to Pramod Kumar; kumar.drpramod@gmail.com

Academic Editor: Nicolo Scuderi

Background. Clinically, scar related complications are observed to be dissimilar in different regions of the body. Unequal distribution of dermal collagen and elastic fibres in different orientations could be one of the multifocal causes of scar related complications, for which this evaluating study has been taken up. *Materials and Method.* 300 skin samples collected in horizontal and vertical orientations were studied histomorphometrically. This study involved image analysis of specially stained histological section using tissue-quant software. The outcome result was termed as quantitative fraction. From the result, various ratio values were also calculated for the ratio analysis. *Results.* The differences in the quantitative fraction of dermal elastic content between 2 directions were statistically significant at joint areas (shoulder joint, wrist, and ankle) ($P < 0.001$) but for collagen, significant difference was observed at shoulder joint and wrist only. Dermis of the forearm and thigh did not show any differences in their collagen content, but for elastic, thigh did show a significant difference while forearm had no change between 2 directions. *Conclusion.* Analysis of unequal content of dermal element in two directions under the perspective of wound healing consequences is subjective depending upon the anatomical position and functional status of the areas.

1. Introduction

Collagen and elastic fibres are the two major dermal connective tissue populations that exhibit their functional significance during wound healing process. Various studies in this aspect have emphasized their complimentary functional attribution in the process of minimizing the scar formation [1]. The scar tissue resulting from the process of wound healing also has similar types of collagen as in normal skin but with a deviated pattern of arrangement and distribution from the normal [2].

For many years, the well-known direction followed to make incisions to obtain aesthetic scar has been Langer's line or cleavage line. There have been many other concepts of lines on the skin which have been put forward and made the concept of Langer's line debatable. Borges studied intensely the lines of skin tension and comprehended with seven best known skin tension lines. According to him, single best choice of line is still questionable to fulfill complete satisfaction of wound healing [3]. Most popular among these is the Langer's line, concept of which lies on the basis of pattern of arrangement of dermal collagen in a particular direction. Previous works on the quantification of dermal collagen and elastic fibres in two different directions of skin samples obtained from the same area of the human body did confirm the asymmetric distribution of them [1, 4, 5]. The results of these studies attempted a hypothetical explanation which possibly explains pleomorphic behaviour of scar in different parts of the body.

Plastic surgeons on the other hand, in their personal experience and observations in the clinical setup, are still in dilemma about the speckled behaviour of scar, even after the incisions are made on the skin according to the standard lines of choice. This made them theorize the possible role of varied quantity and content of dermal collagen together with elastic fibres in different orientations of skin plane in addition to their normal coalition pattern in the dermis. For research purpose, quantification of dermal connective tissue fibres using image analysis technique was reported to be more relevant than the observer's ratings as it is accurate and comparable to polarized light technique [6]. The percentage area occupied by the tissue structures demonstrated by biological stains can be measured by image analysis and its accuracy and reliability have been proved by previous studies [1, 4, 5, 7]. Using similar methodology, histomorphometric analysis of dermal collagen and elastic fibres in two directions from the areas of head and neck [4] and trunk region [5] confirmed its asymmetric distribution as well as diverged content among themselves whose significance was in justification with the observation of life.

2. Materials and Methods

Current study involved 300 skin samples collected in two orientations (horizontal and vertical) from five areas (shoulder joint, wrist, ankle, forearm, and thigh) of extremity region of human cadaver. The skin samples were obtained from 30 formalin embalmed healthy looking human cadavers with the age of approximately 55 ± 5 years. All the samples were immediately immersed in 10% formalin followed by further histological processing. Elliptical skin samples were divided across their long axis before embedding them in the paraffin mould. In the mould, they were oriented in such a way that their cut edges were directed as cutting surfaces. Topographic sites where the skin samples were obtained are illustrated in Figure 1.

2.1. Sample Collection

(i) At shoulder joint, the skin samples were obtained slightly lateral to surface projection overlying the acromion process of scapula. Sections taken along the circumferential line of joint were considered as "horizontal," while perpendicular to it as "vertical."

(ii) Over the wrist area, skin samples in 2 directions were obtained at the side of proximal crease line of flexor surface.

(iii) At ankle area, skin samples were collected at the site immediately above the topographic site of insertion of tendocalcaneous.

(iv) Forearm skin samples were collected over the middle of flexor compartment of the forearm between midpoint of elbow joint and wrist joint.

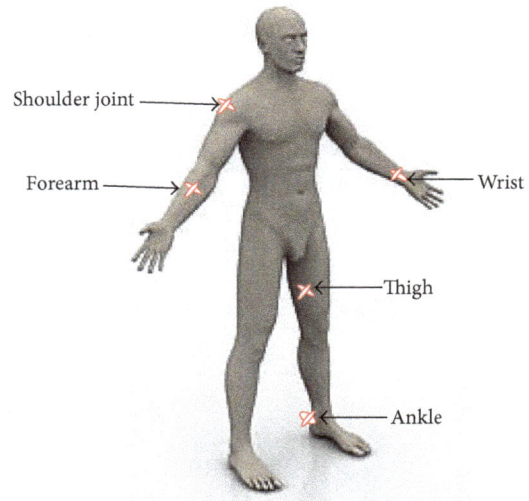

FIGURE 1: Topographic areas of sample collection from extremity region of human body (adapted from http://www.designyourway.net/blog/).

(v) At thigh region, samples were collected along the midpoint on thigh between pubic tubercle and medial condyle of tibia.

2.2. Histological Processing and Image Acquisition. Histological sections were stained by special stain Verhoeff-Van Gieson method for the selective demonstration of collagen and elastic fibres [8]. Digital images were acquired at 20x magnification with the standard resolution of 694×516 VGA using Progress capture Pro 2.1-Jenoptic microscopic camera fitted to inverted phase contrast camera. From each sample three images were obtained in 3 different microscopic fields.

2.3. Image Analysis. Images obtained from special stained slides were subjected to analysis by the software "tissue-quant" version 1.0. This software measures the area occupied by the coloured structure of interest in terms of number of pixels assigned to positively stained area in the image. This measure corresponds to the quantitative fraction of the structure to be analysed. Tissue-quant analysis needs as prerequisites the segmentation of colour and its shades of interest from the rest of the coloured structures (Figure 2). The total number of pixels corresponding to the target area of coloured structure is then converted to percentage value by proper calculation [7].

2.4. Analyzed Morphometric Parameters

2.4.1. Quantitative Fraction Analysis. Image analysis results obtained in terms of percentage area occupied by the collagen and elastic fibres were termed as quantitative fraction. Mean value with standard deviation was calculated and the differences of variables between the samples of two orientations were analysed statistically by employing the paired sample t-test with 95% confidence interval (CI) using SPSS version 5. $P < 0.05$ is considered to be statistically significant.

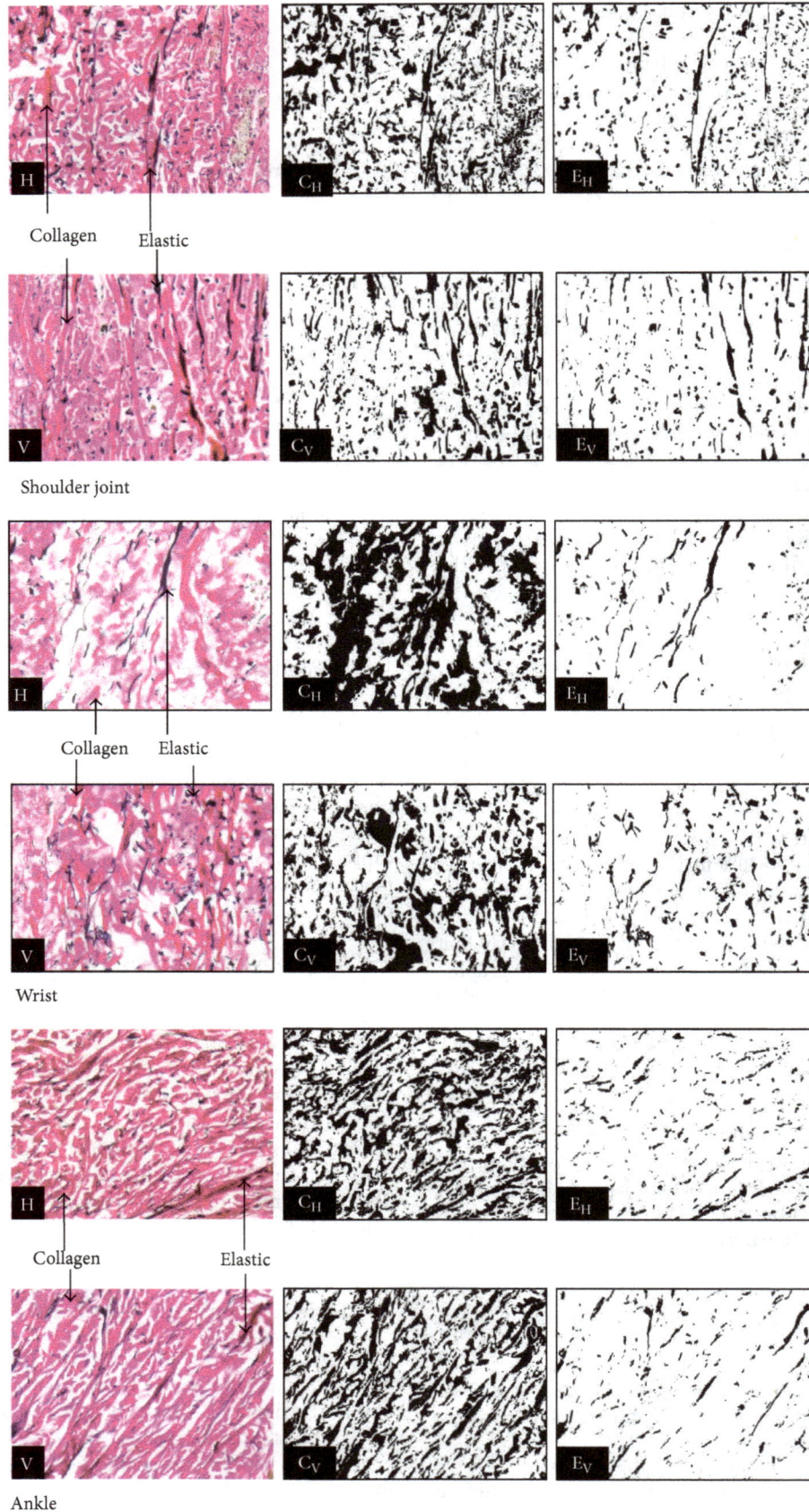

Shoulder joint

Wrist

Ankle

(a)

FIGURE 2: Continued.

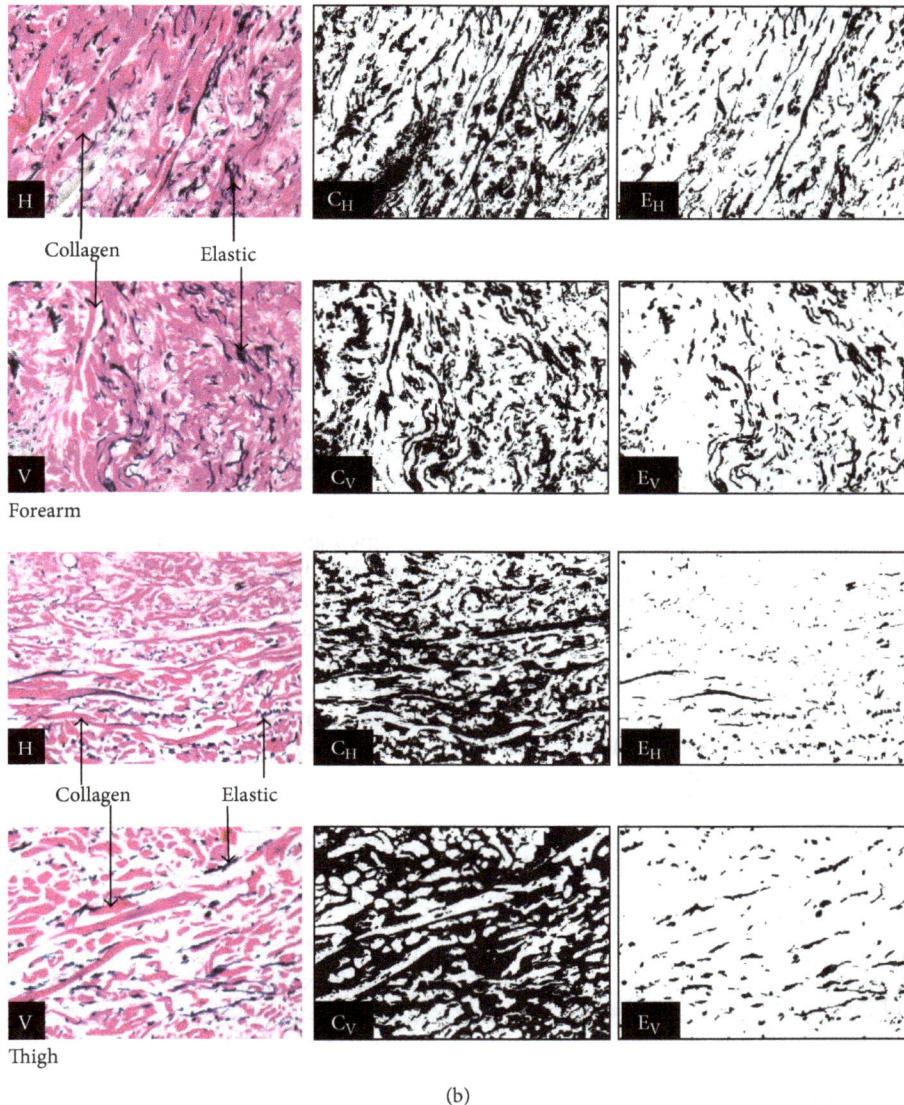

(b)

FIGURE 2: Verhoeff-Van Gieson staining appearance of collagen (pink colour) and elastic fibres (black colour) in horizontal (H) and vertical (V) sections of shoulder joint, wrist, ankle, forearm, and thigh areas. Their pattern of segmentation by tissue-quant software is shown in adjacent photographs. [C_H: collagen in horizontal, C_V: collagen in vertical, E_H: elastic in horizontal, and E_V: elastic in vertical directions].

2.4.2. Ratio Value Analysis. The collagen and elastic fibre content in horizontally obtained sections were denoted as C_H and E_H, respectively, while for their vertical directions as C_V and E_V, respectively. The ratio between C_H and C_V was calculated by dividing the C_V value by C_H and it was denoted by C_V/C_H ratio. Similarly, the ratio between E_H and E_V was calculated by dividing the E_V value by E_H and it was denoted by E_V/E_H ratio. These ratios were expressed in "ratio values" which implies proportionate changes in content of "vertical" with respect to its "horizontal" counterpart [1].

3. Results

3.1. Quantitative Fraction Analysis. The mean quantitative fraction with standard deviation (SD) and mean 95% confidence interval (CI) for collagen in horizontal (C_H) and

collagen in vertical direction (C_V) with the level of statistical significance (P values) between two directions are depicted in Table 1.

The mean C_H of dermis overlying shoulder joint was 53.91% and that of C_V was 49.03% with a significant difference between two directions ($P = 0.005$). The C_H in wrist area was 56.12% and that of its C_V was 60.32%. The wide difference between C_H and C_V confirmed the statistical significance with $P = 0.016$. In the ankle, C_H was 61.61% and $C_V = 62.37$%. The difference in the ankle area was very narrow; thus it was statistically insignificant ($P = 0.640$). The C_H and C_V at forearm were similar to each other, that is, 52.84% and 52.56%, respectively, without any notable difference ($P = 0.856$). Dermis of the thigh area, similar to forearm, also exhibited close ranges of collagen content between horizontal ($C_H = 52.12$%) and vertical ($C_V = 52.06$%) directions. The level

TABLE 1: Descriptive statistics of collagen fibre assay between horizontal (C_H) and vertical (C_V) directions from the areas of extremity region of human cadaver.

Area	Horizontal (C_H) Mean (SD)	Vertical (C_V) Mean (SD)	Mean 95% CI	P value
Shoulder joint	53.91 (12.3)	49.03 (10.6)	4.88	0.005[*]
Wrist	56.12 (12.0)	60.32 (11.2)	−4.19	0.016[*]
Ankle	61.61 (7.7)	62.37 (8.1)	−0.75	0.640
Forearm	52.84 (12.2)	52.56 (12.1)	0.28	0.856
Thigh	52.12 (12.3)	52.06 (14.1)	0.06	0.964

[*]Indicates statistically significant difference of content between horizontal and vertical direction ($P < 0.05$).

of significance in the difference was statistically insignificant ($P = 0.964$).

The mean quantitative fraction with standard deviation (SD) and mean 95% confidence interval (CI) for elastic fibre content between horizontal (E_H) and vertical (E_V) directions with its level of statistical significance of differences (P values) are depicted in Table 2.

The content of elastic fibres in skin of shoulder joint was 10.34% and 13.07% for E_H and E_V, respectively. The difference was statistically significant ($P = 0.011$). In the wrist, E_H was 6.36% and it was much lesser than its E_V (8.20%) making remarkable difference which was statistically significant ($P = 0.014$). In the ankle, E_H was 5.06% and E_V was 8.14% with the statistical significance ($P = 0.001$). Similar to collagen at forearm, the elastic content was also more or less the same, as E_H was 14.38% and E_V was 14.28% ($P = 0.892$). Unlike the collagen, in the thigh, the amount of elastic showed the significant difference in its content ($P = 0.028$) between horizontal ($E_H = 14.68\%$) and vertical ($E_V = 12.32\%$) directions.

3.2. Ratio Value Analysis. Results of various ratio values of collagen and elastic fibres between horizontal and vertical directions are tabulated in Table 3. For description purpose, the ratio values obtained from statistically significant ($P < 0.05$) quantitative fractions were considered.

4. Discussion

A quantitative study of dermal collagen using computerized digital image analysis with comparison of its biochemical analysis was reported to be significantly correlated. The reason for this observation was attributed to the pattern of distribution of collagen irrespective of its type in the dermis [9]. In the human body, the collagen fibres display basket weave like pattern with the random organization [10]. Although the collagen fibre density evaluation normally does not show changes with age, decrease in its content was reported with the observation in individual variations [9]. Even the elastic fibre distribution assay in this aspect was also found to have no variation with respect to sex or age [11].

Stereological analysis of dermal collagen and elastic fibres done by Vitellaro-Zuccarello et al. reported constant volume of collagen throughout the depth of the dermis and increased density of the collagen as age advances in both sexes up to 30–40 years. On the other hand, the elastic fibre's volume and diameter vary in dermal layers and the increment is

observed in reticular dermis particularly in males till first decade of life [12]. The elastin content differs and distribution is dependent on the dermal area as it is different among the subjects [13]. In response to stretch, both elastic and collagen fibre's realignment are observed [14].

Subcutaneous or fascial tensile reduction sutures tend to apply negligible tension that in turn plays an effective role in the reduction of recurrence of keloids or hypertrophic scars [15]. The quantitative fraction evaluation of dermal collagen and elastic fibres in the extremities of the body is highly intricate and subjective due to involvement of joints. The present study involves 3 joint areas (shoulder joint, wrist, and ankle) and two other nonstretchable areas (thigh and forearm). For joint area, the evaluation was made under two factors involving burst force exerted over the stretched skin of flexed/adducted joint (e.g., the shoulder joint) and stretch force over skin during movement at joints that are not acutely bent in rest position (e.g., wrist and ankle joint).

4.1. Shoulder Joint Area. During normal adducted position at rest, the maximum stretch on the shoulder skin over deltoid region causing burst force with the tendency to create wound in vertical direction. To counteract this force in nature, strength is required along horizontal direction. Thus, the collagen deposition (that provides strength) predominates along the horizontal direction. This was evident from our data in which significant higher collagen fibre content in horizontal direction compared to the vertical direction ($C_H = 53.91\%$ versus $C_V = 49.03\%$, $P = 0.005$) was seen. To compensate between excess stretching and laxity on one or another surface of joint during movement, elastic fibres necessitate increased concentration in vertical direction, that is, perpendicular to the joint line. This was confirmed with our findings in which elastic fibre content ($E_V = 13.07\%$) was significantly higher than horizontal ($E_H = 10.34\%$) direction ($P = 0.011$).

Thus, when the scar is placed in vertical direction over deltoid region, the burst force during adducted position tends to exhibit wide and/or hypertrophic scar in due course of time. On the other hand, when the scar is placed along horizontal direction, the elastic content in vertical direction is divided and exerts pull on the wound edge producing stretched and/or hypertrophied scar (gaping). Also, the effect of gravity aggravates the force on the horizontal wound edge exerted by divided elastic fibres. Since surgical incision is made along the horizontal direction, the tension produced by elastic fibres on wound/scar edge is probably weaker than

TABLE 2: Descriptive statistics of elastic fibre assay between horizontal (E_H) and vertical (E_V) direction from the areas of extremity region of human cadaver.

Area	Horizontal (E_H) Mean (SD)	Vertical (E_V) Mean (SD)	Mean 95% CI	P value
Shoulder joint	10.34 (4.5)	13.07 (5.9)	−2.73	0.011*
Wrist	6.36 (2.6)	8.20 (3.5)	−1.84	0.014*
Ankle	5.06 (2.2)	8.14 (4.2)	−3.07	0.001*
Forearm	14.38 (4.7)	14.28 (6.4)	0.10	0.892
Thigh	14.68 (6.7)	12.32 (5.4)	2.36	0.028*

*Indicates statistically significant difference in the content between horizontal and vertical direction ($P < 0.05$).

TABLE 3: Descriptive analysis of ratio values of collagen (C) and elastic (E) fibres with respect to horizontal (H) and vertical (V) directions.

Areas	C_V/C_H ratio value	E_V/E_H ratio value
Shoulder joint	0.90#	1.26#
Wrist	1.07#	1.28#
Ankle	1.01	1.60#
Forearm	0.99	0.99
Thigh	0.99	0.83#

#Ratio values of statistically significant quantitative fraction ($P < 0.05$).

TABLE 4: Force effects at joint areas in anatomical position and during various movements.

Force applicable	Shoulder joint	Wrist area	Ankle area
Burst force due to position	Maximum	Minimum	Moderate
Stretch force due to movement	Minimum	Maximum	Moderate

burst force due to adducted position (rest position); resulting scar will be better if incision is horizontally placed compared to vertically.

4.2. Wrist and Ankle. Similar to shoulder joint area, the functional correlation of elastic fibres in vertical direction is comparable with that of shoulder joint area as the quantitative fraction of elastic fibre was significantly increased at vertical direction at wrist ($E_H = 6.36$ and $E_V = 8.20$ with $P = 0.014$) and at ankle ($E_H = 5.06$ and $E_V = 8.14$ with $P = 0.001$) areas.

However, in terms of collagen content, both wrist and ankle exhibit higher content of collagen in vertical direction which is contrary to shoulder joint area. But the difference was observed to be significant in wrist (C_H versus C_V, $P = 0.016$) and insignificant at ankle (C_H versus C_V, $P = 0.640$). This diverged fact of collagen content may be considered to be anatomical (rest) position of the joint which in turn could be attributed to the facts of burst force versus stretch force as shown in Table 4.

4.3. Forearm and Thigh Area. Since there is a minimal effect of movement and gravity over the thigh and forearm skin, no significant differences in the collagen and elastic fibre content between horizontal and vertical directions were to be expected. The results of current study partially support this

hypothesis in terms of elastic content except that significant difference in the elastic fibre content over horizontal direction of the thigh region was noted. This becomes obligatory due to a possible stretch force produced by the slow circumferential tissue expansion of bulky thigh with growth of the body that necessitates deposition of more elastic along horizontal direction compared to vertical ($E_H > E_V$; $P = 0.028$). Contrary to this, the circumferential growth of forearm is less as compared to that of thigh region; the above mentioned observation of thigh is unseen at forearm. As a result, there was no significant difference in elastic content of forearm between two directions ($E_H = 14.38\%$, $E_V = 14.28\%$, $P = 0.892$).

4.4. Ratio Value Evaluation (Table 3). In the shoulder joint area the C_V/C_H ratio value was less than 1. Horizontal wound edges on this area will often have less distracting force during movements as compared to the burst force on vertical wound edge during rest period. Clinical experience also shows that lower is the value and better is the long term result of horizontally placed scar.

In the wrist area, where the C_V/C_H ratio value was more than 1, burst force produced in horizontal direction during movements (mainly in extension) necessitates providing maximum strength to reduce damage. Due to this, probably collagen content in vertical direction was more.

In the thigh area, where the E_V/E_H ratio value was less than 1, the slow expansion of the tissues causes maximum stretch force in horizontal direction. Therefore elastic content was significantly higher in horizontal direction than in vertical.

In all 3 joint areas (shoulder joint, ankle, and wrist) with the E_V/E_H ratio value more than 1, the constant stretching in vertical direction due to either embryologic growth pattern or gradual growth after birth might have influenced the higher content of elastic fibres along vertical directions (Table 2).

5. Conclusion

The analysis of unequal distribution of dermal collagen and elastic fibres in the region of extremities is a complex process and it is solely dependent on the anatomical perspective of the joints involved. The burst force and the stretch force effects at the joint area and corresponding profiles of quantitative fraction of dermal elements need to be taken into consideration before performing surgical incision. In other areas (forearm and thigh) these factors may have negligible effects.

Authors' Contribution

Naveen Kumar is responsible for integrity and accuracy of the data analysis, Pramod Kumar and Satheesha Nayak Badagabettu are responsible for study concept and design, Keerthana Prasad is responsible for data analysis, Raghuveer Coimbatore Vasudevarao and Ranjini Kudva are responsible for critical revision of the paper, and Pramod Kumar is responsible for study supervision.

Acknowledgment

Thanks are due to Ms. Mellisa Glenda Lewis (Research Scholar, Department of Statistics, Manipal University, Manipal) for the statistical analysis.

References

[1] K. Naveen, K. Pramod, P. Keerthana, and N. B. Satheesha, "A histological study on the distribution of derma l collagen and elastic fibres in different regions of the body," *International Journal of Medicine and Medical Sciences*, vol. 4, no. 8, pp. 171–176, 2012.

[2] J. A. Sherratt, *Mathematical Modelling of Scar Tissue Formation*, Department of Mathematics, Heriot-Watt University, Edinburgh, UK, 2010, http://www.ma.hw.ac.uk/~jas/research-interests/scartissueformation.html.

[3] A. F. Borges, "Relaxed skin tension lines (RSTL) versus other skin lines," *Plastic and Reconstructive Surgery*, vol. 73, no. 1, pp. 144–150, 1984.

[4] K. Naveen, K. Pramod, P. Keerthana, N. B. Satheesha, K. Ranjini, and C. V. Raghuveer, "Histomorphometric analysis of dermal collagen and elastic fibres in skin tissues taken perpendicular to each other from head and neck region," *Journal of the American Academy of Orthopaedic Surgeons*, vol. 4, no. 1, pp. 30–36, 2014.

[5] N. Kumar, P. Kumar, S. N. Badagabettu, K. Prasad, R. Kudva, and C. V. Raghuveer, "Quantitative fraction evaluation of dermal collagen and elastic fibres in the skin samples obtained in two orientations from the trunk region," *Dermatology Research and Practice*, vol. 2014, Article ID 251254, 7 pages, 2014.

[6] P. P. M. van Zuijlen, H. J. C. de Vries, E. N. Lamme et al., "Morphometry of dermal collagen orientation by Fourier analysis is superior to multi-observer assessment," *The Journal of Pathology*, vol. 198, no. 3, pp. 284–291, 2002.

[7] K. Prasad, P. B. Kumar, M. Chakravarthy, and G. Prabhu, "Applications of "TissueQuant"—a color intensity quantification tool for medical research," *Computer Methods and Programs in Biomedicine*, vol. 106, no. 1, pp. 27–36, 2012.

[8] D. B. John, *Theory and Practice of Histological Techniques*, Marilyn Gamble, Churchil Livingstone, Philadelphia, Pa, USA, 5th edition, 2002.

[9] M. C. Branchet, S. Boisnic, C. Frances, C. Lesty, and L. Robert, "Morphometric analysis of dermal collagen fibers in normal human skin as a function of age," *Archives of Gerontology and Geriatrics*, vol. 13, no. 1, pp. 1–14, 1991.

[10] P. P. M. Van Zuijlen, J. J. B. Ruurda, H. A. Van Veen et al., "Collagen morphology in human skin and scar tissue: no adaptations in response to mechanical loading at joints," *Burns*, vol. 29, no. 5, pp. 423–431, 2003.

[11] C. Frances, M. C. Branchet, S. Boisnic, C. L. Lesty, and L. Robert, "Elastic fibers in normal human skin. Variation with age: a morphometric analysis," *Archives of Gerontology and Geriatrics*, vol. 10, no. 1, pp. 57–67, 1990.

[12] L. Vitellaro-Zuccarello, S. Cappelletti, V. dal Pozzo Rossi, and M. Sari-Gorla, "Stereological analysis of collagen and elastic fibers in the normal human dermis: variability with age, sex, and body region," *Anatomical Record*, vol. 238, no. 2, pp. 153–162, 1994.

[13] I. Pasquaili-Ronchetti and M. Baccarani-Contri, "Elastic fiber during development and aging," *Microscopy Research and Technique*, vol. 38, no. 4, pp. 428–435, 1997.

[14] P. D. Verhaegen, H. J. Schouten, W. Tigchelaar-Gutter et al., "Adaptation of the dermal collagen structure of human skin and scar tissue in response to stretch: an experimental study," *Wound Repair and Regeneration*, vol. 20, no. 5, pp. 658–666, 2012.

[15] R. Ogawa, S. Akaishi, C. Huang et al., "Clinical applications of basic research that shows reducing skin tension could prevent and treat abnormal scarring: the importance of fascial/subcutaneous tensile reduction sutures and flap surgery for keloid and hypertrophic scar reconstruction," *Journal of Nippon Medical School*, vol. 78, no. 2, pp. 68–76, 2011.

16

Free Flaps in a Resource Constrained Environment: A Five-Year Experience— Outcomes and Lessons Learned

Wanjala F. Nangole,[1] **Stanley Khainga,**[1] **Joyce Aswani,**[1]
Loise Kahoro,[2] **and Adelaine Vilembwa**[2]

[1]*Department of Surgery (Plastic), University of Nairobi, P.O. Box 30197, Nairobi 00100, Kenya*
[2]*Kenyatta National Hospital, P.O. Box 20723, Nairobi 00202, Kenya*

Correspondence should be addressed to Wanjala F. Nangole; nangole2212@yahoo.com

Academic Editor: Yoshihiro Kimata

Introduction. Free flap surgery is a routine procedure in many developed countries with good surgical outcomes. In many developing countries, however, these services are not available. In this paper, we audit free flaps done in a resource constrained hospital in Kenya. *Objective.* This is a five-year audit of free flaps done in a tertiary hospital in Kenya, between 2009 and 2014. *Materials and Methods.* This was a prospective study of patients operated on with free flaps between 2009 and 2014. *Results.* A total of one hundred and thirty-two free flaps in one hundred and twenty patients were performed during the five-year duration. The age range was eight to seventy-two years with a mean of 47.2. All the flaps were done under loupe magnification. The overall flap success rate was eighty-nine percent. *Conclusion.* Despite the many limitations, free flaps in our setup were successful in the majority of patients operated on. Flap salvage was noted to be low due to infrequent flap monitoring as well as unavailability of theatre space. One therefore has to be meticulous during surgery to reduce any possibilities of reexploration.

1. Introduction

Reconstruction of surgical defects requires a reconstructive surgeon to be well versed in all the reconstructive options. Simple defects could be reconstructed with the use of skin grafts or local flaps. Complex defects however require either regional, distant, or free flaps. Free flaps have been in use since inception about forty years ago [1–3]. Initially, they were practiced only in well established centres, though currently many centres in the developed countries routinely carry out these surgical procedures.

Successful free flaps surgeries require a well motivated and trained surgical team, good perioperative monitoring of the flaps, well equipped and readily available theatre space, good laboratory support services, and availability of intensive care unit beds [4]. The nursing team must also be ready to work for long hours without any reprieve.

The reality in many developing countries is however such that most of the above conditions are not available. Ironically, patients requiring free flap services are probably more than those in the developed countries (Figure 2). In this paper, we audit our work for the last five years in such an environment.

2. Materials and Method

2.1. Setting. The study was carried out at Kenyatta National Hospital, Nairobi, Kenya.

2.2. Study Design. This was a prospective study of patients reconstructed with free flaps.

2.3. Study Duration. Study duration was from August 2009 to December 2014.

2.4. Methodology. Patients reconstructed with free flaps at Kenyatta National Hospital were followed up for a minimum of six months. Data collected included patients' demographic features such as age and sex. Other information

TABLE 1: Summary of the surgical conditions the patients presented with.

Diagnosis	Frequency	Percentage
Cancer of the tongue	31	25.8
Mandibular defect	23	19.2
Neck contracture	8	6.7
Facial/scalp defects	21	17.5
Neck tumours	5	4.1
Leg defects	12	10
Upper limb defects	6	5
Upper limb lymphoedema	2	1.7
Lower limb lymphoedema	6	5
Palatal defects	3	2.5
Penile defects	3	2.5
Total	120	100

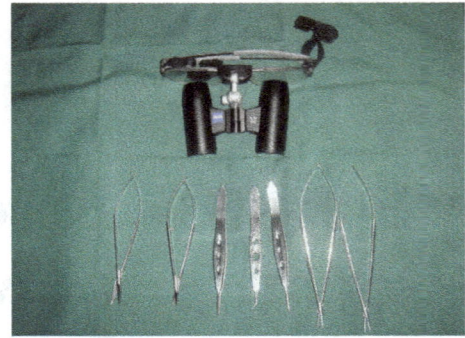

FIGURE 1: Basic instruments used for microsurgery.

gathered included patients current and past medical conditions, anatomical location of the defect, and flaps used to reconstruct the defect (Tables 1 and 2). The surgical techniques employed for the patients during surgery were loupe magnifications for dissection and anastomosis of the vessels, arterial anastomosis before venous anastomosis, end-to-end arterial anastomosis with prolene 9/0 interrupted, end-to-end or end-to-side venous anastomosis with prolene 9/0, and topical application of heparin in a ratio of 100 units/mL of normal saline. Systemic heparin was occasionally utilized after the anastomosis. Postoperatively, patients were nursed in the critical care unit for at least 24 hours if a bed was available. Time taken after surgery and the first postoperative review of the flap and the frequency were noted. Intravenous antibiotics and clexane were given to all patients till the 7th postoperative day.

Flap related complications such as arterial compromise, venous congestion, haematoma, infections, and flap necrosis were documented. Donor site morbidity evaluated included wound dehiscence or skin-graft failure.

3. Results

A total of one hundred and twenty patients were operated on during the study duration of five years. The age range for the patients was eight years to seventy-two years with a median age of 51.4 years and a mean age of 47.2 years. The male-to-female ratio was three to two. Five patients were being managed for diabetes mellitus (4%) while six patients (5%) were HIV positive with one patient's CD4 count at less than 200. Seventy-three percent of the defects managed were in the head and neck region, fifteen percent lower limb, and seven percent upper limb.

Operatively, 16 flaps had two venous anastomoses done (turbocharged). The mean duration from the completion of surgery to the assessment of the flap was 10.35 hours. All flaps were assessed at least once per day in the first week of surgery. Fifteen percent were assessed at least twice per day

in the first 24 hours of surgery. No flap was assessed at four-hourly interval. All the assessments were done with the use of the needle-prick technique. Of the fifteen flaps lost, eight flaps were lost due to venous congestion, five due to arterial occlusion, and two due to infections within one week after surgery. Reexploration was done in eight flaps with only one flap being salvaged. Haematoma was noted in five patients, four of whom had been given intravenous heparin during surgery.

Donor site morbidity was noted in 24 patients. Twenty-one patients had partial graft take that healed with wound dressings alone. These were ten patients with radial forearm donor site, seven patients with free fibula donor site, and four patients with anterior lateral thigh flap donor site. Three patients, one with free fibula donor site and two with anterior lateral thigh donor site, had a repeat skin graft to cover the donor site.

4. Discussions

Free flaps have revolutionized management of complex wounds. With the advent of free flaps, wounds that would otherwise not be managed are now routinely managed with good surgical outcomes [4–6]. Tumours that would otherwise be considered inoperable are now being operated on and defects reconstructed with free flaps. Microsurgery in many cases is now considered the first option in reconstructing complex defects, best in addressing form, function, and aesthetics.

However, the practice of microsurgery has largely remained rudimentary if not nonexistent in many developing countries especially in sub-Saharan Africa. Few centres, if any, practice this important aspect of reconstructive surgery. In spite of this shortcoming, defects requiring free flaps are common; probably more than what is available in the developed countries (Figure 2). The reasons advanced for these are lack of surgical skills and necessary equipment to carry out the surgeries. However, as demonstrated in our series, free flaps could safely be carried out with the use of basic surgical equipment such as loupes which are readily available in many hospitals (Figure 1). Studies have also demonstrated using loupes for anastomosis to be just as effective as the microscope [7–9]. Anybody keen to perform

TABLE 2: Summary of flaps performed and the outcomes.

Flap performed	Frequency	Successful	Failed	Percentage successful
Radial forearm flap	48	43	5	89.5
Free fibula flap	25	22	3	88
Latissimus dorsi flap	19	18	1	94.7
Anterior lateral thigh	25	21	4	84
Parascapular flap	2	1	1	50
Gracilis muscle flap	1	0	1	0
Cervicofacial lymph node	12	12	0	100
Total	132	117	15	89
	100	89	11	

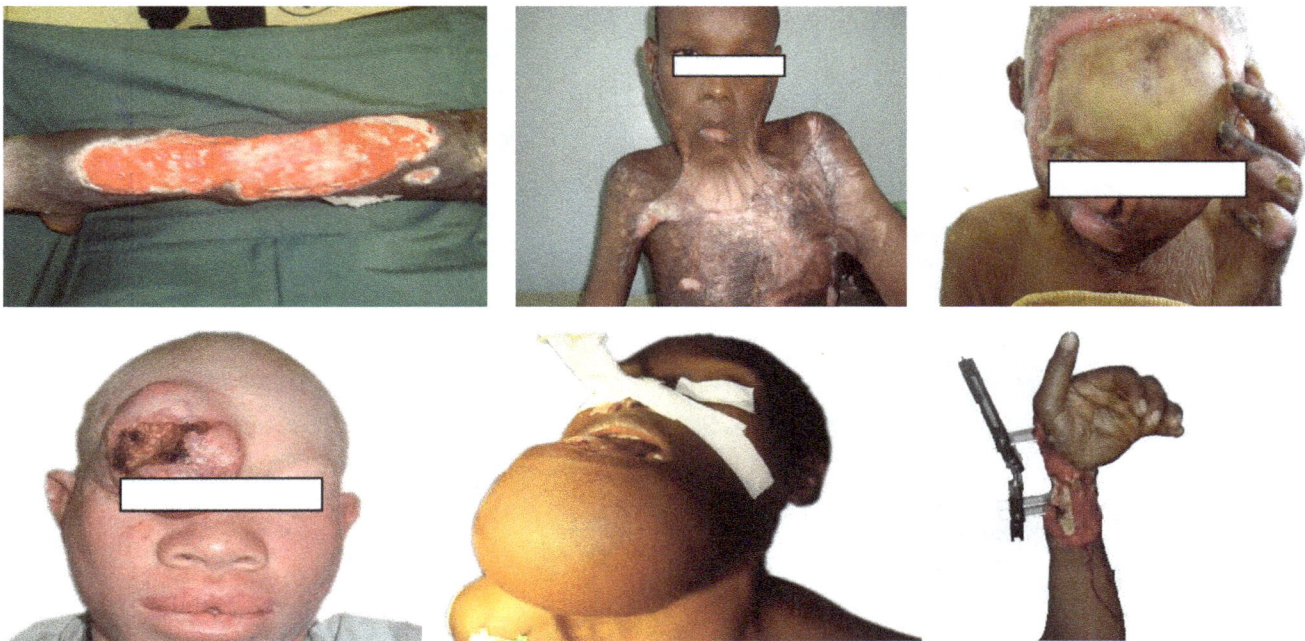

FIGURE 2: Multiple defects requiring free flaps for reconstruction in our hospital.

free flaps could thus get basic training in microsurgery in any centre where it is frequently practiced. The best way to learn microsurgery is by practicing it.

Radial forearm flap in our series accounted for up to a third of the flaps done. The flap was commonly used for tongue reconstruction, penile reconstruction, and majority of the defects of the scalp and the face (Figure 3). It is a relatively easy flap to raise, has a long pedicle, and has relatively large veins allowing for ease of anastomosis. Among the disadvantages of the flap is the donor site morbidity that heals with extensive scarring even after grafting (Figure 3). This flap has been quoted in the literature as the gold standard for tongue, oral cavity, and penile reconstruction [10–12]. Free fibula flap accounted for almost twenty percent of the flaps done. The majority of these were for mandibular reconstruction (Figure 5). Free fibula flap is now considered the gold standard for mandibular reconstruction [13–17]. The

skin paddle in our series was however noted to be unreliable in monitoring the flap.

Latissimus dorsi flap was our workhorse flap for the defects of the extremities (Figure 4). This was either as a musculocutaneous flap or as a muscle flap. Among the advantages of this flap were the large surface area, long and reliable pedicle, and constant anatomical landmarks. The pedicle could also be raised with the nerve for functional reconstruction. It is probably rivaled by no other flap in the covering of extensive defects of the extremities [18–20]. Anterior lateral thigh flap was extensively used in our series for reconstructing large defects in the neck and the scalp region, with very good surgical outcome (Figure 6). The flap has been noted to be very effective for extensive soft tissue reconstruction especially in the head and neck region [5, 6, 21, 22]. The flap however has an unreliable perforator that even with the use of Doppler has to be

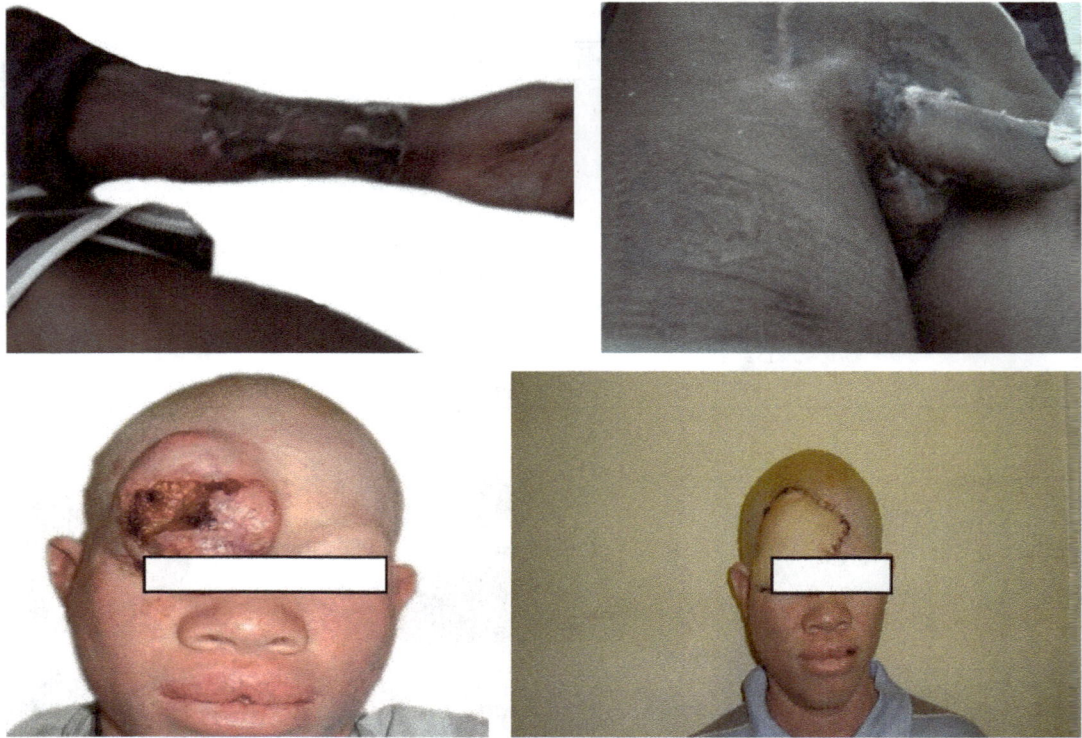

FIGURE 3: Radial forearm flap used for penile reconstruction and forehead reconstruction and its donor site.

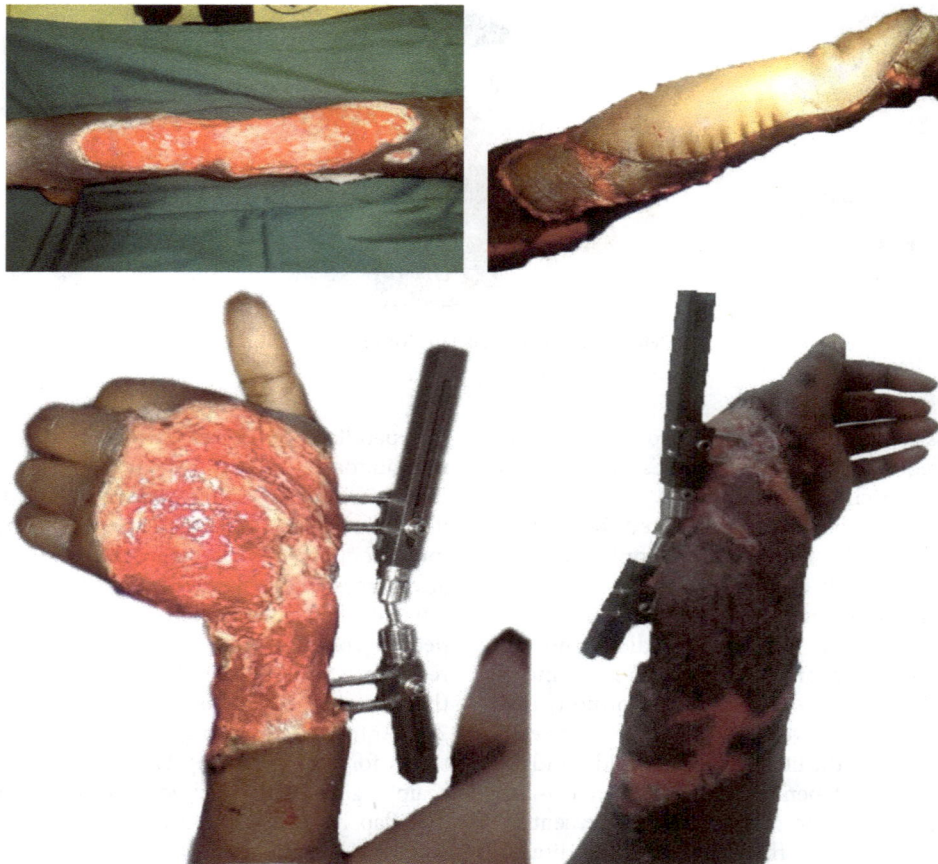

FIGURE 4: Latissimus dorsi flap utilised for reconstructing extensive defects of the extremities.

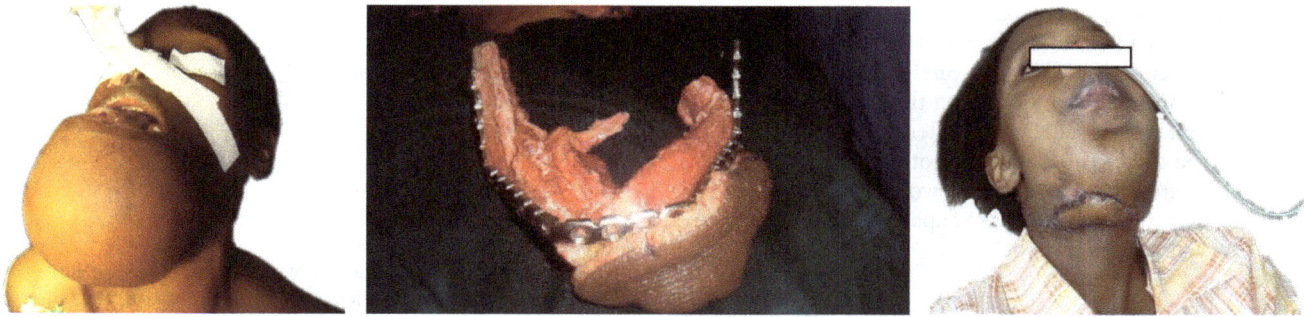

FIGURE 5: Free fibula flap for reconstructing mandibular defect.

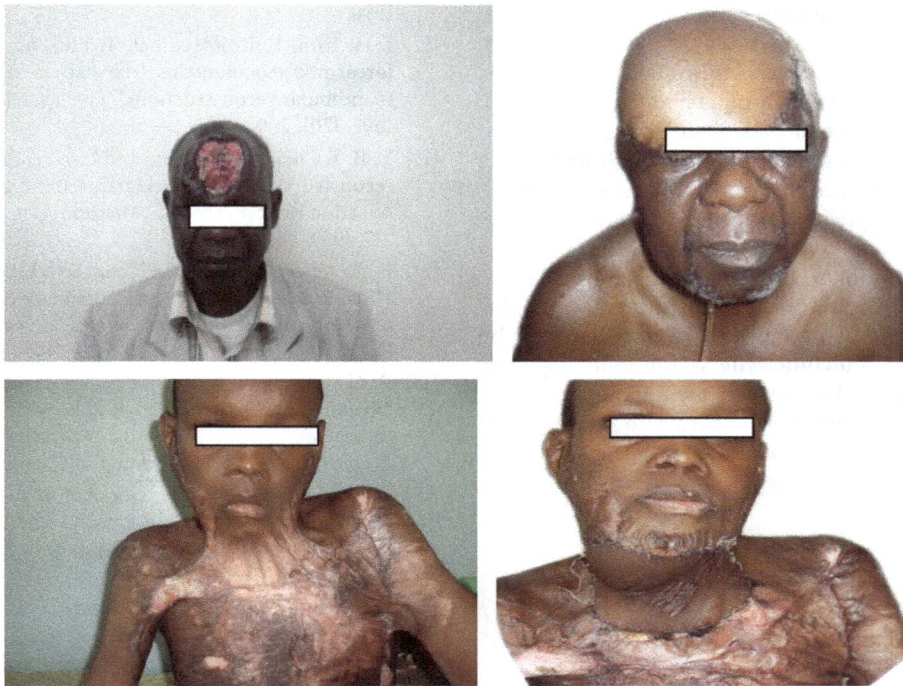

FIGURE 6: Anterior lateral thigh flap utilized in reconstructing extensive scalp and neck defect.

searched for occasionally, extensively, before proceeding with the dissection. In two patients, the procedure had to be abandoned.

Perioperative monitoring of the flap was probably the biggest challenge in doing free flaps in our setup. Though currently there are many innovative ways of monitoring flaps that do not require the physical presence of the surgeon [23, 24], they are expensive and beyond the reach of our hospital. Monitoring was thus based on clinical examination and evaluation of the flap. Majority of the patients had their flaps reviewed for the first time almost twelve hours after surgery. This was due to a few number of staffs that could monitor the flaps, as well as the inability of the surgical team to do frequent monitoring. This probably explains the low flap salvage rate. To counter this, the operating team had to be extra cautious in ensuring flap survival, before reversing the patient from the operating table. Any slightest suggestion that the flap was not perfused well or was congested meant reexploring the anastomosis and starting over again. Another safety precaution taken was by using two venous anastomoses. This has now become our routine precaution measure in ensuring venous competence. Postoperative instructions were also clearly written on the patients dressings (i.e., because one flap was lost by the nursing team tying a dressing around the neck to secure a tracheostomy tube).

Haematoma formation in our patients was noted to be closely related with intravenous injection of heparin. This would later result in compression of the veins resulting in venous congestion. Of the eight flaps lost due to venous congestion, six of them were of patients on intravenous heparin. Routine use of intravenous heparin has since then been stopped and is only used in cases of difficult anastomosis or once a clot forms on the table. Topical irrigation of heparin on the other hand seems to be a safe procedure.

Though majority of our patients were HIV negative, our experience with patients who were HIV positive with low CD4 count was discouraging. In one such patient, one free flap was lost and one abandoned on the table after realizing poor recipient vessels with severe arteritis. A salvage pedicle flap had to be done. Those who do not get arterial or venous compromise are also more prone to wound sepsis, which can result in flap loss. Two of the three flaps lost due to sepsis were of patients who were HIV positive.

Our practice since then has been to be conservative for patients who are HIV positive.

In conclusion, free flaps are a viable option even in resource constrained environment. Good surgical outcomes could be realized by the use of basic surgical equipment such as loupes. The best approach is through a multidisciplinary approach with teams encompassing various related disciplines. The team must ensure adequate training in microsurgery before starting on the surgeries through fellowship programs or by inviting faculties from centres where these surgeries are done frequently. For starters, flaps that are relatively easy to raise and with good calibre vessels may be the best to start with, followed by more complex procedures. Meticulous surgical technique and careful observation of the flaps on the table and soon after surgery is paramount in ensuring good surgical outcome. The saying that "flaps are lost on the table" is probably truer in such an environment than anywhere else. The team must also learn to support each other in the event of flap failure and regroup again to try again, for that is the only sure way of being perfect with free flaps.

References

[1] R. K. Daniel and G. I. Taylor, "Distant transfer of an island flap by microvascular anastomoses," *Plastic and Reconstructive Surgery*, vol. 62, article 111, 1973.

[2] D. H. McClean and H. J. Buncke, "Auto-transplant of omentum to a large scalp defect with micro-surgical re-vascularization," *Plastic and Reconstructive Surgery*, vol. 49, article 268, 1972.

[3] I. A. McGregor and I. T. Jackson, "The groin flap," *British Journal of Plastic Surgery*, vol. 25, pp. 3–16, 1972.

[4] D. Serafin, R. E. Sabatier, R. L. Morris, and N. D. Georgiade, "Reconstruction of the lower extremity with vascularized composite tissue: improved tissue survival and specific indications," *Plastic & Reconstructive Surgery*, vol. 66, no. 2, pp. 230–241, 1980.

[5] I. Koshima, H. Fukuda, H. Yamamoto et al., "Free anterolateral thigh flaps for reconstruction of head and neck defects," *Plastic & Reconstructive Surgery*, vol. 92, no. 3, pp. 421–430, 1993.

[6] A. Mosahebi, J. J. Disa, A. L. Pusic, P. G. Cordeiro, and B. J. Mehrara, "The use of the extended anterolateral thigh flap for reconstruction of massive oncologic defects," *Plastic and Reconstructive Surgery*, vol. 122, no. 2, pp. 492–496, 2008.

[7] S. M. Shenaq, M. J. A. Klebuc, and D. Vargo, "Free-tissue transfer with the aid of loupe magnification: experience with 251 procedures," *Plastic & Reconstructive Surgery* vol. 95, no. 2, pp. 261–269, 1995.

[8] J. M. Serletti, M. A. Deuber, P. M. Guidera et al., "Comparison of the operating microscope and loupes for free microvascular tissue transfer," *Plastic and Reconstructive Surgery*, vol. 95, no. 2, pp. 270–276, 1995.

[9] D. Pieptu and S. Luchian, "Loupes-only microsurgery," *Microsurgery*, vol. 23, no. 3, pp. 181–188, 2003.

[10] D. S. Soutar, L. R. Scheker, N. S. B. Tanner, and I. A. McGregor, "The radial forearm flap: a versatile method for intra-oral reconstruction," *British Journal of Plastic Surgery*, vol. 36, no. 1, pp. 1–8, 1983.

[11] E. D. Vaughan, "The radial forearm free flap in orofacial reconstruction: personal experience in 120 consecutive cases," *Journal of Cranio-Maxillofacial Surgery*, vol. 18, no. 1, pp. 2–7, 1990.

[12] J. H. Kim, E. L. Rosenthal, T. Ellis, and M. K. Wax, "Radial forearm osteocutaneous free flap in maxillofacial and oromandibular reconstructions," *Laryngoscope*, vol. 115, no. 9, pp. 1697–1701, 2005.

[13] Y.-B. T. Chen, H.-C. Chen, and L.-H. Hahn, "Major mandibular reconstruction with vascularized bone grafts: indications and selection of donor tissue," *Microsurgery*, vol. 15, no. 4, pp. 227–237, 1994.

[14] F.-C. Wei, C.-S. Seah, Y.-C. Tsai, S.-J. Liu, M.-S. Tsai, and D. A. Hidalgo, "Fibula osteoseptocutaneous flap for reconstruction of composite mandibular defects," *Plastic and Reconstructive Surgery*, vol. 93, no. 2, pp. 294–306, 1994.

[15] P. G. Cordeiro, J. J. Disa, D. A. Hidalgo, and Q. Y. Hu, "Reconstruction of the mandible with osseous free flaps: a 10-year experience with 150 consecutive patients," *Plastic and Reconstructive Surgery*, vol. 104, no. 5, pp. 1314–1320, 1999.

[16] D. A. Hidalgo, "Fibula free flap mandible reconstruction," *Microsurgery*, vol. 15, no. 4, pp. 238–244, 1994.

[17] K.-C. Yang, J. K. W. Leung, and J.-S. Chen, "Double-paddle peroneal tissue transfer for oromandibular reconstruction," *Plastic and Reconstructive Surgery*, vol. 106, no. 1, pp. 47–55, 2000.

[18] M. Lassen, C. Krag, and I. M. Nielsen, "The latissimus dorsi flap: an overview," *Scandinavian Journal of Plastic & Reconstructive Surgery and Hand Surgery*, vol. 19, no. 1, pp. 41–51, 1985.

[19] N. Franceschi, K. K. Yim, W. C. Lineaweaver et al., "Eleven consecutive combined latissimus dorsi and serratus anterior free muscle transplantations," *Annals of Plastic Surgery*, vol. 27, no. 2, pp. 121–125, 1991.

[20] H. M. Rosen, "Double island latissimus dorsi muscle-skin flap for through-and-through defects of the forefoot," *Plastic & Reconstructive Surgery*, vol. 76, no. 3, pp. 461–463, 1985.

[21] R. S. Ali, R. Bluebond-Langner, E. D. Rodriguez, and M.-H. Cheng, "The versatility of the anterolateral thigh flap," *Plastic and Reconstructive Surgery*, vol. 124, no. 6, pp. e395–e407, 2009.

[22] A. A. Mäkitie, N. J. P. Beasley, P. C. Neligan, J. Lipa, P. J. Gullane, and R. W. Gilbert, "Head and neck reconstruction with anterolateral thigh flap," *Otolaryngology—Head and Neck Surgery*, vol. 129, no. 5, pp. 547–555, 2003.

[23] N. F. Jones, "Intraoperative and postoperative monitoring of microsurgical free tissue transfers," *Clinics in Plastic Surgery*, vol. 19, no. 4, pp. 783–797, 1992.

[24] M. K. Wax, "The role of the implantable doppler probe in free flap surgery," *The Laryngoscope*, vol. 124, supplement 1, pp. S1–S12, 2014.

17

Use of Vein Conduit and Isolated Nerve Graft in Peripheral Nerve Repair: A Comparative Study

Imran Ahmad and Md. Sohaib Akhtar

Post Graduate Department of Burns, Plastic and Reconstructive Surgery, JNMC, AMU, Aligarh, Uttar Pradesh 202002, India

Correspondence should be addressed to Md. Sohaib Akhtar; drsohaibakhtar@gmail.com

Academic Editor: Nicolo Scuderi

Aims and Objectives. The aim of this study was to evaluate the effectiveness of vein conduit in nerve repair compared with isolated nerve graft. *Materials and Methods.* This retrospective study was conducted at author's centre and included a total of 40 patients. All the patients had nerve defect of more than 3 cm and underwent nerve repair using nerve graft from sural nerve. In 20 cases, vein conduit (study group) was used whereas no conduit was used in other 20 cases. Patients were followed up for 2 years at the intervals of 3 months. *Results.* Patients had varying degree of recovery. Sensations reached to all the digits at 1 year in study groups compared to 18 months in control group. At the end of second year, 84% patients of the study group achieved 2-point discrimination of <10 mm compared to 60% only in control group. In terms of motor recovery, 82% patients achieved satisfactory hand function in study group compared to 56% in control group ($P < .05$). *Conclusions.* It was concluded that the use of vein conduit in peripheral nerve repair is more effective method than isolated nerve graft providing good sensory and motor recovery.

1. Introduction

Successful repair of peripheral nerve injury remains a difficult task for the reconstructive surgeons. A small nerve gap can be repaired primarily which is one of the best methods of repair [1]. A large nerve gap may require grafts. The various available options for grafting are autologous nonvascularised nerve graft, autologous vascularised nerve grafts, interposition of venous or arterial segments, or use of muscle or synthetic conduits [2]. Cable grafts for large nerve defects have been universally used for nerve repair [3, 4].

There are various available conduits that have been used for peripheral nerve repair. Use of vein as conduit is well-described in the literature [5]. Many investigators have used vein grafts for peripheral nerve repair that can be used alone or packed with muscle fibres [6, 7]. Vein conduit helps in nerve regeneration by preventing sprouting of nerve fibres at the neurorraphy sites [8, 9]. Besides, there are neurotrophic factors released from the endothelial layer of the vein that provides a more favourable environment for regeneration [10]. Vein conduit also leads to lower inflammatory cells to migrate, higher rate of axonal regeneration under neurotropism, and a thinner epineurium to regenerate [11–13].

In this series, we have used autologous sural nerve for the repair of peripheral nerve with and without vein conduit. To the best of our knowledge, currently there is no study that focuses on comparison between use of nerve graft with conduit and isolated nerve graft.

2. Materials and Methods

This retrospective study included a total of 40 patients who underwent nerve repair between November 2010 and January 2013. The study was approved by the Ethics Committee of the Hospital and informed consent was taken from each patient. All the patients had nerve defect of more than 3 cm and underwent nerve repair using autologous nerve graft from sural nerve. In 20 cases, we used autologous short saphenous vein as conduit (study group) while in other 20 cases, no conduit was used. Information regarding age, etiology of the defects, duration of injury, types of nerve and repair, nerve defect, distance between proximal nerve end and tip of middle finger, associated vascular injury, and comorbidity were recorded from patients' medical records. Participating patients were matched with a randomly selected cohort of

TABLE 1: Baseline characteristics.

Characteristics	Study group = 20 (nerve graft + vein conduit)	Control group = 20 (nerve graft)
Mean age (years)	28 ± 7	25 ± 6
Etiology	Sharp injury—8 (40%) Crush injury—12 (60%)	Sharp injury—9 (45%) Crush injury—11 (55%)
Types of nerve	Ulnar—7 Median—13	Ulnar—8 Median—12
Time since injury	Old injury—5 (25%) Fresh injury—15 (75%)	Old injury—6 (30%) Fresh injury—14 (70%)
Nerve defect	3.5 cm—6 (30%) 4.5 cm—8 (40%) 5.5 cm—6 (30%)	3.5 cm—7 (35%) 4.5 cm—7 (35%) 5.5 cm—6 (30%)
Types of repair	Epineural	Epineural
Mean distance from proximal nerve end to tip of middle finger	10–15—5 15–20—13 >20—2	10–15 cm—6 15–20 cm—12 >20 cm—2
Smoking	3 (15%)	4 (20%)
Associated vascular injury	4 (20%)	3 (15%)
Associated tendon injury	3 (15%)	4 (20%)
Associated co morbidity	None	None

control patients with nerve defects, according to age, etiology of the defects, duration of injury, types of nerve repair, nerve defect, distance between proximal nerve end and tip of middle finger, associated vascular injury, tendon injury, and comorbidity, who were treated by nerve graft without vein conduit (Table 1). Associated tendon or vessel injury was repaired in the standard way. All patients were operated under general anesthesia in supine position with tourniquet control.

2.1. Surgical Technique. Following steps were performed (Figures 1, 2, and 3).

(1) There is exploration of the affected nerve under magnification.

(2) Both the ends were identified.

(3) Neuroma or scar, if present, was excised up to the healthy fascicles while in case of fresh injury, ends were trimmed till bleeding and then defect was measured.

(4) The fascicles from each end were properly oriented and aligned.

(5) Sural nerve graft and short saphanous vein were harvested through same incisions.

(6) Vein was turned inside out.

(7) Sural nerve was turned on itself and packed within the vein (2–5 times depending on diameter of the nerve).

(8) Both the ends were excised to get freshly cut ends.

(9) Then graft was put into the defect.

(10) Tension free repair was done taking interrupted sutures between epineurium and vein wall.

(11) Skin closure was done.

(12) Limb was immobilized in slightly flexed position.

Patients were followed up for 2 years at intervals of 3 months. At the end of 2 years, following scales were used for final evaluation of sensory and motor recovery.

(1) Scale for 2-point discrimination:

normal = 0–5 mm;

fair = 6–10 mm;

poor = 11–15 mm;

protective sensation = 1 point;

anesthetic = no point.

(2) Semmes-Weinstein monofilament test:

normal = 2.83;

diminished = 3.61;

diminished protective = 4.31;

loss of protective = 4.56.

(3) Pain/discomfort evaluation:

0 = function hindered;

1 = disturbed;

2 = moderate;

3 = none (normal).

(4) Power grading of the affected muscles:

grade 0: complete paralysis;

grade 1: flicker of contraction present;

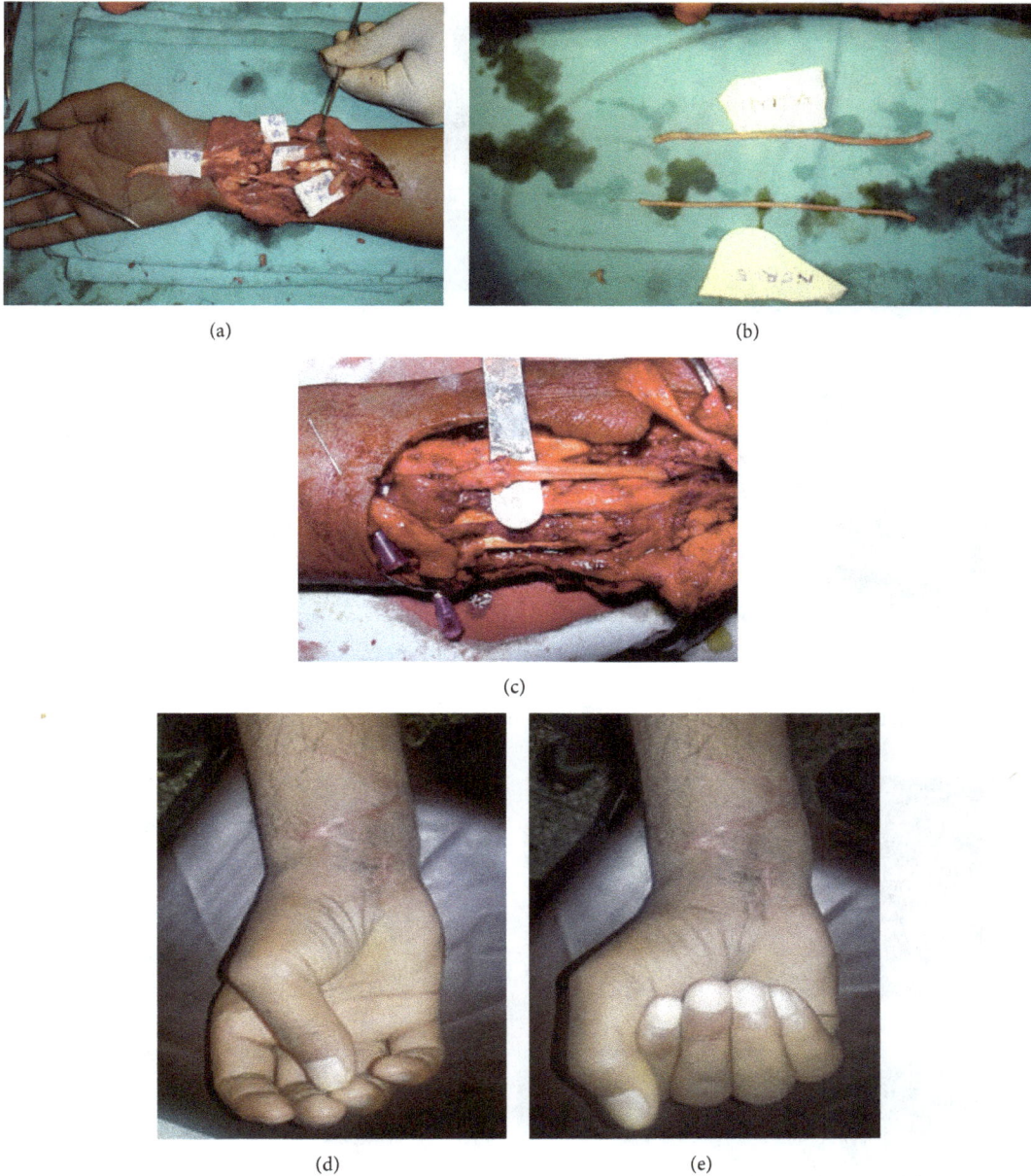

FIGURE 1: (a) Photograph showing median nerve gap. Associated tendon injury is visible. (b) Sural nerve and short saphaneous vein harvested. (c) Graft inerted into the defect after the nerve was packed within the vein. (d) and (e) Follow-up photograph showing good functional recovery.

grade 2: active movement with gravity eliminated;

grade 3: active movement against gravity;

grade 4: active movement against gravity and some resistance;

grade 5: normal power.

(5) Medical research scale (MRC scale):

0 = no atrophy;

1 = mild atrophy;

2 = moderate atrophy;

3 = severe atrophy.

While evaluating sensation at the finger tips, the other uninjured nerve was blocked by local anesthesia.

MRC grading was done by assessing muscle strength and size of the first dorsal interossei (for ulnar nerve evaluation) and flexor pollicis brevis for median nerve evaluation. Atrophy of these muscles was graded as 0, 1, 2, and 3.

All the patients underwent nerve conduction study on follow-up.

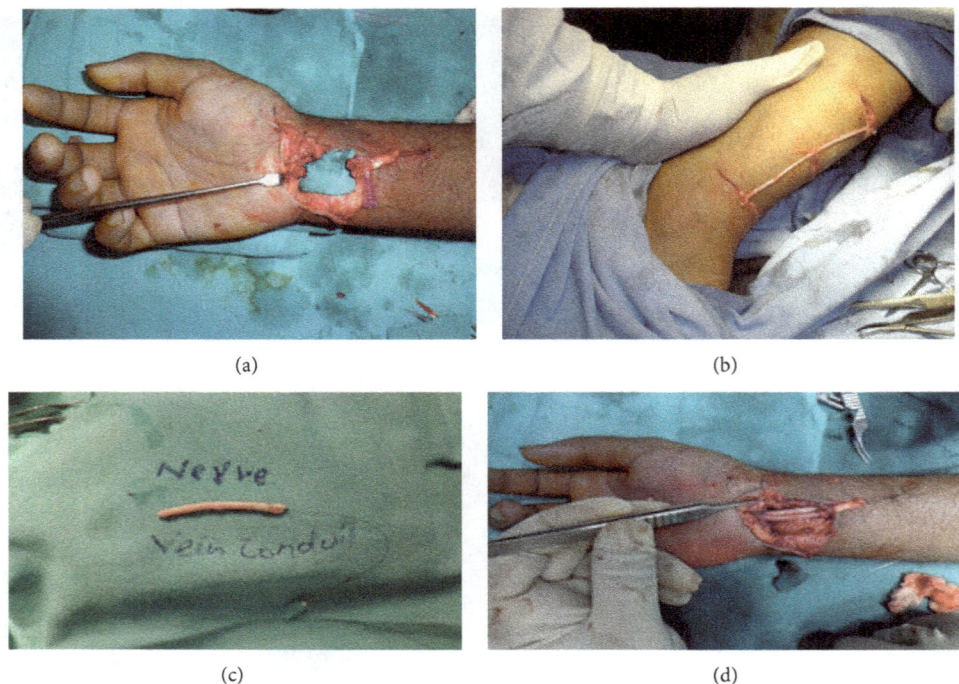

FIGURE 2: (a) Photograph showing median nerve defect. (b) Harvesting of sural nerve and short saphaneous vein through the same incision. (c) Sural nerve packed within the short saphaneous vein after turning on itself. (d) Graft inserted into the defect and anastomosis done.

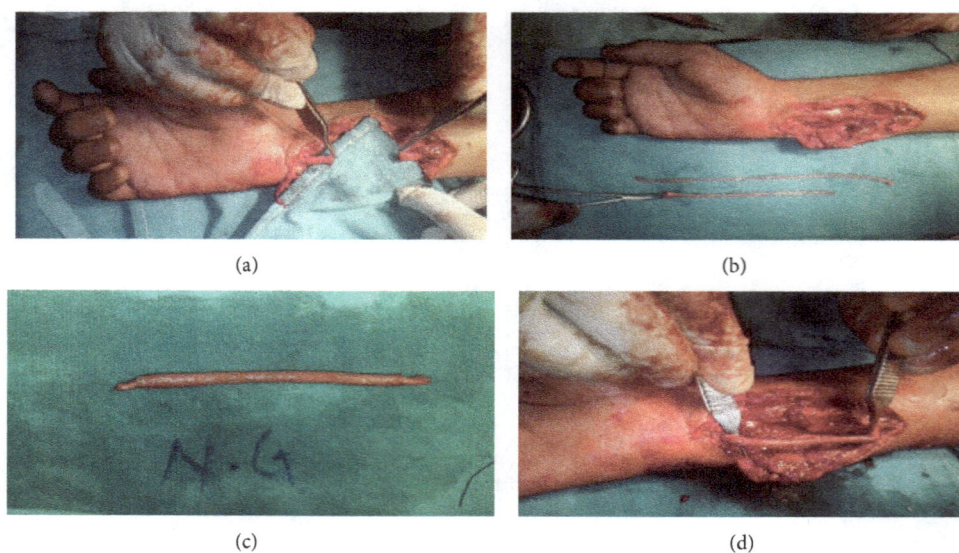

FIGURE 3: (a) Photograph showing ulnar nerve defect right hand. (b) Sural nerve and short saphaneous vein harvested. (c) Sural nerve packed within the short saphaneous vein after turning on itself. (d) Graft put into the defect and anastomosis done.

3. Results

All the patients were evaluated in terms of sensory and motor recovery. Two-point discrimination (2-PD), Semmes-Weinstein monofilament test (SW test) and power of involved muscles, and MRC scale were recorded. Pain/discomfort evaluation was performed for cold intolerance.

Sensations reached to all the digits at 1 year in study groups compared to 18 months in control group.

At the end of second year, 90% patients of study group achieved 2-point discrimination of <10 mm compared to only 60% in control group ($P < 0.05$).

One patient (5%) in the study group had 2-PD more than 15 compared to 5 patients (25%) in the control group (Table 2).

Semmes-Weinstein monofilament test showed a score of ≤2 in 8 patients (40%) in the study group compared to only 2 patients (10%) in the control group ($P < 0.05$) (Table 3).

TABLE 2: Sensory outcome—2 PD.

2 PD (mm)	Study group Number of patients (%)	Control group Number of patients (%)
<5	7 (35%)	4 (20%)
5–10	11 (55%)	8 (40%)
10–15	1 (5%)	3 (15%)
>15	1 (5%)	5 (25%)

$P < 0.05$.

TABLE 3: Sensory outcome—SW exam.

Semmes Weinstein monofilament test	Study group Number of patients (%)	Control group Number of patients (%)
1	3 (15%)	1 (5%)
2	5 (25%)	1 (5%)
3	9 (45%)	8 (40%)
4	3 (15%)	10 (50%)

$P < 0.05$.

TABLE 4: Pain/discomfort evaluation—cold intolerance.

Scale (problem estimation)	Study group Number of patients	Control group Number of patients
0	2 (10%)	6 (30%)
1	3 (15%)	7 (35%)
2	11 (55%)	6 (30%)
3	4 (20%)	1 (5%)

TABLE 5: Motor outcome—power.

Power grade	Study group Number of patients	Control group Number of patients
0	0 (0%)	3 (15%)
1	0 (0%)	3 (15%)
2	3 (15%)	3 (15%)
3	4 (20%)	3 (15%)
4	10 (50%)	6 (30%)
5	3 (15%)	2 (10%)

$P < 0.05$.

Pain/discomfort for cold intolerance was higher in control group as compared to study group (Table 4).

Normal cold intolerance was noticed in 4 (20%) patients in study group as compared to 1 (5%) patients in control group.

In terms of motor recovery, 13 patients (65%) achieved satisfactory hand function (power 4/5) in study group as compared to 8 patients (40%) in control group ($P < 0.05$) (Table 5).

MRC scale was 2 or less than 2 in 85% of patients in study group compared to 60% in control group (Table 6).

TABLE 6: Motor outcome—MRC scale.

MRC scale	Study group Number of patients	Control group Number of patients
0	8 (40%)	2 (10%)
1	5 (25%)	3 (15%)
2	4 (20%)	7 (35%)
3	3 (15%)	8 (40%)

TABLE 7: Nerve conduction findings.

Characteristics	Study group	Control group
Conduction velocity	Normal—14 (70%) Decreased—6 (30%)	Normal—7 (35%) Decreased—13 (65%)
Latency	Normal—19 (95%) Increased—1 (5%)	Normal—10 (50%) Increased—10 (50%)
Amplitude	Normal—14 (70%) Increased—6 (30%)	Normal—8 (40%) Increased—12 (60%)

The nerve conduction findings showed better results in study group as compared to control group (Table 7).

Statistical Analysis. All data analysis was conducted using SPSS software (SPSS Inc.) Significant differences were calculated using Fisher exact test, with $P < 0.05$ considered significant.

4. Discussion

Repair of large nerve gap remains a controversial issue. There are many options available for the reconstruction of these defects. Cable graft has long been considered an ideal option [4, 14–17]. However, continued research leads to the use of many alternative bridging materials in order to avoid donor nerve morbidity. These include the use of vein graft [18, 19], arterial grafts [20], and muscle graft for short nerve gap (less than 3 cm). These options are difficult to use for larger defects. Use of vein and muscle for larger defect may lead to collapse and dispersion of regenerating axons out of the muscle respectively.

Later on, filling of vein with muscle fibre and pieces of nerve was recommended to avoid the collapse of veins when used for large nerve gap [21]. Brunelli et al. report the application of vein conduit filled with muscle fibres in rat model for reconstruction of nerve gap. This technique leads to better functional outcome as compared to isolated vein conduit or muscle graft. Since its description, this method was not widely used for many years till Battiston et al. showed their clinical results on "Nerve repair by means of vein filled with muscle grafts" in 2004 and then they reviewed the literature later and described their clinical experience comparing biological and synthetic conduits for sensory nerve repair [22, 23].

Aly and Azab described a new technique using both cable nerve autograft and autogenous vein conduit to reconstruct wide nerve defects to get the benefits of both the methods [24].

In this series, we have used the similar technique of combined use of cable nerve graft and vein conduit to reconstruct the defects of more than 3 cm in size and compared the results with the use of isolated cable nerve graft technique. We noted a significantly better outcome in our study group where vein conduit was used as compared to control group where no conduit was used. This difference could be due to the prevention of sprouting of nerve fibre at the neurorrhaphy site by vein conduit in the study group.

Aly and Azab used the sural nerve and great saphaneous vein in their study. In our study we have used the sural nerve and short saphenous vein. This allowed us to harvest the nerve and vein through the same incisions leading to lower operating time and donor site scar as compared to Aly and Azab study.

Various researchers have demonstrated that for regeneration and maturation of nerve fibres, autogenous vein grafts are the supportive conduits [25, 26]. The advantages of veins grafts are that these are nonimmunogenic, easy to harvest, and available in variable sizes, have longer half-life, and are less inflammatory [27]. The vein wall is thin, acting as a barrier against scar tissue ingrowing and permeable enough to allow adequate nutrients diffusion and provide a favorable internal environment for nerve regeneration and maturation. Laminin, a glycoprotein, is found in good concentration in all the three layers of vein wall. Laminin promotes neurite and enhances nerve cell adhesion, proliferation, and differentiation thus helping to direct growth cone neurite [28].

There are various modalities for evaluation of nerve recovery. Wong et al. [29] assessed different tools for evaluation of peripheral nerve function. These include the touch moving 2-point discrimination (2PD); Semmes-Weinstein (SW) monofilament test, motor (Medical Research Council (MRC) scale), combined motor and sensory (Dellon modification of the Moberg pick up test; Moberg Recognition test), and pain (visual analogue scale; pinprick-test). They found that the results of the moving 2 PD were comparable with those of the SW monofilaments but having poor correlation and MRC score correlated well with opposition movement of the thumb and muscle wasting ($P < 0.01$). We used 2 PD, Semmes-Weinstein (SW) monofilament test for sensory evaluation and power of the involved muscle and MRC for evaluation of motor recovery.

Aly and Azab found that majority of the patients in their series had adequate and useful 2-PD (60% with 2-PD < 10 mm) and over 82% resumed light touch with variable degrees. The results were comparable to our study where 90% of the patients resumed 2 PD < 10 mm and 85% had SW monofilament score ≥3. In terms of motor recovery, 85% of patients in our study group resumed a power of ≥3 leading to good functional gain.

5. Conclusion

It was concluded that the use of vein conduit in peripheral nerve repair is more effective method than isolated nerve graft providing good sensory and motor recovery.

Ethical Approval

Ethical clearance was taken from ethics committee of the hospital.

Disclosure

The level of evidence is as follows: Level of evidence: II.

References

[1] M. Jabaley, "Primary nerve repair," in *Peripheral Nerve Surgery: Practical Applications in the Upper Extremity*, D. J. Slutsky and V. R. Hentz, Eds., pp. 23–38, Churchill Livingstone Elsevier, Philadelphia, Pa, USA, 2006.

[2] F. Schonauer, S. Marlino, S. Avvedimento, and G. Molea, "Peripheral nerve reconstruction with autologous grafts," in *Basic Principles of Peripheral Nerve Disorders*, InTech, Rijeka, Croatia, 2012.

[3] D. S. Ruch, N. D. Deal, J. Ma et al., "Management of peripheral nerve defects: external fixator-assisted primary neurorrhaphy," *Journal of Bone and Joint Surgery. American Volume*, vol. 86, no. 70, pp. 1405–1413, 2004.

[4] N. K. Daoutis, N. E. Gerostathopoulos, D. G. Efstathopoulos, D. P. Misitizis, G. N. Bouchlis, and S. K. Anagnostou, "Microsurgical reconstruction of large nerve defects using autologous nerve grafts," *Microsurgery*, vol. 15, no. 7, pp. 502–505, 1994.

[5] M. F. Meek and J. H. Coert, "Clinical use of nerve conduits in peripheral-nerve repair: review of the literature," *Journal of Reconstructive Microsurgery*, vol. 18, no. 2, pp. 97-109, 2002.

[6] G. Risitano, G. Cavallaro, and M. Lentini, "Autogenous vein and nerve grafts: a comparative study of nerve regeneration in the rat," *Journal of Hand Surgery B*, vol. 14, no. 1, pp. 102–104, 1989.

[7] D. T. W. Chiu and B. Strauch, "A prospective clinical evaluation of autogenous vein grafts used as a nerve conduit for distal sensory nerve defects of 3 cm or less," *Plastic and Reconstructive Surgery*, vol. 86, no. 5, pp. 928–934, 1990.

[8] J. Xu, D. G. Sotereanos, A. R. Moller et al., "Nerve wrapping with vein grafts in a rat model: a safe technique for the treatment of recurrent chronic compressive neuropathy," *Journal of Reconstructive Microsurgery*, vol. 14, no. 5, pp. 323–330, 1998.

[9] F. Zhang, B. Blain, J. Beck et al., "Autogenous venous graft with one-stage prepared Schwann cells as a conduit for repair of long segmental nerve defects," *Journal of Reconstructive Microsurgery*, vol. 18, no. 4, pp. 295–300, 2002.

[10] J. Xu, S. E. Varitimidis, K. J. Fisher, M. M. Tomaino, and D. G. Sotereanos, "The effect of wrapping scarred nerves with autogenous vein graft to treat recurrent chronic nerve compression," *Journal of Hand Surgery*, vol. 25, no. 1, pp. 93–103, 2000.

[11] B. R. Seckel, S. E. Ryan, R. G. Gagne, T. H. Chiu, and E. Watkins Jr., "Target-specific nerve regeneration through a nerve guide in the rat," *Plastic & Reconstructive Surgery*, vol. 78, no. 6, pp. 793–800, 1986.

[12] S. Stahl and J. A. Goldberg, "The use of vein grafts in upper extremity nerve surgery," *European Journal of Plastic Surgery*, vol. 22, no. 5-6, pp. 255–259, 1999.

[13] M. Acar, A. Karacalar, M. Ayyildiz et al., "The effect of autogenous vein grafts on nerve repair with size discrepancy in rats: an electrophysiological and stereological analysis," *Brain Research*, vol. 1198, pp. 171–181, 2008.

[14] D. S. Ruch, D. N. Deal, J. Ma et al., "Management of pheriperal nerve defects: external fixator-assisted primary neurorrhaphy," *Journal of Bone and Joint Surgery A*, vol. 86, no. 7, pp. 1405–1413, 2004.

[15] S. E. Mackinnon, "New directions in peripheral nerve surgery," *Annals of Plastic Surgery*, vol. 22, no. 3, pp. 257–273, 1989.

[16] H. Millesi, "Techniques for nerve grafting," *Hand Clinics*, vol. 16, no. 1, pp. 73–91, 2000.

[17] T. Trumble, "Overcoming peripheral nerve defects," in *Operative Nerve Repair and Reconstruction*, R. H. Gelberman, Ed., pp. 507–524, JB Lippincott, Philadelphia, Pa, USA, 1991.

[18] V. R. Hentz, J. M. Rosen, S.-J. Xiao, K. C. McGill, and G. Abraham, "The nerve gap dilemma: a comparison of nerves repaired end to end under tension with nerve grafts in a primate model," *The Journal of Hand Surgery*, vol. 18, no. 3, pp. 417–425, 1993.

[19] D. T. W. Chiu and B. Strauch, "A prospective clinical evaluation of autogenous vein grafts used as a nerve conduit for distal sensory nerve defects of 3 cm or less," *Plastic and Reconstructive Surgery*, vol. 86, no. 5, pp. 928–934, 1990.

[20] F. Schonauer, I. La Rusca, and G. Molea, "Homolateral digital artery nerve graft," *Plastic and Reconstructive Surgery*, vol. 117, no. 5, pp. 1661–1662, 2006.

[21] G. A. Brunelli, B. Battiston, A. Vigasio, G. Brunelli, and D. Marocolo, "Bridging nerve defects with combined skeletal muscle and vein conduits," *Microsurgery*, vol. 14, no. 4, pp. 247–251, 1993.

[22] B. Battiston, P. Tos, T. R. Cushway, and S. Geuna, "Nerve repair by means of vein filled with muscle grafts. I. Clinical results," *Microsurgery*, vol. 20, no. 1, pp. 32–36, 2000.

[23] B. Battiston, S. Geuna, M. Ferrero, and P. Tos, "Nerve repair by means of tubulization: literature review and personal clinical experience comparing biological and synthetic conduits for sensory nerve repair," *Microsurgery*, vol. 25, no. 4, pp. 258–267, 2005.

[24] A. M. Aly and A. A. Azab, "Repair of wide nerve gaps using nerve auto-grafts and vein conduits: evaluation of a new technique," *Egypt, Journal of Plastic and Reconstructive Surgery*, vol. 35, no. 1, pp. 65–70, 2011.

[25] D. T. W. Chiu, I. Janecka, T. J. Krizek, M. Wolff, and R. E. Lovelace, "Autogenous vein graft as a conduit for nerve regeneration," *Surgery*, vol. 91, no. 2, pp. 226–233, 1982.

[26] N. Suematsu, Y. Atsuta, and T. Hirayama, "Vein graft for repair of peripheral nerve gap," *Journal of Reconstructive Microsurgery*, vol. 4, no. 4, pp. 313–318, 1988.

[27] M. Foidart-Dessalle, A. Dubuisson, A. Lejeune et al., "Sciatic nerve regeneration through venous or nervous grafts in the rat," *Experimental Neurology*, vol. 148, no. 1, pp. 236–246, 1997.

[28] P. K. Thanos, S. Okajima, and J. K. Terzis, "Ultrastructure and cellular biology of nerve regeneration," *Journal of Reconstructive Microsurgery*, vol. 14, no. 6, pp. 423–436, 1998.

[29] K. H. Wong, J. H. Coert, P. H. Robinson, and M. F. Meek, "Comparison of assessment tools to score recovery of function after repair of traumatic lesions of the median nerve," *Scandinavian Journal of Plastic and Reconstructive Surgery and Hand Surgery*, vol. 40, no. 4, pp. 219–224, 2006.

18

Evaluation of Complication Rates after Breast Surgery Using Acellular Dermal Matrix: Median Follow-Up of Three Years

Felix J. Paprottka,[1] Nicco Krezdorn,[2] Heiko Sorg,[3] Sören Könneker,[4] Stiliano Bontikous,[5] Ian Robertson,[6] Christopher L. Schlett,[7] Nils-Kristian Dohse,[1] and Detlev Hebebrand[1]

[1]*Department of Plastic, Aesthetic, Reconstructive and Hand Surgery, Agaplesion Diakonieklinikum Rotenburg, Elise-Averdieck-Straße 17, 27356 Rotenburg (Wümme), Germany*
[2]*Harvard Medical School, Brigham and Women's Hospital, Department of Surgery, Division of Plastic Surgery, 75 Francis Street, Boston, MA 02115, USA*
[3]*Department of Plastic, Reconstructive, Aesthetic and Hand Surgery, Alfried Krupp Krankenhaus, Hellweg 100, 45276 Essen, Germany*
[4]*Department of Plastic, Aesthetic, Hand and Reconstructive Surgery, Hannover Medical School, Carl-Neubergstraße 1, 30625 Hannover, Germany*
[5]*Department of Pathology, Agaplesion Diakonieklinikum Rotenburg, Elise-Averdieck-Straße 17, 27356 Rotenburg, Germany*
[6]*Department of Surgery, Royal Brompton Hospital, Sydney St, London, UK*
[7]*Department of Diagnostic and Interventional Radiology, University Hospital Heidelberg, Im Neuenheimer Feld 110, 69120 Heidelberg, Germany*

Correspondence should be addressed to Felix J. Paprottka; felix.paprottka@me.com

Academic Editor: Nicolò Scuderi

Introduction. Acellular dermal matrices (ADMs) are now commonly used for breast reconstruction surgery. There are various products available: ADMs derived from human (HADM), porcine (PADM), or bovine (BADM) sources. Detailed long-term follow-up studies are necessary to detect differences in complication rates between these products. *Material and Methods.* From 2010 to 2015, forty-one patients underwent 52 ADM-breast reconstructions in our clinic, including oncologic breast reconstructions and breast augmentation revisions ($n = 52$). 15x HADMs (Epiflex®/DIZG), 21x PADMs (Strattice®/LifeCell), and 16x BADMs (Tutomesh®/RTI Surgical) were implanted. Retrospective data collection with median follow-up of 36 months (range: 12–54 months) was performed. *Results.* Overall complication rate was 17% after ADM implantation (HADM: 7%; PADM: 14%; BADM: 31%). In a composite endpoint of complications and Red Breast Syndrome, a lower event probability was observed between BADMs, PADMs, and HADMs (44%, 19%, and 7%, resp.; $p = 0.01$ for the trend). Furthermore, capsular contracture occurred in 6%, more frequently as compared to the current literature. *Conclusions.* When ADM-based reconstruction is indicated, the authors suggest primarily the use of HADMs and secondary the use of PADMs. It is shown that BADMs have the highest complication probability within our patient cohort; nevertheless, BADMs convey physical advantages in terms of flexibility and better aesthetic outcomes. The indication for the use of ADMs should be filled for each case individually.

1. Introduction

An acellular dermal matrix (ADM) is a decellularized soft tissue material derived from a biological source. In breast surgery, ADMs have been used as an alternative to autologous myocutaneous flap grafts to bridge defects following aesthetic or oncoplastic breast reconstruction [1]. Advantages of this technique include improved implant stabilization as well as a

TABLE 1: Patient collective with ADM-implementation.

ADM	Product	Number of ADM implants used	Number of treated patients	Avg. patient age (years)	Avg. follow-up time (months)
HADM	Epiflex/DIZG	15	12	46 (36–76)	40 (20–50)
PADM	Strattice/LifeCell	21	16	56 (44–66)	43 (30–54)
BADM	Tutomesh/RTI Surgical	16	13	53 (33–74)	20 (12–31)
Total	*All ADMs*	*52*	*41*	*52 (33–76)*	*36 (12–54)*

Listing of matrix, name of ADM-product and its fabricant, amount of breast reconstructions (BR)/augmentations with usage of ADMs, number of patients treated with ADMs, average patient age and range in years, and average follow-up time + range in months of the given patient collective, which received a breast reconstruction with ADM; HADM: human ADM, PADM: porcine ADM, and BADM: bovine ADM.

decrease rate of capsular contracture [1]. Furthermore, ADMs can be used for reconstruction of the inframammary fold (IMF) in order to achieve an improved aesthetic outcome [2].

A variety of human derived ADMs (HADMs) are commercially available: Epiflex by DIZG (Berlin, Germany), Alloderm® by LifeCell Corporation (Bridgewater, NJ, USA), and DermaMatrix® by Synthes CMF (West Chester, PA, USA). However, Alloderm is not currently licensed for use in Germany. Strattice by LifeCell Corporation (Bridgewater, NJ, USA) is derived from porcine dermis/corium (PADM) and Tutomesh by RTI Surgical (Alachua, FL, USA) is derived from bovine pericardium.

Reported complications of ADM reconstruction techniques include skin necrosis, seroma, haematoma, infection, and Red Breast Syndrome (RBS). RBS is erythematous change occurring superficially to the area of ADM implantation without any specific signs of local infection; its mechanism is not well understood [3]. Few documented reports compare the long-term outcomes and associated risks of different types of ADMs [1, 4, 5].

The aim of this study is to assess the incidence of short- and long-term complications of implantation of various kinds of ADMs in our centre.

2. Material and Methods

Our analysis followed 41 female patients with a total of 52 ADM-based breast reconstructions between 2010 and 2015, using matrices such as Epiflex by DIZG (Berlin, Germany), Strattice by LifeCell Corporation (Bridgewater, NJ, USA), and Tutomesh by RTI Surgical (Alachua, FL, USA). Indications for reconstruction included secondary oncologic breast reconstructions (delayed), primary augmentations (in large breasts), or secondary breast augmentations (revision). In further detail, 15 HADMs (Epiflex), 21 PADMs (Strattice), and 16 BADMs (Tutomesh) were applied. Detailed information about the patient demographics with respect to type of ADM used is shown in Table 1. Indications for usage of ADMs within our patient cohort are listed in Table 2. Sixteen patients had a history of radiotherapy prior to ADM implementation; see Table 3. In all cases, ADMs were used in combination with subpectoral implant augmentation (Style 410 implants by Allergan); hereby these matrices were used to expand the pocket. Surgical drains were placed between the ADM and

the implant. A single dose of intravenous antibiotics was administered intraoperatively.

Retrospective data analysis was performed using our hospital information system (HIS), median follow-up of 36 months (range: 12–54 months). Only patients with at least one year of follow-up time were included in our study. Patients were followed up at intervals of one week, two weeks, one month, three months, six months, and one year and then annually thereafter or if complications occurred. Assessment of short-term complications such as infection, seroma, haematoma, or skin necrosis and long-term complications such as capsular contracture (>Baker-St. II), implant malposition, or implant loss was made. Red Breast Syndrome (RBS) was the only complication occurring shortly after ADM usage in which no further medical treatment was indicated, though differential diagnosis might be challenging. Ultrasound imaging was performed in all patients with suspicion of RBS. Histopathological samples of the ADM implementation area were taken in four cases ($n = 4$).

2.1. Statistical Analysis. Continuous variables were expressed as median (range) and categorical variables as percentages (frequencies) if not other specified. Primary endpoints were skin necrosis, seroma, haematoma, infection, recurrence of capsular contracture, implant malposition, and implant loss. The composite endpoint included all complications as well as the Red Breast Syndrome. In order to analyze whether a trend exists regarding the endpoints between HADM, PADM, and BADM, Mantel-Haenszel Chi-Square was applied. Further, Chi-Square analysis allowed direct comparison between two kinds of ADMs. Statistical analysis was performed using the software SAS (Version 9.4, SAS Institute Inc., Cary, NC). A two-sided p value of <0.05 was considered statistically significant.

3. Results

All documented complications after implementations of ADMs occurring during the follow-up interval are demonstrated in Table 3. A relative reduction in probability for complications was observed between BADMs, PADMs, and HADMs, although statistical significance was not achieved (31%, 14%, and 7%, resp.; $p = 0.07$ for the trend). Similarly, the direct comparison between two kinds of the different

TABLE 2: Indications for ADM implementation.

| ADM | Product | BR with ADM (n) | Oncologic indication | | Aesthetic indication | | |
			BR with no capsular contracture[*]	BR with capsular contracture[**]	Primary augmentation[*,***]	Secondary augmentation after capsular contracture[*]	Others[*]
HADM	Epiflex/DIZG	15	1	3	9	2	0
PADM	Strattice/LifeCell	21	6	8	5	2	0
BADM	Tutomesh/RTI Surgical	16	2	5	3	2	4

Listing of kind of matrix used, name of product, number of breast reconstructions with certain ADMs, and indications for ADM usage (breast reconstruction (BR) with no capsular contracture, BR with capsular contracture, primary augmentation, secondary augmentation after capsular contracture). Oncologic patients made up 27% of the HADM group, 67% of the BADM group, and 44% of the BADM group; HADM: human ADM, PADM: porcine ADM, and BADM: bovine ADM; * = no history of radiotherapy; ** = history of radiotherapy; *** = primary augmentation in cases with large breasts.

TABLE 3: Complications after ADM implementation.

ADM	Product	Complication rate*	Skin necrosis	Seroma	Haematoma	Infection	Recurrence of capsular contracture	Implant malposition	Implant loss	RBS***
HADM	Epiflex/DIZG	7%	—	—	—	1	—	—	—	—
PADM	Strattice/LifeCell	14%	1**	1	—	—	1	—	—	1
BADM	Tutomesh/RTI Surgical	31%	1**	—	—	1	2**	—	1	2

Complications following ADM implantation for breast reconstruction with type of matrix, product, complications requiring further medical treatment (in %), infection, seroma, haematoma, skin necrosis, recurrence of capsular contracture, implant malposition, implant loss, and Red Breast Syndrome (RBS); HADM: human ADM, PADM: porcine ADM, and BADM: bovine ADM; * = excluding occurrence of RBS; ** = one pat. with skin necrosis + recurrence of capsular contracture in two separate breasts; *** = not part of complications requiring further medical treatment.

ADM did not achieve statistical significance (all $p > 0.08$). Using a composite endpoint of complications and Red Breast Syndrome, the significant stepwise reduction was observed between BADMs, PADMs, and HADMs (44%, 19%, and 7%, resp.; $p = 0.01$ for the trend). In the direct comparison of two kinds of ADMs, HADMs demonstrated a significant lower probability for the composite endpoint as compared to BADMs (7% versus 44%, resp.; $p = 0.02$), while all other comparisons did not achieve statistical significance (all $p > 0.10$).

Three out of 15 patients, who were treated with Epiflex, required revision breast surgery: three patients received a mastopexy with contralateral breast refinement after 4, 7, or 8 months postoperatively. One month after breast reconstruction with ADM, an infection occurred in a patient with a history of radiotherapy; this was managed conservatively with antibiotics.

Five out of 21 patients, who received a Strattice implant, required revision surgery.

One patient needed revision surgery due to capsular contracture after 11 months postoperatively, and another with a history of radiotherapy had to be surgically revised due to skin necrosis after four months. One patient required ultrasound-guided drainage of a seroma after two months. After 5, 13, and 17 months postoperatively, three patients received a mastopexy with a contralateral mammary adaptation.

Four out of 16 patients, who were treated with Tutomesh, received a surgical revision.

one patient, with a history of chemotherapy, had a skin necrosis plus recurrence of capsular contracture after 6 months postoperatively, resulting in a DIEP-flap coverage. Another had a shell rupture of an implant after two months postoperatively, leading to a breast implant loss. After 10 months postoperatively, one patient with a recurrence of capsular contracture and a history of radiotherapy received a capsulotomy and implant exchange. After two months postoperatively, one patient with infection and loss of IMF underwent a surgical debridement followed by IMF-reconstruction and reaugmentation. In this group, there were no mastopexies with contralateral mammary adaptation during the given follow-up interval. Overall complications, after usage of all three given ADMs, are demonstrated in Table 4. In our study, an increased risk of general complications with 17% after ADM application could be shown. In further detail, complication risk for HADM (Epiflex) was 7% (1/15 patients), for PADM (Strattice) 14% (3/21 patients), and for BADM (Tutomesh) 31% (5/16 patients).

In four patients, who had undergone revision procedures, histopathologic biopsy samples could be taken within HADM-implementation zone (Figures 1 and 2). Furthermore, preoperative and postoperative images of two patient cases after ADM-breast reconstruction are demonstrated in Figures 3-4.

4. Discussion

ADM-based techniques are now well established for breast reconstruction. There are various products available on the

TABLE 4: Overall complication probabilities for used ADMs.

ADM	HADM (Epiflex/DIZG), PADM (Strattice/LifeCell), BADM (Tutomesh/RTI Surgical)
Breasts (total)	52
Avg. follow-up time (in months)	36 (12–54)
Complications (total)	9 (17%)
Short-term complications	
Skin necrosis	2 (4%)
Seroma	1 (2%)
Haematoma	0 (0%)
Infection	2 (4%)
RBS*	3 (6%)*
Long-term complications	
Capsular contracture**	3 (6%)
Implant malposition	0 (0%)
Implant loss	1 (2%)

Short-term (skin necrosis, seroma, haematoma, infection, and Red Breast Syndrome (RBS)) and long-term complications (capsular contracture, implant malposition, and implant loss) for all breasts with usage of ADMs (human ADM (HADM), porcine ADM (PADM), bovine ADM (BADM)), median follow-up time for all patients, total complications of all breasts being reconstructed with ADMs; * = excluded from overall complications, which required further medical treatment; ** = >Baker-St. II.

market: Epiflex is a cell-free dermis allograft, which is up to now the only licensed medicinal HADM product in German-speaking countries; Strattice is a sterile, acellular reconstructive tissue matrix, which is derived from porcine dermis; Tutomesh (BADM) is an avital, acellular, and xenogeneic membrane made from bovine pericardium. All manufacturers advertise their acellular matrices to rapidly integrate into the surrounding tissue without causing any immune response. Due to a special treatment of the human or animal source materials, cells, which may cause an autoimmune reaction, are washed out, leaving only a natural collagen membrane behind. But certainly, ADMs generated out of human, porcine, or bovine tissue might still have different qualities concerning tissue integration and postoperative outcomes.

According to the available literature, several studies have demonstrated reduction of capsular contracture [6, 7]. Long-term follow-up after primary breast augmentation without ADM implementation suggest the risk of capsular contracture formation is around 2%, 15%, and 19% after 3, 6, and 10 years, respectively [8–10]. Secondary augmentation revealed capsular contracture rates of 5%, 21%, and 29% after 3, 6, and 10 years, respectively [8–10]. The rate of capsular contracture occurrence after standard breast reconstruction with implants was 6%, 16%, and 25% after 3, 6, and 10 years, respectively [8–10]. Overall capsular contracture rate in our retrospective study was 6%, including one patient with a history of chemotherapy and one patient with a history of radiotherapy. Within the current literature, capsular contracture rates after ADM implantation differ from 0 up to 3.75% [6, 11–19].

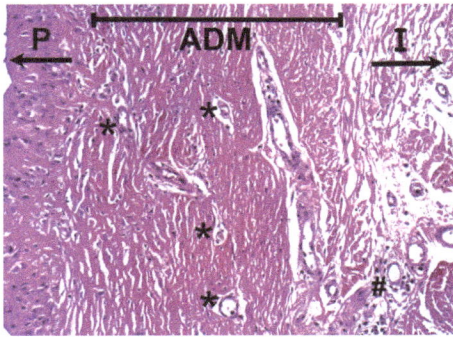

FIGURE 1: Histological slide within area of ADM implementation, H&E stain. Vascular invasion within the BADM (Strattice/LifeCell) after 6 months postoperatively. P = patient's side with breast tissue; ADM = acellular dermal matrix; I = implant side; * = proliferation of new capillaries; # = foreign body response with soft tissue reaction. H&E stain; 200-fold microscopic magnification.

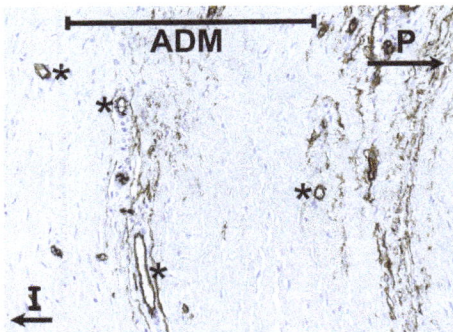

FIGURE 2: Histological slide within area of ADM implementation, CD34 stain. No histological evidence of capsular contracture in sample taken 6 months after BADM-implementation (Strattice/LifeCell). Immunohistochemistry showing strong expression of CD34 in endothelial cells within new grown vessels. P = patient's side with breast tissue; ADM = acellular dermal matrix; I = implant side; * = new vessel formation. CD34 immunohistochemical staining; 200-fold microscopic magnification.

The incidence of RBS in our cohort was 6% (3/52 patients), with one case in the Strattice and two cases in the Tutomesh group.

In comparison to previously published data, we demonstrate a higher overall complication rate after the implantation of ADM summing up to 17%. In detail, BADM (Tutomesh) had the highest complication probability with 31%, followed by PADM (Strattice) with 14%, and HADM (Epiflex) with 7%. A statistically increased complication probability was noted between the HADM and BADM group, if RBS was included to the other complications requiring further medical treatment. The inclusion of oncologic patients with breast reconstruction after/without radio- and/ or chemotherapy may have resulted in greater heterogeneity and therefore increased complication rates.

Furthermore, it has already been shown that radio- or chemotherapy had an influence on implanted ADMs (Alloderm), resulting in a limited ADM modeling [20].

Salzberg et al. listed an overall complication rate of 3.9% in patients treated with prophylactic or oncologic SSM/NSM in combination with direct-to-implant immediate breast reconstruction using Alloderm (median follow-up: 28.9 months) [1]. In a meta-analysis, Newman et al. demonstrated a higher complication rate following HADM implementation with tissue expanders or permanent implants (12%) after therapeutic or prophylactic mastectomy and breast reconstruction [4]. Glasberg and Light published data in 2012, in which the complication rate after mastectomy and breast reconstruction with tissue expander was 6% using Strattice and 21% in patients with Alloderm [6]. Nevertheless, our presented data show an increased risk for complications after application of ADMs. In one of the largest studies, where Alloderm was used for breast reconstruction [1], rate of implant loss, skin necrosis, haematoma, capsular contraction, and infection were 1.3%, 1.1%, 0.4%, and 0.2%, respectively, compared with 2%. 4%, 6%, and 4%, respectively, in our study. However, there were no incidences of haematoma and implant malposition in our study, compared with 1.1% and 0.2%, respectively, in the studies by Salzberg et al. [1]. Seroma rate was 2% in our patient collective, whereas, in the study by Salzberg et al. [1], no information is given. Although Alloderm is made by the same manufacturer as Strattice, it is not available for purchase in Germany; therefore direct comparison of results should be interpreted with caution.

In a recent publication by Mendenhall et al., outcomes from time of tissue expander and HADM placement (Alloderm and DermaMatrix) to definitive reconstruction after simple and total skin and nipple-areola complex-sparing mastectomy were assessed [5]. Many of the treated breast cancer patients received chemo- or radiotherapy [5]. Overall complication rate in the Alloderm group was 33.6% and in the DermaMatrix group 38.8%, summing up to an all-breast complication rate of 36.2% [5]. 19.6% skin necrosis and 15.1% infection were the leading complications in this patient cohort [5]. Therefore, ADM implementation in patients receiving chemo-/radiotherapy seems to severely increase postoperative occurrence of complications [5]. Nevertheless, this data is not completely applicable to our patient cohort.

Other limitations of our study include the relative brevity of follow-up with a mean time period of 36 months. Many of the complications occurred early in the follow-up interval. Statements about the incidence of long-term complications such as capsular contractures are limited. Certainly, a larger patient collective and a longer follow-up interval are needed to obtain statistically significant results concerning complication rates.

As a result, indications for the use of ADMs should be considered on a case-by-case basis. Surely product costs may influence the surgeon's decision from time to time: from all three ADMs compared in our study, Strattice was the most expensive matrix and Tutomesh the one with the lowest price.

In our experience, ADMs are useful to correct these problems: loss of the IMF, implantation of high-volume implants, slight capsular contracture, bottoming-out, or other forms of implant malposition.

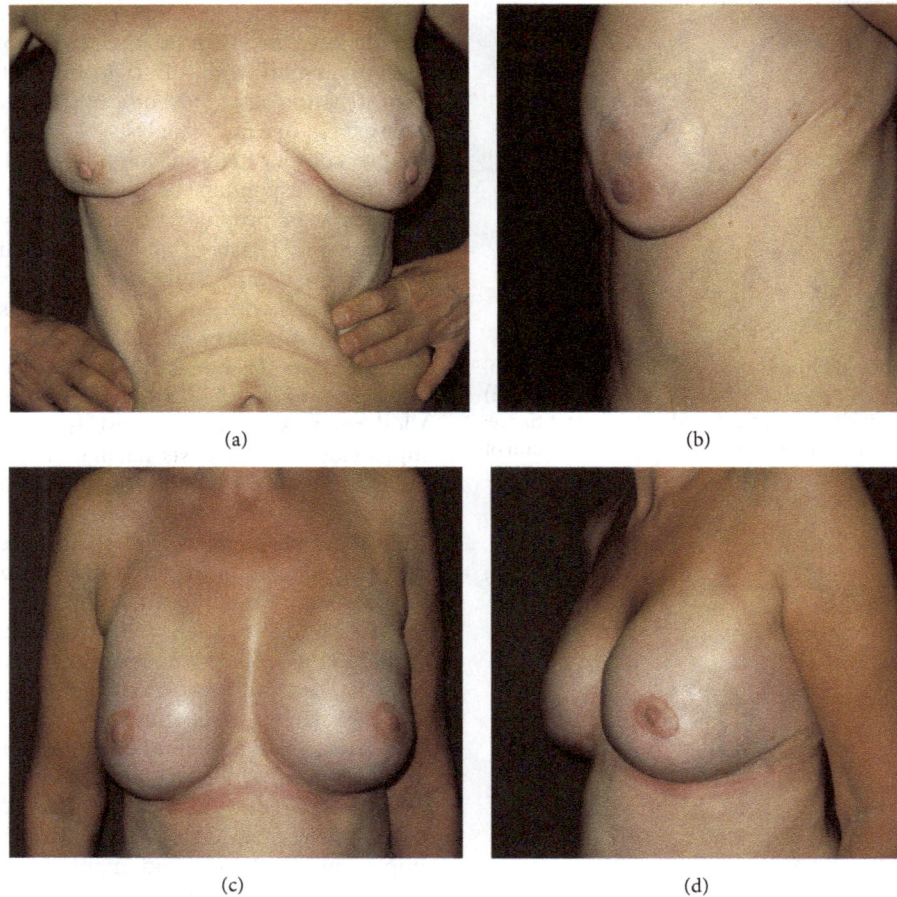

FIGURE 3: Case I: 57-year-old female patient suffering from implant malposition with lateral deviation, bottoming-out, ripping, ptosis with different nipple-areola complex (NAC) and IMF positions preoperatively; (a) frontal view; (b) lateral view; one-year postoperative results after BADM implantation (Strattice/LifeCell) with frontal (c) and lateral view (d).

In this study, Epiflex (HADM) had the lowest complication rate, which may be due to allogenicity; nevertheless our detected total complication rate is greater than rates published within the available literature. In terms of preventing capsular contracture, thicker ADMs, such as Epiflex or Strattice, might be more appropriate for breast reconstruction. This effect could be explained due to prolonged vascular ingrowth time throughout the matrix and a delayed autoimmune response, caused by a longer isolation of the implant from the surrounding tissue. When aesthetic considerations are the greatest concern with loss of the IMF or bottoming-out of the implant, Tutomesh, which is made out of thinner bovine pericardium (offering a greater plasticity), may be favored. But an increased complication rate following BADM application has to be taken into account and should be discussed with the patient preoperatively.

5. Conclusions

Our retrospective study demonstrated that the use of HADMs is associated with the lowest complication risk (7%) among the three ADMs tested. In comparison with the available literature, the total complication rate of 17% was high. In our study, the capsular contracture rate after ADM reconstruction was 6% at a median follow-up interval of 36 months, that is also increased in comparison to other literature. The authors recommend a judicial use of ADM, taking into account costs, condition after radiotherapy, and uncertain long-term results. The flexible properties of BADMs have advantages in tissue handling and aesthetic properties but had the highest complication probability compared to the other subgroups within our study. Treatment of recurring capsular contracture calls for thicker ADMs such as Epiflex or Strattice. Overall, Epiflex (HADM) had the lowest complication rate within our study, whereas Tutomesh (BADM) showed the highest complication rate. In the case of loss of the IMF, large-volume implants, slight capsular contracture, bottoming-out, and implant malposition, the authors recommend in selected cases HADMs as primary and PADM as secondary treatment options. Due to the small amount of patients included in this retrospective study, a larger patient collective is urgently needed for further evaluation; therefore we suggest a prospective randomised study in order to receive more distinct results.

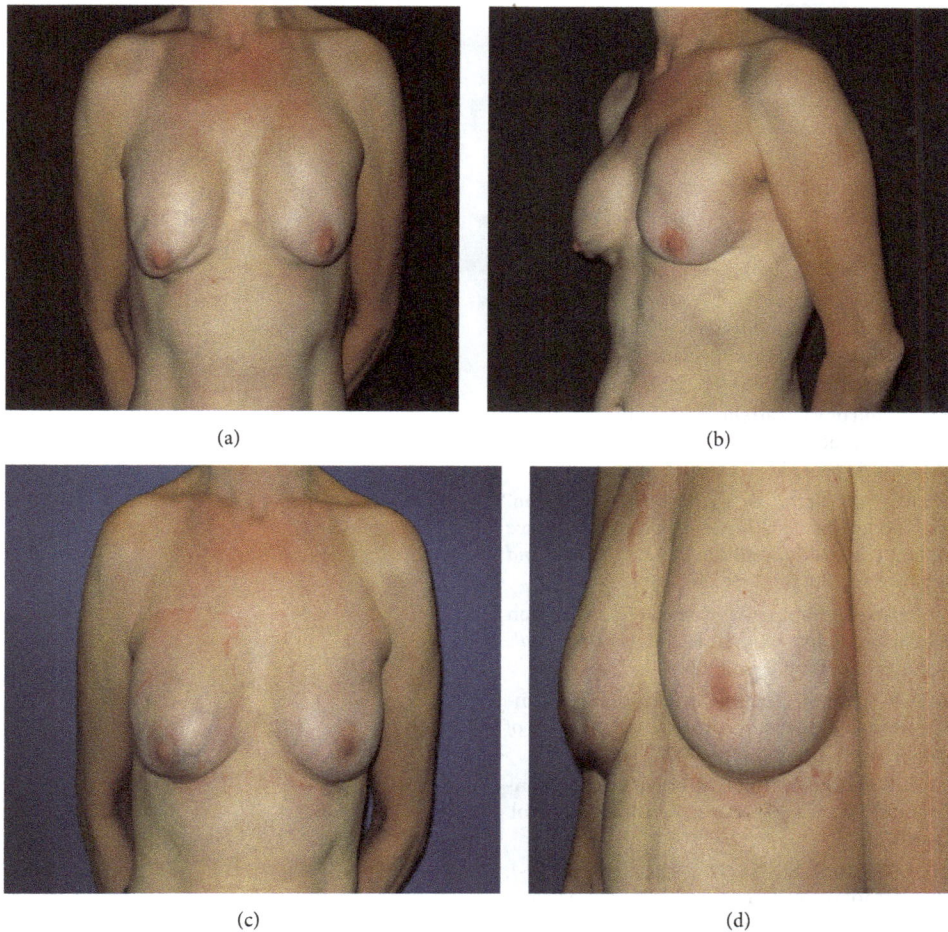

FIGURE 4: Case II: skin sparing mastectomy and breast augmentation performed in 54-year-old female patient with a history of breast carcinoma, complicated by shell rupture of the left-sided implant and subsequent breast-expander implantation; (a) frontal view; (b) lateral view; three-month postoperative results after HADM usage (Epiflex/DIZG) with frontal (c) and lateral view (d).

Ethical Approval

The research project with all its procedures was granted by the Local Ethics Committee (medical association of Lower Saxony, Germany) and is in accordance with national law and the World Medical Association Declaration of Helsinki (1964) with its ethical principles for medical research involving human subjects and subsequent amendments.

Disclosure

The authors received no payment, compensation, or funding for the current study and thus have no conflicts of interest to declare. Highest ethical and scientific standards were applied. After the study was completed and reviewed, DIZG (Berlin, Germany) was approached and agreed to pay the Article Processing Charge for open access publication.

References

[1] C. A. Salzberg, A. Y. Ashikari, R. M. Koch, and E. Chabner-Thompson, "An 8-year experience of direct-to-implant immediate breast reconstruction using human acellular dermal matrix (AlloDerm)," *Plastic and Reconstructive Surgery*, vol. 127, no. 2, pp. 514–524, 2011.

[2] A. M. S. Ibrahim, P. G. L. Koolen, O. Ganor et al., "Does acellular dermal matrix really improve aesthetic outcome in tissue expander/implant-based breast reconstruction?" *Aesthetic Plastic Surgery*, vol. 39, no. 3, article 11, pp. 359–368, 2015.

[3] P. S. Wu, S. Winocour, and S. R. Jacobson, "Red breast syndrome: a review of available literature," *Aesthetic Plastic Surgery*, vol. 39, no. 2, pp. 227–230, 2015.

[4] M. I. Newman, K. A. Swartz, M. C. Samson, C. B. Mahoney, and K. Diab, "The true incidence of near-term postoperative complications in prosthetic breast reconstruction utilizing human acellular dermal matrices: a meta-analysis," *Aesthetic Plastic Surgery*, vol. 35, no. 1, pp. 100–106, 2011.

[5] S. D. Mendenhall, L. A. Anderson, J. Ying et al., "The BREAS-Trial: stage I. outcomes from the time of tissue expander and acellular dermal matrix placement to definitive reconstruction,"

Plastic and Reconstructive Surgery, vol. 135, no. 1, pp. 29e–42e, 2015.

[6] S. B. Glasberg and D. Light, "AlloDerm and strattice in breast reconstruction: a comparison and techniques for optimizing outcomes," *Plastic and Reconstructive Surgery*, vol. 129, no. 6, pp. 1223–1233, 2012.

[7] M. Leong, C. B. Basu, and M. J. Hicks, "Further evidence that human acellular dermal matrix decreases inflammatory markers of capsule formation in implant-based breast reconstruction," *Aesthetic Surgery Journal*, vol. 35, no. 1, pp. 40–47, 2015.

[8] S. L. Spear, D. K. Murphy, A. Slicton, and P. S. Walker, "Inamed silicone breast implant ussg. Inamed silicone breast implant core study results at 6 years," *Plastic and Reconstructive Surgery*, vol. 120, discussion 7S-8S, no. 7, pp. 8S–16S, 2007.

[9] S. L. Spear and D. K. Murphy, "Natrelle round silicone breast implants: core study results at 10 years," *Plastic and Reconstructive Surgery*, vol. 133, no. 6, pp. 1354–1361, 2014.

[10] B. P. Bengtson, B. W. Van Natta, D. K. Murphy, A. Slicton, and G. P. Maxwell, "Style USCCSG. Style 410 highly cohesive silicone breast implant core study results at 3 years," *Plastic and Reconstructive Surgery*, vol. 120, no. 7, pp. 40S–48S, 2007.

[11] C. A. Salzberg, "Nonexpansive immediate breast reconstruction using human acellular tissue matrix graft (AlloDerm)," *Annals of Plastic Surgery*, vol. 57, no. 1, pp. 1–5, 2006.

[12] K. H. Breuing and A. S. Colwell, "Inferolateral AlloDerm hammock for implant coverage in breast reconstruction," *Annals of Plastic Surgery*, vol. 59, no. 3, pp. 250–255, 2007.

[13] R. J. Zienowicz and E. Karacaoglu, "Implant-based breast reconstruction with allograft," *Plastic and Reconstructive Surgery*, vol. 120, no. 2, pp. 373–381, 2007.

[14] V. Bindingnavele, M. Gaon, K. S. Ota, D. A. Kulber, and D.-J. Lee, "Use of acellular cadaveric dermis and tissue expansion in postmastectomy breast reconstruction," *Journal of Plastic, Reconstructive and Aesthetic Surgery*, vol. 60, no. 11, pp. 1214–1218, 2007.

[15] S. L. Spear, P. M. Parikh, E. Reisin, and N. G. Menon, "Acellular dermis-assisted breast reconstruction," *Aesthetic Plastic Surgery*, vol. 32, no. 3, pp. 418–425, 2008.

[16] J. D. Namnoum, "Expander/implant reconstruction with AlloDerm: recent experience," *Plastic and Reconstructive Surgery*, vol. 124, no. 2, pp. 387–394, 2009.

[17] T. R. Hester Jr., B. H. Ghazi, H. R. Moyer, F. R. Nahai, M. Wilton, and L. Stokes, "Use of dermal matrix to prevent capsular contracture in aesthetic breast surgery," *Plastic and Reconstructive Surgery*, vol. 130, no. 5, pp. 126S–136S, 2012.

[18] S. L. Spear, J. C. Sinkin, and A. Al-Attar, "Porcine acellular dermal matrix (strattice) in primary and revision cosmetic breast surgery," *Plastic and Reconstructive Surgery*, vol. 131, no. 5, pp. 1140–1148, 2013.

[19] U. Hille-Betz, N. Kniebusch, S. Wojcinski et al., "Breast reconstruction and revision surgery for implant-associated breast deformities using porcine acellular dermal matrix: a multicenter study of 156 cases," *Annals of Surgical Oncology*, vol. 22, no. 4, pp. 1146–1152, 2015.

[20] T. M. Myckatyn, J. A. Cavallo, K. Sharma et al., "The impact of chemotherapy and radiation therapy on the remodeling of acellular dermal matrices in staged, prosthetic breast reconstruction," *Plastic and Reconstructive Surgery*, vol. 135, no. 1, pp. 43e–57e, 2015.

19

Sensory Recovery with Innervated and Noninnervated Flaps after Total Lower Lip Reconstruction: A Comparative Study

Meltem Ayhan Oral,[1] **Kamuran Zeynep Sevim,**[2] **Metin Görgü,**[3] **and Hasan Yücel Öztan**[4]

[1] İzmir Katip Celebi University, Ataturk Research and Training Hospital, Department of Plastic and Reconstructive Surgery, 35360 Izmir, Turkey
[2] Sisli Hamidiye Etfal Research and Training Hospital, Department of Plastic and Reconstructive Surgery, 34371 Istanbul, Turkey
[3] Abant İzzet Baysal University, Department of Plastic and Reconstructive Surgery, 14280 Bolu, Turkey
[4] Private Practice, Plastic Surgeon, 35590 Izmir, Turkey

Correspondence should be addressed to Kamuran Zeynep Sevim; kzeynep.sevim@gmail.com

Academic Editor: Francesco Carinci

This study compares sensory recovery after total lower lip reconstruction in a wide variety of flaps including bilateral depressor anguli oris flap, submental island flap, bilateral fan flaps, radial forearm flap, and pectoralis major myocutaneous flaps in a large number of patients. Spontaneous return of flap sensation was documented by clinical testing in the majority (3%) of patients who underwent total lower lip reconstruction. Sensory recovery occurred more often in patients with fasciocutaneous free flaps than in those with musculocutaneous flaps. Flap sensation to touch, two-point discrimination, and temperature perception was correlated with age, smoking, and radiation treated patients. We conclude that reasonable sensory recovery may be expected in noninnervated flaps, provided that the major regional sensorial nerve has not been sacrificed, and also provided that the patients age is relatively young and that enough surface contact area of the recipient bed is present without marked scarring. This trial was regestered with Chinese Clinical Trial Registry (Chi CTR) with ChiCTR-ONC-13003656.

1. Introduction

The reconstruction of an extensive lower defect is a difficult surgical challenge since both aesthetics and function of the lower third of the face have to be restored. The lip is a complex anatomical structure which includes a muscular layer which is a part of the oral sphincter, lying between a muscular layer and the overlying skin. In order to restore the three layers, several reconstructive procedures have been described, including local flaps from the cheeks, pedicled flaps from the chin, expanded cervical or jugal flaps, and finally fasciocutaneous free flap transfers [1–4]. Nevertheless, none of them provide an ideal solution regarding the appearance and function.

In this study we present 125 innervated and noninnervated flaps performed in bothclinics in 65 patients with stage 3 and further squamous cell carcinoma of the total lower lip. To date, 80 patients have been followed-up for a minimum of 1 year after the tumor resection and reconstruction with bilateral fan flaps, Karapandzic flaps, Nakajima flaps, Fujimori gate flaps, submental island flaps, bilateral depressor anguli oris myocutaneous flaps, pectoralis major myocutaneous flaps, and noninnervated radial forearm flaps was performed.

The comparative clinical recovery of sensation in these flaps and its relationship to articulation and perioral continence form the basis for this report.

2. Materials and Methods

From January 1, 1999, to August 2010, 80 patients, ranging in age from 7 to 82 years, underwent resection of stage 3 or greater squamous cell carcinoma of the lower lip.

The extent of resection of primary lesions included total lower lip and adjacent oral mucosa. Eighteen patients received postoperative irradiation and 50 patients received no further treatment.

Defects of the lower lip were reconstructed in 16 patients with 30 bilateral fan flaps, in 20 patients with 40 karapandzic flaps, in 5 patients with 10 Nakajima flaps, in 2 patients with 4 Fujimori Gate flaps, in 15 patients with 16 bilateral depressor anguli oris flaps, in 5 patients with submental island flaps, in 14 patients with radial forearm free flaps, and in 3 patients with pectoralis major musculocutaneous flaps.

The selection of the type of flap to be used for reconstruction in a particular patient was based on multiple factors, including size of the defect, the need and lack of bulk, the results of the Allen's test in the nondominant arm of the patients, the patient's preference after preoperative counseling, and preference of the surgeon. In this prospective study, no attempt was made in any patient to anastomose a neural stump in the recipient site to a nerve or nerves in the flap. Fifty of the patients were treated with surgery alone and 18 patients needed subsequent radiation therapy (70 Gy at the primary tumor site) (Table 3).

Surgical resection was combined with neck lymph-node dissection in 27 cases taking into consideration the patient's general health conditions.

All flaps selected for this study were total/near total lower lip defects in an attempt to minimize the confusion that might result from rapid ingrowth of surrounding nerves in smaller flaps.

The lingual and hypoglossal nerves were preserved carefully during neck dissection. Mean operating time was 2.5 hours.

All patients underwent sensory testing by the same examiner at least 3 months after surgery. Sensory function was assessed in the center of the flaps and on the contralateral side cheek as a control group. The tests were performed with the patient blinded. Patients were asked to acknowledge sensation by holding up their fingers depending on the sensation tested.

Superficial touch was tested by touching the flap with a cotton swab, hot and cold temperature discrimination was tested with immersing 2 test tubes in hot and cold water 5 minutes in hot water ($\leq 40°C$), 5 minutes in cold water ($\geq 15°C$), and two point discrimination was tested with Semmes-weinstein monofilaments.

The following factors and their relationship with flap sensory recovery were analyzed: age, smoking, history, size of the defect, and administration of postoperative radiation therapy (Tables 1, 2, and 3). Comparative statistical analysis ($P \leq 0.05$) between the variety of flaps was performed using a Students-t-test for two point discrimination, and light touch sensation, age, smoking, and length of followup.

Fisher's exact test analysis was used to evaluate hot-cold discrimination and the effect of using postoperative radiation therapy. Quality of life questionnaire was performed to assess articulation, oral continence, and aesthetic satisfaction in patients (in the appendix). Patients were evaluated at postoperative 3 and 6 months for the above mentioned tests. The relationship between cigarette smoking and sensory reinnervation has been evaluated and described in Table 2.

TABLE 1: Age and temperature perception on the lower lip with noninnervated flaps.

	Control	Fan flaps	Noninnervated radial forearm flap	Total
<60 yrs	20	10	7	37
>60 yrs	12	6	5	23

TABLE 2: Smoking and temperature perception on the lower lip with noninnervated flaps.

	Control	Fan flaps	Noninnervated radial forearm flaps	Total
NonSmokers	13	12	7	32
Smokers	19	4	5	28

TABLE 3: Radiation therapy and temperature perception on the lower lip with noninnervated flaps.

	Fan flaps	Noninnervated radial forearm flaps	Total
Nonirradiated	4	6	10
Radiated	1	4	5

3. Results

Seventy-three noninnervated flaps showed comparable results with 52 innervated flaps for the lower lip reconstruction at the time of evaluation, a minimum of 6 months after the reconstruction. A statistical difference between innervated and noninnervated flaps was not seen.

Sensory recovery and sensation to touch was followed in order by two point discrimination and warm versus cold discrimination.

The earliest return of sensation to touch was recorded 3 months after surgery in patients with Nakajima fan flaps (Figures 3(a), 3(b), and 3(c)), and in 3 patients with Karapandzic fan flaps, the latest 24 months with radial forearm free noninnervated flap (Figures 4(a), 4(b), 5(a), 5(b), and 5(c)) postoperatively [5, 6].

Five patients failed to regain any flap sensation after followup of 25 and 18 months, respectively especially in patients reconstructed with pectoralis major myocutaneous flaps and radial forearm free flaps.

68% of the patients showed some sensibility to touch in pectoralis major myocutaneous flaps eventually. Overall there was a strong trend for sensory recovery in fasciocutaneous flaps over myocutaneous flaps (depressor anguli oris flap (Figures 5(a), 5(b), and 5(c)), submental is and flap, and pectoralis major myocutaneous flap) (p:0.09). The patients in our study did tend to perceive functional improvement when recipient site sensation was improved.

TABLE 4: Incontinence frequency in noninnervated and innervated flaps.

	Depressor anguli oris	Karapandzic flap	Nakajima flap	Fujimori gate flap	Submental island flap	Fan flap	Pectoralis major flap	Radial forearm flap
Incontinence	2	4	1	1	1	12	3	8

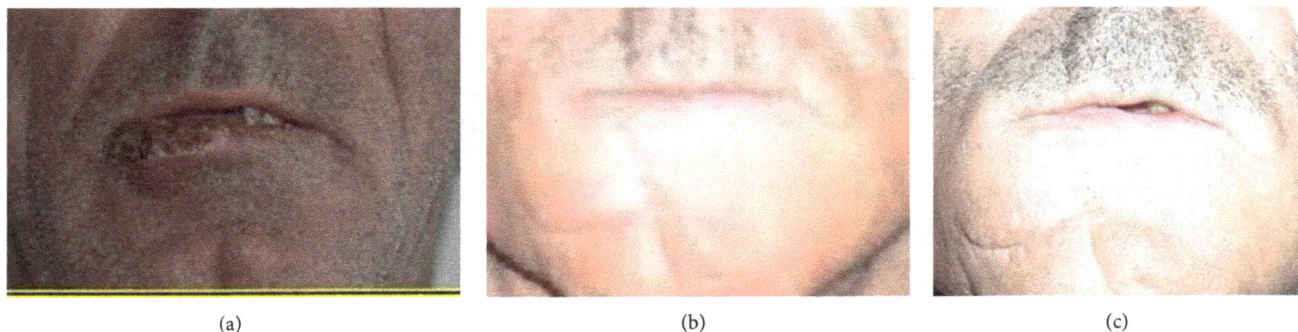

(a)   (b)   (c)

FIGURE 1: (a) Frontal view of patient with lower lip squamous cell carcinoma. (b) Postoperative view of unilateral depressor anguli oris flap. (c) Close-up view of unilateral depressor anguli oris flap.

Two point discrimination tests showed sensibility of the transposed flaps comparable to the original cheek (cheek 2–12 mm), flap average of 10 mm (6–14 mm).

In patients who received radiotherapy, xerostomia was an additional factor complicating oral function since radiotherapy in the head and neck region causes saliva production problems (Table 4).

Touch sensation and temperature perception were significantly decreased when patients had received postoperative radiation therapy ($n = 18$).

Patients had more satisfactory aesthetic results with fan flaps and depressor anguli oris flaps Figures 1(a), 1(b), 1(c), 2(a), 2(b), and 2(c).

We thought that patient age is closely related to postoperative oral function and sensory recovery of the flaps and we tried to demonstrate this relationship in our study.

Patients over the age of 58 showed relatively slower sensory recovery than others. Furthermore, flap thickness, quality of the recipient bed, and regional innervation are thought to play a role in the sensory recovery of noninnervated flaps. In our study we demonstrated this by the recovery rate of pectoralis major myocutaneous flap and submental island, and radial forearm flaps since they showed significantly slower recovery to superficial touch. There was a tendency for younger patients ($P = 0.09$) to have better articulation and oral continence postoperatively.

The results of our study in a fairly large group of patients revealed that there was not a significant sensory recovery in innervated flaps for lower lip reconstruction; these flaps included in this study being depressor anguli oris flaps, karapandzic flaps, nakajima and fujimori flaps, and submental island flaps.

4. Discussion

Nerve regrowth was investigated by several authors throughout the literature [7]. Shindo et al. (1955) investigated the differences in subjective sensibility of facial skin reconstruction versus oral cavity reconstruction with noninnervated skin flaps [8, 9].

Dellon (1988) proposed an association between eventual sensation and the number of sensory fibres connected with the receptor area [10]. The most important factor for natural recovery of noninnervated flaps appears to be the axonal sprouting from the recipient bed to the surface of the flap permitting axonal ingrowth [11].

Although complete recovery over the entire flap does not occur especially in free or pedicled flaps with a thick skin paddle, Hoppenjei et al. reported reinnervation in 5 patients reconstructed with pectoralis major myocutaneous flaps which showed some sensibility to touch [12].

The extent of trigeminal nerve branches that are resected with the tumor is also very important in axonal sprouting. The size of defects is important in sensory recovery. Shindo et al. reported that the degree of natural sensory recovery was greatest when flaps were used for smaller defects because spontaneous reinnervation depends on residual nerve population [7].

Histochemical studies of human skin grafts and flaps provide a basis for an understanding of the mechanism of sensory recovery in noninnervated flaps [13]. Dykes et al. obtained incisional biopsies from nine patients who had undergone skin grafting and found significant histochemical evidence of regenerating nerves at the bed and margins of the skin grafts 3 weeks after surgery [14, 15]. Chemotactic factors in the orientation of neural regeneration are suggested in

(a)

(b)

(c)

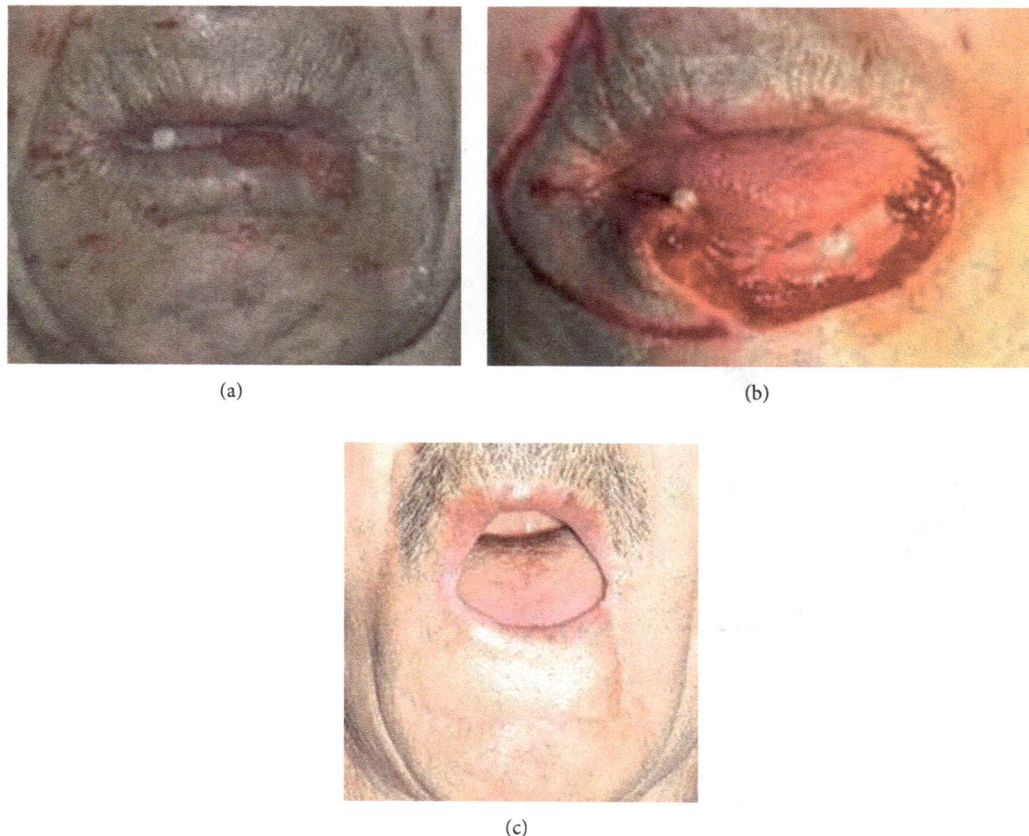

FIGURE 2: (a) Frontal view of patient with lower lip squamous cell carcinoma. (b) Peroperative view of unilateral fan flap. (c) Postoperative mouth-opening of the fan flap.

this phenomenon. The phenomenon of reinnervation by the surrounding tissues has been described by Vriens and Close [16, 17].

The pattern of sensory recovery found in this series of patients of innervated and noninnervated flaps used for total lower lip reconstruction is quite different from others reported in the literature.

For example, the return of sensation to touch in our noninnervated flap patients was comparable and almost equivalent to innervated flaps. In our patients, sensation to touch was noted as soon as 3 months after surgery in patients with Nakajima and Karapandzic fan flaps and as late as 24 months postoperatively in radial forearm free flaps [18].

Similar to the findings in our study, improvement in two point discrimination in transferred flaps compared with that in the donor area has been reported. Cordeiro et al. assumed that this phenomenon was due to the wide cortical representation of these areas [19, 20].

The return of flap sensation in our study did correlate statistically ($P = 0.045$) with both articulation and oral continence. However, multiple factors affected the recovery of articulation and oral continence among which are effects

of postoperative radiation therapy (pain, reduction of saliva), the resolution of postoperative and postradiotherapy edema, and the patient's ability to adapt to their new anatomy.

In our study, sensory recovery was more likely to occur after fan flaps ($n = 86$) than after myocutaneous flaps ($n = 24$). This relative lack of sensory recovery following myocutaneous flaps has been reported by Turkof et al. as well [5]. Turkof tested sensory recovery in 16 free myocutaneous flaps used for the lower extremity reconstruction. After followup of 18 months only 4 patients (25%) had recovery of touch and two point discrimination. Our findings support this observation.

5. Conclusion

This study compares sensory recovery after total lower lip reconstruction in a wide variety of flaps including bilateral depressor anguli oris flap, submental island flap, bilateral fan flaps, radial forearm flap, and pectoralis major myocutaneous flaps in a large number of patients.

We believe that our conclusions will help explain some of the differing reports in the literature on the sensory recovery of noninnervated flaps and will help the surgeons in their

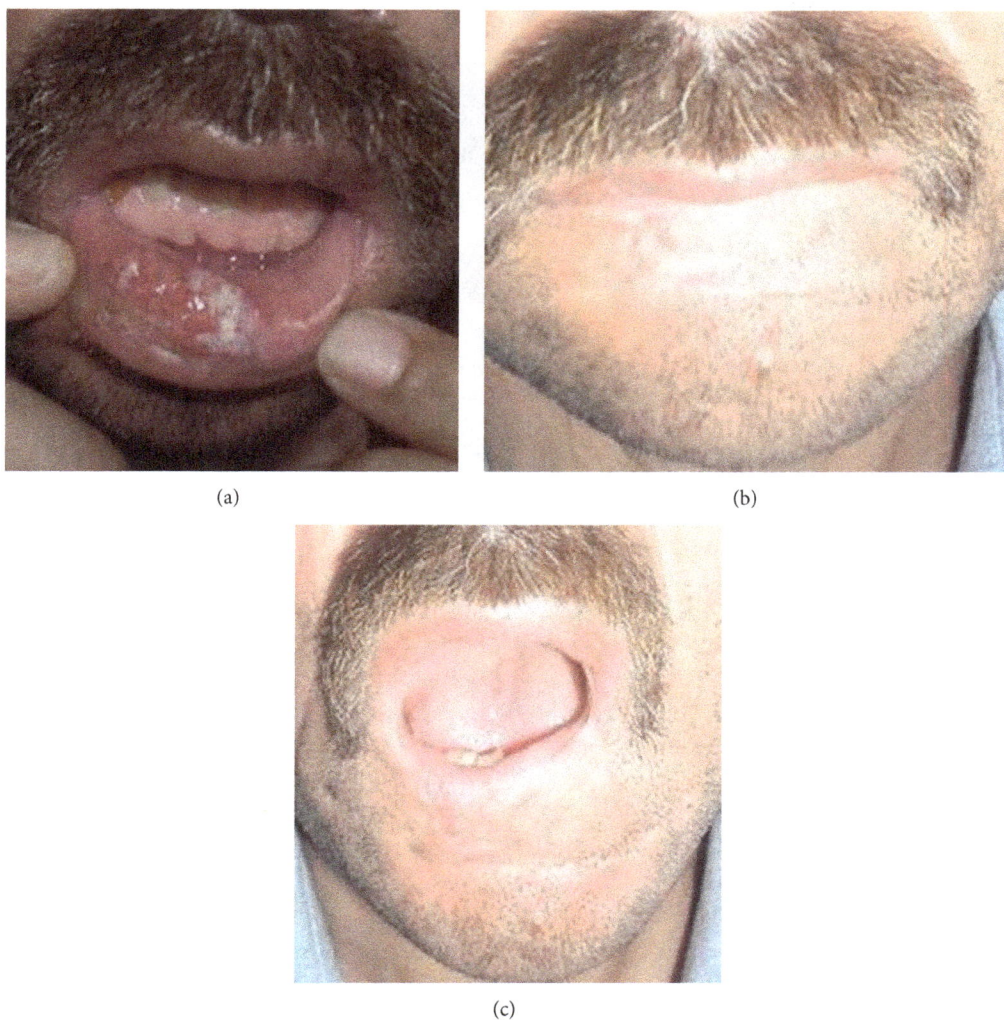

FIGURE 3: (a) Frontal view of patient with lower lip squamous cell carcinoma. (b) Postoperative view of bilateral karapandzic flap. (c) Postoperative mouth-opening of the karapandzic flap.

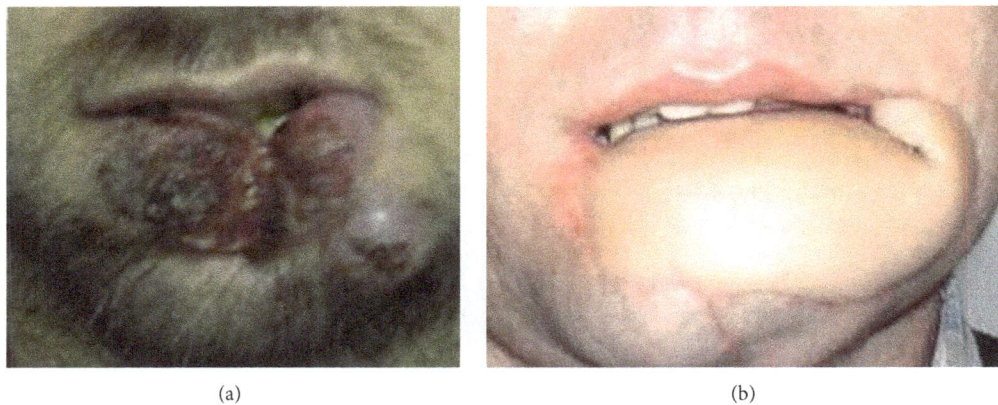

FIGURE 4: (a) Frontal view of patient with lower lip squamous cell carcinoma. (b) Postoperative view of radial forearm free noninnervated flap.

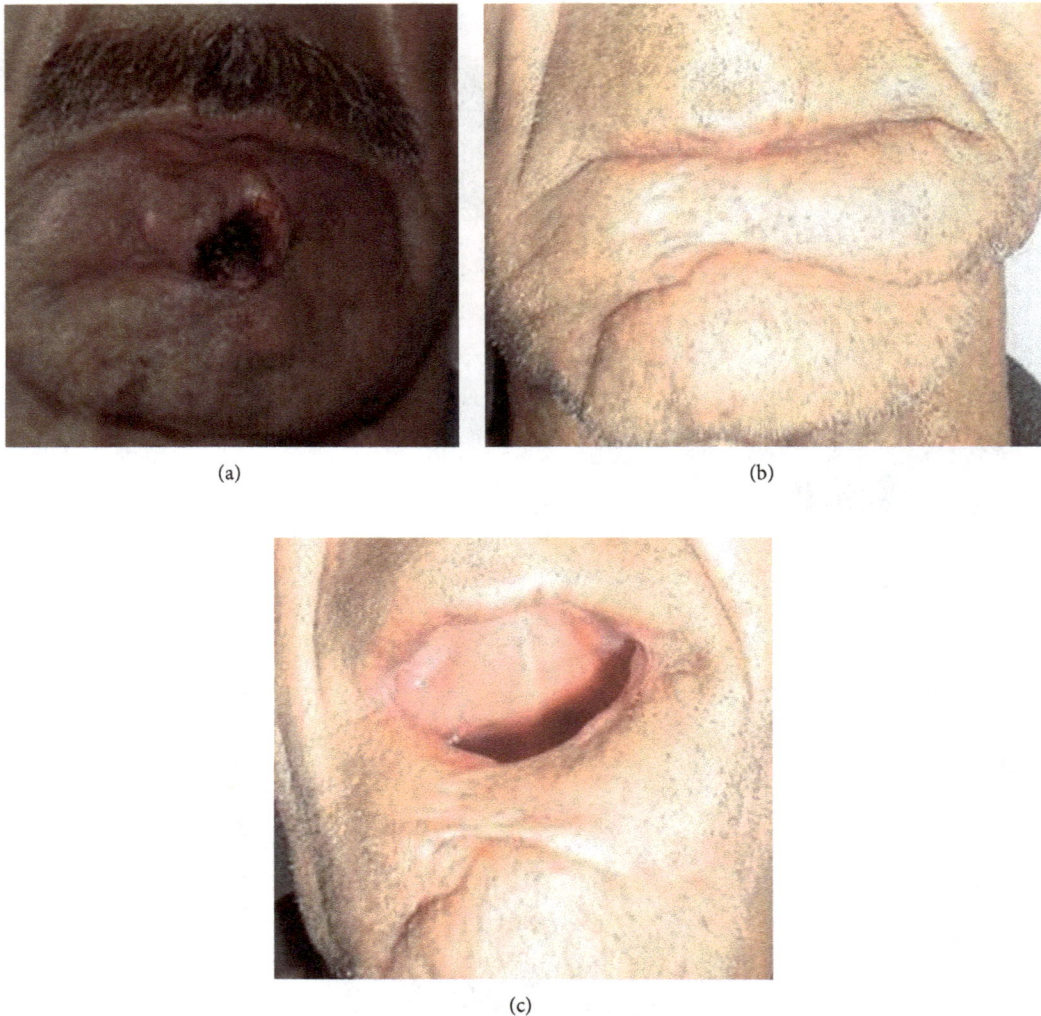

(a)

(b)

(c)

FIGURE 5: (a) Frontal view of patient with lower lip squamous cell carcinoma. (b) Postoperative frontal view of bilateral depressor anguli oris flap. (c) Postoperative mouth-opening in bilateral depressor anguli oris patient.

everyday practice when confronted with a total lower lip reconstruction.

Appendix

Questionnaire

Eating

Do you have trouble with drinking?

To what extent have you changed your meals since the operation?

Do you have a dry mouth?

Do you splutter during speaking?

Do you have problems with drooling? On which side?

Speech

Do you have trouble speaking clearly?

Has your speech changed since the operation?

Can you make yourself comprehensible during a telephone-conversation?

Aesthetics

How would you rate your present appearance?

Do you find the scar(s) in your face annoying?

Does your appearance have a negative effect during your everyday-life?

References

[1] R. Fujimori, "Gate flap for total reconstruction of the lower lip," *British Journal of Plastic Surgery*, vol. 33, pp. 330–340, 1980.

Sensory Recovery with Innervated and Noninnervated Flaps after Total Lower Lip...

127

[2] Y. Ducic and M. Burge, "Nasolabial flap reconstruction of oral cavity defects: a report of 18 cases," *Journal of Oral and Maxillofacial Surgery*, vol. 58, pp. 1104–1108, 2000.

[3] H.-D. Gillies and D.-R. Millard Jr., "Lip trauma," in *Principles and Art of Plastic Surgery*, vol. 2, pp. 496–519, Little Brown, Boston, Mass, USA, 1957.

[4] G.-R. Tobin and T.-G. O'Daniel, "Lip reconstruction with motor and sensory innervated composite flaps," *Clinics in Plastic Surgery*, vol. 17, no. 4, pp. 623–632, 1990.

[5] Y. Kimata, K. Uchiyama, S. Ebinara et al., "Comparison of innervated and noninnervated free flaps in oral reconstruction," *Plastic and Reconstructive Surgery*, vol. 104, no. 5, pp. 1307–1313, 1999.

[6] D. Netscher, A.-H. Armenta, R.-A. Meade, and E.-L. Alford, "Sensory recovery in innervated and non-innervated radial forearm free flaps: functional implications," *Journal of Reconstructive Microsurgery*, vol. 16, pp. 179–180, 2000.

[7] M.-L. Shindo, U.-K. Sinha, and D.-H. Rice, "Sensory recovery in noninnervated free flaps for head and neck reconstruction," *Laryngoscope*, vol. 105, article 1290, 1995.

[8] P.-M. Finlay, F. Dawson, A.-G. Robertson et al., "An evaluation of functional outcome after surgery and radiotherapy for intraoral cancer," *British Journal of Oral and Maxillofacial Surgery*, vol. 30, pp. 14–17, 1992.

[9] K.-L. Woodward and D.-R. Kenshab Sr., "The recovery of sensory function following skin flaps in humans," *Plastic and Reconstructive Surgery*, vol. 79, article 428, 1987.

[10] A.-L. Dellon, *Evaluation of Sensibility and Re-Education of Sensation in the Hand*, John D. Lucas, Baltimore, Md, USA, 1988.

[11] G. Lundborg, Q. Zhao, M. Kanje et al., "Can sensory and motor collateral sprouting be induced from intact peripheral nerve by end-to-side anastomosis?" *Journal of Hand Surgery*, vol. 19, article 277, 1994.

[12] T.-S.-M. Hoppenjei, H.-P.-M. Freihofer, J.-J.-A. Browns et al., "Sensibility and cutaneous reinnervation in pectoralis major myocutaneous island flaps," *Journal of Cranio-Maxillofacial Surgery*, vol. 18, article 237, 1990.

[13] E. Turkof, W. Jurecka, G. Sikos, and H. Piza-Katzer, "Sensory recovery in myocutaneous, noninnervated free flaps: a morphologic, immunohistochemical, and electron microscopic study," *Plastic and Reconstructive Surgery*, vol. 92, article 238, 1993.

[14] R.-W. Dykes, J.-K. Terzis, and B. Strauch, "Sensations from surgically transferred glabrous skin: central versus peripheral factors," *Canadian Journal of Neurological Sciences*, vol. 6, article 437, 1979.

[15] J.-S. Davis and E.-A. Kitlowski, "Regeneration of nerves in skin grafts and skin flaps," *The American Journal of Surgery*, vol. 24, pp. 501–545, 1934.

[16] J.-P.-M. Vriens, R. Acosta, D.-S. Soutar et al., "Recovery of sensation in the radial forearm free flap in oral reconstruction," *Plastic and Reconstructive Surgery*, vol. 98, pp. 649–656, 1996.

[17] L.-G. Close, J.-M. Truelson, R.-A. Milledfe et al., "Sensory recovery in noninnervated flaps used for oral cavity and oropharyngeal reconstruction," *Archives of Otolaryngology*, vol. 121, pp. 967–972, 1995.

[18] A. Ciconetti, C. Matteini, G. Cruccu, and A. Romaniello, "Comparative study on sensory recovery after oral cavity reconstruction by free flaps: preliminary results," *Journal of Cranio-Maxillofacial Surgery*, vol. 28, pp. 74–78, 2000.

[19] H.-S. Matlaub, D.-L. Larson, J.-G. Kuhn, N.-G. Yousif, and J.-R. Sanger, "Lateral arm free flap in oral cavity reconstruction: a functional evaluation," *Head & Neck*, vol. 11, article 205, 1989.

[20] P.-G. Cordeiro, M. Schwartz, R.-I. Neves, and R. Tuma, "A comparison of donor and recipient site sensation in free tissue reconstruction of the oral cavity," *Annals of Plastic Surgery*, vol. 39, article 461, 1997.

20

Nose and Midface Augmentation by Rib Cartilage Grafts: Methods and Outcome in 32 Cases

Adham Farouk and Saad Ibrahiem

Department of Plastic and Reconstructive Surgery, Faculty of Medicine, Alexandria University, Alexandria, Egypt

Correspondence should be addressed to Adham Farouk; mail@adhamfarouk.com

Academic Editor: Nicolo Scuderi

Recession of the midface is a relatively common condition that can have a negative impact on facial and nasal aesthetic appearance, and it poses a challenge to plastic surgeons. In cases with generalized maxillary retrusion and/or malocclusion, bone advancement surgery is required, but in localized cases, mostly seen in cleft lip patients, the quest is for an ideal material and a proper technique that would be used to augment the receding area. Throughout a period of seven years, thirty-two patients with nose and midface retrusion were managed by a construct of rib cartilage grafts designed to compensate the deficiency at the maxillary, piriform, and premaxillary areas. Results were satisfactory for most patients in terms of improved fullness of malar area, improved nasal tip projection and rotation, and improvement of upper lip. The presented technique of rib cartilage grafting is a safe and effective method for nose and midface augmentation.

1. Introduction

A wide variety of pathologic entities causes alteration of midfacial skeletal growth, resulting in varying degrees of midface deficiency presenting as maxillary retrusion with or without malocclusion. These include acquired conditions (posttraumatic and postsurgical) and congenital deformities; best known example (and most common as well) is the patients with cleft lip and palate, in whom the nature of the deformity (deficiency and hypoplasia of maxilla and piriform aperture) and the surgical procedures used to correct it take their toll on the final shape and projection of the midface. This condition is frequently accompanied by other deformities like nasal base recess, nasal tip ptosis, sunken cheeks, and deficient upper lip thrust [1–6].

Many surgical procedures have been suggested and various techniques have been described to address such deformities, with varying degrees of success and complications. These included surgical bone advancement, distraction osteogenesis, autologous osseous and cartilaginous grafts, homologous cartilaginous grafts, and alloplastic implants [1–4, 7–19].

This paper presents a technique of using rib cartilage grafts for nose and midface augmentation in a series of patients.

2. Patients and Methods

Thirty-two patients with maxillary hypoplasia, piriform deficiency, alar base recess, nasal tip ptosis, and deficient upper lip thrust, secondary to cleft lip anomaly, referred for correction of such deformities, throughout the period from 2007 to 2014, were subject to augmentation by rib cartilage grafts.

Adequate preoperative analysis involved detailed history taking, thorough clinical examination, and three-dimensional computed tomography for accurate diagnosis of the skeletal defects (Figure 1(a)), and for adequate planning of the shape and position of the cartilaginous grafts required to augment those skeletal defects (Figure 1(b)).

Surgery was performed under general anesthesia, with local infiltration of the perimeter of the surgical fields (nasolabial and chest wall areas) with 1 : 10000 nore-pinephrine.

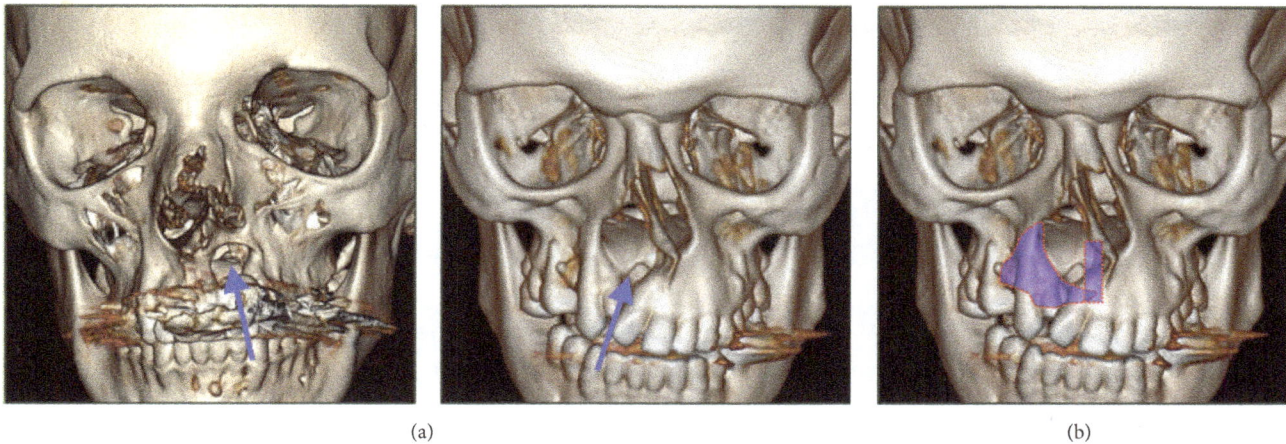

FIGURE 1: (a) Computed tomography pictures of two patients; arrows point to maxillary and piriform deficiency. (b) Computed tomography picture used to fashion the design of the cartilaginous construct (superimposed blue shapes).

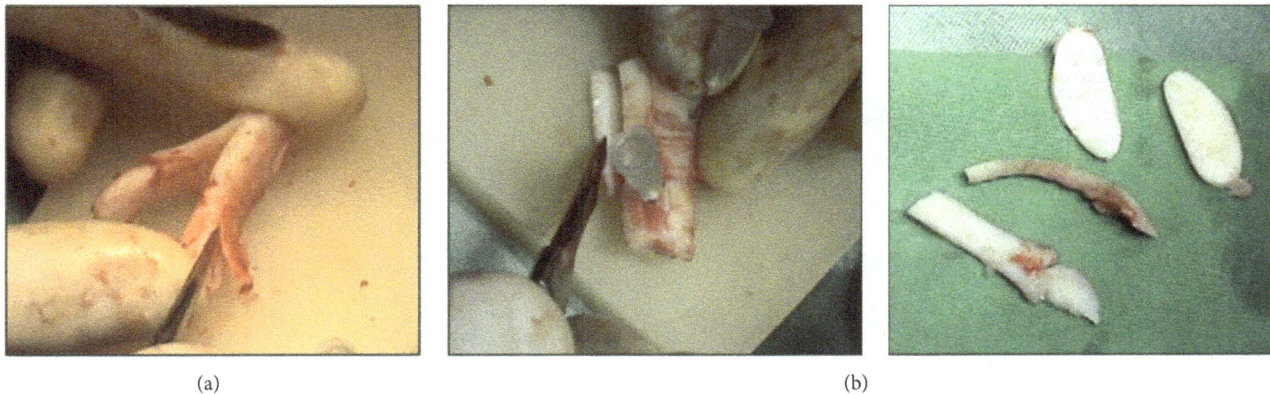

FIGURE 2: Carving rib cartilage grafts. (a) Carving a straight rod out of the central portion of rib cartilage specimen. (b) Carving thin plates out of the peripheral portion of rib cartilage specimen.

The cartilaginous part of the right sixth or seventh rib is harvested (by subperichondrial dissection) through a 5–7 cm transverse incision over the relevant area at the chest wall. Two types of grafts are then sculpted out of the harvested cartilage; the first is a straight (30–40 mm × 5 mm) rod graft carved from the central portion of the rib cartilage (Figure 2(a)), and the second is multiple 1–1.5 mm thickness plates with different shapes and surface areas carved from the remainder of the rib cartilage (Figure 2(b)).

The nasal skeleton was exposed through an external approach, and the piriform aperture and maxilla were exposed through an incision along the border of upper lip and nasal sill (Figure 3(a)). The above-mentioned cartilaginous grafts were then laid into a construct with two components: an anteromedial component comprising a suitable length of the straight rod graft and vertically oriented as a columellar strut and a posterolateral component comprising the plate grafts layered over each other in variable orientations according to the specific pattern needed for each particular case to augment the nasal floor, lateral nasal wall, and maxilla (Figure 3(b)).

The grafts are sutured to each other and fixed to medial crura of lower lateral cartilages, caudal end of septum, periosteum of anterior nasal spine, piriform aperture, and maxilla by permanent sutures (Figure 4). (Note that, in bilateral cases, the cartilaginous graft construct had 3 components: one anteromedial and two posterolateral components.)

Optional additional steps to remodel the nasal skeleton included hump resection, septoplasty, cephalic trims of alar cartilages, lobular alar cartilage incision and overlap, lateral crural steal or overlay, and interdomal tip refining sutures.

All patients received antibiotics for 10 days starting the night before the operation, and wash of surgical fields with gentamycin-saline solution was carried out throughout the surgery. Chest wall and nasal wounds were closed in layers, nasal cavities were packed for 3-4 days, and an external nasal splint was applied for 7–10 days.

3. Results

Out of the 32 patients enrolled for the described technique, 29 patients (90.6%) had unilateral augmentation and 3 patients

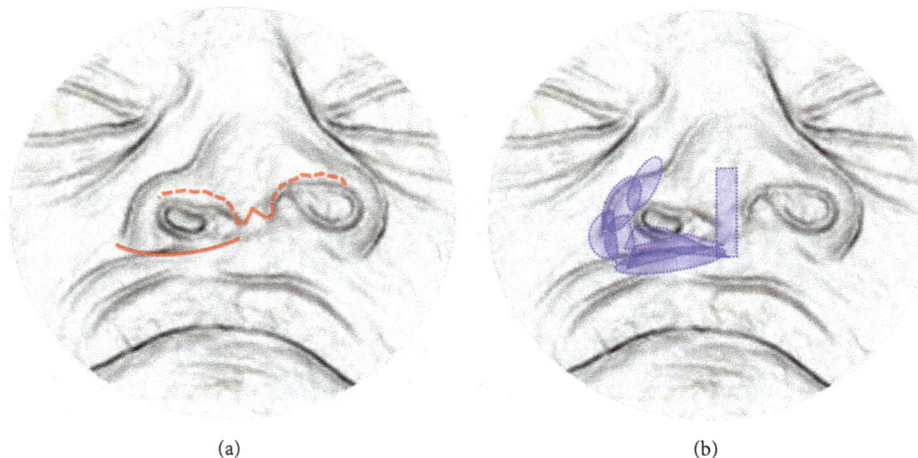

(a)   (b)

FIGURE 3: (a) Diagram illustrating the incision along the border of upper lip and nasal sill to expose the maxilla and piriform aperture, and the transcolumellar infracartilaginous incision to expose the nasal skeleton. (b) Diagram showing the planned shapes and arrangement of the cartilaginous implants.

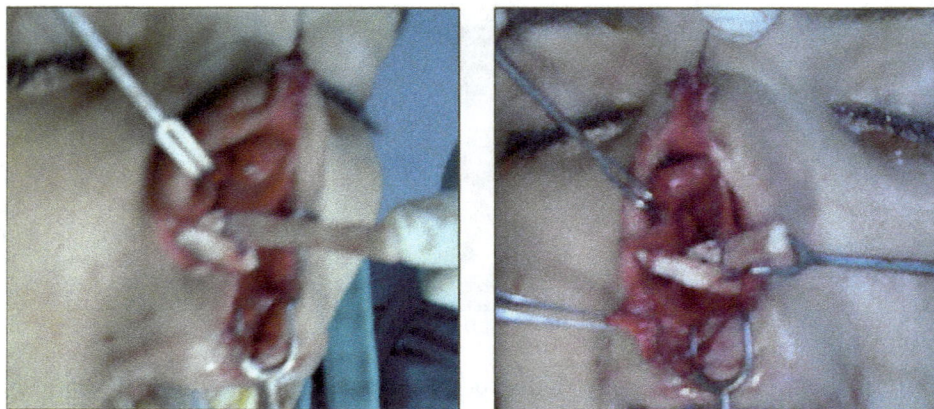

FIGURE 4: Two views during implantation of the rib cartilage construct.

(9.4%) had bilateral augmentation. They were 26 females (81.25%) and 6 males (18.75%). Their age ranged from 18 to 27 years and the mean age at the time of surgery was 21.9 years. The number of previous surgeries (lip/palate/nose) ranged from 1 to 6 surgeries (mean: 2 surgeries).

Throughout the follow-up period that ranged from 6 months to 7 years (mean: 47.5 months), surgical results were satisfactory to most patients and only one case required a revision rhinoplasty for refinement of nasal dorsum after 2 years.

Figures 5–7 depict 3 examples to the outcome of rib cartilage grafts for nose and midface augmentation. These pictures illustrate significant improvement of midface deficiency, nasal tip projection/rotation, and upper lip thrust, and the basal view of Figure 5 demonstrates distinctive improvement of alar base position and nasal sill morphology. Figure 5(c) illustrates the relative size and position of the cartilaginous implants.

Minor complications occurred in 2 patients (6.25%) in the form of hypertrophic scarring of the chest wall wound, which responded well to topical therapy without any need for surgical scar revision, and in 1 patient (3.1%), necrosis at the columellar wound edge occurred and resulted in exposure of a part of the cartilage graft (Figure 8) but did not mandate its extraction and eventually healed by secondary intention.

4. Discussion

Recession of the midface is a relatively common condition that can have a negative impact on facial and nasal aesthetic appearance, and it poses a challenge to plastic surgeons. In the less frequent cases of midface deficiency that exhibits generalized retrusion of the maxilla (retrognathic maxilla) and/or malocclusion, distraction osteogenesis orthognathic surgery, or intraoral maxillary expansion is indicated, but in the more frequent cases exhibiting localized retrusion without malocclusion, characteristically seen in, but not limited to, patients with cleft lip deformity, the quest is for an ideal material and a proper technique that would be used to augment the receding area.

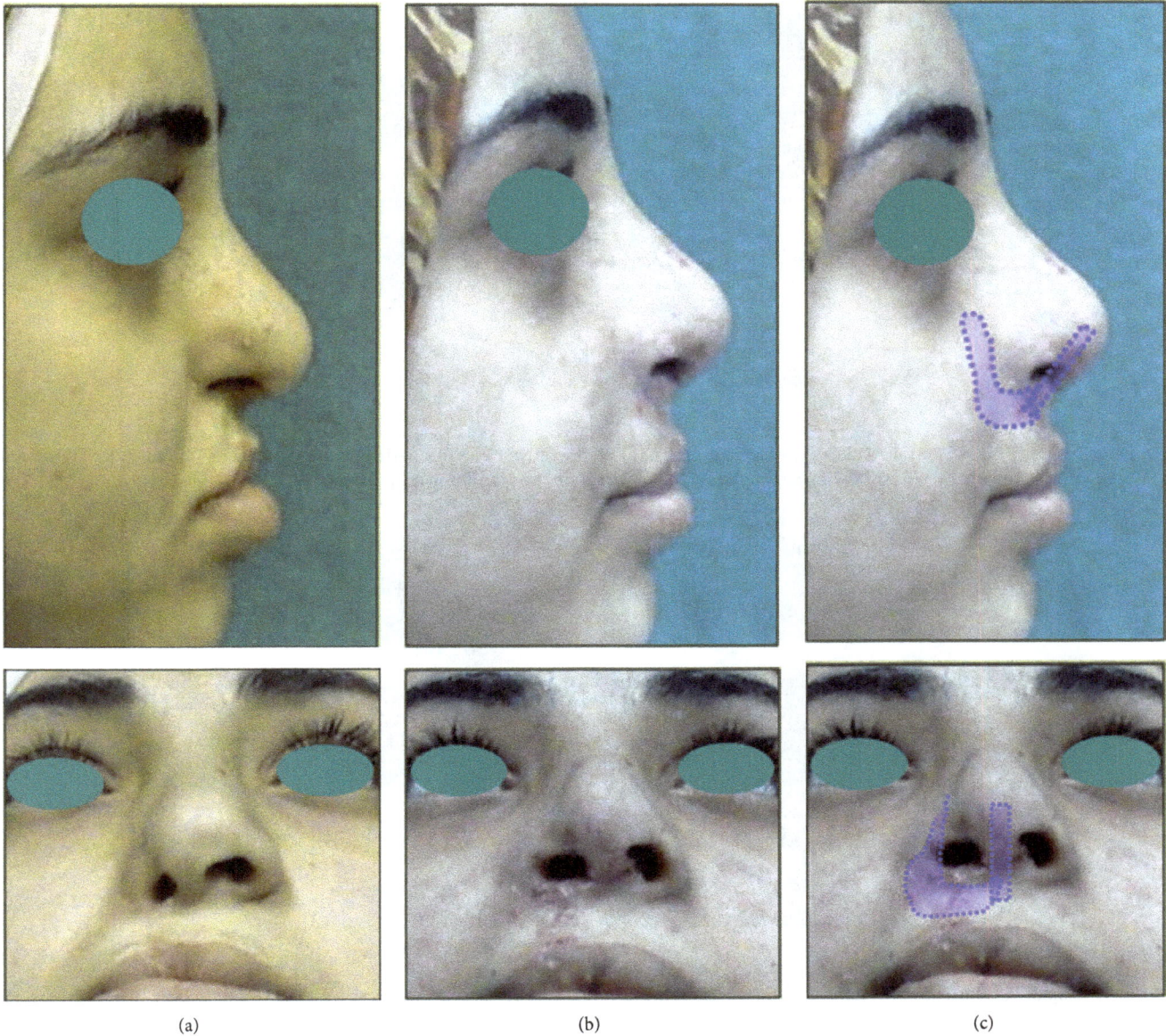

FIGURE 5: Example (1) for clinical results of rib cartilage grafts. (a) Preoperative views of a patient with recession of nasal floor, alar base, and malar area, and obtuse nasolabial angle. (b) Two-week postoperative views showing improved receding elements, nasal tip rotation, and upper lip thrust. (c) Superimposed blue shapes demonstrate the relative size and position of the cartilaginous implants.

Regarding the materials (implants) that can be used for nose and midface augmentation, they fall into three categories according to their source: autologous implants (costal cartilage or calvarial bone), homologous implants (irradiated costal cartilage, acellular dermis), and alloplastic implants (silicone, polyethylene, polytetrafluoroethylene, polyesters, and polyamides). The main advantages of homologous cartilage and alloplastic implants are the unlimited supply and the absence of donor site morbidity, yet the significant disadvantages of possible autoimmune reactions, extrusion, infection, high cost, and patients' concerns about their artificial nature and their safety diminish the odds of their appropriateness for use in this purpose [11, 20–24].

Therefore, the biocompatibility of autologous implants is the main overweighting factor for their selection in this respect.

In comparison to costal cartilage grafts, bone grafts are more difficult to harvest, shape, and fix, are more prone to resorption, and have more potential significant donor site morbidity [23, 24]. This being said, we believe that rib cartilage graft is the most feasible choice for use in the purpose of midface augmentation. It has the lowest rates of rejection, resorption, and infection, is easily harvested and sculpted, and is available in plentiful supply, and our surgical technique adopted specific tactics and precautions that would optimize the results and minimize its drawbacks and side effects.

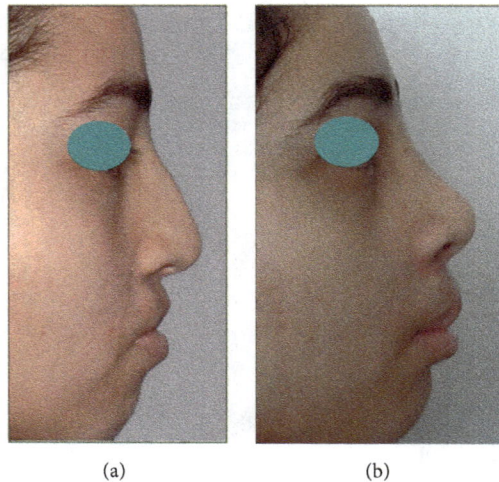

FIGURE 6: Example (2) for clinical results of rib cartilage grafts. (a) Preoperative views of a patient with premaxillary and maxillary retrusion. (b) Three-year postoperative views showing augmented midface, nasal rotation, and upper lip thrust.

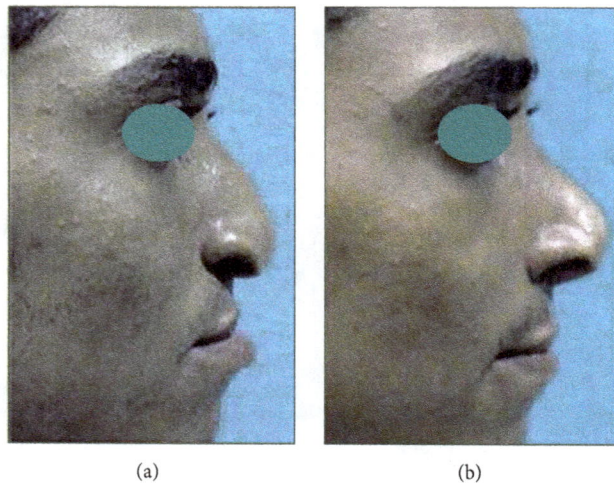

FIGURE 7: Example (3) for clinical results of rib cartilage grafts. (a) Preoperative views of a patient with premaxillary depression and droopy nasal tip. (b) Two-year postoperative views showing augmented midface, nasal rotation, and upper lip thrust.

Strictly aseptic surgical conditions under a strong antibiotic umbrella and liberal wash of surgical fields with gentamycin-saline solution and starting the operation with the process of cartilage graft harvesting, shaping, and soaking in antibiotic-saline solution minimized potential contamination from nasal mucosa and kept infection rate nil in our cases.

Delaying closure of the chest wall wound to allow returning of any remaining pieces of cartilage into the costal defect, and closure of the perichondrium followed by meticulous closure of the wound in layers, prevented the incidence of any significant donor site morbidity.

To maximize survival of the implanted cartilage, and also to make it more amenable to fit onto the irregular defects of the premaxilla, piriform margins, and maxilla, we used thin (1–1.5 mm) slices and stacked them in layers sutured to the periosteum and to each other. Though the most significant drawback of rib cartilage grafts, which is cartilage "warping," is not a big concern in "rough volume augmentation" of midface defect as it would be in "fine shaping" of nasal dorsum, still, the thin slicing can neutralize the mechanical vectors and minimize the impact of any possible warping, and for the columellar strut that is used to correct the droopy nasal tip and nasolabial angle, we employed the most commonly applied method for combating cartilage warping by obtaining balanced cross section from the center of the rib cartilage specimen.

Most of the patients were satisfied by the results and only one of the earlier cases in this series developed a significant complication in the form of exposure of part of the cartilage graft that healed with secondary intention and this complication was attributable to a misfortunate wound edge necrosis (at the most distal part of the columellar flap) and not attributable to an inherent defect in the technique.

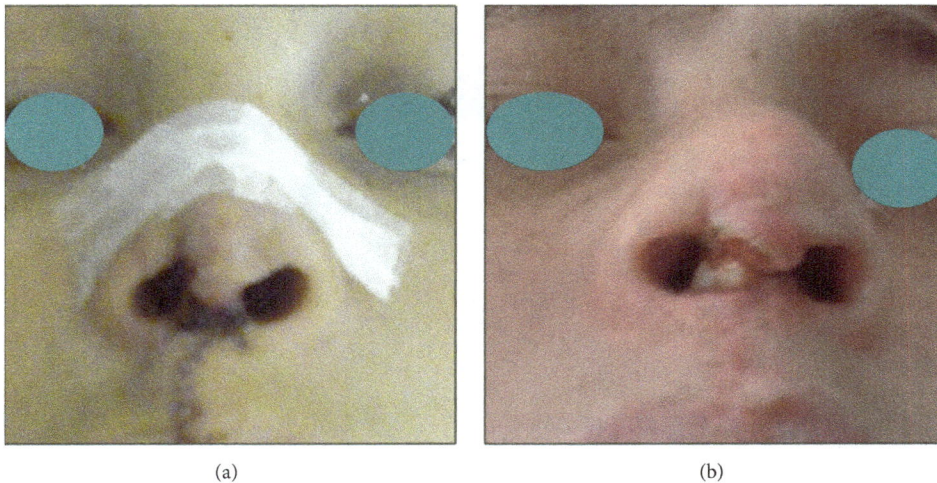

(a)   (b)

FIGURE 8: Picture of a complication which occurred. (a) Skin necrosis at distal part of the columellar flap. (b) Exposure of a part of the rib cartilage graft.

5. Conclusions

The described technique of rib cartilage grafting is a safe, versatile tool for nose and midface augmentation. It can be a good and relatively simple alternative to orthognathic and distraction surgeries in cases of cleft lip deformity without malocclusion, and in cases with malocclusion it can be a complementary procedure to those surgeries when their results are insufficient. The described technique yields not only augmentation of the alar base and malar area retrusion but also improvement of nasal tip projection/rotation and upper lip thrust; that is, it optimizes the aesthetic appearance of all the components of the midface region.

Ethical Approval

All procedures performed in the study involving human participants were in accordance with the ethical standards of the institutional and/or national research committee and with the 1964 Helsinki declaration and its later amendments or comparable ethical standards.

References

[1] S. Menon, R. Sinha, R. Manerikar, and S. K. Roy Chowdhury, "Correction of midface deficiency using intra-oral distraction device," *Journal of Maxillofacial and Oral Surgery*, vol. 9, no. 1, pp. 57–59, 2010.

[2] W. S. Kim, C.-H. Kim, and J.-H. Yoon, "Premaxillary augmentation using autologous costal cartilage as an adjunct to rhinoplasty," *Journal of Plastic, Reconstructive and Aesthetic Surgery*, vol. 63, no. 9, pp. e686–e690, 2010.

[3] N. Fanous and A. Yoskovitch, "Premaxillary augmentation: adjunct to rhinoplasty," *Plastic and Reconstructive Surgery*, vol. 106, no. 3, pp. 707–712, 2000.

[4] J. M. Gurley, T. Pilgram, C. A. Perlyn, J. L. Marsh, and F. J. Menick, "Long-term outcome of autogenous rib graft nasal reconstruction," *Plastic and Reconstructive Surgery*, vol. 108, no. 7, pp. 1895–1907, 2001.

[5] M. D. Fisher, D. M. Fisher, and J. R. Marcus, "Correction of the cleft nasal deformity: from infancy to maturity," *Clinics in Plastic Surgery*, vol. 41, no. 2, pp. 283–299, 2014.

[6] B. Guyuron, "MOC-PS(SM) CME article: late cleft lip nasal deformity," *Plastic and Reconstructive Surgery*, vol. 121, no. 4, supplement, pp. 1–11, 2008.

[7] A. Rachmiel, "Treatment of maxillary cleft palate: distraction osteogenesis versus orthognathic surgery—part one: maxillary distraction," *Journal of Oral and Maxillofacial Surgery*, vol. 65, no. 4, pp. 753–757, 2007.

[8] S. L. Austin, C. R. Mattick, and P. J. Waterhouse, "Distraction osteogenesis versus orthognathic surgery for the treatment of maxillary hypoplasia in cleft lip and palate patients: a systematic review," *Orthodontics & Craniofacial Research*, vol. 18, no. 2, pp. 96–108, 2015.

[9] D. M. Kahn, J. Broujerdi, and S. A. Schendel, "Internal maxillary distraction with a new bimalar device," *Journal of Oral and Maxillofacial Surgery*, vol. 66, no. 4, pp. 675–683, 2008.

[10] W. Smolka, N. Eggensperger, A. Kollar, and T. Iizuka, "Midfacial reconstruction using calvarial split bone grafts," *Archives of Otolaryngology—Head and Neck Surgery*, vol. 131, no. 2, pp. 131–136, 2005.

[11] M. E. Tardy Jr., J. Denneny III, and M. H. Fritsch, "The versatile cartilage autograft in reconstruction of the nose and face," *Laryngoscope*, vol. 95, no. 5, pp. 523–533, 1985.

[12] A. J. C. Burke, T. D. Wang, and T. A. Cook, "Irradiated homograft rib cartilage in facial reconstruction," *Archives of Facial Plastic Surgery*, vol. 6, no. 5, pp. 334–341, 2004.

[13] T. A. Cook, T. D. Wang, P. J. Brownrigg, and V. C. Quatela, "Significant premaxillary augmentation," *Archives of Otolaryngology—Head and Neck Surgery*, vol. 116, no. 10, pp. 1197–1201, 1990.

[14] U. T. Hinderer, "Nasal base, maxillary, and infraorbital implants—alloplastic," *Clinics in Plastic Surgery*, vol. 18, no. 1, pp. 87–105, 1991.

[15] H. S. Byrd and P. C. Hobar, "Alloplastic nasal and perialar augmentation," *Clinics in Plastic Surgery*, vol. 23, no. 2, pp. 315–326, 1996.

[16] E. O. Terino, "Alloplastic midface augmentation," *Aesthetic Surgery Journal*, vol. 25, no. 5, pp. 512–520, 2005.

[17] N. N. Andrade and K. Raikwar, "Medpor in maxillofacial deformities: report of three cases," *Journal of Maxillofacial and Oral Surgery*, vol. 8, no. 2, pp. 192–195, 2009.

[18] L. Schoenrock and A. Reppucci, "Correction of subcutaneous facial defects using Gore-tex," *Facial Plastic Surgery Clinics of North America*, vol. 2, pp. 373–388, 1994.

[19] H. M. T. Foda, "Mersiline mesh in premaxillary augmentation," *Aesthetic Plastic Surgery*, vol. 29, no. 3, pp. 169–173, 2005.

[20] H. D. Vuyk and P. A. Adamson, "Biomaterials in rhinoplasty," *Clinical Otolaryngology & Allied Sciences*, vol. 23, no. 3, pp. 209–217, 1998.

[21] J. P. Porter, "Grafts in rhinoplasty: alloplastic vs autogenous," *Archives of Otolaryngology—Head and Neck Surgery*, vol. 126, no. 4, pp. 558–561, 2000.

[22] P. A. Adamson, "Grafts in rhinoplasty: autogenous grafts are superior to alloplastic," *Archives of Otolaryngology—Head and Neck Surgery*, vol. 126, no. 4, pp. 561–562, 2000.

[23] G. Lin and W. Lawson, "Complications using grafts and implants in rhinoplasty," *Operative Techniques in Otolaryngology*, vol. 18, no. 4, pp. 315–323, 2007.

[24] K. Ansari, J. Asaria, P. Hilger, and P. A. Adamson, "Grafts and implants in rhinoplasty—techniques and long-term results," *Operative Techniques in Otolaryngology*, vol. 19, no. 1, pp. 42–58, 2008.

21

Risk Factors and Surgical Refinements of Postresective Mandibular Reconstruction: A Retrospective Study

Akiko Sakakibara,[1] **Kazunobu Hashikawa,**[2] **Satoshi Yokoo,**[3] **Shunsuke Sakakibara,**[2] **Takahide Komori,**[1] **and Shinya Tahara**[4]

[1] *Department of Oral and Maxillofacial Surgery, Kobe University Graduate School of Medicine, Kobe 650-0017, Japan*
[2] *Department of Plastic Surgery, Kobe University Graduate School of Medicine, Kobe 650-0017, Japan*
[3] *Department of Stomatology and Maxillofacial Surgery, Gunma University Graduate School of Medicine, Gunma 371-8511, Japan*
[4] *Department of Plastic Surgery, Japanese Red Cross Kobe Hospital, Kobe 651-0073, Japan*

Correspondence should be addressed to Akiko Sakakibara; oguni@cool.odn.ne.jp

Academic Editor: Francesco Carinci

Background. Postresective mandibular reconstruction is common in cases of oral and mandibular tumors. However, complications such as infection, plate exposure, or plate fracture can occur. We identified several significant risk factors of complications after reconstructive surgery and compared the effectiveness of different surgical techniques for reducing the incidence of complications. *Methods.* This study is a retrospective analysis of 28 oromandibular cancer cases that required reconstructive surgery between January 1999 and December 2011 at Kobe University Graduate School of Medicine in Japan. All cases were classified using Hashikawa's CAT and Eichner's classification methods. Then, we determined whether these classifications and different treatment or surgical methods were significantly related to complications. *Results.* Complications after mandibular reconstruction occurred in 10/28 patients (36%). Specifically, five patients had plate fractures, four had plate exposures, and one had an infection. Radiation therapy and closure without any flaps were significantly related to infection or plate exposure. The wrap-around technique of securing reconstruction plates was used in 14 cases, whereas the run-through technique was used in two cases. *Conclusions.* The success of mandibular reconstruction depends on both mechanical and biological factors, such as the location of defects, presence of occlusions, and the amount of vascularization of the flap.

1. Introduction

Surgical resection of oral cavity and mandibular tumors often requires postresective mandibular reconstruction. The goals of mandibular reconstruction are primary wound closure, improvement of phonation and deglutition, and aesthetic restoration of the lower face. There are many techniques for mandibular reconstruction, such as soft-tissue free flaps, reconstruction plates, and bone grafts. Bone reconstruction is often the preferred method. For instance, the fibula free flap technique, which involves resection of vascularized bone from the fibula with a free flap of soft tissue and skin, can be used to reconstruct many types of mandibular defects with relative ease and few complications [1, 2]. However, when the donor bone cannot be harvested or the patient's

prognosis is poor, bone reconstruction may not be possible [3, 4]. In such cases, reconstruction plates can be used; however, complications such as infection, plate exposure or fracture, or loosening of the fixation can occur. Minimizing the risk of complications can be challenging, but optimizing the design and fabrication of reconstruction plates and improving surgical techniques may help reduce these risks [5, 6].

For example, the risk of plate exposure can be reduced by wrapping flaps around the reconstruction plate to improve its fit and thereby reduce skin tension and dead space. In our institutions, we have adopted the "wrap-around" and "run-through" techniques in mandibular reconstructions performed using rectus abdominis musculocutaneous flaps. The wrap-around technique involves positioning the flap

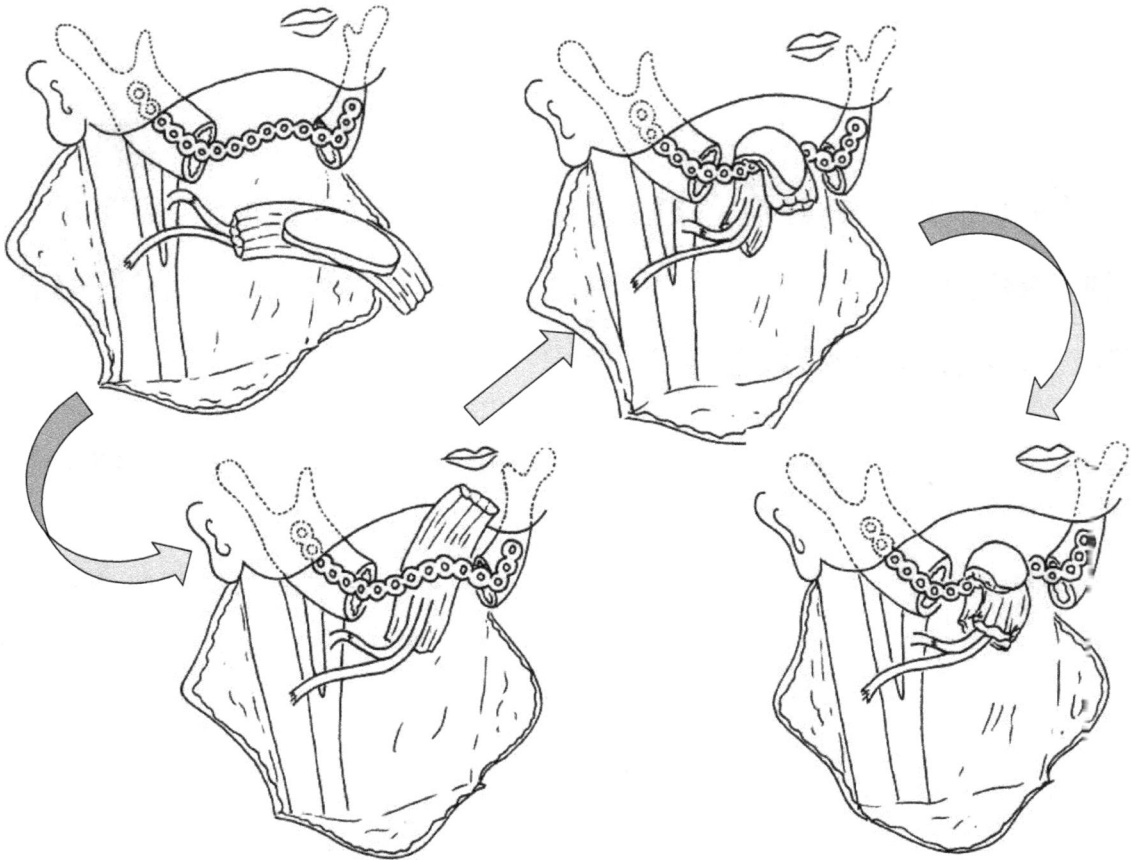

FIGURE 1: The wrap-around technique involves laying the musculocutaneous flap under the reconstruction plate and then wrapping the plate with muscle, fascia, or a denuded island flap.

under the reconstruction plate and then wrapping the plate with muscle, fascia, or denuded island flaps (Figure 1) [7]. The run-through technique (Figure 2), which is used in cases where both the skin of the neck and oral mucosa (e.g., the tongue or mandible) are resected, involves inserting the reconstruction plate through a two-island flap (Figure 3) so that the plate is always covered with skin.

In this study, we identified several risk factors of reconstruction complications and compared the effectiveness of several different treatment methods for reducing their impact in patients who require postresective mandibular reconstruction.

2. Methods

We performed a retrospective analysis of 28 oromandibular cancer cases that required postresective reconstruction between January 1999 and December 2011 at Kobe University Hospital in Japan. Medical protocols conformed to the Declaration of Helsinki; however, since this was a retrospective study, it was granted an exemption by the local ethics committee.

For each case, we used two different classification systems, namely, Hashikawa's CAT classification and Eichner's index, to classify segmental mandibular defects and occlusal

patterns, respectively. Although the HCL or Urken classification system [8, 9] is a well-known system for classifying mandibular defects, we used the CAT system because it is newer than the HCL system and is more suitable for classifying oncological segmental mandibular defects. In the CAT classification system [10] (Figure 4), "C" refers to defects in the condylar head of the mandible, "A" refers to defects in the mandibular angle, and "T" refers to defects in the mental tubercle. In Eichner's classification system [11] (Figure 5), patients are classified into one of six groups based on the presence or absence of occlusal contacts in the premolar and molar regions. After making these classifications, we examined whether radiotherapy or the type of musculocutaneous flaps used during reconstruction was related to the occurrence of infections or plate exposure. We also compared the effectiveness of the wrap-around and run-through techniques.

We identified statistically significant relationships using the chi-square test. P values less than 0.05 were considered statistically significant.

3. Results

The patients in this study consisted of 11 women and 17 men with an average age of 70 years (range: 25–89 years). All

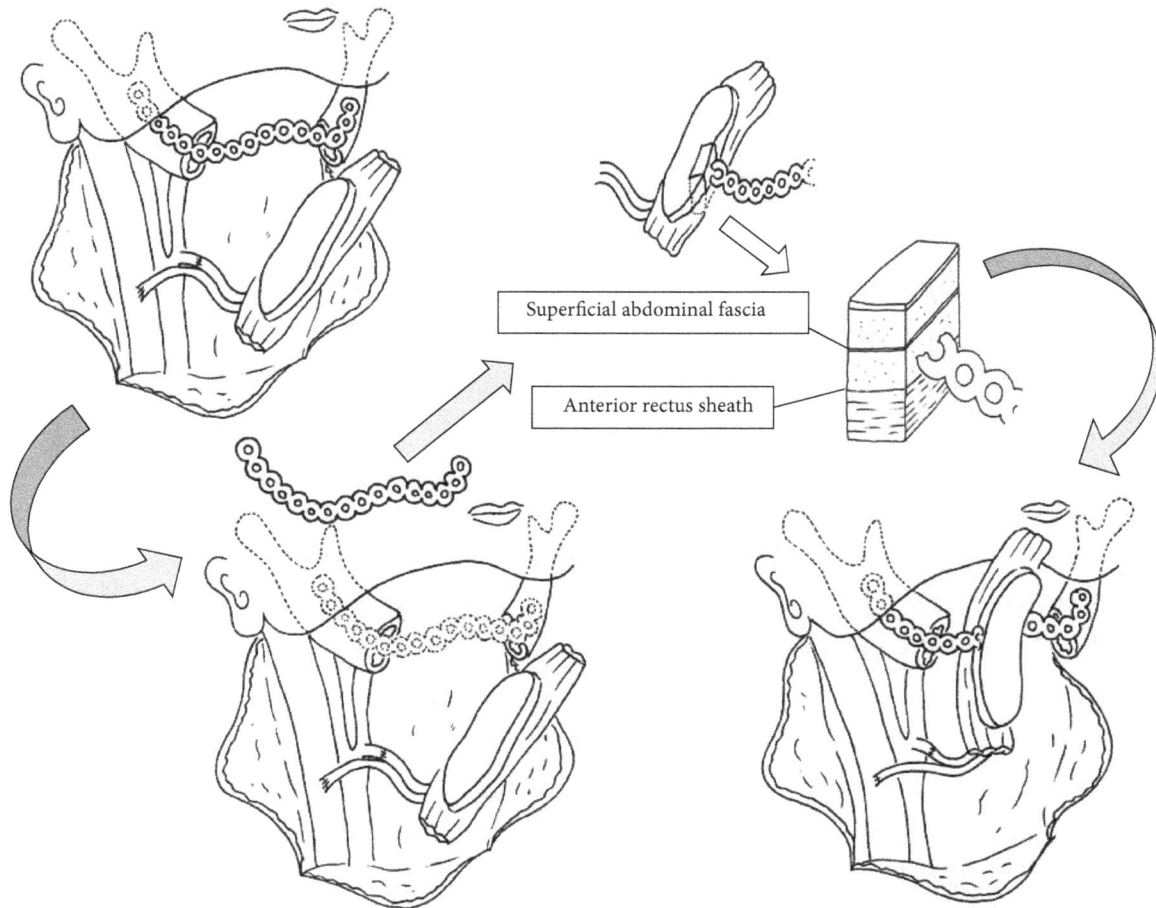

FIGURE 2: The run-through technique involves inserting the reconstruction plate through a two-island flap. Initially, the plate is positioned for fitting to the mandible but subsequently removed. The plate is penetrated into a layer of deep fascia through the rectus abdominis muscle. Finally, part of the reconstruction plate that is penetrated through the flap is fixed to the mandibular bone. Any surplus flap is denuded and buried under the skin of the neck.

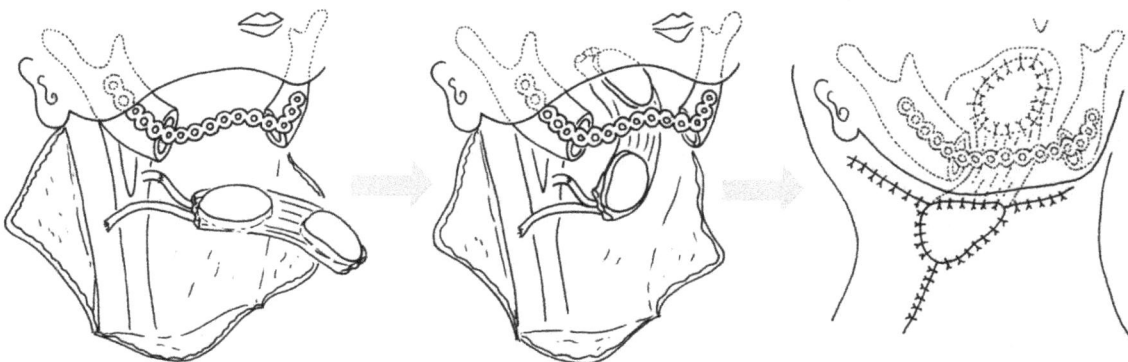

FIGURE 3: Mandibular reconstruction using a two-island flap. The reconstruction plate is placed on top of the muscle and covered with the skin of the neck.

patients were diagnosed with oral or mandibular squamous cell carcinoma (mandibular mucosa (n = 18), oral floor (n = 7), tongue (n = 2), and buccal mucosa (n = 1)) and underwent postresective mandibular reconstruction. Titanium reconstruction plates (Leibinger, Lorenz, or Synthes) were used in all cases.

The distribution of cases according to the CAT and Eichner's classification methods is shown in Tables 1 and 2, respectively. In addition, the relationships between different types of treatment and the occurrence of complications are shown in Tables 3–7. Specifically, five patients received radiation therapy (range: 50–70 Gy). Four of these patients received

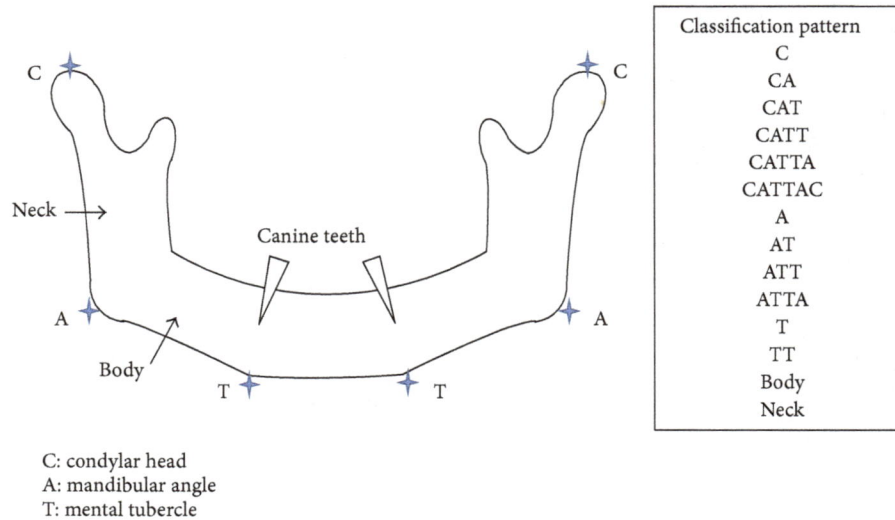

C: condylar head
A: mandibular angle
T: mental tubercle

FIGURE 4: The CAT classification system classifies segmental mandibular defects. "C" refers to defects in the condylar head of the mandible, "A" refers to defects in the mandibular angle, and "T" refers to defects in the mental tubercle. For example, resection of the mandibular angle is classified as "A," resection of the condylar head and mandibular angle is classified as "CA," resection of the entire hemimandible is classified as "CAT," and resection of the mandibular angle and bilateral mental tubercle is classified as "ATT." In addition, the term "body" is used when only the mandibular body is resected, but the mandibular angle and the mental tubercle are preserved. Similarly, the term "neck" is used when only the mandibular ramus is resected, but the condylar head and the mandibular angle are preserved.

radiation therapy within 12 weeks of surgery, while 1 of the patients had recurred after radiation therapy performed ten years previously (Table 3). Although complications occurred regardless of whether radiation therapy was administered, we found a statistically significant relationship between radiation therapy and complications (Tables 3 and 7). In 27 patients, three different types of soft-tissue free flaps were used, while a simple closure was used in the remaining patient (Table 4). Although at least one patient developed either an infection or plate exposure in each technique, only the simple closure technique was significantly related to complications (Tables 4 and 7). Furthermore, among the 28 cases that we examined, 10 patients (36%) developed complications approximately two years after reconstruction (mean: 25.5 months, range: 0.5–82.4 months; Table 5) and nine patients died within 51 months of surgery. However, a Kaplan-Meier analysis showed that there was no specific period when a complication was likely to occur (Figure 6). Among the 10 patients who developed complications, three received radiation therapy and nine reconstructions were performed with a musculocutaneous flap, but all three types of flaps examined in this study were equally common.

Table 5 also shows the CAT classification and Eichner's index for each case. Complications occurred in two type A patients, four type AT patients, two type T patients, and two type TT patients. Furthermore, among 11 cases with at least one occlusal support zone (e.g., B2 and B3), four patients (36%) had a fractured plate. This complication also occurred in 4/14 (28%) cases that involved a mandibular angle defect. Three of six patients with both occlusal support zones and a mandibular angle defect developed a fractured plate. The other two cases of plate fracture occurred in patients without

TABLE 1: Number of cases of plate fracture in each CAT classification. The CAT classification system classifies segmental mandibular defects. "C" refers to defects in the condylar head of the mandible, "A" refers to defects in the mandibular angle, and "T" refers to defects in the mental tubercle.

CAT classification	Patients n (%)	Plate fracture cases
A	3 (10.7)	2
TA	10 (35.7)	3
T	5 (17.9)	1
TT	7 (25.0)	0
ATT	1 (3.8)	0
Body	2 (7.1)	0
Total	28 (100)	6

any occlusions or mandibular angle defects. Chi-square tests showed that only mandibular angle defects and B2 + B3 + B4 occlusions are significantly related to plate fractures (Table 6).

Among the 16 cases that used rectus abdominis musculocutaneous flaps in mandibular reconstructions, the wrap-around technique was used in 14 cases and the run-through technique was used in two cases. Plate exposure only occurred in one patient who had received radiation therapy with the wrap-around technique. No significant relationship was found between plate exposure and the surgical technique used to secure the reconstruction plate ($P = 0.696$).

4. Discussion

Our findings suggest that there are three possible causes of complications of mandibular reconstructions, namely,

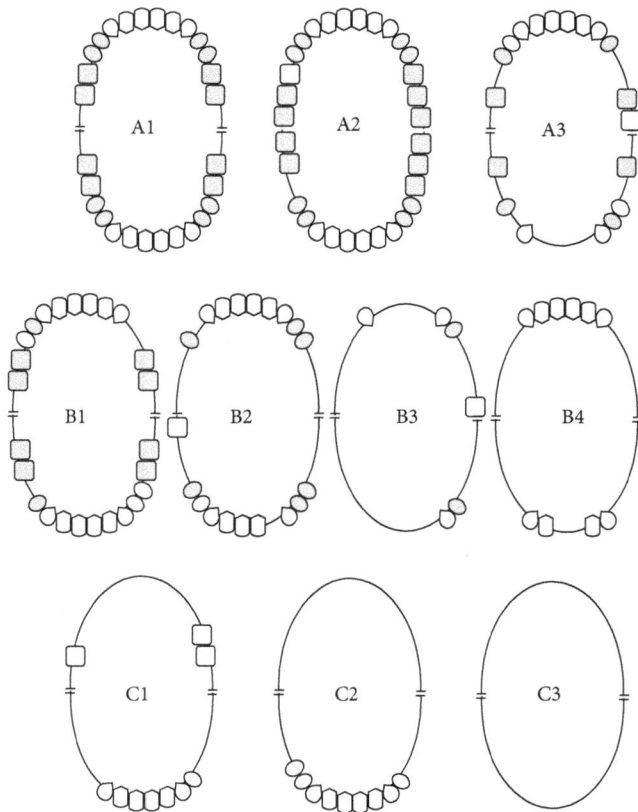

FIGURE 5: Schematic representation of Eichner's index. Shaded teeth indicate occlusal contacts between natural teeth or fixed prostheses in the premolar and molar regions that constitute occlusal support zones (OSZs). Category A contains 4 OSZs. A1: complete dentition. A2: missing teeth in one arch. A3: missing teeth in both arches. Category B contains 1–3 OSZs or contacts in the anterior area only. B1: 3 OSZs. B2: 2 OSZs. B3: 1 OSZ. B4: contacts in the anterior area only. Category C does not have any OSZs. C1: teeth in both arches. C2: teeth in one arch. C3: edentulous.

TABLE 2: Number of cases of plate fracture in each Eichner index. Eichner's classification system groups patients according to the presence or absence of occlusal contacts in different dental zones.

Eichner's classification	Patients n (%)	Plate fracture cases
A1-3	0	0
B1	0	0
B2	5 (17.9)	2
B3	6 (21.4)	3
B4	1 (3.8)	0
C1	1 (3.8)	0
C2	10 (35.7)	1
C3	5 (17.9)	0
Total	28 (100)	6

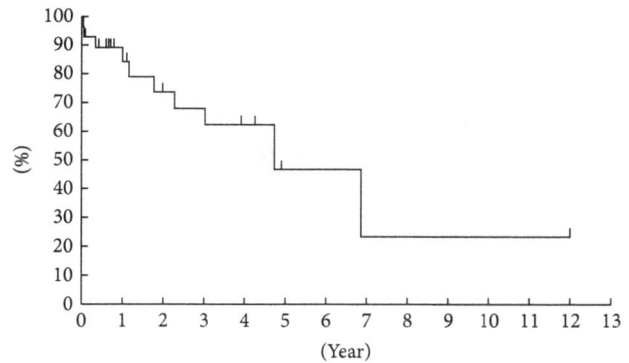

FIGURE 6: Kaplan-Meier plot showing the success rate of mandibular reconstruction in the patients in this study.

TABLE 3: Number of cases with complications in patients who received radiation therapy.

Radiation therapy	Patients n (%)	Number of cases with plate infection or exposure
Yes	5 (17.9)	3
No	23 (82.1)	2
Total	28 (100)	5

TABLE 4: Number of cases with complications in each type of soft-tissue free flap.

Type of flap	Patients n (%)	Number of cases with plate infection or exposure
No flap	1 (3.8)	1
Radial forearm	4 (14.3)	2
RAM	16 (57.1)	1
PMMC	7 (25.0)	1
Total	28 (100)	5

RAM: rectus abdominis musculocutaneous flap and PMMC: pectoralis major musculocutaneous flap.

mechanical stress, infection, and radiation therapy. First, several previous studies have reported that bite force and the type of mandibular defect may play a role in plate fractures and detachments. For example, Shibahara et al. reported plate fractures due to mechanical stress in eight of 110 patients who underwent reconstruction after resection of the mandibular angle [12]. Similarly, Boyd et al. [13] suggested that bite force affects both mechanical stresses on reconstruction plates and the success rate of reconstructive surgery. However, not all plate fractures are caused by occlusal stress; fractures may also be caused by excessive intraoperative bending of titanium reconstruction plates [14].

In this study, among the five cases of plate fracture in their study, four cases involved resection of the mandibular angle and had one or two occlusal support zones (B2 and B3). Our findings that mandibular angle defects and B2 + B3 + B4 occlusions are significantly related to plate fractures are consistent with these studies and the hypothesis that these fractures may be due to bite force or mechanical limitations of reconstruction plates.

TABLE 5: Classification and outcomes of all patients who underwent mandibular reconstruction.

Case number	Age	Sex	Follow-up period (months)	Type of flap	RT	Eichner classification	CAT classification	Complication
1	65	M	13.9	RAM	No	B3	A	Plate fracture
2	64	M	36.3	Radial forearm	No	B2	TA	Plate fracture
3	80	F	82.4	PMMC	No	B2	A	Plate fracture
4	63	M	0.65	PMMC	No	B3	TA	Plate infection
5	61	F	8.5	RAM	No	B2	TA	None
6	54	F	47.1	RAM	No	B2	TA	None
7	68	M	56.8	RAM	No	C2	TA	Plate fracture
8	52	M	12.0	PMMC	No	B3	T	Plate fracture
9	73	F	0.5	None	Yes	C3	TA	Plate exposure
10	70	M	21.2	RAM	Yes	C2	TT	Plate exposure
11	78	M	4.0	Radial forearm	Yes	C2	T	Plate exposure
12	78	F	27.3	Radial forearm	No	C3	TT	Plate exposure
13	26	F	9.5	RAM	Yes	C2	TA	None
14	77	M	7.1	RAM	No	C3	TA	None
15	66	M	7.9	RAM	No	C3	TA	None
16	48	M	2.2	RAM	Yes	C2	ATT	None
17	69	M	43.5	RAM	No	B3	TT	None
18	53	F	47.0	RAM	No	B4	TA	None
19	78	M	48.3	PMMC	No	B3	T	None
20	69	F	50.0	PMMC	No	B3	T	None
21	62	M	5.0	RAM	No	B2	T	None
22	89	F	13.2	PMMC	No	C1	A	None
23	71	M	58.9	RAM	No	C2	TT	None
24	66	F	143.8	RAM	No	C2	TT	None
25	66	M	51.1	RAM	No	C2	TT	None
26	72	F	23.8	Radial forearm	No	C2	Body	None
27	76	M	41.2	RAM	No	C2	TT	None
28	67	F	1.0	PMMC	No	C3	Body	None

RAM: rectus abdominis musculocutaneous flap, PMMC: pectoralis major musculocutaneous flap, and RT: radiation therapy.

Second, infections may displace reconstruction plates. For example, in our study, one patient developed a mandibular infection within one month of reconstructive surgery. As a result, the orocervical fistula enlarged, which eventually dislodged the reconstruction plate. Usually, musculocutaneous flaps, which reduce suture tension and dead space, minimize the occurrence of orocervical fistulas that are associated with these problems [15]. However, heavy pedicles or poor blood flow at the tip of the flap can lead to poor outcomes [16]. We believe that this was the case in this patient, who had poor blood circulation due to diabetes.

Third, radiation therapy has several negative effects, including decreased local tissue vascularity and alteration of the bone-to-metal interface, which increases the risk of plate exposure [17]. In addition, previous studies have shown that titanium can cause a backscatter effect, which may increase the risk of local overdoses around the plate and contribute to screw loosening, osteoradionecrosis, and wound breakdown [17, 18]. Our finding that radiation therapy is significantly associated with plate exposure is consistent with these reports. Collectively, our results suggest that reducing the risk of plate fracture will most likely involve reduction of mechanical and biological stresses on the reconstruction plate and surrounding tissues.

Improved surgical techniques may also mitigate the risk of complications after mandibular reconstruction. For instance, in the run-through technique, even if the skin of the neck is weak, the substructure would be the island of the rectus abdominis musculocutaneous flap, and the plate would not be exposed easily. Therefore, we expected that the run-through technique would reduce the risk of complications, but we did not find any significant relationship between plate exposure and the type of flap used. The sample size might be too small to prove these statements statistically at a significant level. Although improved surgical techniques may not reduce the risk of plate exposure, they may have other structural or aesthetic benefits. More research is needed to verify our findings and advance mandibular reconstruction methods.

TABLE 6: Statistical significance of relationships between plate fracture and CAT and Eichner classifications of patients in this study.

Classification	Chi-square value	P value
Eichner's classification		
B2	1.247	0.246
B3	3.702	0.054
B4	0.283	0.595
C1	0.283	0.595
C2	1.207	0.272
C3	1.247	0.246
B2 + B3 + B4	5.100	0.024*
CAT classification		
A	4.084	0.043*
TA	0.697	0.410
T	0.007	0.932
TT	2.545	0.111
ATT	0.283	0.595
Body	0.643	0.423

*Statistically significant ($P < 0.05$, χ^2 test).

TABLE 7: Statistical significance of relationships between infection or plate exposure, the type of flap used, and radiation therapy in the mandibular reconstruction of patients in this study.

Risc factor	Chi-square value	P value
No flap	4.770	0.029*
Radial forearm	3.287	0.070
RAM	3.429	0.064
PMMC	0.081	0.776
Radiation therapy	7.370	0.007*

*Statistically significant ($P < 0.05$, χ^2 test).
RAM: rectus abdominis musculocutaneous flap and PMMC: pectoralis major musculocutaneous flap.

5. Conclusion

Complications of mandibular reconstruction are significantly related to several risk factors, such as the location of mandibular defects, presence of occlusions, and radiation therapy. Improved surgical techniques may enhance the structural integrity or aesthetics of the reconstruction, but they do not seem to reduce the risk of complications.

References

[1] D. A. Hidalgo, "Fibular free flap: a new method of mandible reconstruction," Plastic and Reconstructive Surgery, vol. 84, no. 1, pp. 71–79, 1989.

[2] J. P. Anthony, J. D. Rawnsley, P. Benham, E. F. Ritter, S. H. Sadowsky, and M. I. Singer, "Donor leg morbidity and function after fibula free flap mandible reconstruction," Plastic and Reconstructive Surgery, vol. 96, no. 1, pp. 146–152, 1995.

[3] J. B. Boyd, "Use of reconstruction plates in conjunction with soft-tissue free flaps for oromandibular reconstruction," Clinics in Plastic Surgery, vol. 21, no. 1, pp. 69–77, 1994.

[4] M. L. Urken, D. Buchbinder, P. D. Costantino et al., "Oromandibular reconstruction using microvascular composite flaps: report of 210 cases," Archives of Otolaryngology: Head and Neck Surgery, vol. 124, no. 1, pp. 46–55, 1998.

[5] R. Lopez, C. Dekeister, Z. Sleiman, and J. R. Paoli, "Mandibular reconstruction using the titanium functionally dynamic bridging plate system: a retrospective study of 34 cases," Journal of Oral and Maxillofacial Surgery, vol. 62, no. 4, pp. 421–426, 2004.

[6] A. Cohen, A. Laviv, P. Berman, R. Nashef, and J. Abu-Tair, "Mandibular reconstruction using stereolithographic 3-dimensional printing modeling technology," Oral Surgery, Oral Medicine, Oral Pathology, Oral Radiology and Endodontology, vol. 108, no. 5, pp. 661–666, 2009.

[7] S. Yokoo, T. Komori, S. Furudoi et al., "Indications for vascularized free rectus abdominis musculocutaneous flap in oromandibular region in terms of efficiency of anterior rectus sheath," Microsurgery, vol. 23, no. 2, pp. 96–102, 2003.

[8] D. D. Jewer, J. B. Boyd, R. T. Manktelow et al., "Orofacial and mandibular reconstruction with the iliac crest free flap: a review of 60 cases and a new method of classification," Plastic and Reconstructive Surgery, vol. 84, no. 3, pp. 391–403, 1989.

[9] M. L. Urken, H. Weinberg, C. Vickery, D. Buchbinder, W. Lawson, and H. F. Biller, "Oromandibular reconstruction using microvascular composite free flaps: report of 71 cases and a new classification scheme for bony, soft-tissue, and neurologic defects," Archives of Otolaryngology—Head and Neck Surgery, vol. 117, no. 7, pp. 733–744, 1991.

[10] K. Hashikawa, S. Yokoo, and S. Tahara, "Novel classification system for oncological mandibular defect: CAT classification," Japanese Journal of Head and Neck Cancer, vol. 34, no. 3, pp. 412–418, 2008.

[11] K. Eichner, "A group classification of missing teeth for prosthodontics," Deutsche Zahnärztliche Zeitschrift, vol. 10, pp. 1831–1834, 1955.

[12] T. Shibahara, H. Noma, Y. Furuya, and R. Takaki, "Fracture of mandibular reconstruction plates used after tumor resection," Journal of Oral and Maxillofacial Surgery, vol. 60, no. 2, pp. 182–185, 2002.

[13] J. B. Boyd, R. S. Mulholland, J. Davidson et al., "The free flap and plate in oromandibular reconstruction: long-term review and indications," Plastic and Reconstructive Surgery, vol. 95, no. 6, pp. 1018–1028, 1995.

[14] W. Knoll, A. Gaida, and P. Maurer, "Analysis of mechanical stress in reconstruction plates for bridging mandibular angle defects," Journal of Cranio-Maxillofacial Surgery, vol. 34, no. 4, pp. 201–209, 2006.

[15] J. Arias-Gallo, P. Maremonti, T. González-Otero et al., "Long term results of reconstruction plates in lateral mandibular defects: revision of nine cases," Auris Nasus Larynx, vol. 31, no. 1, pp. 57–63, 2004.

[16] C. B. Ijsselstein, S. E. Hovius, B. L. ten Have et al., "Is the pectoralis myocutaneous flap in intraoral and oropharyngeal reconstruction outdated?" American Journal of Surgery, vol. 172, no. 3, pp. 259–262, 1996.

[17] J. K. Ryu, R. L. Stern, M. G. Robinson et al., "Mandibular reconstruction using a titanium plate: the impact of radiation therapy on plate preservation," *International Journal of Radiation Oncology, Biology, Physics*, vol. 32, no. 3, pp. 627–634, 1995.

[18] H. Schöning and R. Emshoff, "Primary temporary AO plate reconstruction of the mandible," *Oral Surgery, Oral Medicine, Oral Pathology, Oral Radiology, and Endodontics*, vol. 86, no. 6, pp. 667–672, 1998.

22

The Effectiveness of Modified Cottle Maneuver in Predicting Outcomes in Functional Rhinoplasty

Elaine Fung,[1,2] **Paul Hong,**[1,2] **Corey Moore,**[3] **and S. Mark Taylor**[1,2]

[1] *Department of Surgery, Dalhousie University, 5850 University Avenue, Halifax, NS, Canada B3H 2Y9*
[2] *Department of Surgery, IWK Health Centre, 5850/5920 University Avenue, P.O. Box 9700, Halifax, NS, Canada B3K 6R8*
[3] *Department of Otolaryngology-Head and Neck Surgery, University of Western Ontario, London, ON, Canada N6B 2P2*

Correspondence should be addressed to Paul Hong; paul.hong@iwk.nshealth.ca

Academic Editor: Selahattin Özmen

Objective. To assess the outcomes of functional rhinoplasty for nasal valve incompetence and to evaluate an in-office test used to select appropriate surgical techniques. *Methods.* Patients with nasal obstruction due to nasal valve incompetence were enrolled. The modified Cottle maneuver was used to assess the internal and external nasal valves to help select the appropriate surgical method. The rhinoplasty outcomes evaluation (ROE) form and a 10-point visual analog scale (VAS) of nasal breathing were used to compare preoperative and postoperative symptoms. *Results.* Forty-nine patients underwent functional rhinoplasty evaluation. Of those, 35 isolated batten or spreader grafts were inserted without additional procedures. Overall mean ROE score increased significantly ($P < 0.0001$) from 41.9 ± 2.4 to 81.7 ± 2.5 after surgery. Subjective improvement in nasal breathing was also observed with the VAS (mean improvement of 4.5 (95% CI 3.8–5.2) from baseline ($P = 0.000$)). Spearman rank correlation between predicted outcomes using the modified Cottle maneuver and postoperative outcomes was strong for the internal nasal valve (Rho = 0.80; $P = 0.0029$) and moderate for the external nasal valve (Rho = 0.50; $P = 0.013$). *Conclusion.* Functional rhinoplasty improved subjective nasal airflow in our population. The modified Cottle maneuver was effective in predicting positive surgical outcomes.

1. Introduction

Chronic nasal obstruction can be quite distressing and often has a negative impact on quality of life [1]. Commonly recognized anatomic factors contributing to nasal obstruction include external nasal deformity, septal deviation, turbinate hypertrophy, and nasal tip ptosis [1]. Further, it is crucial that the anatomic areas involving the external and internal nasal valves are evaluated diligently in the preoperative setting to identify the specific area of obstruction.

The nasal valves have been proposed to be a major regulator of nasal airflow, causing resistance and preventing airflow from exceeding the capacity to warm and humidify inspired air [2, 3]. The external nasal valve describes an area of the nasal vestibule bounded by the alar rim, nasal sill, and caudal septum [4, 5]. The internal nasal valve is bounded medially by the nasal septum, superiorly and

laterally by the caudal margin of the upper lateral cartilage, and more laterally by the anterior portion of the inferior nasal turbinate [4, 6]. Many underlying static and dynamic factors can contribute to the obstruction of the nasal valves, including trauma, previous surgery or radiation, congenital weakness of the nasal cartilage, or aging [1, 4]. The Bernoulli principle states that air flowing through a narrow segment accelerates, leading to a decrease in intraluminal pressure [4]. This phenomenon is demonstrated by the collapse of the lateral nasal wall, particularly during deep inspiration. Thus obstruction of the nasal valves may result from varying degrees of static obstruction and dynamic collapse.

Functional rhinoplasty is a well-accepted surgical intervention for correction of nasal airflow obstruction [1–7]. Some commonly used procedures include batten grafts for external valve collapse and spreader grafts for internal valve compromise; other techniques include butterfly onlay grafts, alar rim grafts, suture suspension, and flaring sutures [2–10]. Accurate preoperative diagnosis of the specific anatomic problem and subsequent selection of the appropriate surgical technique will ensure the best possible results for patients undergoing functional rhinoplasty. However, establishing correlation between subjective nasal airflow and physiologic nasal airflow is often difficult [11]. This is certainly observed in many clinic or office settings, where no objective instruments or methods exist to document nasal airflow. Therefore, an easily accessible and reproducible method to examine nasal airflow changes in the clinical setting is needed.

The modified Cottle maneuver [12] may be a simple and easily applied method to determine the presence of external and/or internal nasal valve compromise in an office setting. It may direct surgical planning and lead to improved functional outcomes.

The objectives of the present study are (1) to determine the functional outcomes of rhinoplasty using validated measures and (2) to assess the correlation between the preoperative nasal airflow testing (the modified Cottle maneuver) and postoperative outcomes.

2. Methods

A prospective observational study was conducted at the Queen Elizabeth II Health Centre in Halifax, Nova Scotia. Local Institutional Review Board approval was obtained prior to starting this study.

During the study period of 2002 to 2010, patients with longstanding nasal obstruction evaluated by the senior surgeon (SMT), who met the inclusion criteria, were asked to participate. Inclusion criteria included all patients who were selected for surgical correction of an anatomic nasal defect with minimal benefit from medical therapies. Specifically, failed medical therapies included topical nasal corticosteroid sprays and/or nasal saline rinses. All patients were on at least two-month trial of these medical therapies. Regarding surgical correction, patients deemed to require isolated spreader or batten grafts were selected for the study. Patients were excluded if they underwent a combination of surgical techniques, including septoplasty, inferior turbinate reduction, or tip rhinoplasty. As well, patients who used topical nasal medications or had nasal surgery in the past were also excluded. Informed consent was obtained from the participants.

Prior to physical examination, participants were required to complete the rhinoplasty outcomes evaluation (ROE) form and a 10-point visual analog scale (VAS), which rated the subjective nasal airflow of each nostril on a Likert scale (as shown below). The ROE is a validated quality of life survey that is useful in evaluating rhinoplasty outcomes [13]. The VAS is also a simple and reliable method to assess nasal obstruction [14].

The rhinoplasty outcomes evaluation form and the 10-point visual analog scale for nasal valve obstruction are shown below. On the VAS, a score of 0 indicates complete obstruction, and a score of 10 indicates complete nasal patency.

(1) How well do you like the appearance of your nose?

Not at all	Somewhat	Moderately	Very much	Completely
0	1	2	3	4

(2) How well are you able to breathe through your nose?

Not at all	Somewhat	Moderately	Very much	Completely
0	1	2	3	4

(3) How much do you feel your friends and loved ones like your nose?

Not at all	Somewhat	Moderately	Very much	Completely
0	1	2	3	4

(4) Do you think your current appearance limits your social or professional activities?

Not at all	Somewhat	Moderately	Very much	Completely
0	1	2	3	4

(5) How confident are you that your nasal appearance is the best that it can be?

Not at all	Somewhat	Moderately	Very much	Completely
0	1	2	3	4

(6) Would you like to surgically alter the appearance or function of your nose?

Not at all	Somewhat	Moderately	Very much	Completely
0	1	2	3	4

(7) How well do you breathe through your nose?

No airflow							Perfect airflow			
0	1	2	3	4	5	6	7	8	9	10

(8) Pre-op assessment of baseline, external, and internal nasal valve scores.

Baseline Pre-op   External   Internal   Post-op

Left

Right

The physical examination then commenced, which did not involve the use of topical nasal decongestive medication. Each side of the nose was evaluated independently by occluding the nontest side. All participants were assessed using the modified Cottle maneuver [12]. To test the external valve, an ear curette was used to gently hold the lateral crus of the lower lateral cartilage, and the patient assessed the nasal airflow on the VAS. Another VAS score was obtained for the internal valve when the curette was used to gently lift the upper lateral cartilage of the tested nostril while the patient reassessed the nasal airflow on that side (Figure 1). To improve consistency of this maneuver, only the senior author performed this test with the patients. The modified Cottle maneuver was used to assess nasal valve incompetence and thus select which operative technique was appropriate (batten and/or spreader grafts). Furthermore, the maneuver was used to predict postoperative outcomes.

Spreader grafts were used to correct internal nasal valve collapse; they were all inserted via an open approach. Briefly, the upper lateral cartilages were divided from the septum while preserving the mucoperichondrium to support the spreader graft. A rectangular shaped cartilage graft was then harvested from the nasal septum and placed to span the osteocartilaginous junction to a point caudal to the anterior septal angle. The graft was secured with 5–0 PDS suture (Ethicon, Inc., Somerville, NJ) using a horizontal mattress technique.

Batten grafts were used to strengthen and stabilize the external nasal valves. Briefly, submucosal pockets were dissected in the scroll area just cephalic to the caudal upper lateral cartilage. Cartilage grafts, harvested from the nasal septum, were then placed above the lateral crus and extended laterally toward the piriform aperture. The grafts were secured with 5–0 PDS suture (Ethicon, Inc., Somerville, NJ).

At the 6-month postoperative visit, each patient completed the ROE and VAS as before. The ROE scores were tabulated using the method described by Alsarraf [13]. Both the surgeon and patient were blinded with regard to the preoperative scores. The postoperative nasal patency scores were compared to the preoperative baseline scores, as well as those measuring external and internal valve defects. No surgeon-specific outcome measures were utilized; that is, only the patients assessed the ROE and VAS pre- and postoperatively.

Statistical analysis was carried out using SPSS, version 20 [15]. Overall mean scores were distributed across a wide range and there was statistical evidence that they followed normal distribution, thus allowing the use of the t-test to compare the mean scores. Spearman rank correlation was also used in the analysis.

3. Results

Forty-nine patients completed the pre- and postoperative ROE questionnaires, along with the in-office assessments using the VAS. There were 24 males and 25 females; mean age was 41 years. There were 35 isolated spreader or batten grafts (24 batten grafts, 11 spreader grafts); the remainder required other adjunctive procedures, such as septoplasty or turbinate reduction. Overall, 92% of the patients reported subjective improvement in their nasal breathing, while 8% did not report any improvement.

The overall ROE score, calculated as (ΣPoints/24 $\times$ 100), for each patient was ascertained [13]. The mean ROE score increased from 41.9 to 81.7 ($P < 0.0001$) after surgery.

The mean preoperative and postoperative nasal airflow scores on VAS increased from 3.4 (SD $\pm$ 2.3) to 8.0 (SD $\pm$ 1.8) after surgery, with a mean improvement of 4.5 (95% CI 3.7–5.3) over baseline. This was statistically significant ($P = 0.000$). The range varied from 1 to 9 points ($P < 0.0001$) on a 10-point scale.

The predicted mean improvement in nasal airflow using the modified Cottle maneuver for both internal and external valves and the mean improvement in postoperative outcomes were similar (4.1 (SD $\pm$ 2.3) versus 4.5 (SD $\pm$ 2.2), Table 1). Overall, Spearman rank correlation between the predicted outcomes using the modified Cottle maneuver and the postoperative outcomes showed moderate correlation (Figure 2).

When the nasal valves were assessed independently, there was a statistically significant correlation between the predicted outcomes and the postoperative outcomes. The predicted mean improvement in internal nasal valve assessment using the modified Cottle maneuver and the actual postoperative outcome were 3.0 (SD $\pm$ 1.8) and 5.2 (SD $\pm$ 2.8), respectively, (Table 1). The surgical outcome was slightly better than initially predicted ($P = 0.02$). The Spearman rank correlation was found to be strong (Figure 3).

The predicted outcome using external nasal valve maneuver was 3.7 (SD $\pm$ 2.3). Similarly, the postoperative outcome was 4.3 (SD $\pm$ 1.8) (Table 1). The Spearman rank correlation between the predicted outcome and the postoperative outcome for the external nasal valve was found to be moderate (Rho = 0.50; $P = 0.013$) (Figure 4).

4. Discussion

Patients with chronic nasal obstruction often remain a challenge for the surgeon. During the initial preoperative evaluation, it may be difficult to establish correlation between subjective assessment of nasal airflow and actual physiologic and anatomic characteristics of the patient [16–19]. We have examined the effect of a simple office-based test to assess the nasal valves and its relation to postoperative outcomes.

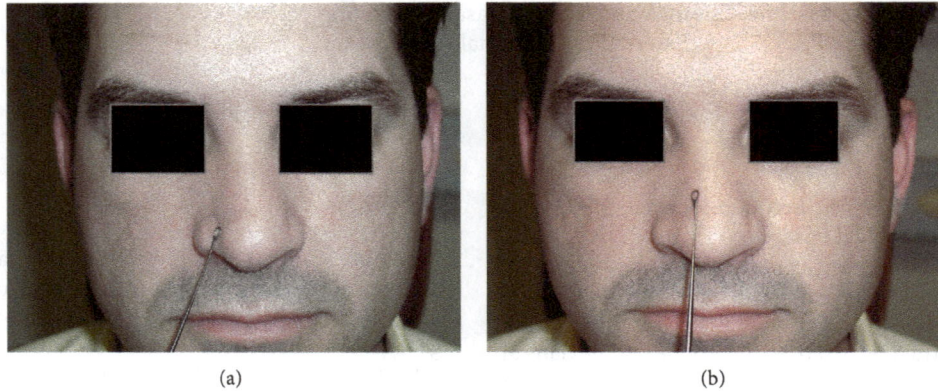

(a)

(b)

FIGURE 1: Demonstration of the modified Cottle nasal valve maneuvers ((a) = external valve; (b) = internal valve), with the curette placed exteriorly only to demonstrate the area to be supported intranasally.

TABLE 1: Comparison of pre- and postoperative nasal airflow improvement scores on a 10-point visual analog scale for batten and spreader grafts. The preoperative score is obtained while performing the modified Cottle maneuver for both the internal and external nasal valve assessments.

Operative technique	Predicted mean improvement	Mean postoperative improvement	Difference in means	Correlation (>0.05 is significant)
Overall ($N = 35$)	4.1 (SD ± 2.3)	4.5 (SD ± 2.2)	$P = 0.23$	0.51 ($P = 0.0016$)
Internal nasal valve spreader graft ($N = 11$)	3.0 (SD ± 1.8)	5.2 (SD ± 2.8)	$P = 0.02^*$	0.80 ($P = 0.0029$)
External nasal valve batten graft ($N = 24$)	3.7 (SD ± 2.3)	4.3 (SD ± 2.0)	$P = 0.17$	0.50 ($P = 0.013$)

* Refers to statistical significance.

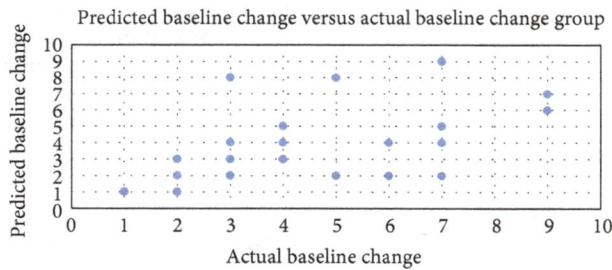

FIGURE 2: Overall outcomes: Spearman rank correlation scatterplot between predicted outcomes using the modified Cottle maneuver and postoperative outcomes ($N = 35$; Rho correlation = 0.51; $P = 0.0016$, with correlation > 0.05 considered significant).

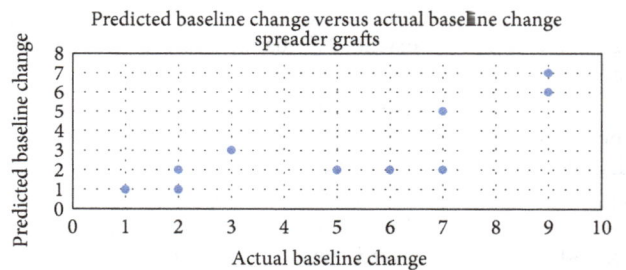

FIGURE 3: Internal nasal valve: Spearman rank correlation between predicted outcomes using the modified Cottle maneuver and postoperative outcomes using spreader grafts ($N = 11$; Spearman rank correlation = 0.80; $P = 0.0029$, with correlation > 0.05 considered significant).

Specifically, we used the modified Cottle maneuver to diagnose internal and external nasal valve incompetence in our study population.

The traditional Cottle maneuver is performed by pulling the cheek laterally to assess ipsilateral nasal patency [12]. The modified Cottle maneuver is more precise in the fact that it assesses the upper and lower lateral cartilage support. We used an ear curette to gently lift the upper and lower lateral cartilages individually to specifically identify internal or external nasal valve insufficiency [12]. Our use of the ear curette and the patient-reported VAS score during the preoperative examination of the functional rhinoplasty patient was a simple and reliable tool in predicting postoperative results for those with nasal valve incompetence, as demonstrated by the good correlation values. The advantage of VAS is that it has been shown to correlate with other objective measures of nasal airflow, such as rhinospirometry [20], and each side of the nasal cavity can be tested independently, and, hence, unilateral symptoms can be assessed. Furthermore,

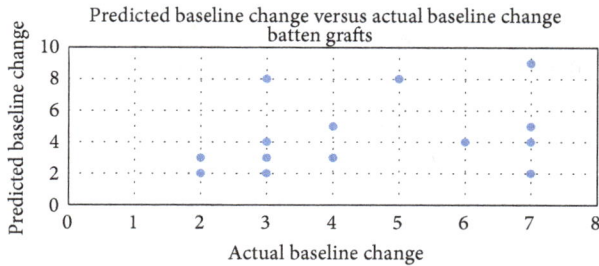

FIGURE 4: External nasal valve: Spearman rank correlation between predicted outcomes using the modified Cottle maneuver and postoperative outcomes using batten grafts (N = 24; Spearman rank correlation = 0.50; P = 0.013, with correlation > 0.05 considered significant).

each nasal valve can be tested independently [21]. Interestingly, several studies have shown better correlation between VAS than some objective measures for nasal obstruction when unilateral VAS is used [21]. Therefore, the modified Cottle maneuver in our study population was an effective predictor of postoperative outcomes, based on the significant correlation of VAS scores and postoperative results for both spreader and batten grafts.

In addition to the VAS, the ROE scores also demonstrated statistically significant improvements in nasal airflow and quality of life after functional rhinoplasty. The mean ROE score improved from 41.9 to 81.7 (P < 0.0001), which is consistent with other published data on primary or revision rhinoplasty procedures [10, 22].

The use of an ear curette to retract the upper lateral cartilage during an evaluation can be uncomfortable for the patient. Hence, introduction of the curette in this sensitive part of the nose may alter the subjective perception of airflow by the patient, and, despite some improvement, it may render the test less reliable in predicting postoperative outcome. However, all patients in our study tolerated this maneuver well and no problems were reported.

A recent systematic review conducted by Rhee and colleagues assessed the evidence supporting functional rhinoplasty and nasal valve repair [10]. Of the 44 articles reviewed, only six (14%) reported outcomes using a validated patient-reported questionnaire and 75% of these studies used adjunctive surgical procedures in combination with nasal valve surgery. Others have noted the difficulty in analyzing outcomes in functional rhinoplasty due to the use of many different surgical techniques, as well as the use of adjunctive procedures, which inevitably leads to confounders [4]. Some surgeons have concluded that patient-oriented measures are generally more effective than objective measures at deducing postoperative outcomes in functional rhinoplasty [4]. Our study is a prospective study using both the ROE and the VAS in isolated batten or spreader graft nasal valve procedures, thus strengthening the evidence for use of these functional rhinoplasty techniques for nasal valve incompetence.

Our study is limited by the nature of the evaluation tool, which is subjective. That is, the modified Cottle maneuver

is a subjective test to administer since the degree of elevation or lift of the nasal structures is operator dependent. For instance, significant lifting may always improve nasal airflow, regardless of the site of obstruction. The use of rhinomanometry, acoustic rhinometry, and other tools to objectively assess nasal airflow may be more helpful in the preoperative assessment [20, 21, 23, 24]. However, there are often practical and logistical difficulties associated with their use, especially in a clinic or office setting. They require specialized equipment and an experienced operator; therefore, these tools are not widely used [21]. In addition, these objective measures typically do not specify the location of the nasal obstruction. Hence, a simple assessment tool, even with its subjective imprecision, may be the most practical in the clinical setting. As well, experienced plastic surgeons may develop consistency with the modified Cottle maneuver that may mimic the surgical changes to be imparted by the rhinoplasty procedure.

5. Conclusion

The modified Cottle maneuver was used to identify the specific site of nasal valve obstruction. Overall, this assessment was well tolerated and was able to predict positive outcomes in patients who underwent functional rhinoplasty in our patient population. Although modified Cottle maneuver is a subjective test and is operator dependent, it may serve as a simple preoperative assessment tool in patients with nasal valve obstruction.

Disclosure

This paper has never been published and is not currently under evaluation in any other peer-reviewed publication.

References

[1] M. B. Constantian and R. B. Clardy, "The relative importance of septal and nasal valvular surgery in correcting airway obstruction in primary and secondary rhinoplasty," *Plastic and Reconstructive Surgery*, vol. 98, no. 1, pp. 38–58, 1996.

[2] P. M. Spielmann, P. S. White, and S. S. M. Hussain, "Surgical techniques for the treatment of nasal valve collapse: a systematic review," *Laryngoscope*, vol. 119, no. 7, pp. 1281–1290, 2009.

[3] D. W. Kim and K. Rodriguez-Bruno, "Functional rhinoplasty," *Facial Plastic Surgery Clinics of North America*, vol. 17, no. 1, pp. 115–131, 2009.

[4] J. S. Rhee, E. M. Weaver, S. S. Park et al., "Clinical consensus statement: diagnosis and management of nasal valve compromise," *Otolaryngology: Head and Neck Surgery*, vol. 143, no. 1, pp. 48–59, 2010.

[5] M. B. Constantian and G. Aiach, "The incompetent external nasal valve: pathophysiology and treatment in primary and

secondary rhinoplasty," *Plastic and Reconstructive Surgery*, vol. 93, no. 5, pp. 919–933, 1994.

[6] J. H. Sheen, "Spreader graft: a method of reconstructing the roof of the middle nasal vault following rhinoplasty," *Plastic and Reconstructive Surgery*, vol. 73, no. 2, pp. 230–239, 1984.

[7] R. J. Schlosser and S. S. Park, "Functional nasal surgery," *Otolaryngologic Clinics of North America*, vol. 32, no. 1, pp. 37–51, 1999.

[8] S. Park, "Treatment of the internal nasal valve," *Facial Plastic Surgery Clinics of North America*, vol. 7, pp. 333–345, 1999.

[9] C. Faris, E. Koury, P. Kothari, and A. Frosh, "Functional rhinoplasty with batten and spreader grafts for correction of internal nasal valve incompetence," *Rhinology*, vol. 44, no. 2, pp. 114–117, 2006.

[10] J. S. Rhee, J. M. Arganbright, B. T. McMullin, and M. Hannley, "Evidence supporting functional rhinoplasty or nasal valve repair: a 25-year systematic review," *Otolaryngology—Head and Neck Surgery*, vol. 139, no. 1, pp. 10–20, 2008.

[11] C. Larsson, E. Millqvist, and M. Bende, "Relationship between subjective nasal stuffiness and nasal patency measured by acoustic rhinometry," *The American Journal of Rhinology*, vol. 15, no. 6, pp. 403–405, 2001.

[12] M. G. Stewart, D. L. Witsell, T. L. Smith, E. M. Weaver, B. Yueh, and M. T. Hannley, "Development and validation of the Nasal Obstruction Symptom Evaluation (NOSE) scale," *Otolaryngology—Head and Neck Surgery*, vol. 130, no. 2, pp. 157–163, 2004.

[13] R. Alsarraf, "Outcomes research in facial plastic surgery: a review and new directions," *Aesthetic Plastic Surgery*, vol. 24, no. 3, pp. 192–197, 2000.

[14] M. Constantinides, S. K. Galli, and P. J. Miller, "Miller simple and reliable method of patient evaluation in the surgical treatment of nasal obstruction," *Ear, Nose & Throat Journal*, vol. 81, pp. 734–737, 2002.

[15] SPSS Version 20, http://www-01.ibm.com/support/knowledge-center/SSLVMB_20.0.0/com.ibm.spss.statistics_20.kc.doc/pv_welcome.html.

[16] J. S. Rhee, D. M. Poetker, T. L. Smith, A. Bustillo, M. Burzynski, and R. E. Davis, "Nasal valve surgery improves disease-specific quality of life," *The Laryngoscope*, vol. 115, no. 3, pp. 437–440, 2005.

[17] D. J. Lam, K. T. James, and E. M. Weaver, "Comparison of anatomic, physiological, and subjective measures of the nasal airway," *The American Journal of Rhinology*, vol. 20, no. 5, pp. 463–470, 2006.

[18] R. J. Schlosser and S. S. Park, "Surgery for the dysfunctional nasal valve. Cadaveric analysis and clinical outcomes," *Archives of Facial Plastic Surgery*, vol. 1, no. 2, pp. 105–110, 1999.

[19] D. M. Toriumi, J. Josen, M. Weinberger, and M. E. Tardy Jr., "Use of alar batten grafts for correction of nasal valve collapse," *Archives of Otolaryngology: Head and Neck Surgery*, vol. 123, no. 8, pp. 802–808, 1997.

[20] J. M. Boyce and R. Eccles, "Assessment of subjective scales for selection of patients for nasal septal surgery," *Clinical Otolaryngology*, vol. 31, no. 4, pp. 297–302, 2006.

[21] D. E. Cannon and J. S. Rhee, "Evidence-based practice: functional rhinoplasty," *Otolaryngologic Clinics of North America*, vol. 45, no. 5, pp. 1033–1043, 2012.

[22] P. W. Hellings and G. J. N. Trenité, "Long-term patient satisfaction after revision rhinoplasty," *Laryngoscope*, vol. 117, no. 6, pp. 985–989, 2007.

[23] R. Vidyasagar, M. Friedman, H. Ibrahim, D. Bliznikas, and N. J. Joseph, "Inspiratory and fixed nasal valve collapse: clinical and rhinometric assessment," *American Journal of Rhinology*, vol. 19, no. 4, pp. 370–374, 2005.

[24] S. Tombu, "Rhinomanometry and acoustic rhinometry in rhinoplasty," *B-ENT*, vol. 6, supplement 15, pp. 3–11, 2010.

23

The Efficiency of Sclerotherapy in the Treatment of Vascular Malformations: A Retrospective Study of 63 Patients

Esko Veräjänkorva,[1] Riitta Rautio,[2] Salvatore Giordano,[1] Ilkka Koskivuo,[1] and Otto Savolainen[1]

[1]Department of Surgery, Division of Plastic Surgery, Turku University Hospital, Turku, Finland
[2]Department of Radiology, Turku University Hospital, Turku, Finland

Correspondence should be addressed to Esko Veräjänkorva; esolve@utu.fi

Academic Editor: Taro Kono

Background and Aims. Vascular malformations are a vast group of congenital malformations that are present at birth. These malformations can cause pain, pressure, and cosmetic annoyance as well as downturn growth and development in a child in the case of *high flow*. Sclerotherapy has become an important tool in the treatment of vascular malformations. However, little is known about the success rate of sclerotherapy. *Material and Methods*. In this study, the efficiency of sclerotherapy in the treatment of vascular anomalies was investigated retrospectively in 63 patients treated in Turku University Hospital between 2003 and 2013. *Results*. Out of the 63 patients investigated, 83% (53) had venous malformations (VMs) and 9% (5) were defined as having arteriovenous malformations (AVMs). Patients with a VM were operated on, in 14% (8) out of all VM cases. Hence 86% (45) of patients with a VM received adequate help to their symptoms solely from sclerotherapy. The duration of treatment for the 14% of the VM patients that needed a surgical procedure was prolonged by 7–9 months, that is, by 41%. *Conclusions*. Sclerotherapy is an effective method in the treatment of VMs with a satisfactory clinical response in patients symptoms in 84% of cases.

1. Introduction

It is estimated that the prevalence of vascular malformations (VMs) in the population is around 4,5% [1]. VMs are congenital vascular malformations (CVMs) that are classified according to anatomical, pathological, and embryological criteria [2]. The most used classification system is the Hamburg classification (also known as the ISSVA classification) from 1988 and it has become the standard system in classification of congenital vascular malformations. This classification has since been updated in Colorado in 1992 and again in Rome in 1996 [3]. This system separates the malformations into arterial malformations (AMs), venous malformations (VMs), arteriovenous malformations (AVMs), lymphatic malformations (LMs), and capillary malformations (CMs) and combined vascular defects. These malformations are known to manifest in all parts of the human body. In addition, these malformations are present at birth; that is, they are congenital, but they usually induce clinical symptoms and findings after childhood, in early adulthood, or in later state of life by the influence of various factors such as trauma, infection, or hormones [4].

Vascular malformations can cause a variety of symptoms depending on their anatomical locations as well as on the flow characteristics of the malformation. It is important to distinguish the different vascular anomalies from each other since the treatment of each type of anomaly differs from the other [5]. A vascular malformation that has an arterial blood pressure (a so-called *high-flow* malformation, AM and AVM) is usually characterized by pain and a sense of pressure. In pediatric patients a high-flow malformation such as AMs and AVMs can cause a downturn of growth and development since the malformation steals blood from the circulation [6]. *Low-flow* malformations such as venous malformations (VMs) and lymphatic malformations (LMs) cause also problems such as dripping of lymphatic fluid or blood through skin and pain, inflict cosmetic annoyance, and exposes the patient to infection [4].

Diagnosis of a vascular malformation is primarily clinical, but ultrasound and especially magnetic resonance imaging (MRI) has an important role [1] in the diagnosis and characterization of the lesion. The treatment of an individual patient is evaluated by a multidisciplinary team that should be centralized in hospitals that have adequate patient population. Treatment options can include minimal therapies such as elevation, compression garments, and aspirin whereas medical management of LMs can require antibiotics and steroids [7]. However, the assessment whether to use surgical or interventional radiologic techniques requires individual evaluation with a multidisciplinary approach and is determined by several factors such as the anatomical site of the lesion, patient expectations, and the facilities at hand in a given hospital. In this judgement the Hamburg classification provides a valuable instrument [8]. Absolute indications for treatment of the CVMs include hemorrhage and hemodynamic problems such as high-output cardiac failure or secondary ischemic complications caused by high-flow AV shunting [9].

Sclerotherapy has become an important tool in the treatment of vascular malformations. However, there has not been presented any evidence that some single sclerosing agent is preponderant if efficiency compared to other products in clinical trials; thus the radiologist personal preference does play a role in the selection of the sclerosant agent [10]. Sclerotherapy is conducted by a radiologist in ultrasound guidance by an injection of a sclerosant substance intravenously, such as polidocanol (Aethoxysklerol®). Polidocanol induces endothelial damage, inflammation, and eventually thrombosis of the vessel. This measure thus causes either a total or partial atrophy of the malformation. The effect of sclerotherapy can be evaluated two months after the injection. Sclerotherapy of VM is in general well tolerated. It can induce some local pain and swelling. In rare cases it can cause necrosis of the skin and nerve injury [11]. LMs are handled by an injection of avirulent *Streptococcus Pyogenes* bacteria (*OK-432*, Picibanil®). The injection of bacteria induces a strong inflammation inside the lymphatic vessel thus inducing atrophy of the vessel. CMs are often treated by light or laser treatment [12].

High-flow malformations such as AMs and AVMs on the other hand are treated with surgical excision. However, prior to surgical excision the high-flow malformation is embolized by a radiologist. In this procedure a sclerosant is injected inside the vessel, for example, gelatin, ethanol, or ethylene vinyl alcohol (Onyx®) [13]. In vast majority this results into tissue necrosis and therefore a surgical resection is mandatory after embolization.

VMs are often complex in structure and penetrate through many tissue structures. Thus radical surgical removal of a vascular malformation would often result in too excessive procedure and tissue morbidity. In addition, the vascular malformation is likely to relapse in case of intralesional excision. Therefore, in the case of VMs, the method of treatment is sclerotherapy. Only if repeated sclerotherapies are unsuccessful, a surgical excision can be performed [14].

Despite the vast research and the number of publications made in the field of sclerotherapies, there is not any study made on the effectiveness of sclerotherapies as a monotherapy in the treatment of vascular malformations. In this study, the success rate of sclerotherapy on the treatment of vascular malformations was investigated retrospectively in patients treated in Turku University Hospital between 2003 and 2013.

2. Materials and Methods

The material for this study was gathered from the patients treated with sclerotherapy for vascular malformation in the Turku University Hospital between 2003 and 2013. The material covers for 63 consecutive patients. The journals of each patient were examined for the following factors: age, medical specialty in charge of treatment, sporadic or familiar malformation, single or multiple and anatomic lesions, any prior treatment, type of radiological imagining, nature of the malformation (venous, lymphatic, venolymphatic, capillary or arteriovenous), smoking, number of sclerotherapies, nature of the sclerosant that was used (polidocanol, OK-432, ethanol, and glue), complications, and duration (follow-up) of treatment.

These factors were recorded in an Excel program and analyzed using the SPSS statistics program. The aim of the analysis was to find predisposing factors that will predict poor outcome in sclerotherapy. Permission for the study was granted by the Head of Department of Surgical Operations and Oncology in the University Hospital of Turku (permission number T182/2013).

3. Results

The 63 patients were divided into two groups: patients that eventually underwent a surgical procedure *versus* patients that did not. Patients were decided to be operated on if the result of the sclerotherapy was regarded as poor. These two patient groups were compared regarding the factors presented above (see Section 2) for statically significant differences.

3.1. Demographics. In the Turku University Hospital there were 63 patients treated with sclerotherapy for vascular malformation between 2003 and 2013.

In this study, neither gender nor age was associated to be a predisposing factor for a poor result in sclerotherapy (Table 1).

3.2. Surgical Specialty. The treatment of the 63 patients was divided between branches of surgical specialties. Majority of the patients, 37 (59%), were treated by plastic surgeons, nine (14%) were treated by pediatric surgeons, six (10%) were treated by hand surgeons, two (3%) were treated by neurosurgeons, and one (2%) was treated by ENT surgeon. The surgical specialty that managed the treatment of the patient was not associated to be a predisposing factor for a poor result in sclerotherapy.

3.3. Family History. There was evidence of family history only in the case of one patient; thus this patient was regarded as having familiar venous malformation. This particular patient

TABLE 1

Gender	
Male	23 (37%)
Female	40 (63%)
Operated on patients (all)	12 (19% out of *high-* and *low-flow* malformations combined)
Operated on males	4 (17% out of women)
Operated on females	8 (20% out of men)
Operated on *low-flow* malformations	8 (14% out of all *low-flow* malformations)
Average age of all patients	36
Median age of all patients	33
Range of age of all patients	3–88
Average age of operated on patients	30
Median age of operated on patients	30
Range of age of operated on patients	6–67

TABLE 2: Anatomical location.

Lower extremity	36 patients (57%)
Upper extremity	15 (24%)
Head and neck	8 (13%)
Torso	3 (5%)
Multiple locations	1 (2%)

TABLE 3: Complications: 10 patients (16%).

Pain	8 (13%)
Fever	1 (2%)
Haematoma	1 (2%)
Finger necrosis	1 (2%)

treatment for their vascular malformation. Out of the patients that were eventually operated on, 50% had a history of previous treatment for their vascular malformation. In all cases the prior treatments were previous attempts of sclerotherapy.

3.8. Identification and Classification of Malformations. Identification of the malformation was done by MRI imaging in 87% (55 patients) of cases whereas ultrasound was used in 13% (8) of cases. Venous malformations covered 83% (52 patients) of all malformations and respectively 9% (5) were classified as arteriovenous malformations. No capillary, lymphatic, or venolymphatic malformations were identified in this study material. However, in 8% (5 patients) of the cases the precise nature of the malformations was left uncertain.

3.9. Sclerotherapy Methodology. Sclerotherapy was conducted 2,39 (median 2, range 1–12) times to patients that were not needed to operate on, but patients who were eventually operated on received sclerotherapy 3,25 (median 3, range 1–12) times. The sclerosant agent used before 2008 was ethanol, after which mainly polidocanol was used.

However, 25% of the patients that eventually were operated on reported also prolonged pain in the operation area. See Table 3 for all complications reported. Majority of patients stayed at the hospital for one night and were discharged on the following morning after sclerotherapy. No general anesthesia was needed to conduct the sclerotherapies in any of the patients.

3.10. Success Rate in Sclerotherapy. From the 63 patients studied in this study, 20% (12) were eventually operated on. This includes also all the patients with a high-flow malformation (5). Patients with a low-flow malformation were operated on, in 14% (8 patients) of cases. Thus 86% of patients with a low-flow malformation received sufficient alleviation to their symptoms from sclerotherapy.

3.11. Duration of Treatment. Duration of treatments (i.e., follow-up) in all patents was 21 months on average (median 17 months, range 2–89). Treatment duration in patients that did not need surgery was 20 months (median 14, range 2–89). Treatment duration in patients that eventually underwent surgery was 29 months (median 24, range 3–72). The difference of treatment duration between operated on and non-operated on patients is therefore 9 months and it infolds a statistically significant difference between these two groups ($p = 0,035$).

was treated altogether by 12 times of sclerotherapies and eventually no surgery was performed. Hence, the nature of the malformation (sporadic *versus* familiar) was not associated to be a predisposing factor for a poor result in sclerotherapy.

3.4. Smoking. The history of smoking was poorly documented in the cases of nearly all patients. Therefore smoking could not be proven to be a predisposing factor for a poor result in sclerotherapy.

3.5. Single versus Multiple Lesions. Single vascular malformations covered 80% (50 patients) out of all patients; that is, in 20% of patients (12) the malformations were multiple. From the patients that were operated on (12), only one had multiple (*low-*flow) lesions. Thus whether the malformation was single or multiple, there was no association for a poor result in sclerotherapy.

3.6. Anatomical Location. The anatomical distribution of the malformations is illustrated in Table 2.

In this study, the anatomical location of the malformation was not associated to be a predisposing factor for a poor result in sclerotherapy.

3.7. History of Previous Treatment. In this study, patient was regarded to have previous medical treatment for vascular malformation, if at least one treatment event could be indicated in their history prior to the latest course of treatment. Out of the patients investigated, 30% had a history of previous

4. Discussion

In this study, the sclerotherapy was found to be an efficient method to relieve the subjective symptoms of a patient with VMs. From the 63 patients studied in this study, 20% (12) were eventually operated on. However this includes also all the patients that had AM or AVM (5). Patients with a VM were operated on, in 14% (8 patients) of cases with a venous malformation. This means that 86% of patients with a VM received adequate help to their symptoms solely from sclerotherapy. This is in level with earlier reports of the efficiency of sclerotherapy in the treatment of VMs [14, 15]. However, all AMs and AVMs did receive preoperative sclerotherapy before operation which is today considered the proper treatment protocol of such malformations [16].

The indication for sclerotherapy in the cases of VMs is mainly the symptoms that the patient has (such as pain or a sensation of a lump or a true deformity); that is, it is rather subjective. However, in the case of AVMs the indication is medically more objective since those malformations are prone to create risks and problems (such as stealing blood from the circulation) but also have more severe symptoms. Consistently the vascular therapy was considered successful if the patient subjectively experienced that the previous symptoms had been discharged through the sclerotherapy.

In this study, there was only one actual complication reported: a necrosis of finger that had to been amputated. This complication occurred as a result of the anatomical fact that there is quite limited vascular supply in fingers. Hence compromising the blood circulation by any means, such as with sclerotherapy, always infolds a risk of tissue necrosis. This is also irrelevant to the type of sclerosant used. This patient was not included in the group of operated on patients. However, there were some adverse events reported in the cases of 10 patients (16%). These included pain (8 patients) and fever (one patient) as well as haematoma in one patient. This result amplifies the consumption of sclerotherapy as a safe treatment option for vascular malformations.

In this study the efficiencies of each individual sclerosant agent were not compared with each other. In a vast review study [17] the efficiencies of different sclerosants used in 1552 patients were compared (from 36 articles). However, despite the strength of that study, the review failed to identify an optimal sclerosant agent. Thus it is not consistent to expect that this notably narrower study (63 patients) could manage to indicate differences between the sclerosants in terms of either efficiency or complication frequency. With similar reasoning, sclerotherapies of the AVMs were not profoundly subanalyzed since there were only five cases of such patients infolded in this study.

Despite the fact that sclerotherapy is not a treatment that radically abolishes a VM, sclerotherapy still manages to reduce the size of a VM, hence reducing symptoms. In addition, sclerotherapy is less invasive procedure than surgical operation, thus causing less tissue morbidity. Sclerotherapy has been estimated to be successful in 75–90% of cases. However, a single sclerotherapy is seldom sufficient for an adequate treatment response. Therefore, sclerotherapy needs often to be applied several times before satisfactory response has been obtained [14]. In this study, sclerotherapy was applied approximately 2,39 (median 2, range 1–12) times to those patients that did not eventually go through surgical procedure; that is, sclerotherapy was considered sufficient. This covers 86% of the patients with a VM. The patients that did not receive adequate treatment response solely with sclerotherapy and underwent surgery received sclerotherapy 3,25 (median 3, range 1–12) times. In this study, no statistical significance of patient age, family history, anatomical localization, the number of malformations, or the number of sclerotherapies could be found to explain or correlate with poor treatment response of sclerotherapy.

In this study the radiological size of the lesion was not marked up. However, this information was not provided in all three-dimensional values and thus the true volume of the malformations could not been calculated. In addition, the radiologist in hand was not always the same as the data had been collected through a period of ten years thus there was reckoned change which also induced imprecision between the reported sizes of the lesions. In future prospective studies with more standardized and systematic volume calculation protocol it may be possible to evaluate whether the size of the lesions predicts bad prognosis for sclerotherapy. However, such a research question will demand a large volume of patients.

The median of treatment durations (i.e., follow-up time) in patients that were successfully treated solely with sclerotherapy was 14 months. In patients that were eventually operated on the median time was 24 months. There is a statistically significant difference in these durations ($p < 0,035$).

In conclusion it can be stated that sclerotherapy is a well tolerated and sufficient method in the treatment of VMs with a success rate of over 86%. In patients that will need complementary surgery, the duration of treatment lengthens by 7–9 moths, that is, by 41%.

Competing Interests

The authors declare that there is no conflict of interests regarding the publication of this paper.

References

[1] A. K. Greene, "Vascular anomalies: current overview of the field," *Clinics in Plastic Surgery*, vol. 38, no. 1, pp. 1–5, 2011.

[2] B. B. Lee, J. Laredo, T. S. Lee, S. Huh, and R. Neville, "Terminology and classification of congenital vascular malformations," *Phlebology*, vol. 22, no. 6, pp. 249–252, 2007.

[3] G. M. Legiehn and M. K. S. Heran, "Classification, diagnosis, and interventional radiologic management of vascular malformations," *Orthopedic Clinics of North America*, vol. 37, no. 3, pp. 435–474, 2006.

[4] R. G. Azizkhan, "Complex vascular anomalies," *Pediatric Surgery International*, vol. 29, no. 10, pp. 1023–1038, 2013.

[5] M. C. Garzon, J. T. Huang, O. Enjolras, and I. J. Frieden, "Vascular malformations. Part I," *Journal of the American Academy of Dermatology*, vol. 56, no. 3, pp. 353–370, 2007.

[6] A. K. Greene and D. B. Orbach, "Management of arteriovenous malformations," *Clinics in Plastic Surgery*, vol. 38, no. 1, pp. 95–106, 2011.

[7] L. M. Buckmiller, "Update on hemangiomas and vascular malformations," *Current Opinion in Otolaryngology and Head and Neck Surgery*, vol. 12, no. 6, pp. 476–487, 2004.

[8] B. B. Lee, "New approaches to the treatment of congenital vascular malformations (CVMs)—a single centre experience," *European Journal of Vascular and Endovascular Surgery*, vol. 30, no. 2, pp. 184–197, 2005.

[9] B.-B. Lee and J. J. Bergan, "Advanced management of congenital vascular malformations: a multidisciplinary approach," *Cardiovascular Surgery*, vol. 10, no. 6, pp. 523–533, 2002.

[10] A. A. de Lorimier, "Sclerotherapy for venous malformations," *Journal of Pediatric Surgery*, vol. 30, no. 2, pp. 188–194, 1995.

[11] J. Dubois, G. Soulez, V. L. Oliva, M.-J. Berthiaume, C. Lapierre, and E. Therasse, "Soft-tissue venous malformations in adult patients: imaging and therapeutic issues," *Radiographics*, vol. 21, no. 6, pp. 1519–1531, 2001.

[12] U. Ernemann, U. Kramer, S. Miller et al., "Current concepts in the classification, diagnosis and treatment of vascular anomalies," *European Journal of Radiology*, vol. 75, no. 1, pp. 2–11, 2010.

[13] J. Pekkola, K. Lappalainen, P. Vuola, T. Klockars, P. Salminen, and A. Pitkäranta, "Head and neck arteriovenous malformations: results of ethanol sclerotherapy," *American Journal of Neuroradiology*, vol. 34, no. 1, pp. 198–204, 2013.

[14] P. E. Burrows and K. P. Mason, "Percutaneous treatment of low flow vascular malformations," *Journal of Vascular and Interventional Radiology*, vol. 15, no. 5, pp. 431–445, 2004.

[15] B. B. Lee, Y. S. Do, H. S. Byun, I. W. Choo, D. I. Kim, and S. H. Huh, "Advanced management of venous malformation with ethanol sclerotherapy: mid-term results," *Journal of Vascular Surgery*, vol. 37, no. 3, pp. 533–538, 2003.

[16] A. K. Greene and A. I. Alomari, "Management of venous malformations," *Clinics in Plastic Surgery*, vol. 38, no. 1, pp. 83–93, 2011.

[17] S. E. Horbach, M. M. Lokhorst, P. Saeed, C. M. de Goüyon Matignon de Pontouraude, A. Rothová, and C. M. van der Horst, "Sclerotherapy for low-flow vascular malformations of the head and neck: a systematic review of sclerosing agents," *Journal of Plastic, Reconstructive & Aesthetic Surgery*, vol. 69, no. 3, pp. 295–304, 2016.

24

Effect of Abdominoplasty in the Lipid Profile of Patients with Dyslipidemia

Guillermo Ramos-Gallardo, Ana Pérez Verdin, Miguel Fuentes, Sergio Godínez Gutiérrez, Ana Rosa Ambriz-Plascencia, Ignacio González-García, Sonia Mericia Gómez-Fonseca, Rosalio Madrigal, Luis Iván González-Reynoso, Sandra Figueroa, Xavier Toscano Igartua, and Déctor Francisco Jiménez Gutierrez

Plastic Surgery Department, Hospital Civil de Guadalajara Fray Antonio Alcalde, Calle Hospital 278, 44280 Guadalajara, JAL, Mexico

Correspondence should be addressed to Guillermo Ramos-Gallardo; guiyermoramos@hotmail.com

Academic Editor: Nicolo Scuderi

Introduction. Dyslipidemia like other chronic degenerative diseases is pandemic in Latin America and around the world. A lot of patients asking for body contouring surgery can be sick without knowing it. *Objective.* Observe the lipid profile of patients with dyslipidemia, before and three months after an abdominoplasty. *Methods.* Patients candidate to an abdominoplasty without morbid obesity were followed before and three months after the surgery. We compared the lipid profile, glucose, insulin, and HOMA (cardiovascular risk marker) before and three months after the surgery. We used Student's *t* test to compare the results. A *P* value less than 0.05 was considered as significant. *Results.* Twenty-six patients were observed before and after the surgery. At the third month, we found only statistical differences in LDL and triglyceride values (*P* 0.04 and *P* 0.03). The rest of metabolic values did not reach statistical significance. *Conclusion.* In this group of patients with dyslipidemia, at the third month, only LDL and triglyceride values reached statistical significances. There is no significant change in glucose, insulin, HOMA, cholesterol, VLDL, or HDL.

1. Introduction

Dyslipidemia is a silent pandemic affecting millions of people around the world. There is more than one factor predisposing this serious problem, where not only diet, exercise, and medications could solve it [1].

The truth is that a lot of people can be sick without knowing it. There is controversy of the possible benefit of liposuction or abdominoplasty in the metabolism of glucose or cholesterol. There are no reports about the effect of abdominoplasty in the metabolism of patients with dyslipidemia.

2. Objectives

Observe any possible change in the lipid profile, weight, cardiovascular risk markers (HOMA), glucose, or insulin of patients with dyslipidemia after an abdominoplasty.

3. Methods

A descriptive observational study was designed to follow up the lipid profile of patients with dyslipidemia candidates to a body contouring surgery as abdominoplasty. The research project was evaluated and approved by the ethics and research committee of the Antiguo Hospital Civil de Guadalajara (file number in the institution 112-11). The ethics and research committee evaluated all the research projects in the decentralized, academic, and public Antiguo Hospital Civil de Guadalajara. It follows the guidelines according to the Health Mexican Norm and the Helsinki ethical principles.

Abdominoplasty or lipoabdominoplasty is offered to women to improve the body images in case of severe skin laxity, excess fat, and flaccidity of the abdominal muscle [2, 3]. We did not operate patients with morbid obesity, where gastric bypass and other bariatric surgeries are suggested.

The following criteria for recruitment were applied patients with recent diagnoses of dyslipidemia with severe laxity of the skin, fat and musculofascial system in the lower and upper abdomen. We excluded patients with negative to participate, alterations in the morphology of abdominal wall (multiples surgical scars and defect on the abdominal wall), pregnancy, systemic illnesses that can put in risk the life of the patient (hepatic, renal or hearth problems), anomalies in the coagulation profile as antiphospholipid syndrome, procoagulants, prothrombotic disorders, primary dyslipidemia, age less than 20 years or more than 60 years and patients that had a previous body countouring surgery as liposuction, fat injection or abdominoplasty.

Demographic variables as age and gender were reported, as well as the fat tissue weight removed after the abdominoplasty. We calculated the sample size taking in account the number of patients operated for an abdominoplasty in one year in the institution (academic, tertiary hospital) with the help of the program in the web page http://www.macorr.com/sample-size-calculator.htm. The sample size was calculated in 17 patients. We collected patients during one year period from October 2010 to September 2011.

We observed before and three months after the surgery any possible change on weight, body mass index, laboratories values as total cholesterol, HDL, LDL, VLDL, triglycerides, hemoglobin, hematocrit, leukocytes, platelet, glucose, urea, creatinine, insulin, albumin, TGO, TGP, and HOMA index (insulin × glucose)/22.5. HOMA index is a cardiovascular risk marker. We used the Student's t test to evaluate any possible change before and three months after the surgery. We considered a P value less or equal to 0.05 as statistical significant.

The patients were followed before and during the postoperative period in junction with the Department of Endocrinology of the same hospital. It was suggested not make any change on diet, exercise, or medications to lower cholesterol or any element in the lipid profile. A questionnaire was applied before and at the third month to evaluate the calorie intake. In the questionnaire, the last three days of food intake were evaluated. The patients were asked about their daily activities in order to identify any possible change in exercise that can increase the calories used. Three months after the surgery, patients continued followup of the dyslipidemia in the Endocrinology Department. They were advised to continue regular consults about cholesterol disorder. Medications and changes in life style as diet and exercise were started.

4. Results

We operated 26 female patients between 26 and 56 years old. The mean age was 39 years old. The mean length was 1.6 meters (1.46–1.75 meters SD 0.32), weight of 69.1 kgs (54–83 kgs, SD 8.09), and body mass index of 27.4 kgs (22–30.8 kgs, SD 1.1).

Before the surgery, the mean glucose value was of 91.45 mg/dL (72–114 mg/dL, SD 9.99), insulin value of 17.11 UI/mL (2–96 UI/mL, SD 23.38), and the HOMA index was 3.96 (0.41–24.33, SD 5.43).

The mean hemoglobin value was 13.99 g/L (11.82–16.3 g/L SD 1.22), hematocrit 42.13 (37.2–47 SD 2.86), leukocytes count 7.33 (4.33–10.7, SD 1.87), and platelets 316 (220–440 SD 56.7).

The mean creatinine value was 0.67 mg/dL (.3–.94 mg/dL, SD 0.54), urea 20.34 mg/dL (10.7–33.2 mg/dL SD 2.2), albumin 4.11 mg/dL (3.9–6.9 mg/dL SD 0.62), DHL 175 (109–283 SD 43.72), TGO 27 mg/dL (16–45 mg/dL SD 6.6), and TGP 28 mg/dL (11–43 mg/dL SD 7.65).

Of the 26 patients, we found 16 of the patients with more than one anomaly in the lipid profile. Sixteen of them had hypercholesterolemia, twelve had hypertriglyceridemia, nine hypoalphalipoproteinemia, and four had hiperprebeta. The results are shown in Figure 1.

The medical treatment, diet and exercise were started by the endocrinologist at the third month of the surgery. Questionnaires were applied in order to evaluate any possible change on diet during the three-month period of time. The patients reported no change on diet. Results are shown in Table 1.

The fat tissue removed weight between 500 and 4000 gr (mean 1700 gr).

The results before and after the surgery in weight, body mass index, total cholesterol, HDL, LDL, VLDL, triglycerides, hemoglobin, hematocrit, leukocytes, platelet, glucose, urea, creatinine, insulin, albumin, TGO, TGP, and HOMA index are shown in Table 2.

5. Discussion

The resection of fat tissue has consequences in the metabolism of patients. It is proved that abdominoplasty improves the metabolism of glucose, lipids, and fatty acid. Andreas and cols showed in this report that body mass index, waist/hip radio, fat mass, fat free mass, fasting plasma glucose, 2-h plasma glucose, triglycerides, total cholesterol, free fatty acids, and systolic and diastolic blood pressure decreased after abdominoplasty [4]. Something important to mention is that the reduction in the values is noticeable and the period of evaluation was longer than one month (40 days). Most of the patients were healthy with no previous impairment in weight, glucose, or any other chronic degenerative diseases. The variables before and after the surgery reached statistical significance and were between normal ranges. The same group evaluated the effect of liposuction in the metabolism of the patients [5]. It is a longer lasting report (followup at the 21 day and 90 day) that showed change in body mass index, waist hip radio, body fat, plasma insulin, triglycerides, total cholesterol, free fatty acid, systolic and diastolic pressure, inflammatory markers, leptin, TNF alfa, adiponectines, resistin, IL6 and IL10 levels. The explanation by the authors is the reduction of fat and consequently the reservoir of cytokines that improved the metabolism of the adiponectines, by decreasing the number of receptors in the fat [5, 6]. When the same group was evaluated in a randomized study, the effect of liposuction and no liposuction positive effect in insulin resistance and circulating markers of vascular inflammation were observed

Lipid profile anomalies

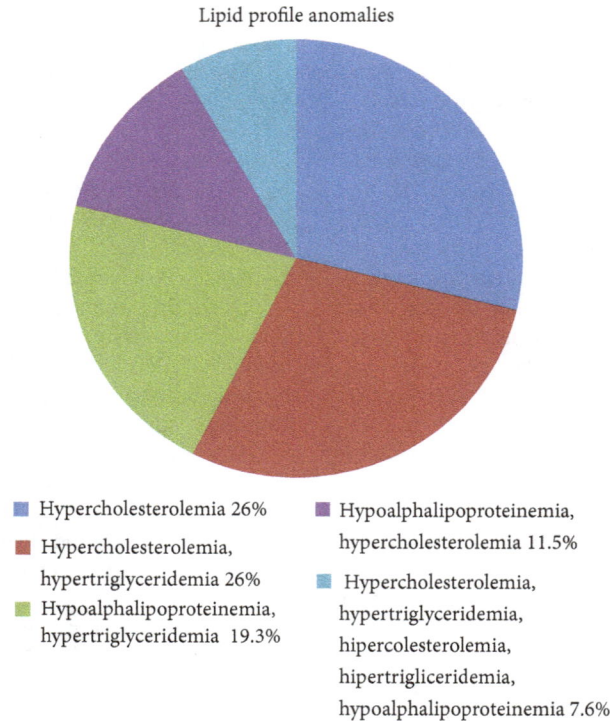

- Hypercholesterolemia 26%
- Hypercholesterolemia, hypertriglyceridemia 26%
- Hypoalphalipoproteinemia, hypertriglyceridemia 19.3%
- Hypoalphalipoproteinemia, hypercholesterolemia 11.5%
- Hypercholesterolemia, hypertriglyceridemia, hipercolesterolemia, hipertrigliceridemia, hypoalphalipoproteinemia 7.6%

FIGURE 1

TABLE 1: Caloric intake estimated.

	Kcal before the surgery	Kcal three months after the surgery	$P < 0.05$
Carbohydrates	893	921	0.67
Lipids	713	732	0.42
Proteins	649	658	0.78
Total	2234	2311	0.85

TABLE 2: It shows media, range, and standard deviation before and three months after the surgery.

Variable	Before the surgery media, range and SD	Three months after the surgery media, range, and SD	P value, standard deviation
Weight	69.1 kgs (54–83 kgs, 8.09)	68.62 kgs (54–83 kgs, 8.07)	0.79 (8.01)
Body mass index	27.4 (22–30.8, 1.1)	27.1 (24.4–28.7, 1.32)	0.81 (1.3)
Glucose	91.45 mg/dL (72–114 mg/dL, 9.99)	90.71 mg/dL (76–106 mg/dL, 8.77)	0.27 (9.32)
Insulin	17.11 UI/mL (2–96 UI/mL, 23.38)	11.79 UI/mL (3–57.4 UI/mL, 11.15)	0.28 (18.3)
HOMA	3.96 (0.41–24.33, 5.43)	2.58 (0.7–10.67, 2.3)	0.22 (4.1)
Hemoglobin	13.99 mg/dL (11.82–16.3 mg/dL, 1.22)	12.79 mg/dL (11–15.3 mg/dL, 1.06)	0.1 (1.2)
Hematocrit	42.1 (37.2–47, 2.86)	42.13 (37–43, 2.8)	0.3 (2.8)
DHL	175 (109–283, 43.72)	178 (110–296, 52.15)	0.83 (47)
TGO	27 mg/dL (16–45 mg/dL, 6.6)	28.32 mg/dL (12–43 mg/dL, 8.05)	0.74 (7.5)
TGP	28 mg/dL (11–43 mg/dL, 7.65)	31.79 mg/dL (14–49 mg/dL, 7.89)	0.33 (8)
Albumin	4.11 mg/dL (3.9–6.9 mg/dL, 0.62)	3.8 mg/dL (2.8–5.3 mg/dL, 0.64)	0.094 (0.64)
Cholesterol	224 mg/dL (134–488 mg/dL, 69.55)	220 mg/dL (128–446 mg/dL, 62.56)	0.84 (65)
Triglycerides	193 mg/dL (61–369 mg/dL, 51.2)	133 mg/dL (26–286 mg/dL, 80.75)	0.03 (73.2)
HDL	44 mg/dL (6–69 mg/dL, 10.99)	49 mg/dL (32–38.6 mg/dL, 29.6)	0.18 (23.2)
VLDL	43 mg/dL (12–133 mg/dL, 26.1)	39.1 mg/dL (11.8–122 mg/dL, 22.04)	0.55 (23.85)
LDL	137 mg/dL (130–390 mg/dL, 68.43)	97.61 mg/dL (26–295 mg/dL, 71.86)	0.04 (72.33)

[6]. Our report includes patients with a previous anomaly in the lipid profile, and we excluded any patient with possible disease that affects glucose, insulin, or any other chronic illness that can bias our results; for example, in the case of medications to control glucose as metformin it can improve the lipid profile and changed our results. As another authors suggested, we had the hypothesis that in patients with lipid profile anomaly the abdominoplasty or liposuction can reduce the metabolism of cholesterol. For us, the explanation can be the effect of resistin, a protein secreted by fat tissue, which increases the production of LDL in human liver cells and also degrades LDL receptors in the liver. Consequently, removing fat tissue from abdominoplasty or liposuction can affect the secretion of resistin and decreased the production of LDL by the liver.

Cholesterol disorders are common and asymptomatic problem in our society. Atherogenesis is strongly related with these anomalies. In Mexico it is estimated that half of the population in some parts can be affected without knowing it [1]. As other authors reported it, we did not find a benefit in other variables of the metabolism of the cholesterol as total cholesterol, VLDL, or HDL. A possible explanation is that our population had disorders of metabolism of cholesterol with higher values than other reports. For this reason, significant statistical change could be more difficult to reach in all the variables.

Most of the patients can feel motivated by a plastic surgery so unconsciousness possible changes on diet, exercise, or life style can be done and that can explaine the positive impact. We estimated the diet before and after the surgery, and we did not find any statistical change. Interestingly, we did not notice any possible statistical change on the weight of the patients. This fact supports the thinking that if we do not modify the habits and costumes of the patients, the remaining fat tissue can hypertrophy and compensated the initial benefit of the surgery. Plastic surgery changes body images of the patients but more complex mechanisms are involved in the metabolism of the cholesterol, and so if we do not modify them plastic surgery benefit can be finished.

We have seen an improvement but the statistical significance was not reached in other variables that were not the primary concern as, for example, insulin and HOMA. A bigger sample can clarify this fact. There are some reports that denied any possible benefit but in some of them the size of the sample is not big enough to rule out any positive benefit [7, 8].

Much of the recent evidence showed a positive impact in these variables [9–12]. We cannot assume that only plastic surgery can improve a complex mechanism of glucose metabolism. As we mentioned before more factors are involved and they should be modified as well. Chronic degenerative diseases are part of the interaction with the environment where less exercise and less healthy food are involved as well as genetics. When we discussed with the patients the evidence of any other possible benefit besides the change in body image we should mention that plastic surgery is not going to change a healthy life style and regular followup with the primary care physician, but that a benefit in the metabolism of glucose and cholesterol has been reported.

In our city, previous reports were done in the case of abdominoplasty, liposuction, or combination of both methods [13, 14]. Significant improvement is noticed. Cholesterol and triglycerides are related with epiandroteniona, and the reduction of the peripheral fat decreased the levels of leptine and as consequence the levels of glucose, insulin, and cholesterol improved. Our observation is unique in evaluating Mexican patients with a documented anomaly in the lipid profile. The followup was longer almost 90 days and the results showed clinical changes with only statistical change on LDL and triglycerides. But not all the reports showed a possible benefit.

Something important to remember is that the most dangerous fat tissue is located inside the body where body contouring surgery does not have any effect [8, 15].

This surgery is not a good choice in morbid obesity patients. But in the case of massive weight lost after a bariatric procedure, the resection of the redundant tissue, besides the functional benefit, can have an extra benefit in reducing inflammatory markers [16]. At the end, we would like to comment on the report of Swanson, one of the biggest reports about this matter. He found a positive effect in liposuction and abdominoplasty in the lipid profile of his patients. He included 322 patients. He found a difference in triglycerides values and leucocytes count. He did not find any benefits in cholesterol, VLDL, LDL, and HDL. The group of patient was a combination of different procedures (no homogeneous about the type of surgery) but the size of the group is one of the biggest reports in the literature [17].

6. Conclusion

We found a reduction in triglycerides and LDL. We did not find any positive benefit in cholesterol, HDL, and VLDL, as well as hemoglobin, hematocrit, leukocytes, glucose, insulin, HOMA index, TGO, TGP, albumin, body mass index, or weight.

Most of the patients in this group have more than one anomaly in the lipid profile. Hypercholesterolemia, hypertriglyceridemia, and hypoalphalipoproteinemia are the most common anomalies, different from reports in Mexican population. Chronic degenerative diseases are pandemic problem, where genetics is not only involved.

Beside the possible motivation after body contouring surgery, the fat tissue that the plastic surgeons remove can have an impact on the cholesterol metabolism (especially in triglycerides and LDL). But we should be careful with this finding. If diet, life style, and exercise are not modified, the remaining fat tissue could increase in size and any positive effect can be finished.

References

[1] A. Aguilar, F. Goméz-Pérez, I. Lerman, C. Vazquez, O. Pérez, and C. Posadas, "Diagnóstico y tratamiento de las dislipidemias

posición de la Sociedad Mexicana de Nutrición y Endocrinología," *Revista de Endocrinologia y Nutrición*, vol. 12, pp. 7–41, 2004.

[2] C. Le Louarn and J. F. Pascal, "The high-superior-tension technique: evolution of lipoabdominoplasty," *Aesthetic Plastic Surgery*, vol. 34, no. 6, pp. 773–781, 2010.

[3] J. Perez-Avalos and G. González, "Experiencia clínica en abdominoplastía," *Cirurgia Plástica*, vol. 9, pp. 112–119, 1999.

[4] F. D'Andrea, R. Grella, M. R. Rizzo et al., "Changing the metabolic profile by large-volume liposuction: a clinical study conducted with 123 obese women," *Aesthetic Plastic Surgery*, vol. 29, no. 6, pp. 472–478, 2005.

[5] M. R. Rizzo, G. Paolisso, R. Grella et al., "Is dermolipectomy effective in improving insulin action and lowering inflammatory markers in obese women?" *Clinical Endocrinology*, vol. 63, no. 3, pp. 253–258, 2005.

[6] G. Giugliano, G. Nicoletti, E. Grella et al., "Effect of liposuction on insulin resistance and vascular inflammatory markers in obese women," *British Journal of Plastic Surgery*, vol. 57, no. 3, pp. 190–194, 2004.

[7] S. Klein, L. Fontana, L. Young et al., "Absence of an effect of liposuction on insulin action and risk factors for coronary heart disease," *New England Journal of Medicine*, vol. 350, no. 25, pp. 2549–2557, 2004.

[8] K. Esposito, G. Giugliano, D. Giugliano et al., "Metabolic effects of liposuction—yes or no?" *New England Journal of Medicine*, vol. 351, no. 13, pp. 1354–1357, 2004.

[9] J. Ybarra, F. Blanco-Vaca, S. Fernández et al., "The effects of liposuction removal of subcutaneous abdominal fat on lipid metabolism are independent of insulin sensitivity in normal-overweight individuals," *Obesity Surgery*, vol. 18, no. 4, pp. 408–414, 2008.

[10] A. S. Rinomhota, D. U. S. Bulugahapitiya, S. J. French, C. M. Caddy, R. W. Griffiths, and R. J. M. Ross, "Women gain weight and fat mass despite lipectomy at abdominoplasty and breast reduction," *European Journal of Endocrinology*, vol. 158, no. 3, pp. 349–352, 2008.

[11] P. Ziccardi, F. Nappo, G. Giugliano et al., "Reduction of inflammatory cytokine concentrations and improvement of endothelial functions in obese women after weight loss over one year," *Circulation*, vol. 105, no. 7, pp. 804–809, 2002.

[12] K. Esposito, G. Giugliano, N. Scuderi, and D. Giugliano, "Role of adipokines in the obesity-inflammation relationship: the effect of fat removal," *Plastic and Reconstructive Surgery*, vol. 118, no. 4, pp. 1048–1057, 2006.

[13] J. A. Robles-Cervantes, S. Yánez-Diaz, and L. Cárdenas-Camarena, "Modification of insulin, glucose and colesterol levels in non obese women undergoing liposuction, is liposuction metabolically safe?" *Annals of Plastic Surgery*, vol. 52, no. 1, pp. 64–67, 2004.

[14] J. A. Robles-Cervantes, M. Espaillat-Pavonessa, L. Cárdenas-Camarena, E. Martínez-Abundis, and M. González-Ortiz, "Dehydroepiandrosterone behavior and lipid profile in non-obese women undergoing abdominoplasty," *Obesity Surgery*, vol. 17, no. 3, pp. 361–364, 2007.

[15] D. Canoy, "Coronary heart disease and body fat distribution," *Current Atherosclerosis Reports*, vol. 12, no. 2, pp. 125–133, 2010.

[16] W. Cintra, M. Modolin, J. Faintuch, R. Gemperli, and M. C. Ferreira, "C-reactive protein decrease after postbariatric abdominoplasty," *Inflammation*, vol. 1, pp. 12–18, 2011.

[17] E. Swanson, "Prospective clinical study reveals significant reduction in triglyceride level and white blood cell count after liposuction and abdominoplasty and no change in cholesterol levels," *Plastic and Reconstructive Surgery*, vol. 228, pp. 182–197, 2011.

25

Maximizing Outcomes While Minimizing Morbidity: An Illustrated Case Review of Elbow Soft Tissue Reconstruction

Adrian Ooi, Jonathan Ng, Christopher Chui, Terence Goh, and Bien Keem Tan

Department of Plastic, Reconstructive and Aesthetic Surgery, Singapore General Hospital, Singapore 169608

Correspondence should be addressed to Bien Keem Tan; bienkeem@gmail.com

Academic Editor: Nicolo Scuderi

Background. Injuries to the elbow have led to consequences varying from significant limitation in function to loss of the entire upper limb. Soft tissue reconstruction with durable and pliable coverage balanced with the ability to mobilize the joint early to optimize rehabilitation outcomes is paramount. *Methods.* Methods of flap reconstruction have evolved from local and pedicled flaps to perforator-based flaps and free tissue transfer. Here we performed a review of 20 patients who have undergone flap reconstruction of the elbow at our institution. *Discussion.* 20 consecutive patients were identified and included in this study. Flap types include local ($n = 5$), regional pedicled ($n = 7$), and free ($n = 8$) flaps. The average size of defect was 138 cm^2 (range 36–420 cm^2). There were no flap failures in our series, and, at follow-up, the average range of movement of elbow flexion was 100°. *Results.* While the pedicled latissimus dorsi flap is the workhorse for elbow soft tissue coverage, advancements in microvascular knowledge and surgery have brought about great benefit, with the use of perforator flaps and free tissue transfer for wound coverage. *Conclusion.* We present here our case series on elbow reconstruction and an abbreviated algorithm on flap choice, highlighting our decision making process in the selection of safe flap choice for soft tissue elbow reconstruction.

1. Introduction

Soft tissue defects of the elbow are commonly encountered by the reconstructive surgeon and can result from causes such as trauma, infection, burns, tumour resection, and radiation injuries. The extent of injury can involve a wide variety of tissues including skin, vessels, nerves, muscle, bone, and joints. Reconstruction of these defects is a challenging conundrum which requires pliable and durable skin that can allow for repetitive flexion and extension. In addition, the elbow joint is prone to develop postinjury stiffness and early mobilization is of paramount importance for optimal recovery [1]. The final outcome in patients with complex elbow injuries is largely dependent on the extent of the initial injury, with larger and more complex injuries involving the bones and joints associated with a higher degree of stiffness [2]. Historically, soft tissue coverage around the elbow has used local and regional pedicled flaps. With advances in microsurgery, free tissue transfer is now the gold standard for composite defects and is often the most favorable choice for early return of function [3]. The option chosen for defect coverage is traditionally based on the exposure of critical structures and the size and location of the defect [4]. Poor decision making can result in reconstructive failure, which may lead to catastrophic outcomes such as osteomyelitis or amputation. Therefore a third dimension that must be considered is the safest path to success. At our institution, we have utilized a variety of flaps to achieve successful coverage while minimizing patient and wound morbidity. Using our clinical cases, this paper aims to review the reconstructive options available and highlight our decision making process which has helped to maximize clinical outcomes for the patient.

2. Methods

20 consecutive patients at our institution underwent soft tissue flap coverage of the elbow for coverage of critical structures. Wounds were classified according to size and location. Flaps types used for reconstruction were divided into three categories: local flaps, regional pedicled flaps, and free flaps.

TABLE 1: Summary of patient data.

Age	Sex	Flap type	Cause	Size (cm²)	Complications	Range of motion (degrees)
			Local flaps			
29	M	Medially based transposition	Trauma	60	Nil	100
37	M	Advancement	Myositis ossificans	50	Nil	120
40	F	Advancement	Prominent plate	40	Nil	130
38	M	Lateral forearm	Trauma	72	Superficial infection	100
50	F	Flexor carpi radialis muscle, flexor carpi ulnaris muscle	Tumour	75	Nil	90
			Regional pedicled flap			
39	M	Extended groin	Trauma	104	Nil	90
30	M	Extended groin	Trauma	117	Nil	Lost to follow-up
30	M	Lateral abdominal perforator	Exposed implant	150	Nil	70
58	M	LD myocutaneous	Postop infection	80	Wound breakdown	85
40	F	LD muscle	Trauma	120	Nil	110
45	M	LD muscle	Tumour	140	Nil	100
50	M	Rectus	Trauma	140	Nil	105
			Free flaps			
40	M	ALT	Trauma	420	Nil	115
35	M	ALT	Trauma	360	Nil	110
40	M	ALT	Trauma	240	Septic arthritis	45
25	M	ALT	Postop infection	120	Wound breakdown	100
61	M	ALT	Postop infection	36	Nil	140
56	M	Rectus	Postop infection	104	Nil	80

Local flaps encompass all perforator-based fasciocutaneous flaps (including cases where tissue expansion was utilized) as well as local muscle flaps. Indications included trauma ($n = 10$), infection ($n = 4$), tumour resection ($n = 3$), exposed orthopedic implants ($n = 2$), and myositis ossificans ($n = 1$). The average defect size was 138 cm² (range 36–420 cm²). The mean age of the patients was 40 years (range 25–61). 16 patients were male and 2 were female. Average time from injury to coverage was 18.8 days (range 11–42).

3. Results

Patient data is summarized in Table 1. Flap types were divided into local ($n = 5$), pedicled ($n = 7$), and free flaps ($n = 8$). Average defect size for the local flaps was 59.4 cm² (range 40–75 cm²). Perforator-based local flaps used included 1 medial rotational and 1 pedicled lateral forearm. We used 1 pedicled flexor carpi radialis (FCR) and flexor carpi ulnaris (FCU) muscle flap. There were 2 cases of tissue expansion and advancement. For the regional pedicled flaps, average defect size was 119 cm² (range 80–150 cm²). This category of flaps included 2 latissimus dorsi (LD) (Figure 1(d)) flaps, 2 extended groin flaps, 1 lateral abdominal perforator flap, and 1 rectus abdominis muscle flap. Average defect size for

the free flaps was 213 cm² (range 36–420 cm²). We used 7 anterolateral thigh (ALT) flaps, 1 free LD myocutaneous flap, and 1 free rectus abdominis flap.

Postoperative complications included 3 cases of wound breakdown, one in a free ALT flap and one in a pedicled LD muscle flap and one superficial infection in the lateral forearm flap. There was one major complication of septic arthritis in a free ALT flap patient, which necessitated the removal of orthopedic implants. There were no flap failures. At an average follow-up of 12 months, the range of movement for 19 patients recorded on a goniometer was an average of 100° (range 45–140°). One patient was lost to follow-up.

3.1. Case Examples

Case 1. An 80-year-old female with multiple comorbidities including ischemic heart disease and chronic renal failure developed an ulcerating squamous cell carcinoma of her right elbow measuring 7 × 5 cm. Radiological studies showed no bony or joint involvement. The resultant wide excision included the skin, subcutaneous tissue, and underlying muscle, with a defect size of 75 cm² exposing the elbow joint capsule and ulnar nerve. To avoid prolonged operative time, the defect was covered with pedicled FCR and FCU muscles

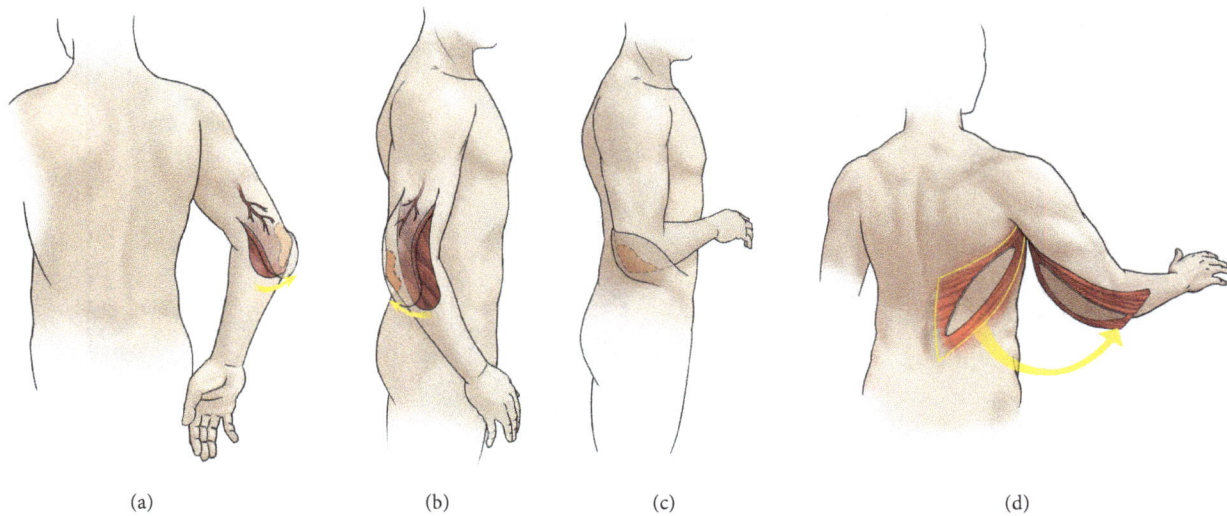

(a)   (b)   (c)   (d)

FIGURE 1: (a) Perforator-based medial fasciocutaneous transposition flap. (b) Perforator-based lateral forearm flap. (c) Pedicled lateral abdominal perforator flap. (d) Pedicled latissimus dorsi flap.

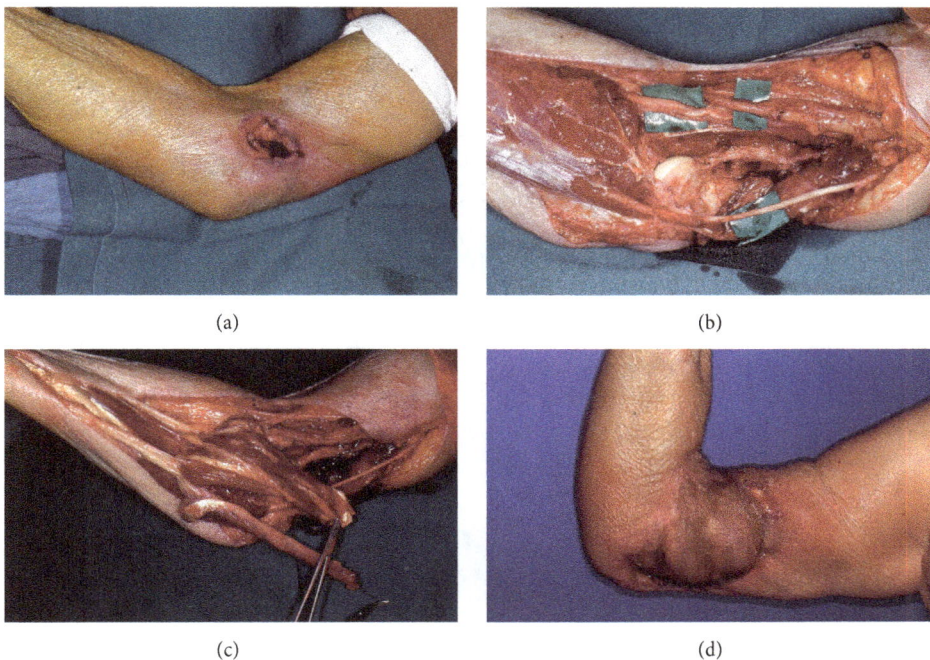

(a)   (b)

(c)   (d)

FIGURE 2: (a) A squamous cell carcinoma measuring 5 × 4 cm over the medial elbow of a 75-year-old female. (b) Defect after resection: the brachial artery, median nerve, ulnar nerve, and elbow joint are exposed. The humeral epicondyle together with the origins of the flexor carpi ulnaris, flexor carpi radialis, and pronator teres was resected. (c) The flexor carpi ulnaris and flexor carpi radialis muscles were transposed to cover the defect and skin grafted. (d) Postoperative result after 4 months.

(Figure 2). The postoperative course was uneventful and in 10 months postoperatively the range of motion (ROM) at the elbow was 90°.

Case 2. A 29-year-old male sustained an open olecranon fracture of the left elbow. Fixation of the fracture was done resulting in a 60 cm^2 soft tissue defect. This was covered with a medial fasciocutaneous transposition flap based on a

medial upper arm perforator. The donor site was skin grafted. Recovery was uneventful, and the patient's ROM at the elbow was recorded as 100° 8 months postoperatively (Figure 3).

Case 3. A 30-year-old male sustained a left elbow fracture with severed brachial artery for which vascular repair of the artery and fixation of the fracture were done. Nine months later he presented with exposure of the implant. He was

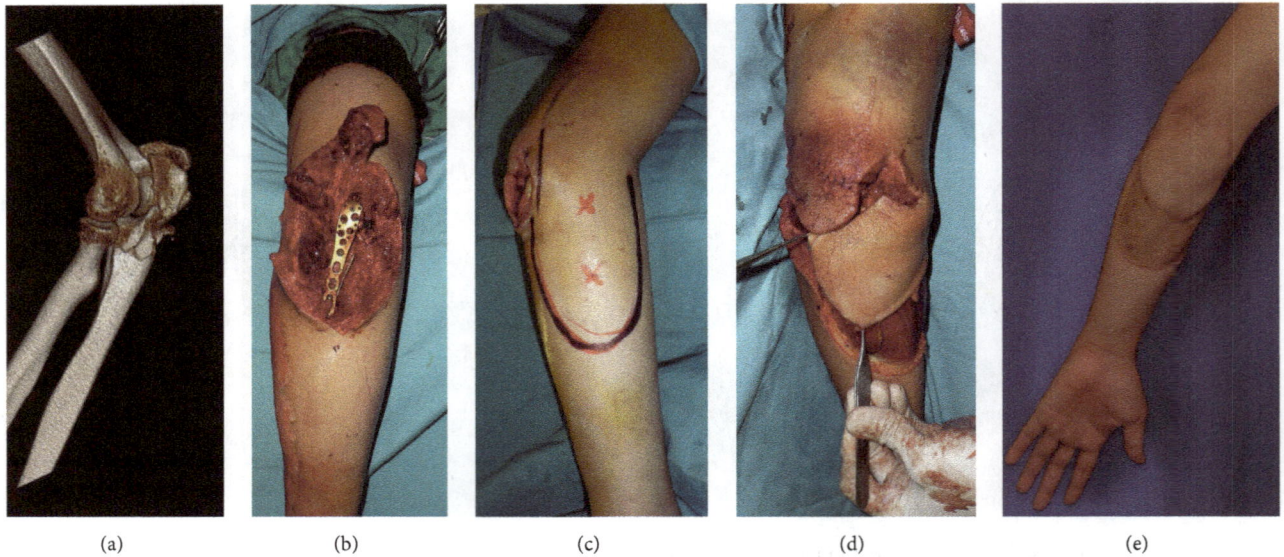

(a) (b) (c) (d) (e)

FIGURE 3: Perforator-based transposition flap. ((a), (b)) A 29-year-old man sustained an open olecranon fracture for which place fixation was done. ((c), (d)) A proximally based medial forearm fasciocutaneous transposition flap was used to cover the elbow defect. (e) Postoperative result in 1 year. The donor site defect was skin grafted.

very thin and had significant heterotopic calcification causing ankylosis of the elbow after injury. Due to the ankylosis and previous brachial artery injury exploration of vessels for free tissue transfer was difficult; therefore lateral abdominal perforator flap was used to cover the defect after implant removal (Figures 4 and 5). The coverage required 2 stages and was completed within 3 weeks. Ten months postoperatively his ROM was 70°, which was similar to his preoperative ROM.

Case 4. A 35-year-old male sustained loss of anterior elbow soft tissue in a workplace accident. This exposed underlying tendons, vessels, and nerves. The large defect was resurfaced with a free ALT fasciocutaneous flap with a cuff of vastus lateralis muscle (Figure 6). In 12 months postoperatively, the patient has excellent contour and 110° ROM.

4. Discussion

Reconstruction of the elbow is a challenging subject. In our series, we were able to achieve a balance of successful pliable soft tissue coverage and early mobilization of the joint which led to good postoperative function. All this was achieved with no flap failures and a small number of complications whose occurrences were independent from flap choice. Flap coverage in our center depended on a number of variables, including size of the wound, patient comorbidities, surgical expertise, and vital structures involved. We successfully applied our abbreviated algorithm presented in Figure 7 to achieve a series of safe and efficacious flap choice in our 20 patients requiring elbow reconstruction.

Local fasciocutaneous flaps are simple and fast, suitable for small shallow defects with healthy adjacent tissue. These flaps enabled the earliest mobilization of the elbow joint in our series of patients and allowed the patients a relatively quicker return to full range of motion. In cases where timing of coverage is not an issue and additional tissue is required, tissue expansion can be carried out as a staged surgery as was done in two of our patients. While local fasciocutaneous flaps were originally of random pattern in nature, the angiosome concept first described by Taylor et al. forms the basis for a predictable axial pattern of blood supply to the skin and fascia via fasciocutaneous or musculocutaneous perforators [5]. Local axial fasciocutaneous flaps have the advantage of a known axial blood supply, which allows for more mobility and a narrower flap base. Axial flaps to the elbow are based on the radial, ulnar, anterior, and posterior interosseous arteries with a rich interconnecting vascular network [5–7]. These vessels give off perforators to the skin and forearm at regular intervals and form the basis for retrograde flaps to the elbow. The most common axial fasciocutaneous flap for elbow coverage in the literature is the radial forearm flap [8]. The radial forearm flap possesses a flexible arc of rotation, reliable vascularity, and possible sensory innervation. In our series we used a perforator-based medial transposition flap (Figures 1(a) and 3) and a perforator-based lateral forearm flap (Figures 1(b) and 4). The drawbacks of these flaps are their limited mobility and size and donor site scarring.

There are numerous local muscle flaps available for coverage, such as the flexor carpi ulnaris, brachioradialis, and anconeus flaps [9–11]. Some flaps, such as the brachioradialis, have been described with a skin island. Each has its benefits and drawbacks, but apart from the anconeus muscle flap ultimately each of these options does sacrifice some level of function. Key to utilizing local muscle is to balance need for local coverage with absence of fasciocutaneous tissue with donor site morbidity. It is not our preference to use local muscle as we feel the donor site morbidity warrants the use of regional pedicled flaps instead. We used pedicled

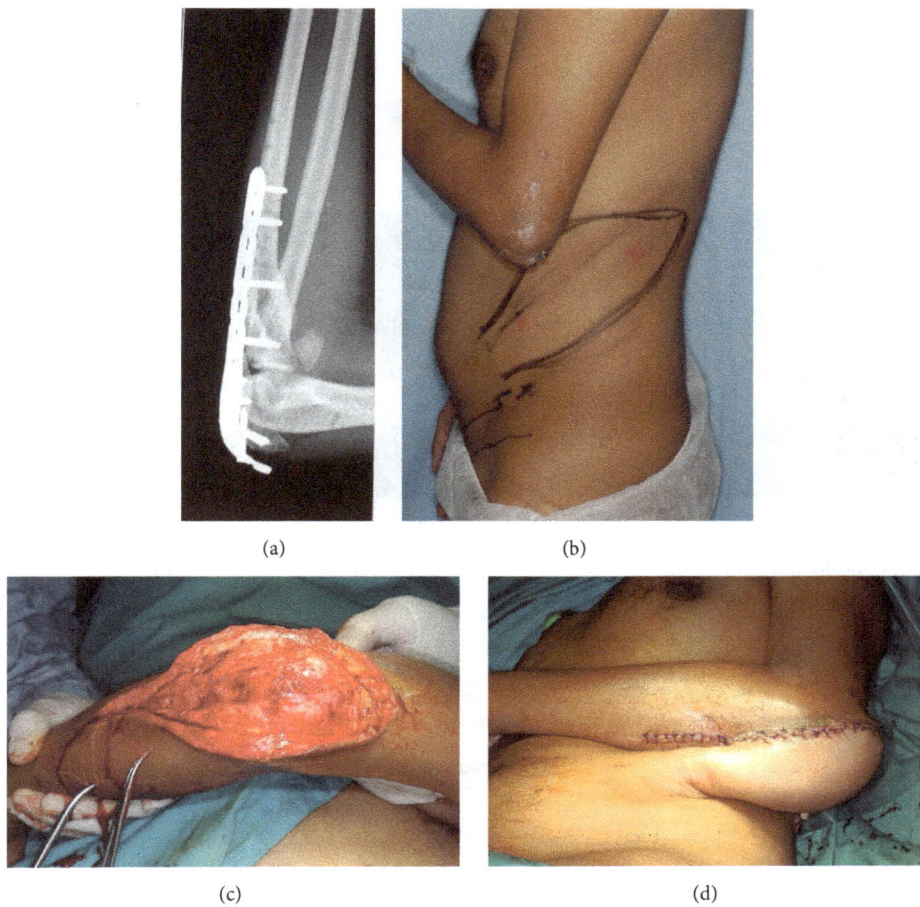

(a)   (b)

(c)   (d)

FIGURE 4: Pedicled lateral abdominal perforator flap. ((a), (b)) 30-year-old male with fixed flexion deformity of the elbow and exposed plate. He had traumatic brachial plexus and brachial artery injuries. (c) Defect after removal of the implant. (d) A pedicled lateral abdominal perforator flap was used to cover the defect.

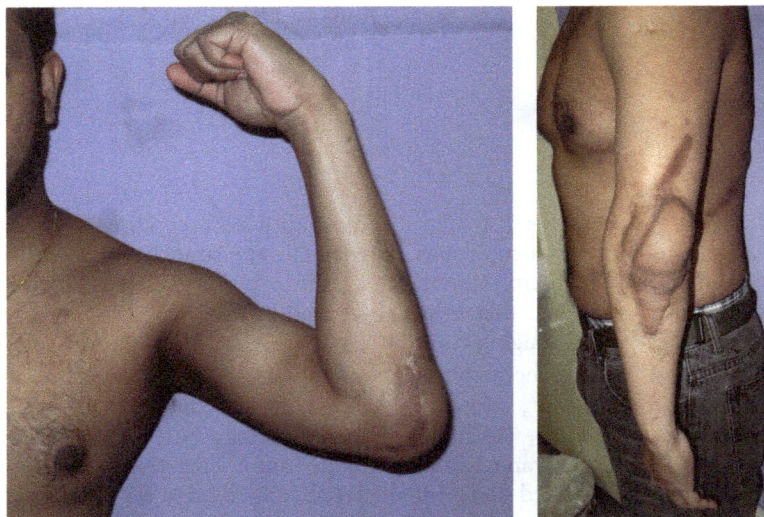

FIGURE 5: Same patient as in Figure 4 in 10 months postoperatively with 70° elbow range of movement, similar to preop.

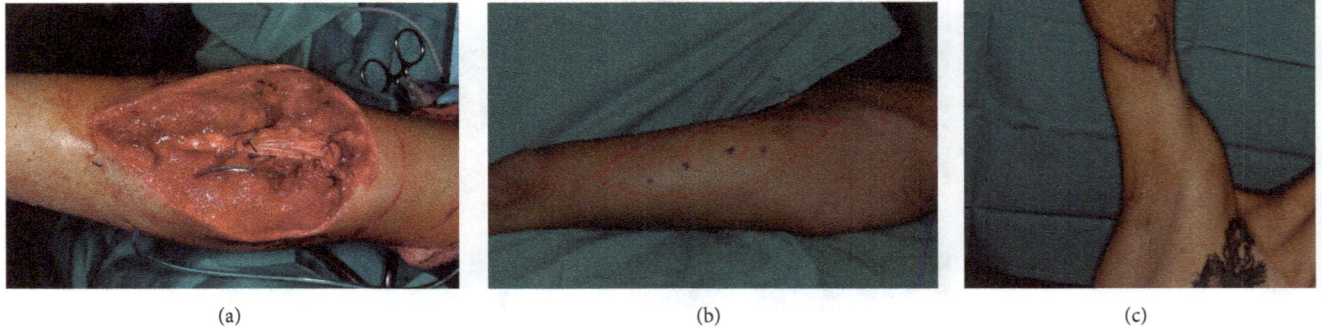

(a)   (b)   (c)

FIGURE 6: (a) Open fracture of the posterior elbow in a 26-year-old male. (b) A left free anterolateral thigh flap was used to resurface the soft tissue defect. (c) Postop result in 8 months.

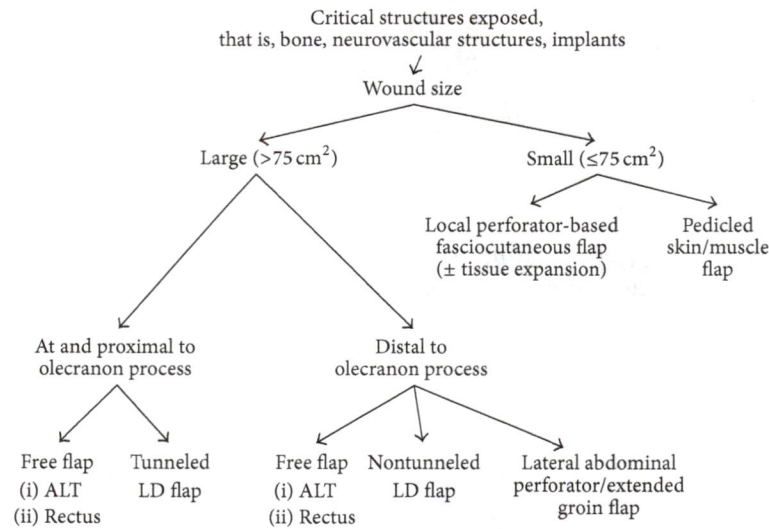

FIGURE 7

FCU and FCR muscles in a single case where a patient with multiple comorbidities and lack of local fasciocutaneous tissue for coverage required a simple and expedient solution to coverage (Figure 1). The literature has shown that local tissue can be used to cover defects averaging ranging from $12\,cm^2$ to $164\,cm^2$, with an average of $55\,cm^2$. The majority of these flaps covered defects less than $80\,cm^2$, with the exception of the ulnar recurrent adipofascial flap, which has been shown to cover defects up to $164\,cm^2$. Stevanovic and Sharpe have recently presented their case based series of elbow reconstructive options with a preference towards local-regional flap options due to their experience with donor site morbidity, such as chronic aching, dysesthesias, and poor cosmetic appearances [12].

Historically, distant fasciocutaneous pedicled flaps were commonly used for elbow coverage [13]. These were usually raised from the groin or chest wall and required multiple operations including division and inset. These flaps have largely been abandoned because of multiple disadvantages including long hospital stay and joint stiffness due to prolonged immobilization. However, we feel that they are still a viable alternative for patients with medium-sized defects and in those who do not have other options of free tissue transfer or local flaps. These patients either have no recipient vessels or previous vessel injury, brachial plexus injuries or have minimally functioning elbow joints with preexisting Volkmann's contracture, thus minimizing the necessity for early mobilization. These regional fasciocutaneous flaps can be made even more reliable with a delay procedure. Examples of flaps that we have used in the past include the extended groin flap based on the superficial circumflex iliac artery (Figures 4 and 5) and the lateral abdominal perforator flap (Figure 1(c)) based on the lateral abdominal wall perforators. The latter was done in a patient where severe elbow joint injury had caused brachial artery injury, making free tissue transfer difficult. In addition to this, he had posthealing heterotopic calcification at the elbow joint which led to severe ankylosis and permanent deformity. On balance, a distant pedicled fasciocutaneous flap provided the simplest method of coverage in a patient with poor elbow rehabilitative function.

Muscle flaps for soft tissue coverage are preferred when infection is present or when muscle bulk is required for obliteration of significant dead space [14]. In addition to providing coverage, flaps such as the pedicled latissimus dorsi or triceps may be transferred to restore elbow flexion. In our experience, we have used tunneled and nontunneled pedicled latissimus dorsi flaps as well as a single case of a pedicled proximally based rectus abdominis flap. The latissimus dorsi muscle flap is the workhorse flap for elbow soft tissue coverage and is preferred because of its size, versatility, ease of use, and reliability [15–18]. It can be mobilized to include either part of the muscle or the entire muscle and can include a skin paddle for cutaneous resurfacing. In addition, the donor site can be closed primarily. However, when used for defects beyond the olecranon it has a propensity for distal tip necrosis, wound breakdown, or failure [18]. The resultant wound edge tension from extension beyond the olecranon may also require extended periods of immobilization.

Microsurgical techniques have revolutionized the field of reconstructive surgery by allowing reliable transfer of free soft tissue to replace muscle, skin, or bone in small or large defects. Although free tissue transfer has become increasingly popular, the literature contains relatively few reports on its use in elbow coverage. Hallock advocated using local flaps for mild injuries around the elbow but maintained that free flaps were necessary in larger or composite defects [19]. Choudry et al. reported using free tissue transfers in only 19 percent of cases in their series of 96 patients requiring soft tissue coverage of the elbow [2].

The advantages of free flaps are manifold. They are versatile and can afford coverage to large wounds. They are especially useful when trauma to surrounding tissues has excluded the use of local flaps or when external fixation precludes local flap use. The flap can be harvested from a multitude of locations in various forms. Other than the ALT flap, fasciocutaneous flaps including the thoracodorsal artery perforator, superficial circumflex iliac artery perforator, scapular, parascapular, and lateral arm flaps offer good skin coverage [20–25]. Some authors advocate the use of muscle flaps when infection is present or significant dead space needs to be filled [13]. Potential donor sites for pure muscle or myocutaneous flaps include the latissimus dorsi,

rectus abdominis, or gracilis. Free flaps are also useful when composite tissue needs to be replaced, such as when tendon reconstruction or vascularized bone is required, for example, in a vascularized tensor fascia lata flap. This allows restoration of both form and function simultaneously. Free tissue transfer also tends to produce donor sites that can be closed primarily. Another advantage of free flaps is the potential for functional muscle transfer to restore elbow flexion. The use of free tissue does, however, relies on the availability of recipient vessels. In our experience, revascularization of the flap is best done end-to-end to the radial or ulnar artery by turning their proximal ends up or end-to-side to the brachial artery if vessels distant to the joint are not available.

Choice of flap is dictated by size of defect, donor site morbidity, and tissue defect. In the past, we have used a rectus abdominis flap to cover a large elbow defect. More recently, Chui et al. reported the use of the anterolateral thigh (ALT) flap in 5 patients from our center [24]. Defects ranging from 36 cm^2 to 450 cm^2 were resurfaced with either fasciocutaneous or musculocutaneous ALT flaps, with no flap failures or major complications. All patients had reasonable and functional return of active elbow motion. The advantages of the ALT flap are large amounts available and the potential to include the vastus lateralis in the flap. The motor nerve to the vastus lateralis can be used as a vascularised nerve graft if required, and fascia lata grafts can be harvested at the time of flap elevation. In addition, the fasciocutaneous flap allows for gliding of tendons and secondary surgery if needed.

We recognize that the above study is limited by its small sample size. However, each case was carefully considered and dissected based on each individual's requirements. In addition to this, our case series and algorithm have been limited to the need for soft tissue reconstruction of the elbow. Patients who require bone or joint reconstruction would need additional considerations besides those mentioned above. In our center, the presence of microsurgical expertise in combination with the versatility of free tissue transfer has now made it our first choice for soft tissue coverage in the reconstruction of large elbow defects. Drawing from our clinical experience and literature review, we have created a clinical algorithm (Figure 7) for soft tissue coverage of the elbow that is based on size and location of the defect which has helped our center make safe yet rehabilitation-optimized flap choices. When critical structures are exposed, soft tissue coverage is paramount and the choice of flap is simply mandated by size. Smaller defects, determined from our experience as those <75 cm^2, can be covered with local skin and/or muscle whilst defects ≥75 cm^2 warrant either pedicled regional or free flap coverage. Though, all of the above reconstructive options may be used for soft tissue reconstruction of the elbow. We have found, when considering the factors presented above, we have been able to provide appropriately sized, durable coverage for our patients, with the additional benefit of availing them to rehabilitative specialists at the earliest possible time, whilst minimizing the risk of complications.

References

[1] R. Sherman, "Soft tissue coverage of the elbow," *Hand Clinics*, vol. 13, p. 291, 1997.

[2] U. H. Choudry, S. L. Moran, S. Li, and S. Khan, "Soft-tissue coverage of the elbow: an outcome analysis and reconstructive algorithm," *Plastic and Reconstructive Surgery*, vol. 119, no. 6, pp. 1852–1857, 2007.

[3] M. Stevanovic, F. Sharpe, and J. M. Itamura, "Treatment of soft tissue problems about the elbow," *Clinical Orthopaedics and Related Research*, no. 370, pp. 127–137, 2000.

[4] M. Jensen and S. L. Moran, "Soft tissue coverage of the elbow: a reconstructive algorithm," *Orthopedic Clinics of North America*, vol. 39, no. 2, pp. 251–264, 2008.

[5] A. Hayashi, Y. Maruyama, M. Saze, and E. Okada, "Ulnar recurrent adipofascial flap for reconstruction of massive defects around the elbow and forearm," *British Journal of Plastic Surgery*, vol. 57, no. 7, pp. 632–637, 2004.

[6] G. I. Taylor, C. M. Caddy, P. A. Watterson, and J. G. Crock, "The venous territories (venosomes) of the human body: experimental study and clinical implications," *Plastic and Reconstructive Surgery*, vol. 86, no. 2, pp. 185–213, 1990.

[7] C. Tiengo, V. Macchi, A. Porzionato et al., "The proximal radial artery perforator flap (PRAP-flap): an anatomical study for its use in elbow reconstruction," *Surgical and Radiologic Anatomy*, vol. 29, no. 3, pp. 245–251, 2007.

[8] N. B. Meland, C. M. Clinkscales, and M. B. Wood, "Pedicled radial forearm flaps for recalcitrant defects about the elbow," *Microsurgery*, vol. 12, no. 3, pp. 155–159, 1991.

[9] B. Elhassan, F. Karabekmez, C.-C. Hsu, S. Steinmann, and S. Moran, "Outcome of local anconeus flap transfer to cover soft tissue defects over the posterior aspect of the elbow," *Journal of Shoulder and Elbow Surgery*, vol. 20, no. 5, pp. 807–812, 2011.

[10] D. E. S. Payne, A. M. Kaufman, R. W. Wysocki, M. J. Richard, D. S. Ruch, and F. J. Leversedge, "Vascular perfusion of a flexor carpi ulnaris muscle turnover pedicle flap for posterior elbow soft tissue reconstruction: a cadaveric study," *Journal of Hand Surgery*, vol. 36, no. 2, pp. 246–251, 2011.

[11] R. W. Wysocki, R. L. Gray, J. J. Fernandez, and M. S. Cohen, "Posterior elbow coverage using whole and split flexor carpi ulnaris flaps: a cadaveric study," *Journal of Hand Surgery*, vol. 33, no. 10, pp. 1807–1812, 2008.

[12] M. Stevanovic and F. Sharpe, "Soft-tissue coverage of the elbow," *Plastic and Reconstructive Surgery*, vol. 132, no. 3, pp. 387e–402e, 2013.

[13] G. L. Farber, K. F. Taylor, and A. C. Smith, "Pedicled thoracoabdominal flap coverage about the elbow in traumatic war injuries," *Hand*, vol. 5, no. 1, pp. 43–48, 2010.

[14] W. Calderon, N. Chang, and S. J. Mathes, "Comparison of the effect of bacterial inoculation in musculocutaneous and fasciocutaneous flaps," *Plastic & Reconstructive Surgery*, vol. 77, no. 5, pp. 785–794, 1986.

[15] A. A. Dorai, A. S. Halim, and W. Zulmi, "Versatility of the latissimus dorsi flap in upper limb salvage tumour surgery," *The Medical journal of Malaysia*, vol. 59, pp. 42–46, 2004.

[16] R. A. Rogachefsky, A. Aly, and W. Brearley, "Latissimus dorsi pedicled flap for upper extremity soft-tissue reconstruction," *Orthopedics*, vol. 25, no. 4, pp. 403–408, 2002.

[17] C.-H. Ma, Y.-K. Tu, C.-H. Wu, C.-Y. Yen, S.-W. Yu, and F.-C. Kao, "Reconstruction of upper extremity large soft-tissue defects using pedicled latissimus dorsi muscle flaps—technique illustration and clinical outcomes," *Injury*, vol. 39, no. 4, pp. 67–74, 2008.

[18] Y. Sajjad, A. Hameed, N. A. Gill, and A. W. Bhutto, "Use of a pedicled flap for reconstruction of extensive soft tissue defects around elbow," *Journal of the College of Physicians and Surgeons Pakistan*, vol. 20, no. 1, pp. 47–50, 2010.

[19] G. G. Hallock, "The utility of both muscle and fascia flaps in severe upper extremity trauma," *Journal of Trauma-Injury Infection & Critical Care*, vol. 53, no. 1, pp. 61–65, 2002.

[20] I. Koshima, Y. Nanba, T. Tsutsui, Y. Takahashi, and A. Kawai, "Vascularized femoral nerve graft with anterolateral thigh true perforator flap for massive defects after cancer ablation in the upper arm," *Journal of Reconstructive Microsurgery*, vol. 19, no. 5, pp. 299–302, 2003.

[21] P. M. Hashmi, "Free scapular flap for reconstruction of upper extremity defects," *Journal of the College of Physicians and Surgeons Pakistan*, vol. 14, no. 8, pp. 485–488, 2004.

[22] F. del Piñal, F. J. García-Bernal, A. Studer, H. Ayala, L. Cagigal, and J. Regalado, "Super-thinned iliac flap for major defects on the elbow and wrist flexion creases," *Journal of Hand Surgery*, vol. 33, no. 10, pp. 1899–1904, 2008.

[23] A. Momeni, Z. Kalash, G. B. Stark, and H. Bannasch, "The use of the anterolateral thigh flap for microsurgical reconstruction of distal extremities after oncosurgical resection of soft-tissue sarcomas," *Journal of Plastic, Reconstructive and Aesthetic Surgery*, vol. 64, no. 5, pp. 643–648, 2011.

[24] C. H.-K. Chui, C.-H. Wong, W. Y. Chew, M.-H. Low, and B.-K. Tan, "Use of the fix and flap approach to complex open elbow injury: the role of the free anterolateral thigh flap," *Archives of Plastic Surgery*, vol. 39, no. 2, pp. 130–136, 2012.

[25] J. T. Kim, B. S. Koo, and S. K. Kim, "The thin latissimus dorsi perforator-based free flap for resurfacing," *Plastic and Reconstructive Surgery*, vol. 107, no. 2, pp. 374–382, 2001.

26

Catastrophic Outcomes in Free Tissue Transfer: A Six-Year Review of the NSQIP Database

David W. Grant,[1] Alexei Mlodinow,[1] Jon P. Ver Halen,[2] and John Y. S. Kim[1]

[1] Division of Plastic and Reconstructive Surgery, Feinberg School of Medicine, Northwestern University, Chicago, IL 60611, USA

[2] Division of Plastic and Reconstructive Surgery, Baptist Cancer Center, Vanderbilt Ingram Cancer Center, St. Jude Children's Research Hospital, Memphis, TN 38139, USA

Correspondence should be addressed to John Y. S. Kim; jokim@nmh.org

Academic Editor: Georg M. Huemer

Background. No studies report robust data on the national incidence and risk factors associated with catastrophic medical outcomes following free tissue transfer. *Methods.* The American College of Surgeons (ACS) multicenter, prospective National Surgical Quality Improvement Program (NSQIP) database was used to identify patients who underwent free tissue transfer between 2006 and 2011. Multivariable logistic regression was used for statistical analysis. *Results.* Over the 6-year study period 2,349 patients in the NSQIP database underwent a free tissue transfer procedure. One hundred and twenty-two patients had at least one catastrophic medical outcome (5.2%). These 122 patients had 151 catastrophic medical outcomes, including 93 postoperative respiratory failure events (4.0%), 14 pulmonary emboli (0.6%), 13 septic shock events (0.5%), 12 myocardial infarctions (0.5%), 6 cardiac arrests (0.3%), 4 strokes (0.2%), 1 coma (0.0%), and 8 deaths (0.3%). Total length of hospital stay was on average 14.7 days longer for patients who suffered a catastrophic medical complication ($P < 0.001$). Independent risk factors were identified. *Conclusions.* Free tissue transfer is a proven and safe technique. Catastrophic medical complications were infrequent but added significantly to length of hospital stay and patient morbidity.

1. Introduction

Since Seidenberg and colleagues reported the first free tissue transfer (FTT) in 1959 for esophageal reconstruction [1], and McLean and Buncke's first report in 1972 [2], free autogenous tissue transfer with microvascular anastomosis has become a safe and effective procedure in many reconstructive settings [3–6]. Its superior patient satisfaction has made it the gold standard in postoncologic breast reconstruction [7, 8], and it is requisite for the reconstruction of many oncologic, traumatic, and congenital defects. Yet while a great deal is known about surgical success and complication rates [3, 4, 9–14], much less is known about medical complications and their specific risk factors, despite the known negative effect of medical complications on recovery time, patient satisfaction, and healthcare system costs [5, 13, 15].

Among the most serious medical complications—rates of death, pulmonary embolism (PE), stroke, or myocardial infarction (MI)—there exists no benchmark to use when counseling patients about the risks of FTT surgery. Only data from individual surgeons operating at single institutions have been reported, and the data are both variable and incomplete [5, 6, 9, 12–22]. It is in this setting that a focused examination of catastrophic outcomes following FTT was undertaken.

The National Surgical Quality Improvement Program (NSQIP) database is a nationally validated, risk-adjusted surgical outcomes database, implemented to improve the quality of care delivered to surgical patients in the United States [23]. The robust cohort of patients undergoing FTT enables a high-powered retrospective analysis to be performed. Our focus was on identifying risk factors independently associated with catastrophic medical outcomes.

2. Patients and Methods

NSQIP was instituted by the American College of Surgeons in 2004 and provides a comprehensive database of 240 pre- and postoperative variables for over 1.3 million patients from over 250 institutions across the United States. Participant Use Data Files for 2006–2011 were downloaded from the ACS NSQIP website (http://www.acsnsqip.org/). The NSQIP database was retrospectively reviewed to obtain data on all patients undergoing free flap procedures with microvascular anastomosis between 2006 and 2011. The data collection methods for NSQIP have been previously described in detail [23–25].

Patients undergoing FTT procedures were identified by the presence of primary or concurrent current procedural terminology (CPT) codes 15756, 15757, 15758, 15842, 19364, 20969, 20970, 20972, 20973, 43496, and 49906, all of which refer to FTT procedures. Patients with incomplete demographic data were excluded.

Descriptive statistics, as well as complication profiles, were calculated for the study population. The primary endpoint was catastrophic medical outcomes (CMO), including the following complications: pulmonary embolism, postoperative respiratory failure (PRF, defined as failure to wean from mechanical ventilation for more than 48 hours and unplanned reintubation [26–28]), coma, stroke, cardiac arrest requiring CPR, myocardial infarction, septic shock, and death. Demographic data included age, body mass index (BMI), gender, and race. The only lifestyle variables included in the analysis were smoking status in the year before admission and whether the patient consumed more than 2 alcoholic drinks per day in the two weeks preceding admission. The following clinical characteristics were tracked: steroid use for chronic conditions, radiotherapy <90 days prior to surgery, chemotherapy <30 days prior to surgery, and a previous operation within 30 days prior to the index operation. The following comorbidities were tracked: diabetes mellitus (controlled with oral agents or insulin), hypertension requiring medication, dyspnea at rest or with moderate exertion, severe chronic obstructive pulmonary disease (COPD), dependence on mechanical ventilation, bleeding disorders, open wound/wound infection, SIRS/systemic sepsis/septic shock, previous cardiac surgery, rest pain/gangrene or revascularization procedure/amputation (peripheral vascular disease, PVD), transient ischemic attack (TIA) or stroke with/without neurological impairment (cerebrovascular disease, CVD), and disseminated cancer. The following surgical variables were tracked: total operation time, wound classification (clean, clean-contaminated, contaminated, and dirty/infected), and ASA classification. Length of total hospital stay was also tracked.

Statistical analyses were performed using SPSS version 20 (IBM Corp., Armonk, NY). Demographics, comorbidities, and outcomes were compared using chi-squared tests or Fisher's Exact Test for categorical variables and ANOVA for continuous variables. Significance level was set at $P < 0.05$. All preoperative variables with $P < 0.2$ and 10 or more occurrences in both groups upon univariate analysis were included in a binomial logistic regression.

3. Results

3.1. Study Population. In total 2,376 patients were identified who underwent FTT between 2006 and 2011. Nine patients (0.4%) had no gender listed and were deleted. An additional eighteen patients (0.8%) had height and/or weight data missing and were deleted. Of the remaining 2,349 patients, most were female (71.4%) and white (73.7%). Seventeen-point-three percent were active smokers in the year before surgery, and 3.2% consumed more than 2 alcoholic drinks per day in the 2 weeks before surgery. The most common comorbidity was hypertension requiring medication (34.3%). Ten percent of patients had open wound infections at the time of surgery, 8.7% of patients had diabetes, 5.6% of patients had dyspnea, and 5.1% had previous surgery within 30 days. All other comorbidities and clinical characteristics occurred in less than 5% of patients (Table 1).

3.2. Catastrophic Medical Outcomes. One hundred and twenty-two patients (5.2%) had a total of 151 CMO. One patient suffered a total of four catastrophic complications, 3 patients (0.1%) had three, 20 patients (0.9%) had two, and the remaining 98 patients (4.2%) had one, accounting for the 151 total CMO.

The most common CMO was postoperative respiratory failure, occurring in 93 patients (4.0%). Other events included 14 pulmonary emboli (0.6%), 13 episodes of septic shock (0.5%), 12 myocardial infarctions (0.5%), 6 cardiac arrests requiring CPR (0.3%), 4 cerebrovascular accidents (0.2%), 1 coma (0.0%), and 8 deaths (0.3%). Of these 8 patients who died, all were ASA class III or IV, only 1 patient had a clean case, 2 patients failed to wean from mechanical ventilation for >48 hours, 1 patient had a PE, 2 had cardiac arrests, 1 had a stroke, and no patients had MI, coma, or septic shock. A complete summary of the catastrophic events is presented in Table 2.

Considering clinical characteristics of the 122 patients who suffered at least 1 CMO, 35 patients (28.7%) were active smokers in the year before surgery, 8 patients (6.6%) had >2 alcoholic drinks/day in the 2 weeks preceding surgery, and 12 patients (9.8%) had a previous surgery within 30 days. Common comorbidities included hypertension (54.1%), diabetes (19.7%), open wound infection (21.3%), cerebrovascular disease (10.7%), dyspnea at rest or with moderate exertion (13.9%), disseminated cancer (9.0%), or a history of cardiac surgery (5.7%). A full summary of demographic and clinical characteristics of this cohort is presented in Table 3.

With respect to operative data, patients with an ASA classification of II or IV were twice as likely to have a CMO (89.9% versus 42.4%; $P < 0.001$) (Table 4). Similarly, patients with wound classification other than clean (i.e., clean-contaminated, contaminated, or dirty/infected) were significantly more likely to have CMO ($P < 0.001$). Length of stay for the CMO cohort was 21.7 days, versus 7.0 for the no-CMO patients ($P < 0.001$). Operative time was just under 2 hours longer in the group that had a catastrophic outcome (601.6 versus 489.3 minutes, $P < 0.001$). While infrequent, emergency cases were significantly associated with CMO

TABLE 1: Population demographics: all free tissue transfers in NSQIP database from 2006 to 2011.

	All patients (n = 2349)	
	n	%
Age (years, mean ± SD)	54.3 ± 12.9	
BMI (kg/m^2, mean ± SD)	27.9 ± 6.3	
Sex		
Female	1678	71.4%
Male	671	28.6%
Race (%)		
White	1732	73.7%
Black	244	10.4%
Asian	61	2.6%
Other	312	13.3%
Clinical characteristics		
Active smoker within one year	406	17.3%
EtOH > 2 drinks/day	76	3.2%
Steroid use for chronic condition	38	1.6%
Radiotherapy <90 days	36	1.5%
Chemotherapy <30 days	94	4.0%
Previous OP <30 days	121	5.1%
Comorbidities		
Diabetes mellitus with oral agents or insulin	204	8.7%
Hypertension	805	34.3%
Dyspnea	132	5.6%
Bleeding disorders	51	2.2%
COPD	66	2.8%
Open wound/wound infection	235	10.0%
Disseminated cancer	88	3.7%
Number of patients with PVD	25	1.1%
Number of patients with CVD	66	2.8%

* denotes significant value, $P < 0.05$.
BMI: body mass index; EtOH: alcohol use; OP: operation; COPD: chronic obstructive pulmonary disease; PVD: peripheral vascular disease; CVD: cerebrovascular disease.

TABLE 2: Catastrophic outcomes.

Postoperative outcome	Total number of patients	% of all patients (n = 2349)	% of catastrophic outcomes (n = 122)
4 outcomes	1	0.0%	0.8%
3 outcomes	3	0.1%	2.5%
2 outcomes	20	0.9%	16.4%
1 outcome	98	4.2%	80.3%
Total	**122**		
Type of outcome			
Pulmonary embolism	14	0.6%	9.3%
PRF	93	4.0%	61.6%
Coma	1	0.0%	0.7%
Stroke	4	0.2%	2.6%
Cardiac arrest requiring CPR	6	0.3%	4.0%
Myocardial infarction	12	0.5%	7.9%
Septic shock	13	0.5%	8.6%
Death	8	0.3%	5.3%
Total	**151**		
Overall catastrophic complications*	122	5.2%	

* Patients can have more than one catastrophic complication.
PRF: prolonged respiratory failure; CPR: cardiopulmonary resuscitation.

4. Discussion

Catastrophic medical outcomes (CMO) are generally defined as any perioperative sudden event that could potentially result in patient death or permanent disability within 30 days of surgery [29, 30]. CMO can occur from a number of specific events, including injury to vessels or nerves, retained devices, visceral perforation, and wrong-site surgery [31]. While the majority of these events are procedure-specific and are thus not tracked in NSQIP, it is possible to use the generic variables available in the dataset to identify CMO. These defined our primary endpoints and included the following complications: pulmonary embolism, postoperative respiratory failure (PRF, defined as failure to wean from mechanical ventilation for more than 48 hours and unplanned reintubation [26–28]), coma, stroke, cardiac arrest requiring CPR, myocardial infarction, septic shock, and death. Reconstructive microsurgery is unique in that it requires prolonged operative times, multiple surgical sites (i.e., flap donor and recipient sites), multiple surgical teams (in many cases), and often significant physiologic insult (e.g., composite head and neck resection, limb salvage after trauma). Thus, patients undergoing FTT are uniquely susceptible to CMO.

This study is the largest and most comprehensive examination to date of catastrophic medical outcomes following FTT. It establishes a benchmark for surgeons to use when

(P = 0.043). Outpatient surgery was not associated with catastrophic outcomes ($P = 0.146$).

3.3. Binomial Regression. A binomial logistic regression analysis was performed using variables that met statistical requirements ($n > 10$ and $P < 0.20$) (Table 5). Five variables were found to be independently associated with CMO: bleeding disorder (OR 3.13, $P = 0.003$), CVD (OR 2.25, $P = 0.021$), wound classification other than clean (OR 2.20, $P = 0.001$), diabetes (OR 1.72, $P = 0.048$), ASA classification of class III or IV (OR 2.17, $P = 0.004$), and total operation time (OR 1.002, $P < 0.001$).

TABLE 3: Population demographics, stratified by catastrophic outcome.

	Catastrophic outcome $n = 122$		No catastrophic outcome $n = 2,227$			P value
	n	%	n	%		
Age (years, mean ± SD)	61.0 ± 14.3		53.9 ± 12.7			0.000*
BMI (kg/m², mean ± SD)	26.4 ± 6.5		27.9 ± 6.3			0.007*
Sex						
Male	73	59.8%	598	26.9%		0.000*
Female	49	40.2%	1629	73.1%		
Race (%)						
White	93	76.2%	1639	73.6%		
Black	6	4.9%	238	10.7%		
Asian	1	0.8%	60	2.7%		
Other	22	18.0%	290	13.0%		
Clinical characteristics						
Active smoker within one year	35	28.7%	371	16.7%		0.001*
EtOH > 2 drinks/day in preceding 2 wks	8	6.6%	68	3.1%	§	0.057
Steroid use	5	4.1%	33	1.5%	§	0.044*
Radiotherapy <90 days	7	5.7%	29	1.3%	§	0.002*
Chemotherapy <30 days	4	3.3%	90	4.0%	§	1.000
Previous OP <30 days	12	9.8%	109	4.9%		0.016*
Comorbidities						
Diabetes	24	19.7%	180	8.1%		0.000*
Hypertension	66	54.1%	739	33.2%		0.000*
Dyspnea	17	13.9%	115	5.2%		0.000*
Bleeding disorder	12	9.8%	39	1.8%	§	0.000*
Ventilator dependent status preop	3	2.5%	3	0.1%	§	0.002*
History of severe COPD	7	5.7%	59	2.6%	§	0.080
Systemic sepsis	8	6.6%	42	1.9%		0.004*
Open wound infection	26	21.3%	209	9.4%		0.000*
Disseminated cancer	11	9.0%	77	3.5%	§	0.005*
History of cardiac surgery	7	5.7%	32	1.4%	§	0.003*
Peripheral vascular disease	2	1.6%	23	1.0%	§	0.376
Cerebrovascular disease	13	10.7%	53	2.4%	§	0.000*

* denotes significant value, $P < 0.05$.
§ Fisher's Exact Test; all others Pearson chi-square.
BMI = body mass index; EtOH = alcohol consumption; OP = operation; COPD = chronic obstructive pulmonary disease.

TABLE 4: Operative data.

	Catastrophic outcome $n = 122$		No catastrophic outcome $n = 2227$			P value
	n	%	n	%		
Outpatient setting	2	1.6%	97	4.4%		0.146
Emergency case	4	3.3%	22	1.0%	§	0.043*
ASA classification III or IV	98	89.9%	945	42.4%		0.000*
Wound classification 2, 3, or 4	86	70.5%	685	30.8%		0.000*
Operative time (minutes ± standard deviation)	601.6 ± 264.6		489.3 ± 217.0			0.000*
Length of total hospital stay (days ± standard deviation)	21.7 ± 17.0		7.0 ± 7.6			0.000*

* denotes significant value, $P < 0.05$.
§ Fisher's Exact Test; all others Pearson chi-square.
ASA: American Society of Anesthesiologists.

TABLE 5: Binomial logistic regression.

Predictor	P value	Odds ratio	95% confidence interval	
Patient age	0.427	1.01	0.99	1.02
Male gender	0.116	1.43	0.92	2.23
BMI	0.135	0.97	0.94	1.01
Active smoker within one year	0.473	1.19	0.74	1.89
Previous OP <30 days	0.146	1.67	0.84	3.32
Wound classification 2, 3, or 4*	**0.001**	**2.20**	1.36	3.57
ASA classification III or IV*	**0.004**	**2.17**	1.27	3.69
Diabetes*	**0.048**	**1.72**	1.01	2.93
Hypertension	0.131	1.40	0.91	2.16
Dyspnea	0.304	1.37	0.75	2.51
Bleeding disorder*	**0.003**	**3.13**	1.49	6.60
Open wound infection	0.275	1.33	0.80	2.22
Disseminated cancer	0.876	1.06	0.52	2.15
Cerebrovascular disease*	**0.021**	**2.25**	1.13	4.49
Total operation time*	**0.000**	**1.002**	1.00	1.00

* denotes significant value, $P < 0.05$.
H-L statistic: 0.736.
c-statistic: 0.815.
Criteria for inclusion into binomial logistic regression included $P < 0.2$ on univariate analysis and $n > 10$. BMI: body mass index; OP: operation; ASA: American Society of Anesthesiologists.

counseling patients about the risks of undergoing FTT surgery. The overall 30-day mortality rate for our cohort was 0.3 percent, and the overall CMO rate was 5.2 percent. Pulmonary complications (PRF and PE) accounted for the majority of CMO (4.6 percent). While every CMO collected by NSQIP occurred at least once, nonpulmonary complications were rare (0.6 percent). These outcomes were independently related to the medical comorbidities of diabetes, CVD, and bleeding disorders. They were also independently related to the surgical indices of ASA class III or IV, and wound class other than clean (i.e., clean-contaminated, contaminated, and dirty/infected). An important (although unsurprising) additional result of this study was that CMO extended LOS by approximately 14.7 days ($P < 0.001$).

Advantages of the NSQIP database include a large cohort of 2,349 patients from geographically diverse inpatient and outpatient centers, with a large number of surgeons over 6 years. The above attributes make this paper an important contribution to the current literature on medical outcomes following FTT, which previously consisted primarily of single-institution, single-surgeon experiences, which did not completely evaluate catastrophic outcomes [5, 6, 9, 12–21, 32]. The data presented here is valid for generalization by institutions that do not themselves perform internal quality analyses and hence establishes a national benchmark for CMO following FTT. The limitations of NSQIP have been previously described [33–35]. Specific to this study, NSQIP only reports data for 30 days after surgery, leading to a likely

underreporting of complications [36]. However, it is unlikely that CMO occur beyond 30 days postoperatively. The other limitation specific to this study is that some preoperative risk factors, like COPD, sepsis, or preoperative chemotherapy or radiotherapy, occurred too infrequently for inclusion in regression analysis, and so larger studies using NSQIP data from forthcoming years will aid in further defining independent risk factors for catastrophic outcomes. Finally, NSQIP does not track the specific type of free flap used for reconstruction, which can have implications for the type of CMO incurred with a given surgery [37]. Regardless of these limitations, the data presented in the paper is the most robust analysis of CMO after FTT.

Our study found an overall 30-day mortality of 0.3 percent, redemonstrating the safety of FTT. Mortality rates reported in the literature are quite variable, from as low as zero percent [13] to as high as 6.3 percent [9], likely reflecting the result of single-institution, single-surgeon studies. The data presented here indicate that the free flap mortality rate in the United States is less than estimates of overall surgical mortality in developed nations, at 0.4–0.8 percent [38], indicating that FTT is a safe surgical procedure. The overall CMO rate was 5.2 percent. Pulmonary complications (postoperative respiratory failure (PRF) and PE) occurred most frequently, at 4.6 percent. Other nonpulmonary complications were much rare at 0.6 percent.

In our study, PRF was the most common catastrophic outcome following FTT: it occurred in 93 patients (4.0 percent) and represents 61.6 percent of all 151 catastrophic outcomes. PRF is defined as failure to wean mechanical ventilation for >48 hours or unplanned reintubation [26–28]. PRF is one of the most serious pulmonary complications, and decreasing its incidence will have a large effect on outcomes and costs associated with FTT. PRF is known to increase morbidity and mortality [39] as well as to increase length of stay (LOS) and costs [40]. An analysis of Medicare data showed that PRF occurred in 73,136 patients (17.18 patients per 1000 hospitalized at-risk patients) over 2007–2009, had a mortality of 20.6 percent, and costed Medicare $1.96 billion US dollars [41]. PRF is thus a major burden on healthcare resources. Indeed, another study using the NSQIP database found PRF was associated with the largest attributable cost among the top 4 postoperative complications [40]. The Agency for Healthcare Research and Quality has identified PRF as 1 of 20 patient safety indicators to track healthcare outcomes [42], and in 2014 it will be included in the proposed rule for hospital value-based purchasing program for Medicare inpatient services [41]. Our report is the first to identify the national rate of PRF following FTT, at four percent. Adequate understanding of its risk factors, prevention, and treatment are thus important areas for future investigation.

Pulmonary embolism was the second most common CMO, occurring in 0.6 percent of all patients undergoing FTT and accounting for 9.3 percent of all 151 CMO. The 14 cases of PE occurred throughout the 30 days of available data (range POD 1–24; data not shown) and thus were not clustered in the immediate postoperative period. Rates of PE reported in the literature vary from near zero percent [13, 43] to 3.8 percent [12], again likely reflecting single-institution, single-surgeon studies. Our data again provide an important benchmark of the national multi-institutional rate of PE after FTT and establish PE as the second most common CMO following FTT. In addition, DVT or thrombophlebitis occurred in 6 of the 122 patients (4.9 percent) who suffered a CMO, compared to 11 of the 2,227 patients who did not (0.5 percent) ($P < 0.001$, Fisher's Exact Test; data not shown), suggesting insufficient DVT prophylaxis among patients who suffer CMO following FTT. Indeed, studies of anticoagulation in head and neck FTT patients reveal that less than half of patients achieve therapeutic anticoagulation [19]. Taken together, these findings underscore the importance of adequate VTE prophylaxis in FTT patients. Similar to PRF, postoperative PE or DVT occurred in 130,927 patients from 2007 to 2009 and costed Medicare $1.42 billion in excess costs. For these reasons, it is also included in the proposed rule for hospital value-based purchasing program for Medicare inpatient services [41].

While the overall CMO rate was low at 5.2 percent, an important finding of this study was that such outcomes were significantly associated with a longer length of total hospital stay (LOS), by an average of just over 2 weeks ($P < 0.001$). Thus, while FTT is in general safe, the financial impact of CMO is tremendous. We did not examine this directly, but Fischer and colleagues recently reported that medical complications added about $350,000 of direct costs following FTT for breast reconstruction [13]. Their medical complications were less severe, adding an average of only 1.72 days to their patients' hospital stay, contrasting to 14.7 days added for patients who suffered a CMO in the present report. Preventive strategies targeted at these CMO could thus result in substantial healthcare savings and further optimize the safety of these procedures.

Our regression analysis identified preoperative risk factors that independently predicted CMO, including bleeding disorders, diabetes, and cerebrovascular disease. Wound classification of anything *other than* a clean case (i.e., clean-contaminated, contaminated, dirty/infected) and ASA class of III or IV also independently predicted CMO. Total operation time was also an independent predictor, as reported elsewhere [44]. While the impact of each individual minute was small (OR 1.002), it is understandable how increased operative times of 1-2 hours (or more) could result in clinically significant CMO. The authors thus argue that every effort should be made to maximize efficiency in the operating room and minimize operative time (without sacrificing patient safety or best medical practice).

A number of factors associated with adverse events are well described in the literature, but their association with CMO merits special mention. ASA scores have been utilized as a substitute for overall physical fitness [45]. The potential subjectivity of this value has been a topic of controversy in outcomes studies, yet these results continue to demonstrate its association with outcomes. Consistent with these findings, our study found a significant association between ASA class III or IV and CMO. Diabetes mellitus is associated with a long list of postoperative surgical and medical complications, including stroke, myocardial infarction, and wound infection

[46, 47]. Such findings argue for thorough preoperative optimization of patients before undergoing FTT, particularly with regard to ASA class. We have further adopted a strict protocol for evaluation of diabetic patients. Patients with hemoglobin A1C levels above 7% undergo preoperative medical evaluation to ensure that they have an adequate regimen for diabetic control. All patients abstain from oral hypoglycemic agents the day of surgery but receive one-half of their regular insulin dose. Postoperatively, all patients are started on intravenous insulin drips with continuous titration and resume oral hypoglycemics (if tolerating oral medications and diet) on postoperative day one. Finally, a history of cerebrovascular disease (CVD) has previously been associated with adverse events, presumably owing to issues with airway protection and postoperative mobilization [48, 49]. While a history of CVD is not routinely recognized in single-center outcomes studies as a factor associated with AEs, it has repeatedly appeared in large-database studies, presumably owing to the power of these studies to find significant associations in large numbers of patients. Pursuant to this finding, we routinely request speech therapy evaluations prior to oral intake in patients with difficult speaking or swallowing and rigorously follow positioning, hygiene, physical and occupational therapy, and venous thromboembolic prevention protocols for patients with impaired mobility.

An association between contaminated wounds and adverse events after surgery is well documented. A 2011 study by Lee et al. showed a direct relationship between wound contamination with oral flora and postoperative wound infection, while other studies have found that patients undergoing mandibulectomy, glossectomy, tonsillectomy, and laryngectomy had a significant risk for postoperative pneumonia compared to those undergoing pharyngectomy and esophagectomy, further increasing the length of hospitalization and mortality [50, 51]. Such findings are consistent with the current study, showing increased CMO in the setting of contaminated surgical wounds, and, in cases of head and neck surgery, posit a causative mechanism. Given that contaminated wound status is associated with CMO, what can be done about it? The role of prophylactic antibiotics in preventing surgical site infection in head and neck procedures has been extensively studied at single institutions [52–55]. Studies in the general surgery literature suggest that 24 hours of antibiotic therapy is an adequate treatment period [56, 57]. In the head and neck literature, there has been some evaluation of optimal duration of antibiotic usage, but there is a lack of multi-institutional studies evaluating this. The use of prophylactic antibiotics in clean-contaminated cases has been shown to reduce the risk of wound infection from ranges of 30–80% to 22–47%. A prospective, randomized trial by Righi et al. of 192 patients undergoing aerodigestive or laryngeal surgery through a cervical skin incision was divided into groups receiving either 1 or 3 days of antibiotic prophylaxis. The study failed to show a significant difference in the rate of wound infection, regardless of antibiotic duration. Finally, the principals of debridement of all necrotic or devitalized material and timely surgical intervention before significant infection can be established (as with extremity salvage or sternal wound infection), or of delaying reconstruction until wounds are free of surgical infection are considerations highlighted by our study.

Of the presurgical comorbidities, a history of bleeding disorders was independently associated with catastrophic outcomes and was found to have the highest associated odds ratio (OR 3.13, $P = 0.003$). Bleeding disorders are defined by NSQIP as "any condition that places the patient at risk for excessive bleeding requiring hospitalization due to a deficiency of blood clotting elements (e.g., vitamin K deficiency, hemophilias, thrombocytopenia, chronic anti-coagulation therapy that has not been discontinued prior to surgery). Patients are not included who are on chronic aspirin therapy." Few papers describe the implications of hematologic disorders in free tissue transfer [58–61]. These patients typically suffer postoperative bleeding at the sites of vascular anastomoses or donor site and reoperation [58–60]. Given the focus of our study, we did not include these complications for analysis, but we did identify that, in addition to well-known surgical complications, bleeding disorders are also independent predictors of catastrophic medical complications following FTT. A major limitation of the NSQIP database is that further information regarding the type and nature of a patient's bleeding disorder is not available. Possible explanations are that patients with hematological disease often have other medical problems [58] which could complicate their surgery, that is, hematological malignancies causing thrombocytopenia and/or pancytopenias, predisposing to infection, sepsis, and death [58, 62]. NSQIP also categorizes patients who have not withheld their chronic anticoagulation before surgery as having a bleeding disorder. However, most microsurgeons report the use of anticoagulants in their routine practice [10, 19], although this is controversial [22, 63]. While most discussions of anticoagulation and bleeding disorders focus on flap loss, our study adds an important contribution that bleeding disorders are also associated with CMO. Further research focusing on patients with bleeding disorders, with reference to specific disorders, is needed to clarify this relationship. It has also been estimated that over 95% of clinical hematologic abnormalities can be screened by simply asking the patient, "Have you, or anyone in your family, had and history of bleeding or clotting disorders?" [64]. For patients who respond affirmatively to this question, we routinely send patients for preoperative hematology evaluations. While this may seem to be an onerous burden to patients, physicians, and payers alike, data linking hematologic abnormalities to both free flap loss and now CMO after FTT makes this evaluation worthwhile.

Of note, patients with pulmonary comorbidities before surgery, including dependence on mechanical ventilation and dyspnea at rest or with moderate exertion, were all significantly associated with CMO on univariate analysis. Seventeen of the 122 patients who suffered a CMO had dyspnea at rest or with moderate exertion. Dyspnea was included in the logistic regression but was found not to be an independent predictor of catastrophic outcomes ($P = 0.304$). Severe COPD and ventilator dependence were too infrequent to be included in regression analysis, so we cannot determine if they are independently associated with catastrophic

outcomes. Other studies have found that COPD is independently associated with medical complications (ranging from minor to severe) following FTT, with odds ratios as high as 17.2 [13]. Considering that the majority (4.6 of the total 5.2 percent) of CMO following FTT were pulmonary in nature, preoperative optimization strategies are an excellent target for intervention. These include at the minimum preoperative PA and lateral chest X-rays but more reasonably include a formal respiratory evaluation with a pulmonary specialist and perhaps either pulmonary function tests or CT scans based on the severity of the patient's disease. Based on the results of this study, we have developed same-day extubation protocols for patients undergoing FTT and aggressive postoperative pulmonary toilet (both on and off the ventilator) and are a part of our routine management. While it was not found to be independently associated with CMO after FTT, smoking is a well-documented predictor of surgical complications and surgical failure following reconstructive surgery [17, 32, 35]. The authors still consider it prudent to counsel patients to quit several months before any major surgery [65, 66] and now routinely request preoperative consultations for patients with any smoking history greater than 15 pack-years and for all patients with a smoking history associated with any pulmonary comorbidity.

5. Conclusion

This is the largest single clinical study examining catastrophic outcomes following FTT. The data suggest that FTT is safe, with a 30-day mortality of 0.3 percent. Overall, catastrophic medical complications occurred in 5.2 percent of patients and were associated with a two-week delay in hospital discharge on average. Independent risk factors for catastrophic medical outcomes included wound classification of clean-contaminated, contaminated, or dirty/infected, ASA classification of class III or IV, bleeding disorders, diabetes, and CVD. The results presented in the study provide the microsurgeon with useful risk-stratifying criteria to improve patient outcomes and indicate directions to reduce healthcare costs.

Disclosure

The level of evidence for this study is Level III, prognostic/risk study.

References

[1] B. Seidenberg, S. S. Rosenak, E. S. Hurwitt, and M. L. Som, "Immediate reconstruction of the cervical esophagus by a revascularized isolated jejunal segment," *Annals of Surgery*, vol. 149, no. 2, pp. 162–171, 1959.

[2] D. H. McLean and H. J. Buncke Jr., "Autotransplant of omentum to a large scalp defect, with microsurgical revascularization,"

Plastic and Reconstructive Surgery, vol. 49, no. 3, pp. 268–274, 1972.

[3] W. W. Shaw, "Microvascular free flaps. The first decade," *Clinics in Plastic Surgery*, vol. 10, no. 1, pp. 3–20, 1983.

[4] R. K. Khouri, "Free flap surgery: the second decade," *Clinics in Plastic Surgery*, vol. 19, no. 4, pp. 757–761, 1992.

[5] A. O. Momoh, S. Colakoglu, T. S. Westvik et al., "Analysis of complications and patient satisfaction in pedicled transverse rectus abdominis myocutaneous and deep inferior epigastric perforator flap breast reconstruction," *Annals of Plastic Surgery*, vol. 69, no. 1, pp. 19–23, 2012.

[6] K. Seidenstuecker, B. Munder, A. L. Mahajan, P. Richrath, P. Behrendt, and C. Andree, "Morbidity of microsurgical breast reconstruction in patients with comorbid conditions," *Plastic and Reconstructive Surgery*, vol. 127, no. 3, pp. 1086–1092, 2011.

[7] A. K. Alderman, E. G. Wilkins, J. C. Lowery, M. Kim, and J. A. Davis, "Determinants of patient satisfaction in postmastectomy breast reconstruction," *Plastic and Reconstructive Surgery*, vol. 106, no. 4, pp. 769–776, 2000.

[8] J. H. Yueh, S. A. Slavin, T. Adesiyun et al., "Patient satisfaction in postmastectomy breast reconstruction: a comparative evaluation of DIEP, TRAM, latissimus flap, and implant techniques," *Plastic and Reconstructive Surgery*, vol. 125, no. 6, pp. 1585–1595, 2010.

[9] E. A. Lueg, "Comparing microvascular outcomes at a large integrated health maintenance organization with flagship centers in the United States," *Archives of Otolaryngology—Head and Neck Surgery*, vol. 130, no. 6, pp. 779–785, 2004.

[10] L. Salemark, "International survey of current microvascular practices in free tissue transfer and replantation surgery," *Microsurgery*, vol. 12, no. 4, pp. 308–311, 1991.

[11] R. K. Khouri, "Avoiding free flap failure," *Clinics in Plastic Surgery*, vol. 19, no. 4, pp. 773–781, 1992.

[12] S. O. P. Hofer, T. H. C. Damen, M. A. M. Mureau, H. A. Rakhorst, and N. A. Roche, "A critical review of perioperative complications in 175 free deep inferior epigastric perforator flap breast reconstructions," *Annals of Plastic Surgery*, vol. 59, no. 2, pp. 137–142, 2007.

[13] J. P. Fischer, B. Sieber, J. A. Nelson et al., "Comprehensive outcome and cost analysis of free tissue transfer for breast reconstruction: an experience with 1303 flaps," *Plastic and Reconstructive Surgery*, vol. 131, no. 2, pp. 195–203, 2013.

[14] S. L. Spear, I. Ducic, F. Cuoco, and C. Hannan, "The effect of smoking on flap and donor-site complications in pedicled TRAM breast reconstruction," *Plastic and Reconstructive Surgery*, vol. 116, no. 7, pp. 1873–1880, 2005.

[15] S. Colakoglu, I. Khansa, M. S. Curtis et al., "Impact of complications on patient satisfaction in breast reconstruction," *Plastic and Reconstructive Surgery*, vol. 127, no. 4, pp. 1428–1436, 2011.

[16] M. Y. Nahabedian, B. Momen, G. Galdino, and P. N. Manson, "Breast reconstruction with the free TRAM or DIEP flap: patient selection, choice of flap, and outcome," *Plastic and Reconstructive Surgery*, vol. 110, no. 2, pp. 466–475, 2002.

[17] J. C. Selber, J. E. Kurichi, S. J. Vega, S. S. Sonnad, and J. M. Serletti, "Risk factors and complications in free TRAM flap breast reconstruction," *Annals of Plastic Surgery*, vol. 56, no. 5, pp. 492–497, 2006.

[18] B. J. Mehrara, T. D. Santoro, E. Arcilla, J. P. Watson, W. W. Shaw, and A. L. Da Lio, "Complications after microvascular breast reconstruction: experience with 1195 flaps," *Plastic and Reconstructive Surgery*, vol. 118, no. 5, pp. 1100–1109, 2006.

[19] K. A. Eley, R. J. Parker, and S. R. Watt-Smith, "Low molecular weight heparin in patients undergoing free tissue transfer following head and neck ablative surgery: review of efficacy and associated complications," *British Journal of Oral and Maxillofacial Surgery*, vol. 51, no. 7, pp. 610–614, 2013.

[20] M. Gerressen, C. I. Pastaschek, D. Riediger et al., "Microsurgical free flap reconstructions of head and neck region in 406 cases: a 13-year experience," *Journal of Oral and Maxillofacial Surgery*, vol. 71, no. 3, pp. 628–635, 2013.

[21] J. C. Grotting, M. M. Urist, W. A. Maddox, and L. O. Vasconez, "Conventional TRAM flap versus free microsurgical TRAM flap for immediate breast reconstruction," *Plastic and Reconstructive Surgery*, vol. 83, no. 5, pp. 828–841, 1989.

[22] J. Fosnot, S. Jandali, D. W. Low, S. J. Kovach III, L. C. Wu, and J. M. Serletti, "Closer to an understanding of fate: the role of vascular complications in free flap breast reconstruction," *Plastic and Reconstructive Surgery*, vol. 128, no. 4, pp. 835–843, 2011.

[23] "Resources: ACS NSQIP data: participant use data file," vol. 2012, American College of Surgeons National Surgical Quality Improvement Program, 2012.

[24] J. D. Birkmeyer, D. M. Shahian, J. B. Dimick et al., "Blueprint for a New American College of Surgeons: national surgical quality improvement program," *Journal of the American College of Surgeons*, vol. 207, no. 5, pp. 777–782, 2008.

[25] K. S. Rowell, F. E. Turrentine, M. M. Hutter, S. F. Khuri, and W. G. Henderson, "Use of national surgical quality improvement program data as a catalyst for quality improvement," *Journal of the American College of Surgeons*, vol. 204, no. 6, pp. 1293–1300, 2007.

[26] A. M. Arozullah, J. Daley, W. G. Henderson, and S. F. Khuri, "Multifactorial risk index for predicting postoperative respiratory failure in men after major noncardiac surgery The National Veterans Administration Surgical Quality Improvement Program," *Annals of Surgery*, vol. 232, pp. 242–253, 2000.

[27] H. Gupta, P. K. Gupta, X. Fang et al., "Development and validation of a risk calculator predicting postoperative respiratory failure," *Chest*, vol. 140, no. 5, pp. 1207–1215, 2011.

[28] R. G. Johnson, A. M. Arozullah, L. Neumayer, W. G. Henderson, P. Hosokawa, and S. F. Khuri, "Multivariable predictors of postoperative respiratory failure after general and vascular surgery: results from the patient safety in surgery study," *Journal of the American College of Surgeons*, vol. 204, no. 6, pp. 1188–1198, 2007.

[29] G. L. Kaluza, J. Joseph, J. R. Lee, M. E. Raizner, and A. E. Raizner, "Catastrophic outcomes of noncardiac surgery soon after coronary stenting," *Journal of the American College of Cardiology*, vol. 35, no. 5, pp. 1288–1294, 2000.

[30] S. K. Vora, R. A. Asherson, and D. Erkan, "Catastrophic antiphospholipid syndrome," *Journal of Intensive Care Medicine*, vol. 21, no. 3, pp. 144–159, 2006.

[31] A. Marquez-Lara, S. V. Nandyala, H. Hassanzadeh, M. Noureldin, S. Sankaranarayanan, and K. Singh, "Sentinel events in cervical spine surgery," *Spine*, vol. 39, no. 9, pp. 715–720, 2014.

[32] C. M. McCarthy, B. J. Mehrara, E. Riedel et al., "Predicting complications following expander/implant breast reconstruction: an outcomes analysis based on preoperative clinical risk," *Plastic and Reconstructive Surgery*, vol. 121, no. 6, pp. 1886–1892, 2008.

[33] L. M. Mioton, J. T. Smetona, P. J. Hanwright et al., "Comparing thirty-day outcomes in prosthetic and autologous breast reconstruction: a multivariate analysis of 13,082 patients?" *Journal of Plastic, Reconstructive and Aesthetic Surgery*, vol. 66, no. 7, pp. 917–925, 2013.

[34] M. S. Gart, J. T. Smetona, P. J. Hanwright et al., "Autologous options for postmastectomy breast reconstruction: a comparison of outcomes based on the American College of Surgeons National Surgical Quality Improvement Program," *Journal of the American College of Surgeons*, vol. 216, pp. 216–229, 2013.

[35] S. W. Jordan, L. M. Mioton, J. Smetona et al., "Resident involvement and plastic surgery outcomes: an analysis of 10,356 patients from the american college of surgeons national surgical quality improvement program database," *Plastic and Reconstructive Surgery*, vol. 131, no. 4, pp. 763–773, 2013.

[36] A. A. Ogunleye, C. De Blacam, M. S. Curtis, S. Colakoglu, A. M. Tobias, and B. T. Lee, "An analysis of delayed breast reconstruction outcomes as recorded in the American College of Surgeons National Surgical Quality Improvement Program," *Journal of Plastic, Reconstructive and Aesthetic Surgery*, vol. 65, no. 3, pp. 289–295, 2012.

[37] K. J. Shultz, S. Don, R. C. Mahabir, and C. N. Verheyden, "Pulmonary function after pedicled transverse rectus abdominis musculocutaneous flap breast reconstruction," *Annals of Plastic Surgery*, 2014.

[38] A. B. Haynes, T. G. Weiser, W. R. Berry et al., "A surgical safety checklist to reduce morbidity and mortality in a global population," *The New England Journal of Medicine*, vol. 360, no. 5, pp. 491–499, 2009.

[39] S. F. Khuri, W. G. Henderson, R. G. DePalma et al., "Determinants of long-term survival after major surgery and the adverse effect of postoperative complications," *Annals of Surgery*, vol. 242, no. 3, pp. 326–343, 2005.

[40] J. B. Dimick, S. L. Chen, P. A. Taheri, W. G. Henderson, S. F. Khuri, and D. A. Campbell Jr., "Hospital costs associated with surgical complications: a report from the private-sector National Surgical Quality Improvement Program," *Journal of the American College of Surgeons*, vol. 199, no. 4, pp. 531–537, 2004.

[41] *The Eighth Annual HealthGrades Patient Safety in American Hospitals Study*, HealthGrades Inc., 2011.

[42] Agency for Healthcare Research and Quality, 2013, http://www.qualityindicators.ahrq.gov/.

[43] S. Vega, J. M. Smartt Jr., S. Jiang et al., "500 Consecutive patients with free TRAM flap breast reconstruction: a single surgeon's experience," *Plastic and Reconstructive Surgery*, vol. 122, no. 2, pp. 329–339, 2008.

[44] A. Rambachan, L. M. Mioton, S. Saha, N. Fine, and J. Y. S. Kim, "The impact of surgical duration on plastic surgery outcomes," *European Journal of Plastic Surgery*, vol. 36, no. 11, pp. 707–714, 2013.

[45] S. R. Schwartz, B. Yueh, C. Maynard, J. Daley, W. Henderson, and S. F. Khuri, "Predictors of wound complications after laryngectomy: a study of over 2000 patients," *Otolaryngology—Head and Neck Surgery*, vol. 131, no. 1, pp. 61–68, 2004.

[46] S. E. Kahn, M. E. Cooper, and S. del Prato, "Pathophysiology and treatment of type 2 diabetes: perspectives on the past, present, and future," *The Lancet*, vol. 383, no. 9922, pp. 1068–1083, 2014.

[47] H. Young, B. Knepper, E. E. Moore, J. L. Johnson, P. Mehler, and C. S. Price, "Surgical site infection after colon surgery: National healthcare safety network risk factors and modeled rates compared with published risk factors and rates," *Journal of the American College of Surgeons*, vol. 214, no. 5, pp. 852–859, 2012.

[48] B. Dhungel, B. S. Diggs, J. G. Hunter, B. C. Sheppard, J. T. Vetto, and J. P. Dolan, "Patient and peri-operative predictors of morbidity and mortality after esophagectomy: American College of Surgeons National Sugical Quality Improvement Program (ACS-NSQIP), 2005–2008," *Journal of Gastrointestinal Surgery*, vol. 14, no. 10, pp. 1492–1501, 2010.

[49] R. Ricciardi, P. L. Roberts, T. E. Read, J. F. Hall, P. W. Marcello, and D. J. Schoetz, "Which adverse events are associated with mortality and prolonged length of stay following colorectal surgery?" *Journal of Gastrointestinal Surgery*, vol. 17, no. 8, pp. 1485–1493, 2013.

[50] D. H. Lee, S. Y. Kim, S. Y. Nam, S.-H. Choi, J. W. Choi, and J.-L. Roh, "Risk factors of surgical site infection in patients undergoing major oncological surgery for head and neck cancer," *Oral Oncology*, vol. 47, no. 6, pp. 528–531, 2011.

[51] Y. R. Semenov, H. M. Starmer, and C. G. Gourin, "The effect of pneumonia on short-term outcomes and cost of care after head and neck cancer surgery," *Laryngoscope*, vol. 122, no. 9, pp. 1994–2004, 2012.

[52] N. Penel, C. Fournier, D. Lefebvre, and J.-L. Lefebvre, "Multivariate analysis of risk factors for wound infection in head and neck squamous cell carcinoma surgery with opening of mucosa. Study of 260 surgical procedures," *Oral Oncology*, vol. 41, no. 3, pp. 294–303, 2005.

[53] N. Penel, D. Lefebvre, C. Fournier, J. Sarini, A. Kara, and J.-L. Lefebvre, "Risk factors for wound infection in head and neck cancer surgery: a prospective study," *Head and Neck*, vol. 23, no. 6, pp. 447–455, 2001.

[54] L.-X. Man, D. M. Beswick, and J. T. Johnson, "Antibiotic prophylaxis in uncontaminated neck dissection," *Laryngoscope*, vol. 121, no. 7, pp. 1473–1477, 2011.

[55] M. Righi, R. Manfredi, G. Farneti, E. Pasquini, and V. Cenacchi, "Short-term versus long-term antimicrobial prophylaxis in oncologic head and neck surgery," *Head and Neck*, vol. 18, no. 5, pp. 399–404, 1996.

[56] T. C. Fabian, M. A. Croce, L. W. Payne et al., "Duration of antibiotic therapy for penetrating abdominal trauma: a prospective trial," *Surgery*, vol. 112, no. 4, pp. 788–794, 1992.

[57] S. R. Goldberg, R. J. Anand, J. J. Como et al., "Prophylactic antibiotic use in penetrating abdominal trauma: an eastern association for the surgery of trauma practice management guideline," *Journal of Trauma and Acute Care Surgery*, vol. 73, no. 5, pp. S321–S325, 2012.

[58] Ö. Özkan, H.-C. Chen, S. Mardini et al., "Microvascular free tissue transfer in patients with hematological disorders," *Plastic and Reconstructive Surgery*, vol. 118, no. 4, pp. 936–944, 2006.

[59] C. Carroll, M. J. Yaremchuk, W. R. Bell, D. F. Martin, J. R. Moore, and A. J. Weiland, "Treatment of hemophilic pseudotumor with radical debridement and free tissue transfer. A case report," *Orthopedics*, vol. 12, no. 4, pp. 561–565, 1989.

[60] P. D. Knott, S. S. Khariwala, and J. Minarchek, "Hemophilia B and free tissue transfer: medical and surgical management," *Annals of Plastic Surgery*, vol. 54, no. 3, pp. 336–338, 2005.

[61] T. Y. Wang, J. M. Serletti, A. Cuker et al., "Free tissue transfer in the hypercoagulable patient: a review of 58 flaps," *Plastic and Reconstructive Surgery*, vol. 129, no. 2, pp. 443–453, 2012.

[62] J. Verhoef, "Prevention of infections in the neutropenic patient," *Clinical Infectious Diseases*, vol. 17, supplement 2, pp. S359–S367, 1993.

[63] C. M. Chen, P. Ashjian, J. J. Disa, P. G. Cordeiro, A. L. Pusic, and B. J. Mehrara, "Is the use of intraoperative heparin safe?" *Plastic and Reconstructive Surgery*, vol. 121, no. 3, pp. 49e–53e, 2008.

[64] J. Michaels, D. Coon, C. L. Mulvey, and J. P. Rubin, "Venous thromboembolism prophylaxis in the massive weight loss patient: relative risk of bleeding," *Annals of Plastic Surgery*, 2014.

[65] K. Myers, P. Hajek, C. Hinds, and H. McRobbie, "Stopping smoking shortly before surgery and postoperative complications: a systematic review and meta-analysis," *Archives of Internal Medicine*, vol. 171, no. 11, pp. 983–989, 2011.

[66] C. K. Chow and P. J. Devereaux, "The optimal timing of smoking cessation before surgery," *Archives of Internal Medicine*, vol. 171, no. 11, pp. 989–990, 2011.

27

Skin Sparing Mastectomy with Preservation of Nipple Areola Complex and Immediate Breast Reconstruction in Patients with Breast Cancer: A Single Centre Prospective Study

Debarati Chattopadhyay,[1] **Souradip Gupta,**[2] **Prabir Kumar Jash,**[2]
Marang Buru Murmu,[3] **and Sandipan Gupta**[2]

[1] *Department of Plastic Surgery, IPGME&R, Kolkata, India*
[2] *Department of Plastic Surgery, Medical College Kolkata, 88 College Street, Kolkata, West Bengal 700073, India*
[3] *Department of Surgery, Midnapore Medical College, India*

Correspondence should be addressed to Debarati Chattopadhyay; debarati1981@gmail.com

Academic Editor: Georg M. Huemer

Background. Skin and nipple areola sparing mastectomy (NASM) has recently gained popularity as the management of breast cancer. This study aims to evaluate the aesthetic outcome, patient satisfaction, and oncological safety of NASM. *Methods.* The study prospectively analyzes the results of NASM and immediate breast reconstruction in 34 women with breast cancer. The criteria for inclusion were core biopsy-proven, peripherally located breast cancer of any tumor size and with any "N" status, with documented negative intraoperative frozen section biopsy of retroareolar tissue, and distance from the nipple to tumor margin >2 cm on mammography. *Results.* The median age of the patients was 45 years. The majority had either stage II or stage III breast cancer. The median mammographic distance of tumor from nipple areola complex (NAC) was 3.8 cm. The overall operative morbidity was minimal. The NAC could be preserved in all the patients. There was no local recurrence of tumor at median follow-up of 28.5 months. The aesthetic outcomes were satisfactory. *Conclusion.* NASM and immediate breast reconstruction can be successfully achieved with minimal morbidity and very low risk of local recurrence in appropriately selected breast cancer patients, with acceptable aesthetic results and good patient satisfaction.

1. Introduction

Modified radical mastectomy is a disfiguring operation that is associated with considerable psychological trauma for the affected woman. A woman diagnosed with breast cancer fears not only for her life but also the mutilation of her body. On the other hand women undergoing breast conserving surgery (BCS) live with constant anxiety of harbouring the residual malignancy within. Research to find a feasible alternative has led to the renewal of interest in skin sparing and nipple areola complex sparing mastectomy (NASM) which entails the removal of the breast tissue while preserving the natural skin envelope as much as possible.

First described by Freeman in the 1960s, NASM was traditionally utilized for benign breast lesions [1]. Although there were sporadic reports of mastectomy with NAC preservation

for breast cancer treatment in the 1980s the technique fell into disuse during subsequent years due to controversies about its oncologic safety [1–3].

The resurgence of this procedure as the primary management in breast cancer has been made possible by a number of studies which have concluded that the nipple areola complex involvement by breast cancer has been overestimated in the past. The results of studies worldwide suggest that preservation of the nipple areola complex with immediate breast reconstruction is oncologically safe in carefully selected patients, with superior aesthetic outcome. However, review of the literature has revealed scarcity of data from India on this subject.

The present study prospectively analyzed the results of skin sparing mastectomy with nipple areola complex preservation and immediate breast reconstruction in women with breast cancer in a teaching hospital in India. A total of 34 patients were studied with assessment of the aesthetic outcomes, patient satisfaction with the results of surgery, and evaluation of the oncological safety of the surgical procedure in terms of local recurrence of breast cancer.

1.1. Aims and Objectives of the Study

(1) To evaluate the aesthetic outcome in women undergoing nipple areola and skin sparing mastectomy (NASM) for breast cancer and immediate breast reconstruction.

(2) To assess patient satisfaction after the surgical procedure.

(3) To evaluate the oncological safety of the surgical procedure in terms of local recurrence of breast cancer.

2. Materials and Methods

The present study prospectively analyzed the results of NASM and immediate breast reconstruction in 34 patients with breast cancer attending the Department of Plastic Surgery, Medical College Kolkata, India, over a period of twenty-one months between April 2011 and December 2012. The criteria for inclusion were core biopsy-proven, peripherally located breast cancer of any tumour size and with any "N" status, located >2 cm away from margin of areola, with documented negative intraoperative frozen section biopsy of retroareolar tissue, and distance from the nipple to tumour margin >2 cm on mammography or high-resolution ultrasonography. Patients having a central quadrant tumour, a tumour encroaching within 2 cm of areolar margin, a tumour fixed to the chest wall, clinical suspicion of nipple areola involvement, or inflammatory breast cancer were excluded from the study.

The parameters to be studied were prefixed as follows:

(1) aesthetic outcome: this was stratified by subscales according to Lowery et al. [4]. Volume, contour, placement of breast mound, and inframammary fold were evaluated with zero to 2 points for each parameter. Results were defined as excellent: 7 to 8 points, good: 6 to 6.9 points, fair: 5 to 5.9 points, and poor: <5 points;

(2) patient satisfaction: the scoring was done by the patient along a scale of 1 to 10 where score 1 to 4 was categorized as poor, 5 to 6 as fair, 7 to 8 as good, and 9 to 10 as excellent;

(3) oncological safety: local recurrence was defined as histologically proven recurrent tumor occurring in either the ipsilateral breast skin or the nipple areola complex.

2.1. Study Tools and Technique

2.1.1. Operative Technique. For nipple areola sparing and skin sparing mastectomy (NASM), either lateral incision or

inframammary incision was used. In case of inframammary incision the axillary nodal dissection was done through a separate vertical or inverted hockey stick like incision in the axilla. After skin incision, the breast tissue was dissected from the pectoralis fascia by sharp dissection. The dissection was then carried in the subdermal plane. The skin flap thickness varied from 2 to 5 mm and consisted of 1-2 mm of intact dermis and a thin layer of subcutaneous fat. The base of the nipple was divided sharply. The nipple papilla was not cored out.

2.1.2. Frozen Section Biopsy. Intraoperative frozen section biopsy was taken from two sites. A total of 5 samples were taken in each case:

(i) two samples from the glandular tissue under the areola,

(ii) one sample from the nipple base,

(iii) two samples from the subcutaneous tissue overlying the tumour.

All the frozen section biopsy samples were interpreted by the same pathologist in the Department of Pathology, Medical College Kolkata. The NAC was preserved only when palpation, shape, and color of the nipple were normal and when intraoperative frozen section biopsy from under the NAC was tumor-free. If the subcutaneous tissue overlying the tumor was found to be positive on frozen section biopsy an incision was placed over the tumor site and a skin island was dissected with the breast specimen to achieve distant tumor-free margins.

2.1.3. Breast Reconstruction. After the completion of the mastectomy and appropriate axillary clearance, all patients underwent immediate breast reconstruction with either (i) autologous tissue: the transverse rectus abdominis myocutaneous (TRAM) flap or the latissimus dorsi myocutaneous flap, or (ii) by the placement of a permanent silicone gel implant.

2.1.4. Follow-Up. Adjuvant systemic treatment was administered according to the NCCN guidelines. The final aesthetic results were evaluated at 6 months postoperatively and stratified by subscales according to Lowery et al. [4]. The patients were followed up regularly for at least 18 months after surgery.

3. Results

The median age of the patients was 45 years (range: 28–61 years). Majority of patients (55.9%) were in the age group of 41 to 50 years. At the time of diagnosis 13 patients had TNM stage IIIA breast cancer, 19 patients had stage II cancer, and only one patient had stage I cancer. All the patients had invasive ductal carcinoma, except a single patient who had ductal carcinoma in situ (DCIS) (Table 1). The distance of tumour from the nipple areola complex as seen on mammography was between 2 cm and 4 cm in about two-thirds of the patients in our study, and the median distance of

TABLE 1: Breast cancer stage at diagnosis.

Stage of breast cancer	Number of cases	Percentage
0 (DCIS)	1	2.9
I	1	2.9
IIA	7	20.6
IIB	12	35.3
IIIA	13	38.3
Total	34	100

TABLE 2: List of complications in postoperative period.

Complication	Number of patients	Percentage
Seroma	2	5.8%
Partial desquamation of NAC	1	2.9%
Wound infection	1	2.9%
Partial umbilical necrosis (after TRAM flap)	1	2.9%

TABLE 3: Results of aesthetic outcome in terms of Lowery scale.

Lowery score	Number of patients	Percentage
Excellent (score 7-8)	17	50%
Good (score 6–6.9)	14	41.2%
Fair (score 5–5.9)	3	8.8%
Poor (score < 5)	0	0
Total	34	100

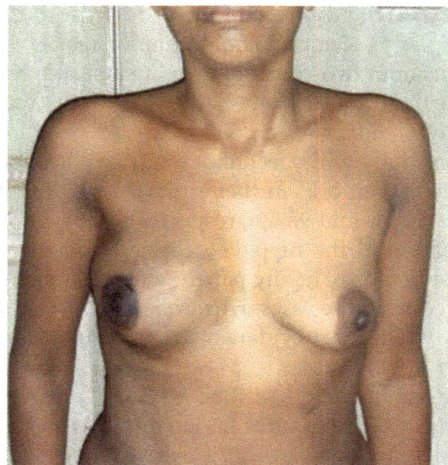

FIGURE 1: Follow-up of patient after NASM and TRAM flap reconstruction of right breast.

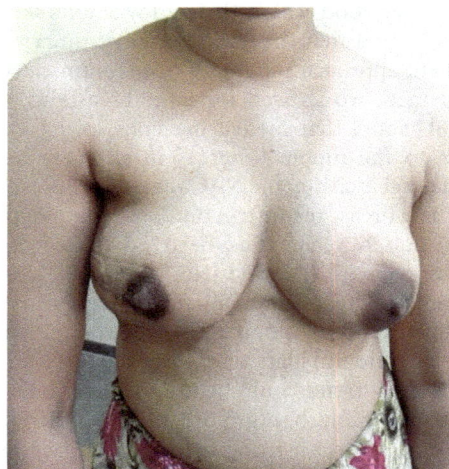

FIGURE 2: Follow-up of patient after NASM and implant reconstruction of right breast.

the tumour from NAC was 3.8 cm (range: 2.4–5.2 cm). Intra-operative frozen section studies of retroareolar tissue and the subcutaneous tissue immediately above the tumour were performed to decide whether the NAC should be preserved or not. No involvement of the nipple core or areola was found on frozen section biopsy in any patient. Frozen section biopsy was positive from the subcutaneous tissue immediately above the tumour in 5 cases (14.7%). The mastectomy incisions used were mainly inframammary (67%) and lateral (17.6%) incisions. Immediate breast reconstruction using autologous tissue was performed in more than 90% of cases (TRAM flap in 55% and latissimus dorsi myocutaneous flap in 36% cases), whereas silicone implants were used in 8.8% of cases only. The patients received adjuvant systemic treatment as per standard practice guidelines. The overall operative morbidity was minimal with only a few minor complications. The nipple areola complex could be preserved in all the cases (Table 2).

The median follow-up was 28.5 months (range: 18–38 months). There was no local recurrence of tumour at follow-up. The aesthetic outcome was excellent in 50% of cases and good in 41.2% of cases (Table 3). Patient satisfaction with results of surgery was excellent in 35.3% of cases and good in 50% of cases. Figures 1 and 2 depict the aesthetic outcome of nipple areola and skin sparing mastectomy after 6 months.

4. Discussion

The technique of NASM involves a combination of a skin sparing mastectomy with preservation of the NAC [5]. There have been various attempts over the years to define the selection criteria for NSM [1, 6–12]. There is still no consensus on the indications for this procedure [1]. Recent multivariate models for patient selection for NASM have reported tumour size, stage, and tumour distance from the nipple as some factors predictive of occult nipple involvement [13, 14]. We followed the criteria used by Garcia-Etienne et al. [1]. However, further studies and longer follow-up are necessary to refine the selection criteria for NASM.

Loewen et al. have shown that mammographic distance between the tumor and the nipple is independently predictive of NAC involvement [12]. Some authors have excluded patients from undergoing NASM if imaging (mammography or MRI) showed evidence of tumour within 2 cm of the nipple [15]. The distance of the tumour from the nipple areola complex as seen on mammography was between 2 cm and 4 cm in about two-thirds of the patients, and the median distance of the tumour from NAC was 3.8 cm (range: 2.4–5.2 cm) in our study.

The sensitivity and specificity for frozen section biopsy to detect malignant cells in the retroareolar region has been reported as 90.9% and 98.5%, respectively [16]. In our study, no involvement of the nipple core or areola was found on frozen section biopsy in any patient. Hence, the NAC could be preserved in all the cases. However, frozen section biopsy was positive from the subcutaneous tissue immediately above the tumour in 14.7% cases.

The inframammary incision was used for skin sparing mastectomy in 67.7% of cases in our study. A lateral incision was used in 17.6%, and in those patients who had positive frozen section biopsy of the subcutaneous tissue immediately above their tumour, an additional incision in the skin overlying the tumour was required. Various incisions have been used for NASM by different authors in their reported series [5, 15, 17, 18]. Garwood et al. in their study of total skin sparing mastectomy found that the use of inframammary incisions is an excellent approach for small- or medium-sized breasts and, if enlarged, works well for large breasts as well [19]. Crowe et al. noted that medial incisions may compromise blood flow to the nipple, whereas in all cases performed through a lateral incision, the NAC remained fully intact [18].

Immediate breast reconstruction using autologous tissue and/or silicone implants has been advocated for breast reconstruction after NASM in various studies [20, 21]. In our study, more than 90% of the patients underwent immediate breast reconstruction with autologous tissue (either TRAM or LDMC flap) and implants were used in only few cases. The reason for such a trend could be the financial issues related to the socioeconomic background of our patients. Use of implants for breast reconstruction in our study was preferred mainly in younger patients with nonptotic breasts and in those with early breast cancer where radiotherapy would not be required.

The overall incidence of complications in the study was minimal, and there were few minor complications like seroma, wound infection, and partial umbilical necrosis after TRAM flap in one case each. There was no flap necrosis in any patient. Necrosis of the NAC is a known complication of NASM, with reported rates of 6.7% to 15.8% for any degree of necrosis [22]. In our study only one patient developed partial desquamation of the nipple areola complex, and there was no NAC loss.

All the patients in our study were followed up for at least 18 months after surgery, and the median follow-up period was 38.5 months (range: 18–38 months). There was no local recurrence of tumour in the present study at a median follow-up of 28.5 months. This low rate of local recurrence is supported by the results of previous studies which have confirmed the oncological safety of NASM. For example, in the single centre study of NASM in 95 patients with early breast cancer reported by Omranipour et al. (2008), local recurrence was seen only in one patient (1.1%) and systemic recurrence was seen in two patients (2.1%) at a median

follow-up of 69 months, and the authors concluded that NSM is oncologically safe for early breast cancer (stages 0–II) [23]. Sookhan et al. successfully preserved the NAC in 18 cases with no local recurrence at a median follow-up of 10.8 months [5]. Caruso et al. reported only 2% local recurrence rate within the NAC in a series of fifty NASMs for breast cancer after a mean follow-up of 5.5 years [24]. Garcia-Etienne et al. reviewed 1826 procedures of NASM performed for breast cancer treatment published in the recent literature and found only three local recurrences (0.6%) within the NAC [1]. Ubirubu et al. reported three cases of local recurrence at the needle biopsy site in patients treated with SSM whose diagnoses were obtained through stereotactic needle biopsy [25]. Fortunately, there was no evidence of tumour recurrence at the site of needle biopsy in any of our patients. Rusby et al. have published the most recent review of NASM in the literature [14]. They also found recurrence rates of less than 5% in properly selected patients undergoing NASM for breast cancer treatment. Kim et al. (2010) in their retrospective study of 520 patients further widened the indications of NASM [26]. The indications for NASM in their study were any stage, any tumor size, and any tumor areola distance, provided the shape, color, and palpation of the nipple were normal. The locoregional recurrence rates were similar for NASM and mastectomy patients. Salhab et al. found that skin sparing mastectomy and immediate breast reconstruction for operable breast cancer are associated with a high level of patient satisfaction and low morbidity [27]. The procedure seems to be oncologically safe, even in patients with high-risk (T3 or node-positive) carcinoma.

The aesthetic outcomes of skin sparing mastectomy with NAC preservation in our study were evaluated by clinical and photography-based assessments. The aesthetic result was stratified by subscales proposed by Lowery et al. [4]. Volume, contour, placement of breast mound, and inframammary fold were evaluated, and results were defined as excellent, good, fair, and poor according to the total score. Various subjective and objective scores have been used evaluating aesthetic outcomes after immediate breast reconstruction following NASM. Salhab et al. assessed the patient's satisfaction with the outcome of surgery with a detailed questionnaire including a linear visual analogue scale ranging from 0 (not satisfied) to 10 (most satisfied) [27]. Salgarello et al. evaluated the reconstructive and aesthetic outcomes by clinical examinations and by reviewing the clinical pictures of the breasts [28]. More than 90% of patients in our study had good or excellent Lowery scores at 6 months of follow-up. Moreover, the patient satisfaction as assessed by questioning the patients about their satisfaction with the aesthetic results of surgery was acceptable in all the cases.

5. Conclusion

We conclude that skin sparing mastectomy with preservation of nipple areola complex and immediate breast reconstruction can be successfully achieved with minimal morbidity and very low risk of local recurrence in appropriately selected breast cancer patients, with acceptable aesthetic results and good patient satisfaction.

Abbreviations

BCS: Breast conserving surgery
NASM: Nipple areola and skin sparing mastectomy
NAC: Nipple areola complex
TRAM: Transverse rectus abdominis myocutaneous.

References

[1] C. A. Garcia-Etienne, H. S. Cody III, J. J. Disa, P. Cordeiro, and V. Sacchini, "Nipple-sparing mastectomy: initial experience at the memorial sloan-kettering cancer center and a comprehensive review of literature," *The Breast Journal*, vol. 15, no. 4, pp. 440–449, 2009.

[2] M. W. Kissin and A. E. Kark, "Nipple preservation during mastectomy," *British Journal of Surgery*, vol. 74, no. 1, pp. 58–61, 1987.

[3] C. P. Hinton, P. J. Doyle, R. W. Blamey, C. J. Davies, H. W. Holliday, and C. W. Elston, "Subcutaneous mastectomy for primary operable breast cancer," *British Journal of Surgery*, vol. 71, no. 6, pp. 469–472, 1984.

[4] J. C. Lowery, E. G. Wilkins, W. M. Kuzon, and J. A. Davis, "Evaluations of aesthetic results in breast reconstruction: an analysis of reliability," *Annals of Plastic Surgery*, vol. 36, no. 6, pp. 601–606, 1996.

[5] N. Sookhan, J. C. Boughey, M. F. Walsh, and A. C. Degnim, "Nipple-sparing mastectomy-initial experience at a tertiary center," *The American Journal of Surgery*, vol. 196, no. 4, pp. 575–577, 2008.

[6] C. Laronga, B. Kemp, D. Johnston, G. L. Robb, and S. E. Singletary, "The incidence of occult nipple-areola complex involvement in breast cancer patients receiving a skin-sparing mastectomy," *Annals of Surgical Oncology*, vol. 6, no. 6, pp. 609–613, 1999.

[7] R. M. Simmons, M. Brennan, P. Christos, V. King, and M. Osborne, "Analysis of nipple/areolar involvement with mastectomy: can the areola be preserved?" *Annals of Surgical Oncology*, vol. 9, no. 2, pp. 165–168, 2002.

[8] A. Banerjee, S. Gupta, and N. Bhattacharya, "Preservation of nipple-areola complex in breast cancer: a clinicopathological assessment," *Journal of Plastic, Reconstructive & Aesthetic Surgery*, vol. 61, no. 10, pp. 1195–1198, 2008.

[9] R. Y. Afifi and A. El-Hindawy, "Analysis of nipple-areolar complex involvement with mastectomy: can the nipple be preserved in Egyptian patients receiving skin-sparing mastectomy?" *Breast Journal*, vol. 10, no. 6, pp. 543–545, 2004.

[10] Z. Vlajcic, R. Zic, S. Stanec, S. Lambasa, M. Petrovecki, and Z. Stanec, "Nipple-areola complex preservation: predictive factors of neoplastic nipple-areola complex invasion," *Annals of Plastic Surgery*, vol. 55, no. 3, pp. 240–244, 2005.

[11] V. Sacchini, J. A. Pinotti, A. C. S. D. Barros et al., "Nipple-sparing mastectomy for breast cancer and risk reduction: oncological or technical problem?" *Journal of the American College of Surgeons*, vol. 203, no. 5, pp. 704–714, 2006.

[12] M. J. Loewen, J. A. Jennings, S. R. Sherman et al., "Mammographic distance as a predictor of nipple-areola complex involvement in breast cancer," *The American Journal of Surgery*, vol. 195, no. 3, pp. 391–395, 2008.

[13] A. K. Schecter, M. B. Freeman, D. Giri, E. Sabo, and J. Weinzweig, "Applicability of the nipple-areola complex-sparing mastectomy: a prediction model using mammography to estimate risk of nipple-areola complex involvement in breast cancer patients," *Annals of Plastic Surgery*, vol. 56, no. 5, pp. 498–504, 2006.

[14] J. E. Rusby, E. F. Brachtel, M. Othus, J. S. Michaelson, F. C. Koerner, and B. L. Smith, "Development and validation of a model predictive of occult nipple involvement in women undergoing mastectomy," *British Journal of Surgery*, vol. 95, no. 11, pp. 1356–1361, 2008.

[15] A. Wijayanayagam, A. S. Kumar, R. D. Foster, and L. J. Esserman, "Optimizing the total skin-sparing mastectomy," *Archives of Surgery*, vol. 143, no. 1, pp. 38–45, 2008.

[16] K. P. Benediktsson and L. Perbeck, "Survival in breast cancer after nipple-sparing subcutaneous mastectomy and immediate reconstruction with implants: a prospective trial with 13 years median follow-up in 216 patients," *European Journal of Surgical Oncology*, vol. 34, no. 2, pp. 143–148, 2008.

[17] J. K. Harness, T. S. Vetter, and A. H. Salibian, "Areola and nipple-areola-sparing mastectomy for breast cancer treatment and risk reduction: report of an initial experience in a community hospital setting," *Annals of Surgical Oncology*, vol. 18, no. 4, pp. 917–922, 2011.

[18] J. P. Crowe Jr., J. A. Kim, R. Yetman, J. Banbury, R. J. Patrick, and D. Baynes, "Nipple-sparing mastectomy: technique and results of 54 procedures," *Archives of Surgery*, vol. 139, no. 2, pp. 148–150, 2004.

[19] E. R. Garwood, D. Moore, C. Ewing et al., "Total skin-sparing mastectomy: complications and local recurrence rates in 2 cohorts of patients," *Annals of Surgery*, vol. 249, no. 1, pp. 26–32, 2009.

[20] S. E. Singletary and G. L. Robb, "Oncologic safety of skin-sparing mastectomy," *Annals of Surgical Oncology*, vol. 10, no. 2, pp. 95–97, 2003.

[21] R. M. Simmons and T. L. Adamovich, "Skin-sparing mastectomy," *Surgical Clinics of North America*, vol. 83, no. 4, pp. 885–899, 2003.

[22] A. L. Komorowski, V. Zanini, L. Regolo, A. Carolei, W. M. Wysocki, and A. Costa, "Necrotic complications after nipple- and areola-sparing mastectomy," *World Journal of Surgery*, vol. 30, no. 8, pp. 1410–1413, 2006.

[23] R. Omranipour, J. Y. Bobin, and M. Esouyeh, "Skin Sparing Mastectomy and immediate breast reconstruction (SSMIR) for early breast cancer: eight years single institution experience," *World Journal of Surgical Oncology*, vol. 6, article 43, 2008.

[24] F. Caruso, M. Ferrara, G. Castiglione et al., "Nipple sparing subcutaneous mastectomy: sixty-six months follow-up," *European Journal of Surgical Oncology*, vol. 32, no. 9, pp. 937–940, 2006.

[25] J. L. Uriburu, H. D. Vuoto, L. Cogorno et al., "Local recurrence of breast cancer after skin-sparing mastectomy following core needle biopsy: case reports and review of the literature," *The Breast Journal*, vol. 12, no. 3, pp. 194–198, 2006.

[26] H. J. Kim, E. H. Park, W. S. Lim et al., "Nipple areola skin-sparing mastectomy with immediate transverse rectus abdominis musculocutaneous flap reconstruction is an oncologically safe procedure: a single center study," *Annals of Surgery*, vol. 251, no. 3, pp. 493–498, 2010.

[27] M. Salhab, W. A. Sarakbi, A. Joseph, S. Sheards, J. Travers, and K. Mokbel, "Skin-sparing mastectomy and immediate breast reconstruction: patient satisfaction and clinical outcome," *International Journal of Clinical Oncology*, vol. 11, no. 1, pp. 51–54, 2006.

[28] M. Salgarello, G. Visconti, and L. Barone-Adesi, "Nipple-sparing mastectomy with immediate implant reconstruction: cosmetic outcomes and technical refinements," *Plastic and Reconstructive Surgery*, vol. 126, no. 5, pp. 1460–1471, 2010.

28

Does Acellular Dermal Matrix Thickness Affect Complication Rate in Tissue Expander Based Breast Reconstruction?

Jessica F. Rose, Sarosh N. Zafar, and Warren A. Ellsworth IV

Division of Plastic Surgery, Department of Surgery, Houston Methodist Hospital, Medical Office Building, 118400 Katy Freeway, Suite 500, Houston, TX 77094, USA

Correspondence should be addressed to Warren A. Ellsworth IV; waellsworth@houstonmethodist.org

Academic Editor: Nicolo Scuderi

Background. While the benefits of using acellular dermal matrices (ADMs) in breast reconstruction are well described, their use has been associated with additional complications. The purpose of this study was to determine if ADM thickness affects complications in breast reconstruction. *Methods*. A retrospective chart review was performed including all tissue expander based breast reconstructions with AlloDerm (LifeCell, Branchburg, NJ) over 4 years. We evaluated preoperative characteristics and assessed postoperative complications including seroma, hematoma, infection, skin necrosis, and need for reintervention. We reviewed ADM thickness and time to Jackson-Pratt (JP) drain removal. *Results*. Fifty-five patients underwent 77 ADM-associated tissue expander based breast reconstructions, with average age of 48.1 years and average BMI of 25.9. Average ADM thickness was 1.21 mm. We found higher complication rates in the thick ADM group. Significant associations were found between smokers and skin necrosis ($p < 0.0001$) and seroma and prolonged JP drainage ($p = 0.0004$); radiated reconstructed breasts were more likely to suffer infections ($p = 0.0085$), and elevated BMI is a significant predictor for increased infection rate ($p = 0.0037$). *Conclusion*. We found a trend toward increased complication rates with thicker ADMs. In the future, larger prospective studies evaluating thickness may provide more information.

1. Introduction

Implant based breast reconstruction is the most common type of breast reconstructions performed in the United States [1]. According to the American Society of Plastic Surgery, 83,149 implant based breast reconstructions were performed in 2014 (81.3% of breast reconstructions), with 74,694 utilizing tissue expanders (73.1% of all reconstructions) [2]. Implant based reconstruction may be chosen because of faster recovery, lack of donor site morbidity, or patient comorbidities that may preclude autologous reconstruction [3]. Implant based breast reconstruction often requires placement of a tissue expander (TE) to enlarge the mastectomy skin envelope enough to fit the desired size of breast implant and ensure successful survival of the often thin mastectomy flaps. In the senior authors' practice, tissue expanders are often used after mastectomy as a bridge to autologous reconstruction, especially when there is a possibility of needing adjuvant therapy including postmastectomy radiation therapy (PMRT). Tissue expanders are most commonly placed in the subpectoral plane with coverage of the lower and lateral poles of the expander with acellular dermal matrices (ADMs) [1].

ADMs are biologic material initially used in revision breast surgery to fix contour deformities, rippling, and malposition. Their use in tissue expander based breast reconstruction has grown exponentially over the past decade. The ADM is placed in the inframammary and lateral mammary folds as a sling to reinforce and support the expander or implant [3–8]. It aids in covering the lower pole of the TE while supporting the position of the prosthesis shaping the breast, and preventing device exposure in the setting of mastectomy flap necrosis [1, 6, 7]. ADM coverage of the lower pole helps to recreate lost anatomic landmarks after mastectomy, provide support, and allow for increased intraoperative fill volume [7–9]. It may also help prevent the formation of a capsule by decreasing local inflammation [10]. Despite these benefits, their use may increase complication rates particularly regarding seroma [5]. There are many types of ADM products on the market; however AlloDerm (LifeCell, Branchburg, NJ) is the most commonly used product in the senior authors practice and the United States today [4].

In contrast, total submuscular placement results in the expander preferentially filling the superior pole, creating a less natural appearing breast. To create a natural, ptotic breast shape, the inferior pole of the expander can be left without muscle coverage, leaving a significant exposure risk [3]. Incorporating ADM can help recreate natural breast structure and ptosis, while simultaneously providing suitable expander coverage. Typically, the use of an ADM also allows the expander to be filled to a larger volume intraoperatively, decreasing requirements for postoperative visits and expansions [1, 3, 10]. Greater initial fill translates to fewer expansions and less time until definitive reconstruction with an implant or flap [5, 11]. Some authors feel that the use of ADM instead of total submuscular placement decreases postoperative pain and pain during expansion, although a randomized trial by Nguyen et al. failed to substantiate that claim [5, 11]. Other advantages include a suggested decreased capsular contracture rate, less revisions, and overall improved aesthetic outcome [5]. Hanna et al. compared expander based reconstruction with ADMs versus total submuscular placement including a patient satisfaction survey [12]. They showed higher mean scores for the ADM group regarding overall satisfaction, shape of the reconstruction, and ease of the expansion experience [12].

Anecdotally, we felt that patients in whom thicker ADMs were used were more likely to develop seromas or prolonged Jackson-Pratt (JP) drain output. Thus, we decided to evaluate our data retrospectively to delineate causation. To our knowledge, there have been no studies specifically looking at ADM thickness and development of complications (particularly seroma) or prolonged drain times.

2. Methods

We retrospectively analyzed records of all consecutive patients over approximately a four-year time period, from January 1, 2011, through April 1, 2015, who underwent breast reconstruction utilizing tissue expander and ADM by the senior author at our institution. Ninety percent of the mastectomies were performed by one of two fellowship trained breast surgical oncologists, with whom the senior author routinely collaborates. We included only those patients who were reconstructed with AlloDerm (LifeCell, Branchburg, NJ) and only included data of one plastic surgeon for consistency in technique of ADM, drain placement, and postoperative drain management and removal.

Multiple factors in the study group were examined: patient age, body mass index (BMI), presence of diabetes, smoking status, postoperative radiation treatment, development of complications (seroma, hematoma, infection, and skin necrosis), need for reintervention, time to Jackson-Pratt (JP) drain removal, thickness of the ADM, and eventual outcome (final breast reconstruction with DIEP flap or implant). Seroma and hematoma were both clinically defined as increasing breast size with fluid collections containing either serous fluid or blood, respectively. Infection was defined by

the need for antibiotics, whether oral or intravenous, as determined clinically by the senior author. JP drain removal time was rounded to the nearest week and averaged per drain. We defined "thick" ADM as greater than or equal to 1.2 mm and "thin" ADM as less than 1.2 mm in thickness. This thickness was chosen, as it was the mean and median thickness of products utilized.

The aim of the study was, first, to assess differences in seroma rate and JP drain time in patients with thick versus thin ADMs. We postulated that thicker ADMs would produce more fluid, prolong integration time, and therefore lengthen time until drain removal. Second, we assessed complication rates between the two groups and risk factors for complication development (radiation, BMI, diabetes, and smoking).

2.1. Operative Technique. Our operative technique is as follows. The patient undergoes a mastectomy by the breast surgeon. The pectoralis major is elevated off of the chest wall using Bovie electrocautery and is disinserted to the 3 o'clock or 9 o'clock position, depending on laterality. AlloDerm is soaked for 10 minutes in a bacitracin and normal saline bath, gloves are changed, and the surgeon then places the ADM in the mastectomy cavity. It is sutured in place using interrupted 2-0 polydioxanone (PDS; Ethicon US, LLC, Somerville, NJ) from the 3 o'clock to 9 o'clock position. Tissue expanders are prepared on the back table and soaked in triple antibiotic solution. The operating team's gloves are exchanged for new gloves. The air from the TEs is removed and the expander is filled with 150 cc of injectable saline with methylene blue. The expander is placed under the pectoralis muscle and ADM, and its tabs are sutured in place using 2-0 PDS "U" stitches. The ADM and muscle are sutured together using 2-0 PDS for total expander coverage. Two 15-French round JP drains are placed: one deep to and one superficial to the ADM. If possible, we add more fluid to the expander until the cavity is filled with minimal tension on the mastectomy closure. We use the SPY Elite (NOVADAQ Technologies Inc., Huntington, NY) with indocyanine green to assess the viability of the mastectomy flaps when concern arises over perfusion. Once complete, we debride the edges of the wound to healthy tissue and close the skin using interrupted 3-0 poliglecaprone 25 (Monocryl; Ethicon US, LLC, Somerville, NJ) deep dermal and 4-0 poliglecaprone 25 subcuticular sutures, followed by Dermabond. Patients are admitted for 23-hour observation for pain control and drain care teaching. They are kept on appropriate antibiotic prophylaxis for 7 days.

All patients had at least 2 drains placed per breast (those with an axillary dissection had a 3rd drain in the axilla). Patients were seen in the office at least weekly until the drains were removed. Drains were removed when the output remained less than 30 cc per day, but their drains were removed by week 5 regardless of the output to decrease retrograde infection potential. All drains were dressed with Biopatch covered with Tegaderm, and this dressing was changed weekly.

2.2. Statistical Methods. Data for continuous variables are reported as the mean ± standard deviation. The Kolmogorov-Smirnov test was used for testing normal distribution of

TABLE 1: Patients' characteristics comparing thick and thin ADMs.

	Thin ADMs (36)	Thick ADMs (41)	p value
Average age (±SD)	50.2 (±12.33)	46.24 (±12.85)	0.2419
Average BMI (±SD)	25.8 (±5.09)	26.1 (±4.90)	0.6321
Number of patients with DM	5 (13.9%)	0 (0%)	**0.0136**
Number of patients requiring radiation	7 (19.4%)	13 (31.7%)	0.2208
Number of smokers	6 (16.7%)	4 (9.8%)	0.3681

TABLE 2: Development of complications comparing thick and thin ADMs.

	Thin ADMs (36)	Thick ADMs (41)	p value
Developed seroma	4 (11.1%)	6 (14.6%)	0.6463
Developed hematoma	1 (2.8%)	0 (0%)	0.2827
Developed infection	3 (8.3%)	7 (17.1%)	0.2550
Developed skin necrosis	4 (11.1%)	6 (14.6%)	0.6463
Required intervention	3 (8.3%)	7 (17.1%)	0.2550
Average drain weeks (±SD)	2.43 (±0.9)	2.45 (±1.0)	0.8523

continuous variables. The independent Mann-Whitney test was used to compare the average drain times between groups of patients with different characteristics or complications. Between-group differences for dichotomous variables, including number of patients with DM, number of patients with radiation, number of smokers, number of patients with thick ADMs (thickness was dichotomized to thick and thin using cutoff of 1.2 mm), number of patients who developed seroma, hematoma, infection, and skin necrosis, number of patients who needed reoperation, and number of patients with complications, were examined using analysis of variance and the Fisher exact test or χ^2 test, as appropriate.

To identify which factors may affect average drain time, we used a linear regression model with average drain time as a dependent variable and age, BMI, DM, radiation, and smoking as independent variables. Also, to identify independent predictors for presence of complications at the conclusion of the study, we used a logistic backward regression model with presence of complications as the dependent variable and the independent variables mentioned above. A p value of ≤0.05 was considered statistically significant. Statistical analyses were performed using R version 3.1.3 software (Bell Laboratories, Madison, WI).

3. Results

Over a 4-year time period, 55 patients underwent 77 ADM/tissue expander breast reconstructions using AlloDerm. Patients' ages ranged from 23 to 76 (average 48.1) with an average BMI of 25.9. Five patients (6.5%) of the population were diabetic, 10 (13.0%) patients were smokers, and 20 (26.0%) patients required radiation treatment.

ADM thickness ranged from 0.86 mm to 2.18 mm (average 1.21 mm; median 1.21 mm). We defined thick ADM as 1.2 mm and above. Forty-one breasts were reconstructed with thick ADMs, while 36 breasts were reconstructed with thin ADMs. Further analysis to determine if the threshold for thick ADMs did not yield statistical significance for any value,

so we maintained our original definition of a thick ADM. Table 1 shows patient characteristics with thin versus thick ADMs, showing well-matched groups with the exception of diabetes.

Complications were more prevalent in the thick group, although not statistically significant (Table 2). We looked at our patient population for the development of complications by ADM thickness and by risk factor, mainly to make sure that our patient population behaved as predicted.

We compared patient characteristics to see how they impacted the development of complications. Smokers were more likely to develop skin necrosis ($p < 0.0001$) and require reintervention ($p = 0.0064$) than other patients. Diabetic patients were more likely to be older, had higher BMIs, and did not have thick ADMs. Patients who were radiated after expander placement were more likely to develop infections ($p = 0.0085$).

We also compared groups by presence or absence of complications. Presence of seroma was a risk factor for prolonged JP drainage (3.53 weeks versus 2.28 weeks, $p = 0.0004$) and was also a risk of other complications such as hematoma ($p = 0.0092$), infection ($p = 0.0002$), skin necrosis ($p = 0.0064$), and the need for reintervention ($p < 0.0001$) (see Table 3).

Patients with and without infections were also compared. Significant risk factors for infection included increased BMI (25.3 versus 30.2 with infection, $p = 0.0037$), radiation (60% of patients who were infected were radiated, $p = 0.0085$), hematoma (the one patient with a hematoma developed an infection, $p = 0.0091$), and seroma (50% of infected patients had seromas versus 7.5% who did not, $p = 0.0002$). Those with infection were also more likely to have prolonged drain times (2.28 weeks versus 3.50 weeks, $p = 0.0001$) and require reintervention (60% of infected patients versus 5.8% of those without infections, $p < 0.0001$). Younger patients were more likely to have developed an infection, average age 41.3 with infections versus 49.1 ($p = 0.0273$).

TABLE 3: Characteristics of patients with and without seromas.

	− Seroma (67)	+ Seroma (10)	p value
Average age (±SD)	48.0 (±12.81)	48.9 (±12.44)	0.7732
Average BMI (±SD)	26.1 (±4.98)	25.0 (±4.97)	0.5437
Number of patients with DM	5 (7.5%)	0 (0%)	0.3717
Number of patients with radiation	16 (23.9%)	4 (40.0%)	0.2782
Number of smokers	8 (11.9%)	2 (20.0%)	0.4794
Number of thick ADMs	35 (52.2%)	6 (60.0%)	0.6463
Developed hematoma	0 (0%)	1 (10.0%)	**0.0092**
Developed infection	5 (7.5%)	5 (50.0%)	**0.0002**
Developed skin necrosis	6 (9.0%)	4 (40.0%)	**0.0064**
Required intervention	4 (6.0%)	6 (60.0%)	**<0.0001**
Average drain weeks (±SD)	2.28 (±0.8)	3.53 (±1.0)	**0.0004**

Patients who did and did not develop skin necrosis were also compared. Smoking was a significant risk factor ($p < 0.0001$). Patients with skin necrosis were prone to other complications like seroma ($p = 0.0064$) and hematoma ($p = 0.0092$) and were more likely to require reintervention ($p < 0.0001$). As anticipated, those requiring reoperation were more likely to be smokers ($p = 0.0064$), have seromas ($p < 0.0001$), hematomas ($p = 0.0092$), and infections ($p < 0.0001$), and require drains longer (2.33 weeks versus 3.20 weeks, $p = 0.0024$).

When ADM thickness was evaluated as a continuous variable, there was no significant threshold for the development of complications. However, patients with thicker ADMs were more likely to have infections ($p = 0.0178$) and skin necrosis ($p = 0.0046$) and require reoperation ($p = 0.0022$). Those with an elevated BMI were more likely to have infections ($p = 0.0035$) and skin necrosis ($p = 0.0279$), and BMI was the only significant risk factor for prolonged drain times ($p = 0.0136$).

When comparing those with thick versus thin ADMs, those with thick ADMs were more likely to still have drains at the 2-week mark (Figure 1). We observed a positive correlation between thickness of ADMs and average drain time without statistical significance (Figure 1).

We found statistical significance in patients with higher BMIs to have prolonged drain times (Figure 2). A linear regression model identified BMI as a significant independent predictor for average drain time. One-unit increase in BMI would lead to a 0.0712 ± 0.0225-week increase in average drain time ($p = 0.002$). Also, logistic regression identified radiation ($p = 0.006$) as independent predictor for overall development of complications.

Overall, 42.0% of our patients went on to have autologous reconstruction after expansion, 40.6% had permanent implants placed, 1.4% had TE removal and no reconstruction, and the rest are pending definitive reconstruction.

4. Discussion

Despite all of their advantages, studies have linked the use of ADMs in TE based breast reconstruction to higher complication rates compared to total submuscular expander

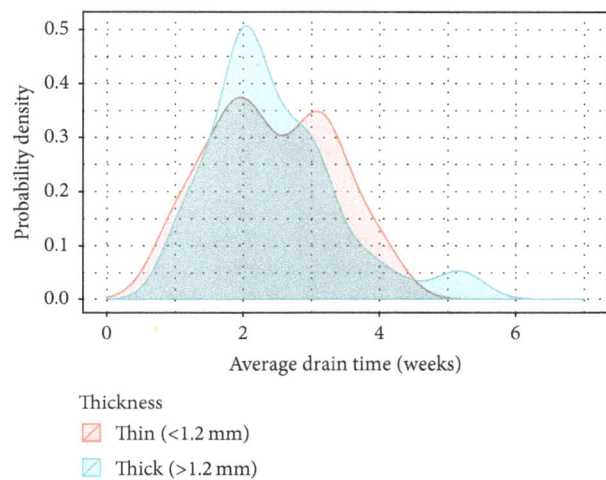

Thickness
◪ Thin (<1.2 mm)
◪ Thick (>1.2 mm)

FIGURE 1

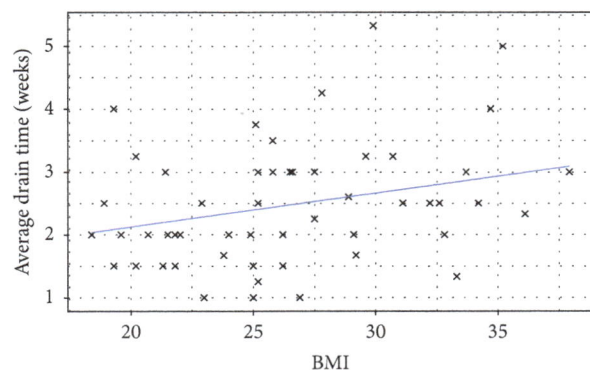

FIGURE 2

placement. The use of AlloDerm in a series by Chun et al. was associated with a fourfold increase in seroma rate and a fivefold increase in infection rate when compared to the non-ADM group [1]. One-third of patients in another study developed a post-op seroma within 72 hours of drain removal [13]. A meta-analysis performed by Ho et al. showed a higher likelihood of seroma, infection, and reconstructive failure when compared to patients who had a tissue expander with myofascial flap coverage [14]. Other studies, such as the analysis by Vardanian et al., showed no difference between patients with and without ADM in regard to infections or development of seroma/hematoma [15]. Clearly, the literature is divided with regard to the complications associated with TE based breast reconstruction using ADM.

The ability to better identify risk factors for major complications may allow us to choose better candidates to undergo breast reconstruction with an ADM and/or modify risks and technique accordingly [13]. There is a paucity of literature regarding details of complication development, particularly with specific ADM choice and characteristics. However, some characteristics have been ascertained. Fenestrated ADMs theoretically help reduce seroma formation by allowing better effacement of the product against the mastectomy skin, increasing surface area to allow revascularization, and making it easier for fluid to drain [16]. Some studies have suggested that particular ADMs are more prone to complications [16]. Generally, the complication rate between FlexHD and AlloDerm is similar, although Ranganathan et al. found increased infections with FlexHD [17]. Drs. Vu et al. found that using a deep dermal ADM with increased porosity decreased complication rates [18]. The difference between the ready to use (RTU) AlloDerm, which is sterile, and the freeze-dried (FD) AlloDerm, which is aseptic, was also studied and no difference in complication profiles was found between either product [19]. Lastly, appropriately placed closed suction drains and prolonged drainage may help prevent seroma in ADM based prosthetic reconstruction [14].

To our knowledge, this is the first study to consider the complication rates of TE reconstruction with an ADM sling as a function of thickness of the ADM. We noticed a trend toward thicker ADMs being associated with higher complication rates. Patients with thicker ADMs had more seromas (14.6% versus 11.1%), infections (17.1% versus 8.3%), skin necrosis (14.6% versus 11.1%), and need for reintervention (17.1% versus 8.3%). While some of our data failed to reach statistical significance, assessing these complications as a function of increasing thickness was statistically significant. This suggests that ADM thickness is a risk factor for seroma and prolonged JP drain times, but our study was underpowered to reach statistical significance.

While some studies suggest that ADM use increases risk of seroma and complication rate, the exact mechanism remains unknown. Since AlloDerm incorporates into tissue by neovascularization [20, 21], we proposed that the thickness of ADM is directly related to its speed of incorporation and therefore length of drain placement. As with any graft, thicker tissue requires a longer time for incorporation and is at higher risk for failure of integration. Also, drain times were averaged to the nearest week based on available data and presentation to the clinic for removal. Statistical significance may have been achieved if we removed each drain on the exact day when output was less than 30 cc/day. However, for practical reasons, patients could not return to the outpatient setting for drain removal on the exact day when ready for removal.

Reasons for complication development are multifactorial. Poor quality mastectomy skin flaps and smoking are known

risks [13]. Common problems are skin flap necrosis, infections, and seromas. A triad of these factors frequently occurs, but their precise relation to each other is yet to be determined [13]. This held true with our patient population, as those with one complication were more likely to have another complication. Increased BMI is a risk factor for seroma, likely due to increased dead space and redundant skin flaps [13]. Seroma may also be attributed to drain specific protocols and the presence of increased dead space where the ADM is placed [15].

Infectious complications are multifactorial; however, the ADM itself can act as a nidus for bacterial colorization and can lead to an infection before the tissue incorporates and revascularizes [3]. Prolonged drain use may also be a risk factor for infection, as the drain can seed an infection [13]. When skin necrosis or breakdown occurs it can lead to infection and eventual exposure [3, 11, 15]. Since seroma rates are higher for ADM based reconstructions, secondary infections are also more frequent. ADM is essentially a foreign body, and the addition of a foreign body with a prosthetic is also an infection risk [15].

Ultimately, it is best to prevent seroma occurrence, but if it develops it needs to be managed appropriately [13]. Many factors, such as patient comorbidities (BMI, diabetes, and smoking) and impaired vascularity of the mastectomy flaps, are outside of the plastic surgeon's control [13]. Some studies have suggested avoiding ADM use in obese patients, where increased dead space and poorly perfused flaps can increase the complication rate [22]. The TE itself can be used to help prevent seroma formation. It is our opinion that the TE should be filled intraoperatively to a point where it approximates the ADM to the mastectomy skin, but without placing excess pressure on the overlying skin, which could lead to ischemia of the mastectomy flaps [3].

One interesting finding in our study is that BMI is an independent risk factor for prolonged drain time. It is well known that patients with increased BMI have a higher complication rate. However, patients with increased BMI and increased breast size are more likely to have infections and mastectomy skin flap necrosis. Likely, this is due to increased dead space and poor apposition of vascularized tissue to the ADM, predisposing it to failure of incorporation.

5. Conclusion

Increased BMI was found to be a statistically significant risk factor for maintaining JP drainage for a longer period of time. There is a clear trend toward increased complication rates when thicker ADMs were chosen; however this did not reach statistical significance. Larger, prospective studies comparing those with thick and thin ADMs are warranted in the future for more thorough characterization of associated risks and to quantify an ideal ADM thickness.

Disclosure

This paper has been seen and approved by all authors, and the material is previously unpublished. The authors wish to disclose that Dr. Warren A. Ellsworth is a speaker and consultant for LifeCell and a consultant for Allergan.

Competing Interests

The authors declare that they have no competing interests.

Acknowledgments

The authors would like to thank Yue (Joy) Duan for her hard work and assistance with the data analysis.

References

[1] Y. S. Chun, K. Verma, H. Rosen et al., "Implant-based breast reconstruction using acellular dermal matrix and the risk of postoperative complications," *Plastic and Reconstructive Surgery*, vol. 125, no. 2, pp. 429–436, 2010.

[2] American Society of Plastic Surgeons, *Report of the 2014 Plastic Surgery Statistics*, 2014, http://www.plasticsurgery.org/Documents/news-resources/statistics/2014-statistics/plastic-surgery-statsitics-full-report.pdf.

[3] S. T. Lanier, E. D. Wang, J. J. Chen et al., "The effect of acellular dermal matrix use on complication rates in tissue expander/implant breast reconstruction," *Annals of Plastic Surgery*, vol. 64, no. 5, pp. 674–678, 2010.

[4] A. Cheng and M. Saint-Cyr, "Comparison of different ADM materials in breast surgery," *Clinics in Plastic Surgery*, vol. 39, no. 2, pp. 167–175, 2012.

[5] T. J. Nguyen, J. N. Carey, and A. K. Wong, "Use of human acellular dermal matrix in implant- based breast reconstruction: evaluating the evidence," *Journal of Plastic, Reconstructive and Aesthetic Surgery*, vol. 64, no. 12, pp. 1553–1561, 2011.

[6] C. A. Salzberg, A. Y. Ashikari, R. M. Koch, and E. Chabner-Thompson, "An 8-year experience of direct-to-implant immediate breast reconstruction using human acellular dermal matrix (AlloDerm)," *Plastic and Reconstructive Surgery*, vol. 127, no. 2, pp. 514–524, 2011.

[7] R. J. Zienowicz and E. Karacaoglu, "Implant-based breast reconstruction with allograft," *Plastic and Reconstructive Surgery*, vol. 120, no. 2, pp. 373–381, 2007.

[8] K. E. Weichman, S. C. Wilson, A. L. Weinstein et al., "The use of acellular dermal matrix in immediate two-stage tissue expander breast reconstruction," *Plastic and Reconstructive Surgery*, vol. 129, no. 5, pp. 1049–1058, 2012.

[9] S. Brooke, J. Mesa, M. Uluer et al., "Complications in tissue expander breast reconstruction: a comparison of AlloDerm, DermaMatrix, and FlexHD acellular inferior pole dermal slings," *Annals of Plastic Surgery*, vol. 69, no. 4, pp. 347–349, 2012.

[10] C. B. Basu, M. Leong, and M. J. Hicks, "Acellular cadaveric dermis decreases the inflammatory response in capsule formation in reconstructive breast surgery," *Plastic and Reconstructive Surgery*, vol. 126, no. 6, pp. 1842–1847, 2010.

[11] C. M. McCarthy, C. N. Lee, E. G. Halvorson et al., "The use of acellular dermal matrices in two-stage expander/implant reconstruction: a multicenter, blinded, randomized controlled trial," *Plastic and Reconstructive Surgery*, vol. 130, no. 5, supplement 2, pp. 57s–66s, 2012.

[12] K. R. Hanna, B. R. DeGeorge Jr., A. F. Mericli, K. Y. Lin, and D. B. Drake, "Comparison study of two types of expander-based breast reconstruction: acellular dermal matrix-assisted versus total submuscular placement," *Annals of Plastic Surgery*, vol. 70, no. 1, pp. 10–15, 2013.

[13] M. A. Brzezienski, J. A. Jarrell, and R. C. Mooty, "Classification and management of seromas in immediate breast reconstruction using the tissue expander and acellular dermal matrix technique," *Annals of Plastic Surgery*, vol. 70, no. 5, pp. 488–492, 2013.

[14] G. Ho, T. J. Nguyen, A. Shahabi, B. H. Hwang, L. S. Chan, and A. K. Wong, "A systematic review and meta-analysis of complications associated with acellular dermal matrix-assisted breast reconstruction," *Annals of Plastic Surgery*, vol. 68, no. 4, pp. 346–356, 2012.

[15] A. J. Vardanian, J. L. Clayton, J. Roostaeian et al., "Comparison of implant-based immediate breast reconstruction with and without acellular dermal matrix," *Plastic and Reconstructive Surgery*, vol. 128, no. 5, pp. 403e–410e, 2011.

[16] D. A. Palaia, K. S. Arthur, A. C. Cahan, and M. H. Rosenberg, "Incidence of seromas and infections using fenestrated versus nonfenestrated acellular dermal matrix in breast reconstructions," *Plastic and Reconstructive Surgery—Global Open*, vol. 3, no. 11, article e569, 2015.

[17] K. Ranganathan, K. B. Santosa, D. A. Lyons et al., "Use of acellular dermal matrix in postmastectomy breast reconstruction: are all acellular dermal matrices created equal?" *Plastic and Reconstructive Surgery*, vol. 136, no. 4, pp. 647–653, 2015.

[18] M. M. Vu, G. S. Jr. De Oliveira, K. E. Mayer, J. T. Blough, and J. Y. Kim, "A prospective study assessing complication rates and patient-reported outcomes in breast reconstructions using a novel, deep dermal human acellular dermal matrix," *Plastic and Reconstructive Surgery—Global Open*, vol. 3, no. 12, article e585, 2015.

[19] V. Rawlani, D. W. Buck II, S. A. Johnson, K. S. Heyer, and J. Y. S. Kim, "Tissue expander breast reconstruction using prehydrated human acellular dermis," *Annals of Plastic Surgery*, vol. 66, no. 6, pp. 593–597, 2011.

[20] O. Garcia Jr. and J. R. Scott, "Analysis of acellular dermal matrix integration and revascularization following tissue expander breast reconstruction in a clinically relevant large-animal model," *Plastic and Reconstructive Surgery*, vol. 131, no. 5, pp. 741e–751e, 2013.

[21] G. M. Gamboa-Bobadilla, "Implant breast reconstruction using acellular dermal matrix," *Annals of Plastic Surgery*, vol. 56, no. 1, pp. 22–25, 2006.

[22] B. F. Michelotti, S. Brooke, J. Mesa et al., "Analysis of clinically significant seroma formation in breast reconstruction using acellular dermal grafts," *Annals of Plastic Surgery*, vol. 71, no. 3, pp. 274–277, 2013.

29

Versatility of Pedicled Tensor Fascia Lata Flap: A Useful and Reliable Technique for Reconstruction of Different Anatomical Districts

Md. Sohaib Akhtar, Mohd Fahud Khurram, and Arshad Hafeez Khan

Post Graduate Department of Burns, Plastic and Reconstructive Surgery, JNMC, AMU, Aligarh, India

Correspondence should be addressed to Md. Sohaib Akhtar; drsohaibakhtar@gmail.com

Academic Editor: Nicolo Scuderi

Aims and Objectives. The aim of this study was to evaluate the versatility of pedicled tensor fascia lata flap for reconstruction of various anatomical regions. *Materials and Methods*. In this retrospective study a total of 34 patients with defects over various anatomical regions were included. The defects were located over the trochanter ($n = 12$), groin ($n = 8$), perineum ($n = 6$), lower anterior abdomen ($n = 6$), gluteal region ($n = 1$), and ischial region ($n = 1$). The etiology of defects included trauma ($n = 12$), infection ($n = 8$), pressure sores ($n = 8$), and malignancy ($n = 6$). Reconstruction was performed using pedicled tensor fascia lata flaps. Patients were evaluated in terms of viability of the flap and donor site morbidity. The technical details of the operative procedure have also been outlined. *Results*. All the flaps survived well except 5 patients in which minor complications were noted and 1 who experienced complete flap loss. Of those with minor complications, 1 patient developed distal marginal necrosis and 1 developed infection which subsided within three days by dressings and antibiotics and in 2 patients partial loss of the skin graft occurred at the donor site out of which 1 required regrafting and another one healed completely with dressing and antibiotics. All the patients were followed up for an average period of 6 months, ranging from 1 to 12 months. Donor site morbidity was minimal. *Conclusion*. It was concluded that the pedicled tensor fascia lata flap is a versatile, reliable, easy, and less time consuming procedure for the coverage of defects around trochanter, groin, lower anterior abdomen, perineum, and ischial region.

1. Introduction

Wangensteen first reported the tensor fascia lata flap for abdominal wall reconstruction [1]. Later, in 1978, Hill et al. and Nahai et al. described it as free musculocutaneous flap. Since then it has widely been used for reconstruction of various anatomical regions as pedicled or free flaps [2, 3].

This is a myofasciocutaneous flap that can be used as a pedicled flap for a wide variety of regions including trochanter, groin, perineum, ischium, and lower abdomen that can occur following trauma, infection, orthopaedic intervention, and pressure sores and after resection of malignant lesions/lymph node dissection.

These regions are usually associated with exposure of vital structures including bone or vessels. Therefore these anatomical districts almost always require flap cover.

Currently there are many options available for the reconstruction of these regions. Tensor fascia lata flap is one of the good alternatives.

Due to various features of tensor fascia lata flap, it is considered as a reliable flap for the reconstruction of many challenging defects [4, 5]. This includes the fact that this flap can be used as motor and sensory innervated; it has adequate and different types of soft tissues [4–7].

In this series we present our experience with the use of pedicled tensor fascia lata flap for the reconstruction of various anatomical regions.

2. Materials and Methods

In this retrospective study a total of 34 patients with defects over various anatomical regions were included. The defects were located over the trochanter ($n = 12$), groin ($n = 8$), perineum ($n = 6$), lower anterior abdomen ($n = 6$), gluteal region ($n = 1$), and ischial region ($n = 1$). The etiology of defects included trauma ($n = 12$), infection ($n = 8$), pressure sores ($n = 8$), and malignancy ($n = 6$). Reconstruction was performed using pedicled tensor fascia lata flaps. The technical details and operative time of the procedure have also been outlined.

All of the flaps were harvested from the lateral thigh regions and the raw area created was covered with a split thickness skin graft or closed primarily. The size of the flaps was slightly bigger to those of the defects. All flaps were based on a single dominant pedicle of ascending branch of lateral circumflex artery. The following operative steps were performed.

(1) First of all, anterior border of the flap was delineated by drawing a line from anterior superior iliac spine and lateral condyle of tibia.

(2) The posterior border of the flap was represented by greater trochanter, superior border by iliac crest, and inferior border within 8 cm from joint line.

(3) Location of perforators was marked with hand held doppler at the junction of proximal and middle third.

(4) Recipient site was prepared and actual size of the defect was measured.

(5) Size and location of the flap was designed by following principle of planning in reverse.

(6) Lower border of the flap was incised first followed by anterior and posterior border.

(7) Dissection was performed in distal to proximal direction in the subfascial plane.

(8) The vascular pedicle was identified at the preoperatively marked site at anterior aspect (8–10 cm distal to anterior superior iliac spine).

(9) Flap was then transferred to the recipient site and finally in setting and suturing of the flap was done into the defect.

(10) Donor site was skin grafted or primarily closed.

3. Results

Patients were evaluated in terms of viability of the flap and donor site morbidity. All the flaps survived well except 5 patients in which minor complications were noted and 1 who experienced complete flap loss.

Of those with minor complications, 1 patient developed distal marginal necrosis and 1 developed infection which subsided within three days by dressings and antibiotics and in 2 patients partial loss of the skin graft occurred at the donor site out of which 1 required regrafting and another one healed completely with dressing and antibiotics.

The length of the flap ranged from 14 to 22 cm and the width from 6 to 12 cm with mean operating time 1 hr.

Out of thirty-four patients, 28 were males and 6 were females. The average age of the patients was 30.4 years (range, 14 to 58 years).

All the patients were followed up for an average period of 6 months, ranging from 1 to 12 months. Donor site morbidity was minimal. No newly developed functional deficit of the lower limb was noted in any patient.

4. Discussion

Reconstruction of soft tissue defects around trochanter, groin, perineum, ischium, and lower abdomen remains a challenging task for the plastic surgeon. These regions often require flap cover due to associated exposure of bones or vessels or other vital structures. The flap can be harvested from local or remote areas. The local flaps can be taken from abdomen or thigh. Many local flaps have been described in the literature.

The various muscle flaps used for groin regions are rectus abdominis flap [8], rectus femoris flap, sartorius flap, internal oblique flap, and vastus lateralis flap [9–11].

For lower abdominal wall reconstruction, the available options are rectus abdominis muscle flap [12], tissue expansion [13], and medial mobilization of abdominal wall muscle [14].

Similarly, for perineal defects, the various reconstructive options are gracilis myocutaneous flap [15], rectus abdominis flaps [16], deep inferior epigastric perforator (DIEP) flap [17], superior gluteal artery perforator (SGAP) flap [18], and gluteal (split) flaps [19].

For ischial regions, gluteus maximus muscle flap [20], myocutaneous or fasciocutaneous posterior thigh flap [21], and gracilis muscle flap [22] have been well described in the literature.

Out of these numerous surgical techniques used for reconstruction of above-mentioned anatomical districts, each has its own advantages and disadvantages.

Use of rectus abdominis muscle flap may lead to abdominal weakness [11] or hernia, rectus femoris may cause knee weakness [23], and gluteus maximus may lead to gait disturbance [24].

Size of the internal oblique muscle is small and its dissection can be difficult and bloody [9].

Medial mobilization of abdominal muscle is difficult to use in the field of surgical oncology and tissue expansion takes a longer time [25]. Functional deficit may follow with the use of gracilis muscle flap.

The tensor fascia lata flap is a reliable flap having good vascularity and composed of skin, subcutaneous tissue, fascia, and muscle. Besides the fact that that this muscle is expendable, it causes minimal donor site morbidity without any knee weakness [26].

In this study we have used tensor fascia lata flap in different anatomical soft tissue defects. We observed a high success rate of this flap. All the flaps survived well except 5 patients in which minor complications were noted and 1 who experienced complete flap loss.

Six flaps in this series were used for abdominal wall reconstruction (Figure 1). We found no complication in terms of herniation or abdominal wall weakness. This corresponds to literature as described by some authors who reported that

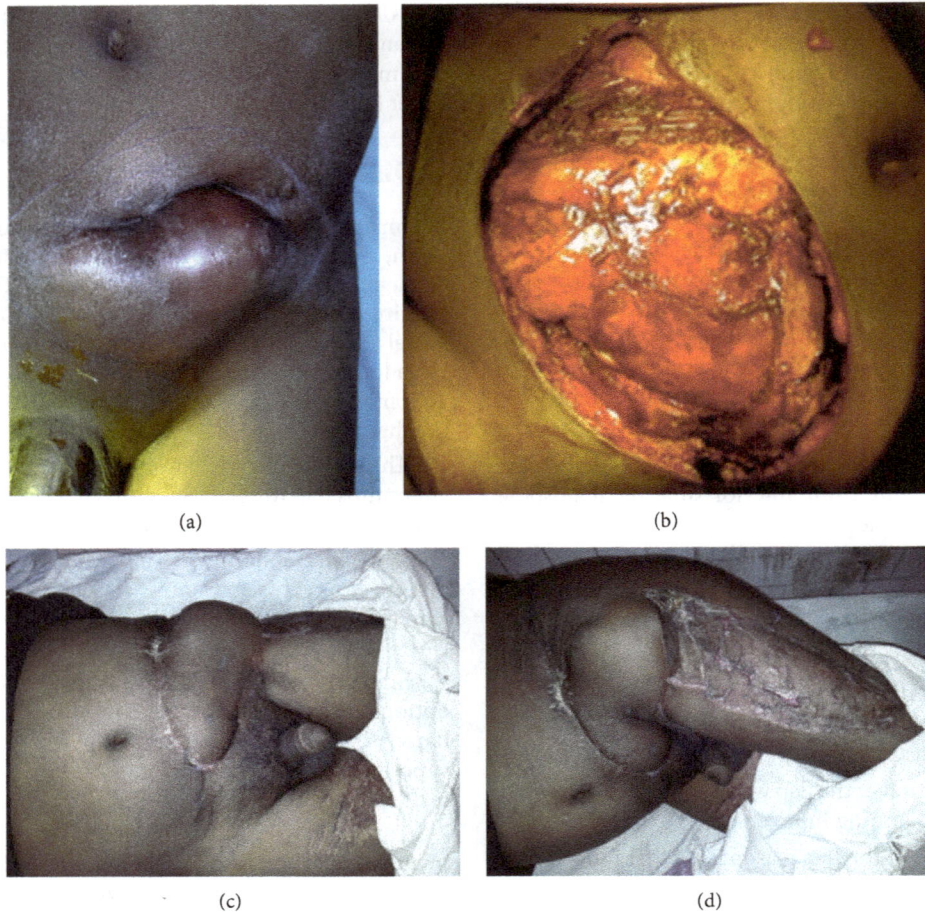

FIGURE 1: (a) Left lower abdominal wall malignancy (dermatofibrosarcoma). (b) Defect after local wide excision of tumour. (c) Follow-up photograph showing well set flap. (d) Follow-up photograph showing well set flap and well taken-up skin graft.

fascia lata is an effective flap that avoids the use of mesh and having a low incidence of recurrent herniation [27, 28].

We performed groin reconstruction in 8 patients, out of which 4 underwent lymph node dissection due to malignancy in different regions, 2 had traumatic soft tissue loss, and 2 had postinfectious soft tissue loss.

Agarwal et al. [29] performed pedicled tensor fascia lata thigh flap after block dissection of inguinal lymph nodes for malignant deposits in 15 patients. They observed that there were two cases of marginal flap necrosis, three cases developed lymphoedema which was managed by stockings, there were two cases of infection which were settled by antibiotics, and there were three cases of loss of a small area of skin graft at the donor site. They concluded that pedicled tensor fascia lata flap is a good and reliable option for groin reconstruction.

Pedicled tensor fascia lata flap was performed in majority of the patients with defects over trochanter totalling around 30% (12 patients) (Figures 2 and 3).

Karabeg et al. [30] used 39 pedicled TFL flaps for reconstruction of trochanteric pressure sore defects in 34 patients. The size of the flaps used ranged from 15 × 6 cm to 30 × 15 cm. All flaps survived with distal tip necrosis occurred in 4 cases where very large flap was used beyond the safe

limit. They found that tensor fascia lata flap is reliable flap but problem with the flap can be encountered if the flap is harvested beyond the safe limits and improperly designed. Only 1 patient in our study underwent distal tip necrosis. The reason of low complication is that we kept the size of the flap within the safe limit.

One of the good alternatives for ischial sore reconstruction is tensor fascia lata flap [3]. We used TFL flap in 1 patient in ischial sore reconstruction. All flaps survived well.

For perineal reconstruction, TFL can be safely used for lateral defects including inguinal regions [2, 31]. The size and consequently reach of the flap can be increased when used in combination with anterolateral thigh flap [32].

A total of 6 patients with perineal defects were included in this study, 2 with defects in the medial side and 4 having lateral defects. In those with medial defects TFL was used in combination with ALT flap. One flap in this group sustained complete necrosis. Compression or twisting of the pedicle could be the possible reason of total loss of the flap.

Contedini et al. [33] reported 11 cases of soft tissue reconstruction firstly planned with the ALT flap and then converted into TFL perforator flap. They concluded that result

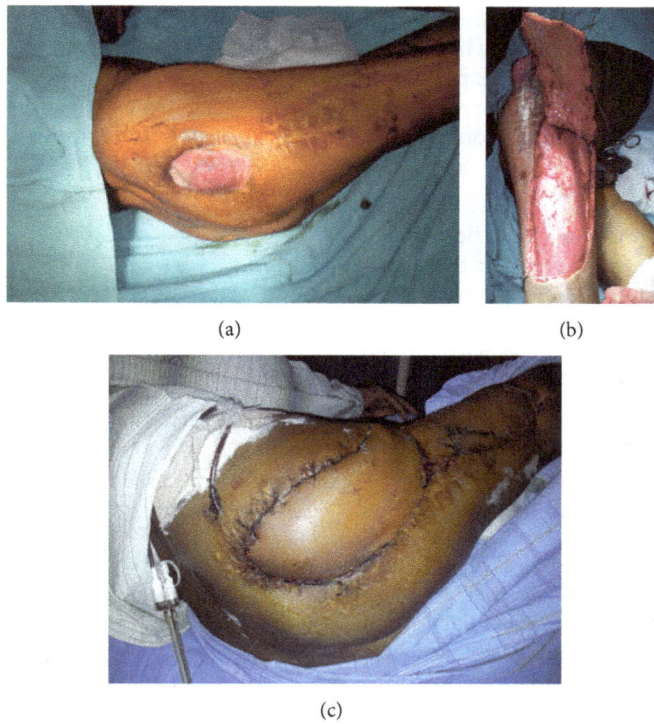

FIGURE 2: (a) Postarthroplasty soft tissue defect over right trochanteric region. (b) Photograph showing TFL flap elevation and arc of rotation of the flap. (c) Postoperative photograph after 2 weeks showing well set flap and well taken-up graft at donor site.

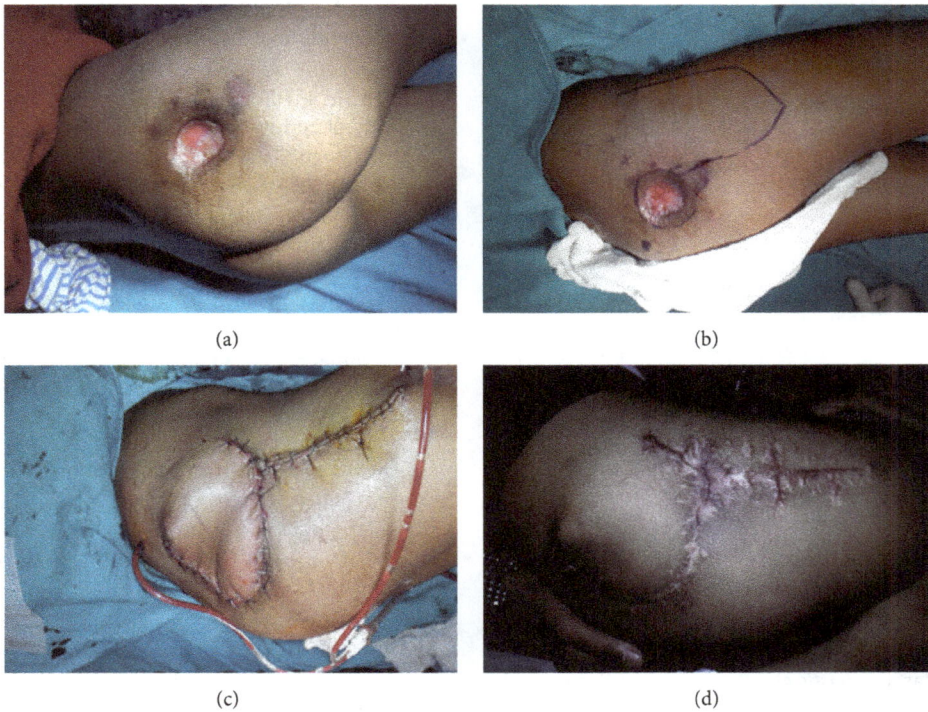

FIGURE 3: (a) Postinfection soft tissue defect over right gluteal region. (b) Photograph showing markings and TFL flap design. (c) Immediate postoperative photograph showing flap inset into the defect and donor site primarily closed. (d) Long term follow-up photograph.

was always satisfactory in terms of the donor site morbidity and reconstructive outcome. The main disadvantage of anterolateral thigh flap is its anatomical variability in number and location of perforators. They found that TFL perforator flap can be a good alternative. Some other researchers reported the similar possibility [34, 35]. The anatomy of TFL is more constant than ALT flap [36].

Aesthetic problem at the donor site could be avoided by using free flaps. However free flaps have their own limitations including high anaesthesia risk, long operating time, demands of microsurgical expertise, and a costly well equipped microsurgical set-up. Besides that, we have limited facility of microsurgery at our centre.

Main advantage of this flap is that it is very fast and reliable, so it is a good technique for critical patients who require a fast operation and cannot tolerate a lengthy operation that may lead to higher rate of complication. Other advantage of TFL flap is that it consist of highly vascular skin, subcutaneous tissue, fascia, and muscle and can be used to cover even irradiated tissues. Other advantage of this flap is that the donor site grafted site is hidden and less visible as compared to other donor sites from abdomen and groin thus minimising aesthetic concerns.

We acknowledge the limitation of our study. In some instances, TFL was used despite the availability of other options.

5. Conclusion

It was concluded that the pedicled tensor fascia lata flap is a versatile, reliable, easy, and less time consuming procedure for the coverage of defects around trochanter, groin, lower anterior abdomen, perineum and ischial region.

References

[1] O. H. Wangensteen, "Repair of recurrent and difficult hernias and other large defects of the abdominal wall employing the iliotibial tract of fascia lata as a pedicled flap," *The Journal of Surgery, Gynecology and Obstetrics*, vol. 59, pp. 766–780, 1934.

[2] H. L. Hill, F. Nahai, and L. O. Vasconez, "The tensor fascia lata myocutaneous free flap," *Plastic and Reconstructive Surgery*, vol. 61, no. 4, pp. 517–522, 1978.

[3] F. Nahai, J. S. Silverton, H. L. Hill, and L. O. Vasconez, "The tensor fascia lata musculocutaneous flap," *Annals of Plastic Surgery*, vol. 1, no. 4, pp. 372–379, 1978.

[4] S. Deiler, A. Pfadenhauer, J. Widmann, H. Stutzle, K.-G. Kanz, and W. Stock, "Tensor fasciae latae perforator flap for reconstruction of composite Achilles tendon defects with skin and vascularized fascia," *Plastic and Reconstructive Surgery*, vol. 106, no. 2, pp. 342–349, 2000.

[5] K. G. Krishnan, P. A. Winkler, A. Müller, G. Grevers, and H.-J. Steiger, "Closure of recurrent frontal skull base defects with vascularized flaps—a technical case report," *Acta Neurochirurgica*, vol. 142, no. 12, pp. 1353–1358, 2000.

[6] P. Brenner and C. Krebs, "Brachial plexus innervated, functional tensor fasciae latae muscle transfer for controlling a utah arm after dislocation of the shoulder caused by an electrical burn," *Journal of Trauma—Injury, Infection and Critical Care*, vol. 50, no. 3, pp. 562–567, 2001.

[7] K. Ihara, K. Doi, M. Shigetomi, and S. Kawai, "Tensor fasciae latae flap: alternative donor as a functioning muscle transplantation," *Plastic and Reconstructive Surgery*, vol. 100, no. 7, pp. 1812–1816, 1997.

[8] W. G. Payne, M. S. Walusimbi, M. L. Blue, G. Mosiello, T. E. Wright, and M. C. Robson, "Radiated groin wounds: pitfalls in reconstruction," *American Surgeon*, vol. 69, no. 11, pp. 994–997, 2003.

[9] S. S. Ramasastry, J. W. Futrell, S. L. Williams, and D. J. Hurwitz, "Internal oblique muscle pedicle flap for coverage of a major soft tissue defect of the groin," *Annals of Plastic Surgery*, vol. 15, no. 1, pp. 57–60, 1985.

[10] R. Rayment and D. M. Evans, "Use of an abdominal rotation flap for inguinal lymph node dissection," *British Journal of Plastic Surgery*, vol. 40, no. 5, pp. 485–487, 1987.

[11] P. Russo, E. F. Saldana, S. Yu, T. Chaglassian, and D. A. Hidalgo, "Myocutaneous flaps in genitourinary oncology," *The Journal of Urology*, vol. 151, no. 4, pp. 920–921, 1994.

[12] S. J. Mathes and J. Bostwick III, "A rectus abdominis myocutaneous flap to reconstruct abdominal wall defects," *British Journal of Plastic Surgery*, vol. 30, no. 4, pp. 282–283, 1977.

[13] W. M. Jacobsen, P. M. Petty, U. Bite, and C. H. Johnson, "Massive abdominal-wall hernia reconstruction with expanded external/internal oblique and transversalis musculofascia," *Plastic and Reconstructive Surgery*, vol. 100, no. 2, pp. 326–335, 1997.

[14] O. M. Ramirez, E. Ruas, and A. L. Dellon, "'Components separation' method for closure of abdominal-wall defects: an anatomic and clinical study," *Plastic and Reconstructive Surgery*, vol. 86, no. 3, pp. 519–525, 1990.

[15] I. Ducic, J. H. Dayan, C. E. Attinger, and P. Curry, "Complex perineal and groin wound reconstruction using the extended dissection technique of the gracilis flap," *Plastic and Reconstructive Surgery*, vol. 122, no. 2, pp. 472–478, 2008.

[16] S. W. Bell, N. Dehni, M. Chaouat, J. C. Lifante, R. Parc, and E. Tiret, "Primary rectus abdominis myocutaneous flap for repair of perineal and vaginal defects after extended abdominoperineal resection," *British Journal of Surgery*, vol. 92, no. 4, pp. 482–486, 2005.

[17] G. Muneuchi, M. Ohno, A. Shiota, T. Hata, and H. H. Igawa, "Deep inferior epigastric perforator (DIEP) flap for vulvar reconstruction after radical vulvectomy: a less invasive and simple procedure utilizing an abdominal incision wound," *Annals of Plastic Surgery*, vol. 55, no. 4, pp. 427–429, 2005.

[18] P. N. Blondeel, K. Van Landuyt, M. Hamdi, and S. J. Monstrey, "Soft tissue reconstruction with the superior gluteal artery perforator flap," *Clinics in Plastic Surgery*, vol. 30, no. 3, pp. 371–382, 2003.

[19] W. L. Gould, N. Montero, J. Cukic, R. C. Hagerty, and T. R. Hester, "The "split" gluteus maximus musculocutaneous flap," *Plastic and Reconstructive Surgery*, vol. 93, no. 2, pp. 330–336, 1994.

[20] S. Parkash and S. Banerjee, "The total gluteus maximus rotation and other gluteus maximus musculocutaneous flaps in the treatment of pressure ulcers," *British Journal of Plastic Surgery*, vol. 39, no. 1, pp. 66–71, 1986.

[21] Y. Yamamoto, A. Tsutsumida, M. Murazumi, and T. Sugihara, "Long-term outcome of pressure sores treated with flap coverage," *Plastic and Reconstructive Surgery*, vol. 100, no. 5, pp. 1212–1217, 1997.

[22] G. B. Wingate and J. A. Friedland, "Repair of ischial pressure ulcers with gracilis myocutaneous island flaps," *Plastic and Reconstructive Surgery*, vol. 62, no. 2, pp. 245–248, 1978.

[23] J. Bostwick III, H. L. Hill, and F. Nahai, "Repairs in the lower abdomen, groin, or perineum with myocutaneous or omental flaps," *Plastic and Reconstructive Surgery*, vol. 63, no. 2, pp. 186–194, 1979.

[24] A. Hurbungs and H. Ramkalawan, "Sacral pressure sore reconstruction—the pedicled superior gluteal artery perforator flap," *The South African Journal of Surgery*, vol. 50, no. 1, pp. 6–8, 2012.

[25] P. M. Chevray and N. K. Singh, "Abdominal wall reconstruction with the free tensor fascia lata musculofasciocutaneous flap using intraperitoneal gastroepiploic recipient vessels," *Annals of Plastic Surgery*, vol. 51, no. 1, pp. 97–102, 2003.

[26] J. K. Williams, G. W. Carlson, T. DeChalain, R. Howell, and J. J. Coleman, "Role of tensor fasciae latae in abdominal wall reconstruction," *Plastic and Reconstructive Surgery*, vol. 101, no. 3, pp. 713–718, 1998.

[27] H. L. Hill, R. Hester, and F. Nahai, "Covering large groin defects with the tensor fascia lata musculocutaneous flap," *British Journal of Plastic Surgery*, vol. 32, no. 1, pp. 12–14, 1979.

[28] Y.-R. Kuo, M.-H. Kuo, B. S. Lutz et al., "One-stage reconstruction of large midline abdominal wall defects using a composite free anterolateral thigh flap with vascularized fascia lata," *Annals of Surgery*, vol. 239, no. 3, pp. 352–358, 2004.

[29] A. K. Agarwal, S. Gupta, N. Bhattacharya, G. Guha, and A. Agarwal, "Tensor fascia lata flap reconstruction in groin malignancy," *Singapore Medical Journal*, vol. 50, no. 8, pp. 781–784, 2009.

[30] R. Karabeg, V. Dujso, and M. Jakirlić, "Application of tensor fascia lata pedicled flap in reconstructing trochanteric pressure sore defects," *Medicinski arhiv*, vol. 62, no. 5-6, pp. 300–302, 2008.

[31] J. C. McGregor and A. C. Buchan, "Our clinical experience with the tensor fasciae latae myocutaneous flap," *British Journal of Plastic Surgery*, vol. 33, no. 2, pp. 270–276, 1980.

[32] I. Koshima, H. Fukuda, R. Utunomiya, and S. Soeda, "The anterolateral thigh flap; variations in its vascular pedicle," *British Journal of Plastic Surgery*, vol. 42, no. 3, pp. 260–262, 1989.

[33] F. Contedini, L. Negosanti, V. Pinto et al., "Tensor fascia latae perforator flap: an alternative reconstructive choice for anterolateral thigh flap when no sizable skin perforator is available," *Indian Journal of Plastic Surgery*, vol. 46, no. 1, pp. 55–58, 2013.

[34] I. Koshima, K. Urushibara, K. Inagawa, and T. Moriguchi, "Free tensor fasciae latae perforator flap for the reconstruction of defects in the extremities," *Plastic and Reconstructive Surgery*, vol. 107, no. 7, pp. 1759–1765, 2001.

[35] O. K. Coskunfirat and Ö. Özkan, "Free tensor fascia lata perforator flap as a backup procedure for head and neck reconstruction," *Annals of Plastic Surgery*, vol. 57, no. 2, pp. 159–163, 2006.

[36] M. G. Hubmer, N. Schwaiger, G. Windisch et al., "The vascular anatomy of the tensor fasciae latae perforator flap," *Plastic and Reconstructive Surgery*, vol. 124, no. 1, pp. 181–189, 2009.

30

A Systematic Review of the Evolution of Laser Doppler Techniques in Burn Depth Assessment

Manaf Khatib, Shehab Jabir, Edmund Fitzgerald O'Connor, and Bruce Philp

St. Andrews Centre for Plastic Surgery and Burns, Broomfield Hospital, Chelmsford CM1 7ET, UK

Correspondence should be addressed to Shehab Jabir; shihab.jabir@googlemail.com

Academic Editor: Bishara S. Atiyeh

Aims. The introduction of laser Doppler (LD) techniques to assess burn depth has revolutionized the treatment of burns of indeterminate depth. This paper will systematically review studies related to these two techniques and trace their evolution. At the same time we hope to highlight current controversies and areas where further research is necessary with regard to LD imaging (LDI) techniques. *Methods.* A systematic search for relevant literature was carried out on PubMed, Medline, EMBASE, and Google Scholar. Key search terms included the following: "Laser Doppler imaging," "laser Doppler flow," and "burn depth." *Results.* A total of 53 studies were identified. Twenty-six studies which met the inclusion/exclusion criteria were included in the review *Conclusions.* The numerous advantages of LDI over those of LD flowmetry have resulted in the former technique superseding the latter one. Despite the presence of alternative burn depth assessment techniques, LDI remains the most favoured. Various newer LDI machines with increasingly sophisticated methods of assessing burn depth have been introduced throughout the years. However, factors such as cost effectiveness, scanning of topographically inconsistent areas of the body, and skewing of results due to tattoos, peripheral vascular disease, and anaemia continue to be sighted as obstacles to LDI which require further research.

1. Introduction

Burn wounds that heal within a 3-week window have improved aesthetic and functional outcomes with a reduced degree of scarring [1]. This has meant that early accurate assessment of burn depth is essential in burn patients in order to decide between conservative treatment and surgical excision of the burn and grafting in order to achieve healing within this 2-3-week timeframe. Bedside clinical assessment is usually effective when the burns are either superficial or full thickness. However, in partial thickness burns where the burn depth is not well defined, clinical assessment is not as accurate. Overall, clinical assessment of burn depth when dealing with a burn of indeterminate depth has been shown to be accurate in only 65–70% of cases even when performed by an experienced burns surgeon [2]. For this reason a number of adjuncts to aid the clinician in making an accurate burn depth assessment were devised. Foremost among these techniques, and by far, the one that received unanimous approval by the burn community was laser Doppler technique to assess burn wound depth. Laser Doppler techniques utilize the Doppler effect described by the Austrian physicist Christian Doppler. In the case of laser Doppler techniques to assess burn depth, laser light is directed at moving blood cells in sampled tissue. The frequency change of the waves of laser light observed is proportional to the amount of perfusion in the tissue.

In this systematic review of the use of laser Doppler in assessing burn wounds we will trace the evolution of this technique and its application to burn depth assessment. Furthermore, the evidence for laser Doppler assessment will also be reviewed. Alternative techniques to determine burn depth will also be reviewed and compared to laser Doppler techniques. Finally, we intend to highlight current controversies and areas where further clarification and research are necessary.

2. Methods

Initially a study protocol was formulated with relevant inclusion and exclusion criteria defined for studies to be included in the systematic review (Table 1).

TABLE 1: Inclusion and exclusion criteria for this systematic review.

Inclusion Criteria

(i) Studies involving humans

(ii) English language publication

(iii) Studies published from inception of database to February 2014

Exclusion Criteria

(i) Use of LD techniques on animal models

(ii) Non-English language publication

(iii) Purely technical descriptions of the use of LD techniques with no analysis of outcomes

A literature search was then carried out on PubMed, Medline, Embase, and Google Scholar and the Cochrane databases from inception to February 2014 for studies on the topic of laser Doppler in burn depth assessment. The following key words were used: "laser Doppler imaging," "laser Doppler flow," and "burn depth." The search terms were combined with the Boolean operator "and." The references of selected studies were also perused for papers that may have been missed via the electronic search.

The title and abstract of all identified studies were examined by two reviewers (Manaf Khatib and Shehab Jabir). In cases where suitability of a study for inclusion in the review was unclear, the entire paper was obtained and assessed for suitability. Eligibility as mentioned above was determined by the criteria listed in Table 1. Any issues pertaining to eligibility of studies were solved via discussion with the senior author (Bruce Philp).

3. Results

A total of 53 studies were retrieved following the search. 27 studies were excluded following review of the title and abstract. The remaining 26 papers were reviewed to establish suitability for inclusion. The remaining 26 papers all met the inclusion criteria and were included in the review (Table 2).

4. Discussion

4.1. LD Flowmetry. Following Stern et al.'s proposal for the use of laser Doppler technology in burn depth assessment in 1975, a number of studies investigating and validating its use in clinical practice took place [3]. Green et al. published a landmark paper on this technology in 1988 and paved the way for forthcoming research [4]. The authors investigated the use of laser Doppler flowmetry on 13 burn wounds from 10 patients. Measurements were recorded twice daily after every dressing change in the first 72 h from the onset of the burn. Seven wounds healed conservatively within 21 days (healing group) and 6 wounds required excision and grafting (nonhealing group). The authors found statistically significant differences in laser Doppler measurements in the two groups ($P < 0.02$) at each 24 h interval measured. The authors did allude to several limitations in the study design, including; uncontrolled environmental factors and lack of

knowledge of the effect of different dressings applied [4]. Despite the presence of limitations in the study and lack of description of the device and exact measurement of the laser Doppler values, the study was a pioneering study that instigated the development of further trials.

O'Reilly et al. soon followed the works of Green et al. and conducted a prospective cohort study in which they investigated the use of laser Doppler Flowmetry in 59 burns from 10 different patients [5]. LD assessment was compared to clinical assessment at initial presentation of the burn wound. Wounds deemed to require excision and grafting also underwent biopsies and histological assessment. LD values had no effect on the decision making of the burn surgeons and subsequent management. A cut-off point of 1.4 (arbitrary value of laser Doppler flow) was established and values above 1.4 had a 98.4% positive predictive value to heal within 21 days [5]. A substantial limitation to the study was that only burns that required surgery underwent biopsies and hence we have no way to determine the histological assessment of the wounds that healed conservatively [6]. This is especially important as the authors state that there was a "very poor correlation between LD values and the histologic depth in millimetres" [5]. The results obtained in view of the limitations do not support the strong conclusion of the authors that "LD flowmetry can diagnose accurately and early this critical level of thermal injury in burns of indeterminate depth" [5].

In another prospective cohort study by Waxman et al., 51 burn wounds from 33 patients were investigated [7]. Only patients with burns of indeterminate depth by clinical assessment and patients presenting within 48 h of the onset of burn were included in the study. The study not only investigated the accuracy of prediction of healing by LD flowmetry but also investigated the effect of different generated temperatures on the sensitivity and specificity of the assessment technique. The authors placed the measurement probe on different areas of burn wounds at temperatures of 35, 38, 41, and 44°C. All burns were managed conservatively, and burns that healed within 3 weeks were deemed as superficial partial thickness and burns that did not heal within this timeframe were deemed as deep dermal burns. 18 of the 51 burn wounds did not heal and required subsequent excision and grafting. The authors showed that burns with LD flow values of more than 6 mL/100 g/min at temperature of 35°C would heal in three weeks (100% specificity but poor sensitivity). Increasing the temperature to 44°C increased the sensitivity to 94% but decreased specificity [7]. A substantial limitation in the presentation of the result was that the authors failed to present the total body surface area (TBSA) of the burn wounds, as different sizes of burns will have different physiological consequences that could alter both core and peripheral surface temperatures.

Atiles et al. conducted a prospective cohort study that investigated 86 burn wounds from 21 different patients [8]. LD flowmetry was used with a contact probe heated to 39°C. Daily measurements were taken at days 0–3. Wounds were classified as either healed or not healed at 3 weeks after the burn. The study showed that burn wounds with more than 80 perfusion units (PU) will heal within 3 weeks with a

TABLE 2: Summary of retrieved studies in the literature.

Authors country	Year	Type of study	Patient n	Burns n	Type of laser Doppler device	Surgery needed	Findings	Limitation
Green et al. [4], USA	1988	Observational Study	10	13	LD flowmetry Nonspecified type of LD scanner	6	Statistically significant difference in LD value between healing and nonhealing group	Lack of description of methodology of measurement
O'Reilly et al. [5], USA	1989	Prospective cohort *LD measurements did not influence clinical judgement*	41	59	LD flowmetry Laser flow blood perfusion monitor BPM403	8	LD < 1.4 PPV 98.4%, LD > 1.4 deemed superficial and will heal within 21 days	43 > 1.4 LD burned areas excised and grafted Day of measurement not specified
Waxman et al. [7], USA	1989	Prospective cohort *LDI within 48 h of burn Indeterminate depth only*	33	51	LD Flowmetry Laser flow blood perfusion monitor BPM403	18	100% specificity re: healing if flow >6 mL/100 g/min NPV 75%	TBSA not specified
Niazi et al. [9], UK	1993	Prospective cohort *Burns of indeterminate depth Children excluded*	13	13	LD imaging Newcastle laser Doppler scanner	7	Good correlation of LDI with histological assessment	No statistical analysis
Atiles et al. [8], USA	1995	Prospective cohort	21	86	LD flowmetry Perimed PF4000	33	<40 PU; Sen: 0.46, Spec: 1.0, PPV:1.0, NPV: 0.85 >80 PU; Sen: 0.85, Spec: 0.82, PPV: 0.79, NPV: 0.87	No histological assessment. No burn cause identified
Park et al. [10], Korea	1998	Prospective cohort	44	100	LD flowmetry Periflux system 4001	Not specified	Primary outcome; healing at 2 weeks >100 PU 90% PPV 10–100 PU 96% PPV <10 100% PPV	Surgery not specified—just said not healed 2 weeks
Banwell et al. [11], UK	1999	Prospective cohort	30	n/a	LD flowmetry and LD imaging Moor LDI scanner	Not specified	Good correlation LDI results and histology	No stats
Pape et al. [12], UK	2001	Prospective cohort *Intermediate depth 48–72 h of presentation*	48	76	LD imaging Moor LDI scanner	25	97% PPV of LDI compared with 70% of clinical assessment	
Kloppenborg et al. [13], Netherlands	2001	Prospective cohort	16	22	LD imaging PIM 1.0 laser Doppler perfusion imager (Lisca development AB)	6	Sensitivity 100% and specificity 93.8% on day 4	Invalid statistical analysis

TABLE 2: Continued.

Authors country	Year	Type of study	Patient n	Burns n	Type of laser Doppler device	Surgery needed	Findings	Limitation
Holland et al. [14], Australia	2002	Prospective cohort *Paediatric burns only 12 days cut-off point for healing*	57	57	LD imaging Moor LDI V 3.1	17	Deep dermal; partial thickness Clinical examination 66% LDI 90%; clinical 71%, LDI 96%	Mobility of children No validated endpoint
Jeng et al. [15], USA	2003	Prospective blinded trial *Burns of indeterminate depth*	23	41	LD imaging Moor LDI-VR	7	56% agreement between clinician and LDI 71.4% accuracy of surgeon compared to histological diagnosis	8/18 burns deemed superficial by LDI but required grafting
Mileski et al. [16], USA	2003	Prospective cohort	56	159	LD flowmetry PF 4001 laser Doppler flowmeter	53	Sensitivity: 68% Specificity: 88% PPV: 81% NPV: 76%	Clinical assessment once versus serial LDI
Riordan et al. [17], USA	2003	Prospective blinded trial *Surgeon blinded to LDI result*	22	35	PIM #II LISCA	24	At threshold value of 1.3 Sensitivity: 95% Specificity: 94%	
La Hei et al. [18], Australia	2006	Prospective blinded trial *No clinical assessment done Assessment by images and LDI only*	31	50	LD imaging Moor LDI V2	22	Sensitivity: 97% Specificity: 100%	Statistical analysis and small number
McGill et al. [19], UK	2007	Prospective blinded comparison	20	27	LD imaging Moor LDI versus PW Allen videomicroscope: transcutaneous microscopy	10	LDI: sensitivity 100% VM: sensitivity for SPT 100%	No histological assessment Expert user of VM VM not tolerated by children
Hoeksema et al. [20], Belgium	2009	Prospective blinded trial *Early assessment of burns using LDI Intermediate depths Day 0, 1, 3, 5, 8, and 21*	40	40	LD imaging Moor LDI	12	Sensitivity increases with days after burn. Statistically significantly better than clinical assessment from day 3 Sensitivity: 100% Specificity: 92.3%	2 cases that required surgery and histology showed that burn wound was superficial in nature
Cho et al. [21], Republic of Korea	2009	Prospective cohort study *Paediatric burns Only burns of indeterminate depth 48–72 h*	103	181	LD imaging Periscan PIM 3	n/a	Healing by 14 days at PU of 250 Sensitivity 80.6% and Specificity 76.9%	No confirmation of superficial nature of burn with histology

TABLE 2: Continued.

Authors country	Year	Type of study	Patient n	Burns n	Type of laser Doppler device	Surgery needed	Findings	Limitation
Mill et al. [22], Australia	2009	Prospective cohort study *Paediatric burns Testing different effect of dressings*	48	85	LD imaging Moor LDI2	6	Scans within 24 h accurately predict outcome Colour palette corresponds to healing time. Cut-off of 14 days	No blinding Wide range of scanning time 0–120 h
Kim et al. [23], Australia	2010	Case-control trial *Only patients requiring grafting <16 years*	196	196	LD imaging Moor LDI2	196	Reduction in decision for surgery in LDI group 8.9 days versus 11.6 days in control group (P = 0.01)	No randomisation
Merz et al. [24], Germany	2010	Retrospective cohort study	28	173	LD flowmetry Laser Doppler O2C	88	Sensitivity: 80.6% Specificity: 88.2% PPV: 93.1% NPV: 69.8%	No histological assessment
Nguyen et al. [25], Australia	2010	Prospective cohort *Paediatric population Two groups; < and >48 h presentation*	400	637	LD imaging Moor LDI2-BI	89	<48 h Sensitivity: 78% Specificity: 74% >48 h Sensitivity: 75% Specificity: 85%	No histological assessment in patients operated on
Lindahl et al. [26], Sweden	2013	Prospective cohort	14	45	LD imaging Laser Speckle contrast imager (Perimed AB)	n/a	Higher perfusion in burns healing in less than 14 days compared to more than 14 days from day 0 from burn.	Small sample of patients No gold standard to compare to
Menon et al. [27], Australia	2012	Retrospective cohort *Friction burns in paediatric population*	36	36	Not specified	12	64% accuracy of LDI predicting burn outcome	Small sample of patients No gold standard to compare to
Pape et al. [28], Multicentre	2012	Prospective cohort	137	433	LD Imaging Moor LDI	ns	Development of validated colour code for interpretation and link to burn outcome	
Park et al. [29], Korea	2013	Retrospective cohort	96	101	LD imaging Periscan PIM3 (Perimed AB)	46	Cut-off point of 154.7PU Sensitivity: 78.3 Specificity: 92.7	
Stewart et al. [30], Canada	2012	Prospective blinded control trial	38	105	LD imaging Moor LDI 2-BI	64	LDI has PPV > 90% accurate in determining need for grafting	

sensitivity of 85%, specificity of 82%, positive predictive value (PPV) of 79%, and negative predictive value (NPV) of 87%. A PU of less than 40 predicted nonhealing at 3 weeks with a sensitivity of 46%, specificity of 100%, PPV of 100%, and NPV of 85% [8]. In the study there was no histological assessment to confirm that the nonhealing wounds were in fact deep at presentation. Confounding factors such as infection and cause of burn were not discussed and hence weakened the results of the study.

In a prospective cohort study by Park et al. in 1998, 100 burn wounds from 44 patients were investigated using LD flowmetry [10]. The primary outcome measure set by the authors was healing at 14 days. Only patients presenting within 72 h of injury were included. A value of more than 100 PU yielded a 90% PPV that the burn wound will heal within 14 days, and a value of <10 yielded a 100% PPV that the wound will not heal within 14 days. Values between 10 and 100 PU yielded a 96% PPV that healing will occur with scarring [10]. A criticism of the study is that the 14-day threshold to categorise burns into a healing and nonhealing group is not validated, the reason for choosing such threshold is not discussed and elaborated upon.

In a short report by Banwell et al., they used the same technique employed by Park et al. and found similar results and agreed that a 100 PU threshold was an accurate cut-off to predict wound healing [11]. They found good correlation between LD assessment and histological assessment. However, the authors discouraged the use of contact LD flowmetry due to the requirement of multiple measurements and contact with the burn wound. They shed some light on the Moor LDI device and touted it as a superior alternative to LD flowmetry due to the noncontact nature of measurement and the ability to cover a larger area [10]. Despite some bold conclusions in the report, there is no presentation of raw data or statistical analysis. However, this short report by Banwell et al. in 1999 set off the LDI revolution in motion and paved the way for the landmark paper on the use of LDI in burn depth assessment by Pape et al. (discussed below) in 2001.

Finally in 2003 Mileski et al. attempted to revive the use of LD flowmetry with a further study on the use of contact LD flowmetry in the assessment of burn wound depth [16]. Fifty six patients with 159 burn wounds were assessed. LD flowmetry was conducted daily from day 1 to 4 after burn. The results of the study showed 88% specificity and an 81% PPV for the identification of wounds that will not heal within 21 days [16]. The authors concluded what has already been established in the literature that LD assessment is more accurate than clinical assessment alone. However, by this time LDI had already superseded LD flowmetry and thus the results of this study added very little to this field.

The aforementioned studies all used LD flowmetry; this requires the direct contact of the laser Doppler probe to a burn wound which of course has inevitable negative implications, namely:

(i) patient comfort;

(ii) need for patients to be still-implications in the paediatric population;

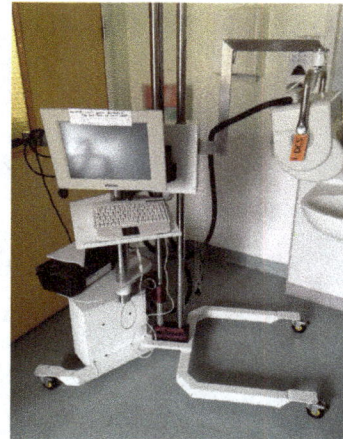

FIGURE 1: The Moor LDI system used by Pape et al. in their study and in our burns unit at St. Andrews Centre for Plastic Surgery and Burns.

(iii) infection and cross contamination due to contact of the instrument;

(iv) small area of measurement and need for several readings to cover a burn wound.

4.2. LD Imaging. Niazi et al. were the first to study the noncontact laser Doppler imaging device in 1993 [9]. The authors studied 13 burn wounds that were scanned at 24, 48, and 72 h after injury. Only burns of indeterminate depth were included and all children were excluded. In contrast to LD flowmetry, the scans were conducted at a distance of 160 cm. LD assessment was compared to both clinical and histological assessment. They found a 100% correlation between LD assessment and histological assessment, compared to 70% correlation between LD assessment and clinical assessment and 40% correlation between clinical assessment and histological assessment [9]. The study did not include any statistical analysis and LD values were not explained and no cut-off point was defined.

In a prospective cohort study, Pape et al. assessed 76 wounds from 48 patients using LDI (Figures 1 and 2) [12]. They recorded LDI values between 48 and 72 h after injury and compared LD evaluation to both clinical assessment in all wounds and histological assessment in wounds that underwent surgery. Wounds that were deemed to be hyperperfused were managed conservatively with daily dressings and wounds deemed to be hypoperfused were managed surgically within the first 24 h of presentation. They found that the accuracy of LD assessment was 97% compared to 70% by clinical assessment [12]. It is imperative to mention that in 4 cases, the clinician ignored the judgement of the LD assessment, which judged the wound to heal within 21 days, and the cases were taken to theatre for excision and grafting. Histological assessment in those 4 wounds supported the clinical judgement. This illustrates that despite the high accuracy of LD assessment in this study, results should be correlated carefully with clinical judgement.

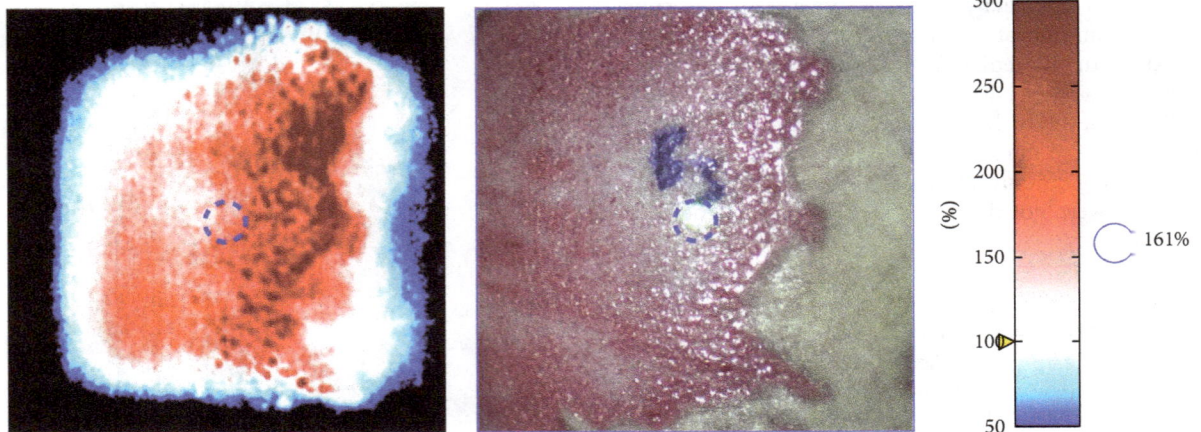

FIGURE 2: Appearance of a burn wound using the Aimago EasyLDI technology. It enables visualization of the microcirculation and the blood flow in small vessels with the increasingly red regions indicating greater blood flow.

Kloppenberg et al. further assessed the use of LDI in burn depth assessment [13]. The authors studied 22 wounds from 16 patients. Only patients with a burn <10% TBSA were investigated in the study. The results of their study showed a 93.8% sensitivity and 100% specificity of day 4 after burn LD assessment prediction of healing within 21 days [13]. The results supported the new studies advocating the superiority of LD imaging over LD flowmetry.

In 2002, Holland et al. focused their study of LD assessment on the paediatric population only [14]. Critics of LDI have argued that accurate measurement of LD values in children will be difficult due to the need for the patient to remain still during the course of the assessment. The authors aimed to investigate if the results of their study on the paediatric population correlate with previous study findings in the adult population. 57 patients were studied over a 10 month period and patients were scanned 36–72 h after injury. They reviewed patients at 12 days to assess if wound healing has occurred or patients required surgery. At that time period, 17 of the patients required excision and grafting. In the deep dermal/full thickness cohort of patients, clinical examination and LDI assessment were 66% and 90% accurate, respectively. In the superficial partial thickness group the accuracy of clinical assessment was 71% and LD assessment was 96% [14]. The study represented an important landmark that proved the efficacy of this technique in the paediatric population despite the difficulties encountered with patient cooperation. A shortcoming of the study, however, is the 12-day threshold for determination of wound healing as it is a nonvalidated cut-off point and the authors do not elaborate on their choice.

Jeng et al. conducted a prospective blinded trial in 2003 [15]. The authors enrolled 23 patients with 41 different wounds of indeterminate depth. Daily assessment and decision of need for grafting were done by a clinician and recorded. LD scans were simultaneously conducted; however, the clinician remained blind to the LD assessment. The results of the study showed that clinical assessment agreed with LD assessment 56% of the time. In 21 wounds

that were histologically analysed, burn depth assessment by clinicians was 71%. The authors further showed 100% agreement between histological analysis and LD assessment when wounds were hypoperfused. They calculated that LDI assessment would have saved a median of 2 days for every patient in determination for need of operating; this has some important implications on cost and reduced patient morbidity [15]. Despite an accurate assessment of need for grafting when the LD showed hypoperfusion, it is important to mention that 8/18 wounds that were deemed to be hyperperfused by LD assessment required grafting and deemed to be deep dermal or full thickness by histological assessment. The shortcoming raises some concerns and triggers the need for further assessment of LD thresholds for stratification of burn wounds.

In another prospective blinded trial, Riordan et al. studied 35 burn wounds from 22 patients using noncontact LDI [17]. The study focused on assessment of wounds to the upper and lower extremities. Scans were conducted at 48 h after the burn and all burn wounds had biopsies taken for histological assessment. A device-specific perfusion index showed a statistically significant inverse relationship between perfusion and burn depth. At a threshold of 1.3 perfusion index, LD assessment had 95% sensitivity and 94% specificity for prediction of wound healing at 21 days [17]. The sound methodology of the study yielded very positive results and further strengthened the argument for the use of LDI in assessment of burns of indeterminate depth.

La Hei et al. conducted another prospective blinded trial in a paediatric population [18]. 50 LD images from 31 patients were taken 72 h after injury. Two experienced burn surgeons were provided with clinical photographs of the wounds, relevant history, and LDI image. Another clinician blinded to the LD values determined on regular intervals if a wound is healing or will require grafting. LD assessment showed a 97% correlation with clinical outcome. All wounds deemed to be deep by LDI did not heal within 21 days or required excision and grafting [18]. The study further dispels the concerns of the reliability of LD assessment in the paediatric population and strengthens the evidence for the use of LD assessment as an adjunct to clinical assessment.

In a comparison between two different modalities, McGill et al. assessed the benefit of videomicroscopy over LDI in the assessment of burn wound depth. Videomicroscopy (VM) was touted as a cheap alternative to LDI [19]. 27 wounds from 20 different patients presenting less than 72 h after a burn were assessed. LDI and VM assessments were carried out on all patients and the results were blinded to the clinical team. Three endpoints were established: healing within 21 days, early surgery, and delayed healing with need for grafting. VM assessment had had strong correlation with both LDI assessment and clinical outcome ($P < 0.001$). The authors concluded that VM is able to accurately assess burn depth and is comparative to LDI assessment with the advantage of being cheaper [19]. However, the results must be analysed with caution, as there was no histological assessment of the wounds that had early surgery and there is no way to find out if any of those wounds would have healed conservatively. Furthermore, VM assessment was carried out by an expert user and the results of the study may not be reproduced in other centres. VM assessment was also not tolerated well by children in the study. All the disadvantages of contact modalities in burn depth assessment still apply and hence its use over LDI is far-fetched.

In 2009, Hoeksema et al. aimed to identify the best day for LD assessment to be carried out and investigate at which day is LD assessment most accurate when being compared to clinical assessment [20]. In a prospective cohort study, the authors studied 40 burn wounds of intermediate depth. Both clinical and LD assessment were carried out in days 0, 1, 3, 5, and 8 after the burn. The two clinicians conducting the clinical assessment were blinded to the LD values. The outcome to compare to was healing within 21 days. For LD assessment the threshold for stratification of wounds in healing and nonhealing categories was 220 PU. On days 0, 1, 3, 5, and 8 LDI assessment was 54%, 79.5%, 95%, 97%, and 100% accurate, respectively. In clinical assessment it was 40.6%, 61.5%, 52.5%, 71.4%, and 100%, respectively. It was deemed that on day 3 LD assessment was significantly better than clinical assessment ($P < 0.001$) and also better on day 5 ($P = 0.005$) [20]. The study was the first to assess the relative benefit of LD assessment over clinical assessment on different days and provided important information to both clinicians in this field and for future research.

Cho et al. aimed to investigate a LDI cut-off that will allow prediction of healing and nonhealing at 14 days [21]. Patients less than 15 years of age with partial thickness wounds were recruited. LD scanning was conducted 48–72 h after the burn. Clinical assessment was conducted by two blinded clinicians. Healing was judged by observation of the wound on regular intervals for evidence of reepithelialisation. From the 181 wounds investigated, when using 250 PU as a cut-off point the sensitivity for healing within 14 days was 80.6% with a specificity of 76.9%. The mean PU for the healing group was 380 compared to 185 in the nonhealing group ($P < 0.001$) [21]. The lower sensitivity and specificity of LD assessment compared to previous studies, for prediction of healing within 14 days, illustrate the difficulty in predicting an outcome at such a short interval and the need for further research is necessary.

In another study focusing on the paediatric population, Mill et al. aimed to assess the validity of LD assessment in burn wounds in children [22]. A total 85 burns from 48 patients were investigated, time for wound healing and need for surgery were recorded. The different dressings used were also recorded. An important finding was that the use of Silver based dressings such as Acticoat did not interfere with the LD assessment. The use of another Silver based dressing, Silvazine, did however underestimate the perfusion in some wounds. The authors found congruence between the LDI colour palette of perfusion and the healing time [22]. A substantial limitation to the study is the lack of control over the time of scanning as the range of scanning was 0–120 h.

Kim et al. aimed to assess if LDI use helped in reducing the decision for operating on burn wounds [23]. A case-control trial was conducted, with patients undergoing LD scanning and clinical assessment (Group 1) and patients only being clinically assessed (Group 2). 196 patients were enrolled of which 49% underwent LD assessment. The mean time for decision to operate was 8.9 and 11.6 days in Groups 1 and 2, respectively, ($P < 0.05$) [23]. The reduction in decision to operate is inevitably beneficial in reducing length of stay, cost, and patient morbidity. The results of the study would have been more significant if randomisation was done; the reason for not randomising the population sample was not alluded to by the authors.

In a retrospective cohort study by Merz et al. they investigated the ability of LD flowmetry to accurately predict wound depth and healing potential in the first 24 h from the burn injury [24]. Twenty-eight patients with 173 wounds were retrospectively analysed. Regarding healing within 21 days, assessment at <24 h by LD flowmetry yielded a 93.1% accuracy when the values were >100 PU, and a value of <100 PU accurately predicated nonhealing in 88.2%. Further LD assessment at 3 and 6 days showed no significant reduction in perfusion [24]. The results are in disagreement Hoeksema et al.'s findings. The findings would have been strengthened if histological assessment was done on the 88 wounds that underwent surgery.

In a large prospective cohort study by Nguyen et al., 637 wounds from 400 patients were studied [25]. Paediatric patients were divided into two groups: presentation before (Group 1) and after (Group 2) 48 h. The sensitivity and specificity of LD assessment were 78% and 74% in Group 1, respectively. In Group 2, it was 75% and 85%, respectively. The difference was not statistically significant [25]. The findings support Merz et al.'s findings and illustrate the beneficial role of LD assessment in the acute phase.

Lindahl et al. operated the laser speckle imaging device in their study of 45 burns from 14 patients [26]. The speckle technology differs from the traditional laser Doppler technology. The device is composed of a source of laser and a detector camera. The emitted laser forms a speckle pattern once it contacts the skin; the contrast of the detected speckle image is affected by the underlying microcirculation and variation in flow. As opposed to LDI any artefact from movement is averaged out the speckle image [26]. The study showed a higher mean perfusion in wounds that healed in 14 days compared to wounds that did not heal. The difference between perfusion in those two groups was highest in 4–7 days after the injury [26].

In an interesting study by Menon et al., they investigated if the success of LD assessment in prediction of scald-burn healing potential is reproducible in friction burns [27]. A retrospective review was carried out on 36 friction burns. LD assessment accurately predicted wound healing in 64% of cases. The differences in the mechanism of burn were attributed to the lower accuracy compared to the literature [27].

Pape et al. conducted a large multicentre study that evaluated 433 burn wounds from 137 patients [28]. The aim of the study was to develop a validated colour code for LDI palette interpretation. They were able to correlate the colour palette with healing potential [28] as follows:

(i) healing within 14 days: red colour >600 PU;

(ii) overlap area, healing within 21 days: pink colour 440–600 PU;

(iii) healing between 14 and 21 days: yellow colour 260–440 PU;

(iv) overlap area, healing most likely within 14–21 days: green colour 200–260 PU;

(v) healing >21 days: light blue colour <200 PU;

(vi) nonhealing at 21 days: dark blue colour <140 PU.

In 2013, Park et al. aimed to analyse if LD assessment can expedite decisions regarding the need for excision and grafting in burn wounds of indeterminate depth [29]. A retrospective cohort study of 101 burn wounds was conducted. Patients were divided into a nonsurgical group (Group 1) and a surgical group (Group 2). There was a significant difference in mean PU between the groups ($P < 0.001$). A cut-off point of 154 PU yielded a sensitivity of 78.3% and 92.7% for prediction of need for surgery [29]. The results add further evidence for the support of LDI in burn depth assessment.

Finally, Stewart et al. conducted a prospective blinded control trial aiming to compare LDI assessment and clinical assessment in decision to operate on a burn wound [30]. The authors studied 105 burn wounds from 38 people. Using histological assessment as a gold standard, LD assessment was found to have a PPV of >90% [30]. The findings are in concurrence with previous studies aimed at assessing the benefit of LD assessment in prediction of need for surgery.

4.3. Alternative Techniques to Assess Burn Depth

4.3.1. Fluorescein Dye. The use of dyes in the assessment of burn wound depth was first proposed by Lang and Boyd in 1942 [31]. As previously mentioned, in 1943 Dingwall studied the use of fluorescein dye to assess burn wound depth in animal models. He demonstrated that fluorescein would only reach areas with patent cutaneous circulation and thereby deeper burn areas can be marked [32]. However, the method was criticized due to the dynamic nature of a burn wound

and the evolution of a burn in the first 24–48 hours [33]. The use of fluorescein dye was not adopted by many burn surgeons and the first study to be published in the literature that applied its use in human burns was not until 1961 [34]. Its use remained unpopular as quantifying the amount of dye in the circulation in certain parts of a burn was not possible before the invention of the fluorometer in the 1970s.

The fluorometer provided a method of quantification of fluorescein dye in the cutaneous circulation [35], and several studies investigated its use in both free flap monitoring [35–37] and burn wounds [38, 39]. Gatti et al. evaluated the ability of the fluorometer to distinguish partial thickness from full thickness burns after injection of fluorescein dye. They used this technique in 63 burn sites and showed that partial thickness burns exhibited the dye within 10 minutes of injection compared to full thickness burns where no dye penetrated the area [38]. Despite encouraging preliminary findings, the technique was regarded as cumbersome and nondefinitive in the assessment of burn depth. Black et al. assessed 59 and 37 burn sites in rats and human models, respectively, readings using a fluorometer were taken at different intervals. Actual depth of burn was judged by healing within 21 days. The results showed no significant difference of fluorescein uptake between partial and full thickness burns with large variability in both human and rat models [39].

Further research led to the discovery of indocyanine green (ICG) and its use in burns depth assessment. This was first described in 1992 by Green et al. who demonstrated the technique in a rat model [40]. They detected ICG fluorescence emission after administering intravenous ICG in partial and full thickness burns in rat skin. Different depths of burn were determined based on the intensity ratios compared to normal skin. An application of this technique in clinical practice was conducted by Still et al. in 2001 [41]. Fifteen burn wounds were assessed using the ICG method of assessment; fluorescence detected after intravenous injection of ICG correlated with the depth of burn as determined by biopsies from the burn sites and histological analysis. As expected, fluorescence was inversely related to burn depth. Cutaneous circulation and different degrees of brightness are demonstrated in the images. Another development in this field is the use of videoangiography to translate the fluorescence images into a colour-coded perfusion image indicating levels of tissue perfusion.

Despite some evidence supporting the use of ICG fluorometer, the method received criticism due to the extravasation of ICG dye in tissue which will inevitably render the method as inaccurate and yield false readings [42]. Moreover, reports of various side effects and anaphylaxis [43] and unknown safety of use in pregnant and breastfeeding women [44] has curtailed its use.

4.3.2. Spectrophotometry. Spectrophotometry relies on the principle that partial thickness burn wounds still maintain their vasculature and capillary architecture whereas in full thickness burn wounds the blood vessels are thrombosed and damaged [34]. Anselmo and Zawacki were the first to describe the use of spectrophotometry in burn depth assessment [45], and infrared light was used to distinguish patent from thrombosed vessels and hence determine burn depth.

More recently, Tehrani et al. in 2008 used a noncontact spectrophotometry scope that uses polarised light from 400 to 1000 nm wavelengths. The scope detects any remitted light yielding images showing relative concentrations of haemoglobin, melanin, and collagen in a burn wound [46]. The authors compared the use of spectrophotometric intracutaneous analysis with LDI in the assessment of burn depth. Nine patients had their burn wounds imaged with both LDI and spectrophotometric techniques.

Results obtained from both modalities in the study were comparative and encouraging. Superficial burns had increased haemoglobin concentrations and lack of melanin compared to normal skin, whereby deep dermal burns had even higher concentrations of haemoglobin and a relative increase in melanin. Deriving absolute conclusions from the study is not possible though, due to the small number of burn wounds investigated.

4.3.3. Thermography.

Thermography is based on the principle that cutaneous circulation of a burn wound and hence temperature are inversely related to the depth of a burn wound [34]. In the 1960s, devices able to record differences in surface temperatures were used in monitoring the viability of flaps [47]. This was first applied to burn depth assessment by Mladick et al. in 1966 [48] and preliminary studies investigating its use found that the surface temperature of full thickness and partial thickness wounds differ by an average of 2 degrees Celsius [49]. In 1974, Hackett used this technique in assessing more than 100 burn wounds, yielding an accuracy of 90% [50]. Critics of this technique argue that temperature of a burn wound is a compound of various variable elements: room temperature, intravenous fluid resuscitation, blood flow, anatomical area, and other factors. Critics specifically argue that evaporative cooling will also lead to overestimation of burn wounds and hence inaccurate assessment and inappropriate management [51].

In 2005 Renkielska et al. investigated the correlation between static thermography and burn depth in an animal model [52]. They investigated the difference in temperature between a burn wound and an unaffected reference area of skin. Thermography was 93.8% accurate in predicting burn wounds that will heal in 21 days compared to 62.5% accuracy in the clinical method alone, this yielded a sensitivity of 97.7% and specificity of 85.8%. In a follow-up study by the same authors in 2006, they investigated the use of active dynamic thermography in burns depth assessment in an animal model. They studied 23 burn wounds of different depths that were inflicted on pigs. Comparing the method to clinical assessment, it had an accuracy of 100% in predicting burn wounds that will heal conservatively in 21 days compared to an accuracy of 61% via clinical assessment alone [53].

Hardwicke et al. recently investigated the role of high resolution digital thermal imaging in burns depth assessment. They studied 11 patients presenting with burns of different depths. Thermographic images were recorded 42 h and 5 days after a burn. They found that full thickness burns compared to normal skin are 2.3°C colder with strong statistical significance ($P < 0.001$), deep dermal burns were also found to be 1.2°C colder ($P < 0.05$), and superficial partial thickness burns were only 0.1°C colder [54]. This technique is presented as a safe, noncontact, inexpensive, and reliable adjunct in burns depth assessment that needs further evaluation and validation in large scale studies before drawing any solid conclusions.

This method of burn depth assessment relies on the principle that the more superficial a burn wound is the more present the dermal circulation is. This method allows a clinician to obtain close-up microscopic images of the underlying tissue and enable them to assess the presence or absence of blood vessels [44]. A contact near-infrared laser is applied on areas of concern and light reflected is captured and processed allowing visualisation of tissue planes up to 350 micrometers. In 2009, Altintas et al. used this method to assess 24 patients presenting with a burn. The wounds were investigated at 12, 36, and 72 h after the onset of a burn. After microscopy the burn wounds were divided into wounds predicted to heal within 3 weeks and wounds that will not heal within that timeframe. Several factors were assessed: presence of inflammatory cells, thickness of basal layer, and blood flow. Results showed an increase in blood flow in the group of burns that healed within 3 weeks compared to the nonhealing group at the different intervals measured. Moreover the thickness of the basal layer was preserved in the healing group compared to the obliteration of the basal layer in the nonhealing group at 36 h of measurement. The preliminary study showed some important findings and paved way for further research [55].

In 2011, Mihara et al. aimed to investigate the critical time for application of reflectance-mode confocal microscopy. This was an essential question to be answered due to the dynamic nature of a burn, and validation of the critical time for measurement is essential in preventing underestimation of burn wound depth and increased patient morbidity. They studied 41 patients with 44 different burn wounds. The use of videomicroscopy was compared to clinical assessment and showed a statistically significant superiority in accuracy of burn wound depth estimation ($P = 0.001$). The accuracy of videomicroscopy was found to be highest 24 h after onset of the burn injury [56].

Further research by the same authors in 2012 was conducted to develop a classification of burn depth and reliability of videomicroscopy. Forty-four patients with 56 burn wounds were investigated and results of videomicroscopy were compared to clinical outcome. This yielded an accuracy of 93% (sensitivity 81.8% and specificity 100%) [57]. Although research has showed positive results, opponents of this technique argue that the use of microscopy is cumbersome and painful to patients as contact between the wound surface and the scope is needed. Furthermore, due to the small surface area visualised by the scope, accurate measurement will require several measurements especially due to the heterogeneous nature of burn wounds [44]. Despite the limitations of its use, it remains an important adjunct that must be honed and developed to circumvent the criticisms received by this modality.

4.3.4. Ultrasonography. Ultrasound techniques are used widely in both diagnostic and therapeutic techniques in different specialties. Goans et al. was the first to propose the notion of using ultrasound in assessing burn depth. The notion was based on the principle that ultrasound can detect the remaining dermal layer available above the subcutaneous tissue after a burn [58]. Preliminary studies in animal models showed that ultrasound techniques can be effective in determining which burn wounds will heal within 21 days and which will require excision and grafting [59, 60]. However, lack of translatable results in humans [61] coupled with limitations such as the need for contact with a burn and need for training in the interpretation of results deterred the acceptance of this modality in burn depth assessment [34].

Developments in the field of ultrasonography and the introduction of Doppler ultrasound led to further research in the field of burn depth assessment. In 2000, Seed et al. studied 78 burn wounds from 15 different patients. The noncontact Doppler ultrasound was used to visualise the different layers of skin within a burn wound: epidermis, dermis, and dermal-fat interface. Burns were deemed to be deep in nature if destruction of the dermal-fat interface is visualised. The accuracy of this method when compared to clinical outcome in the study was 96% [62]. Despite the promising findings, there is a lack of studies investigating the validity and reliability of this technique in burn depth assessment.

5. Conclusion

The need for an adjunct to clinical assessment of burn depth has instigated the development of a wide range of modalities aiming to improve our assessment of burn depth and patient care. It is clear from the discussion above that many of the other alternatives to LD techniques are either more cumbersome and more expensive or more difficult to adapt to the clinical setting resulting in LD techniques coming to the vanguard. Laser Doppler flowmetry and subsequently LDI has come to the forefront of technological adjuncts and several studies have illustrated the objective benefit of the use of LDI in conjunction with clinical assessment. The studies discussed have shown a significant improvement in prediction of burn healing and reduction of time for decision to operate when comparing LD assessment to clinical assessment only. The results indicate that the use of LD technology will reduce costs, length of stay, patient morbidity, and unnecessary surgery. Furthermore, studies with sound methodology have validated the optimal time for LD scanning.

From the available literature, it was apparent that studies did not agree on certain cut-off points of perfusion values. It is imperative for burn centres to validate the LD devices in use at their centres independently in order to find the most suitable cut-off points and levels of burn wound depth stratification.

Despite the positive results attained with the use of LDI, the studies in the literature have given rise to concerns that will need to be addressed in future technological developments and research projects. Opponents of the use of LDI

technology argue that the commercial cost of the device [44] will render it unattainable to many burn units. This must drive further cost-benefit analyses to illustrate the potential cost saving of the technology. Moreover, the topographical artefacts that occur from scanning curved areas such as on flanks and extremities have challenged developers to innovate and design methods to circumvent such obstacles. Skewing of LD assessment results due to tattoos [63], presence of infection, and patient comorbidities such as peripheral vascular disease anaemia and patient use of systemic medication that may alter blood flow [44] have been shown in the literature. However, despite the shortcomings it must be stressed that LD assessment should contribute to the entire clinical picture and should be used as an aid rather than a replacement to clinical assessment.

An important point to shed light upon is the absence of any randomised controlled trials in this field. The paucity of randomised trials and absence of level I evidence in this field of research should drive large centres to conduct randomised studies and answer the research questions that arise regarding the use of LDI technology. In conjunction with the technological developments of the LD devices due to both clinical need and commercial competition, the plethora of research indicates that the age-old difficulty in assessing burn depth is a surmountable challenge. Developments in this field will inevitably lead to an improvement in clinical ability and ultimately patient care.

References

[1] T. C. S. Cubison, S. A. Pape, and N. Parkhouse, "Evidence for the link between healing time and the development of hypertrophic scars (HTS) in paediatric burns due to scald injury," *Burns*, vol. 32, no. 8, pp. 992–999, 2006.

[2] S. Monstrey, H. Hoeksema, J. Verbelen, A. Pirayesh, and P. Blondeel, "Assessment of burn depth and burn wound healing potential," *Burns*, vol. 34, no. 6, pp. 761–769, 2008.

[3] M. D. Stern, "*In vivo* evaluation of microcirculation by coherent light scattering," *Nature*, vol. 254, no. 5495, pp. 56–58, 1975.

[4] M. Green, G. A. Holloway, and D. M. Heimbach, "Laser Doppler monitoring of microcirculatory changes in acute burn wounds," *Journal of Burn Care & Rehabilitation*, vol. 9, no. 1, pp. 57–62, 1988.

[5] T. O'Reilly, R. Spence, R. Taylor, and J. Scheulen, "Laser Doppler flowmetry evaluation of burn wound depth," *Journal of Burn Care & Rehabilitation*, vol. 10, no. 1, pp. 1–6, 1989.

[6] J. S. Chatterjee, "A critical evaluation of the clinimetrics of laser doppler as a method of burn assessment in clinical practice," *Journal of Burn Care and Research*, vol. 27, no. 2, pp. 123–130, 2006.

[7] K. Waxman, N. Lefcourt, and B. Achauer, "Heated laser doppler flow measurements to determine depth of burn injury," *The American Journal of Surgery*, vol. 157, no. 6, pp. 541–543, 1989.

[8] L. Atiles, W. Mileski, G. Purdue, J. Hunt, and C. Baxter, "Laser Doppler flowmetry in burn wounds," *Journal of Burn Care & Rehabilitation*, vol. 16, no. 4, pp. 388–393, 1995.

[9] Z. B. M. Niazi, T. J. H. Essex, R. Papini, D. Scott, N. R. McLean, and M. J. M. Black, "New laser doppler scanner, a valuable adjunct in burn depth assessment," *Burns*, vol. 19, no. 6, pp. 485–489, 1993.

[10] D.-H. Park, J.-W. Hwang, K.-S. Jang, D.-G. Han, K.-Y. Ahn, and B.-S. Baik, "Use of laser Doppler flowmetry for estimation of the depth of burns," *Plastic & Reconstructive Surgery*, vol. 101, no. 6, pp. 1516–1523, 1998.

[11] P. E. Banwell, M. P. H. Tyler, A. M. I. Watts, A. H. N Roberts, and D. A. McGrouther, "Burn depth estimation: use of laser Doppler flowmetry," *Plastic & Reconstructive Surgery*, vol. 103, no. 1, pp. 334–335, 1999.

[12] S. A. Pape, C. A. Skouras, and P. O. Byrne, "An audit of the use of laser Doppler imaging (LDI) in the assessment of burns of intermediate depth," *Burns*, vol. 27, no. 3, pp. 233–239, 2001.

[13] F. W. H. Kloppenberg, G. I. J. M. Beerthuizen, and H. J. ten Duis, "Perfusion of burn wounds assessed by Laser Doppler Imaging is related to burn depth and healing time," *Burns*, vol. 27, no. 4, pp. 359–363, 2001.

[14] A. J. A. Holland, H. C. O. Martin, and D. T. Cass, "Laser Doppler imaging prediction of burn wound outcome in children," *Burns*, vol. 28, no. 1, pp. 11–17, 2002.

[15] J. C. Jeng, A. Bridgeman, L. Shivnan et al., "Laser Doppler imaging determines need for excision and grafting in advance of clinical judgment: a prospective blinded trial," *Burns*, vol. 29, no. 7, pp. 665–670, 2003.

[16] W. J. Mileski, L. Atiles, G. Purdue et al., "Serial measurements increase the accuracy of laser Doppler assessment of burn wounds," *Journal of Burn Care & Rehabilitation*, vol. 24, no. 4, pp. 187–191, 2003.

[17] C. L. Riordan, M. McDonough, J. M. Davidson et al., "Non-contact laser Doppler imaging in burn depth analysis of the extremities," *Journal of Burn Care & Rehabilitation*, vol. 24, no. 4, pp. 177–186, 2003.

[18] E. R. La Hei, A. J. A. Holland, and H. C. O. Martin, "Laser Doppler Imaging of paediatric burns: burn wound outcome can be predicted independent of clinical examination," *Burns*, vol. 32, no. 5, pp. 550–553, 2006.

[19] D. J. McGill, K. Sørensen, I. R. MacKay, I. Taggart, and S. B. Watson, "Assessment of burn depth: a prospective, blinded comparison of laser Doppler imaging and videomicroscopy," *Burns*, vol. 33, no. 7, pp. 833–842, 2007.

[20] H. Hoeksema, K. van de Sijpe, T. Tondu et al., "Accuracy of early burn depth assessment by laser Doppler imaging on different days post burn," *Burns*, vol. 35, no. 1, pp. 36–45, 2009.

[21] J. K. Cho, D. J. Moon, S. G. Kim, H. G. Lee, S. P. Chung, and C. J. Yoon, "Relationship between healing time and mean perfusion units of laser Doppler imaging (LDI) in pediatric burns," *Burns*, vol. 35, no. 6, pp. 818–823, 2009.

[22] J. Mill, L. Cuttle, D. G. Harkin, O. Kravchuk, and R. M. Kimble, "Laser Doppler imaging in a paediatric burns population," *Burns*, vol. 35, no. 6, pp. 824–831, 2009.

[23] L. H. C. Kim, D. Ward, L. Lam, and A. J. A. Holland, "The impact of laser doppler imaging on time to grafting decisions in pediatric burns," *Journal of Burn Care and Research*, vol. 31, no. 2, pp. 328–332, 2010.

[24] K. M. Merz, M. Pfau, G. Blumenstock, M. Tenenhaus, H. E. Schaller, and H. O. Rennekampff, "Cutaneous microcirculatory assessment of the burn wound is associated with depth of injury and predicts healing time," *Burns*, vol. 36, no. 4, pp. 477–482, 2010.

[25] K. Nguyen, D. Ward, L. Lam, and A. J. A. Holland, "Laser Doppler Imaging prediction of burn wound outcome in children: is it possible before 48 h?" *Burns*, vol. 36, no. 6, pp. 793–798, 2010.

[26] F. Lindahl, E. Tesselaar, and F. Sjöberg, "Assessing paediatric scald injuries using laser speckle contrast imaging," *Burns*, vol. 39, no. 4, pp. 662–666, 2013.

[27] S. Menon, D. Ward, J. G. Harvey, E. L. Hei, and A. J. A. Holland, "Friction burns in children: does laser doppler imaging have a role?" *Journal of Burn Care and Research*, vol. 33, no. 6, pp. 736–740, 2012.

[28] S. A. Pape, R. D. Baker, D. Wilson et al., "Burn wound healing time assessed by laser Doppler imaging (LDI). Part 1: derivation of a dedicated colour code for image interpretation," *Burns*, vol. 38, no. 2, pp. 187–194, 2012.

[29] Y. S. Park, Y. H. Choi, H. S. Lee et al., "The impact of laser Doppler imaging on the early decision-making process for surgical intervention in adults with indeterminate burns," *Burns*, vol. 39, no. 4, pp. 655–661, 2013.

[30] T. L. Stewart, B. Ball, P. J. Schembri et al., "The use of laser doppler imaging as a predictor of burn depth and hypertrophic scar postburn injury," *Journal of Burn Care and Research*, vol. 33, no. 6, pp. 764–771, 2012.

[31] K. Lang and L. Boyd, "The use of Fluorescein to determine the adequacy of ciculation," *Medical Clinics of North America*, vol. 26, article 943, 1942.

[32] J. Dingwall, "A clinical test for differentiating second from third degree burns," *Annals of Surgery*, vol. 118, no. 3, pp. 427–429, 1943.

[33] D. M. Jackson, "The diagnosis of the depth of burning," *British Journal of Surgery*, vol. 40, no. 164, pp. 588–596, 1953.

[34] A. D. Jaskille, J. W. Shupp, M. H. Jordan, and J. C. Jeng, "Critical review of burn depth assessment techniques: Part I. historical review," *Journal of Burn Care and Research*, vol. 30, no. 6, pp. 937–947, 2009.

[35] D. G. Silverman, D. D. LaRossa, C. H. Barlow, T. G. Bering, L. M. Popky, and T. C. Smith, "Quantification of tissue fluorescein delivery and prediction of flap viability with the fiberoptic dermofluorometer," *Plastic and Reconstructive Surgery*, vol. 66, no. 4, pp. 545–553, 1980.

[36] B. H. Graham, R. L. Walton, V. B. Elings, and F. R. Lewis, "Surface quantification of injected fluorescein as a predictor of flap viability," *Plastic and Reconstructive Surgery*, vol. 71, no. 6, pp. 826–833, 1983.

[37] J. C. Denneny III, R. A. Weisman, and D. G. Silverman, "Monitoring free flap perfusion by serial fluorometry," *Otolaryngology: Head and Neck Surgery*, vol. 91, no. 4, pp. 372–376, 1983.

[38] J. E. Gatti, D. LaRossa, D. G. Silverman, and C. E. Hartford, "Evaluation of the burn wound with perfusion fluorometry," *Journal of Trauma*, vol. 23, no. 3, pp. 202–206, 1983.

[39] K. S. Black, C. W. Hewitt, D. M. Miller et al., "Burn depth evaluation with fluorometry: Is it really definitive?" *Journal of Burn Care & Rehabilitation*, vol. 7, no. 4, pp. 313–317, 1986.

[40] H. A. Green, D. Bua, R. R. Anderson, and N. S. Nishioka, "Burn depth estimation using indocyanine green fluorescence," *Archives of Dermatology*, vol. 128, no. 1, pp. 43–49, 1992.

[41] J. M. Still, E. J. Law, K. G. Klavuhn, T. C. Island, and J. Z. Holtz, "Diagnosis of burn depth using laser-induced indocyanine

green fluorescence: a preliminary clinical trial," *Burns*, vol. 27, no. 4, pp. 364–371, 2001.

[42] H. Ishihara, N. Otomo, A. Suzuki, K. Takamura, T. Tsubo, and A. Matsuki, "Detection of capillary protein leakage by glucose and indocyanine green dilutions during the early post-burn period," *Burns*, vol. 24, no. 6, pp. 525–531, 1998.

[43] R. Benya, J. Quintana, and B. Brundage, "Adverse reactions to indocyanine green: a case report and a review of the literature," *Catheterization and Cardiovascular Diagnosis*, vol. 17, no. 4, pp. 231–233, 1989.

[44] M. Kaiser, A. Yafi, M. Cinat, B. Choi, and A. J. Durkin, "Noninvasive assessment of burn wound severity using optical technology: a review of current and future modalities," *Burns*, vol. 37, no. 3, pp. 377–386, 2011.

[45] V. Anselmo and B. Zawacki, "Infrared photography as a diagnostic tool for the burn ward," *Proceeding Society of Photo-Optical Instrumentation Engineers*, vol. 8, p. 181, 1973.

[46] H. Tehrani, M. Moncrieff, B. Philp, and P. Dziewulski, "Spectrophotometric intracutaneous analysis: a novel imaging technique in the assessment of acute burn depth," *Annals of Plastic Surgery*, vol. 61, no. 4, pp. 437–440, 2008.

[47] F. L. Thorne, N. G. Georgiade, and R. Mladick, "The use of thermography in determining viability of pedicle flaps," *Archives of Surgery*, vol. 99, no. 1, pp. 97–99, 1969.

[48] R. Mladick, N. Georgiade, and F. Thorne, "A clinical evaluation of the use of thermography in determining degree of burn injury," *Plastic and Reconstructive Surgery*, vol. 38, no. 6, pp. 512–518, 1966.

[49] A. C. Watson and C. Vasilescu, "Thermography in plastic surgery." *Journal of the Royal College of Surgeons of Edinburgh*, vol. 17, no. 4, pp. 247–252, 1972.

[50] M. E. J. Hackett, "The use of thermography in the assessment of depth of burn and blood supply of flaps, with preliminary reports on its use in Dupuytren's contracture and treatment of varicose ulcers," *British Journal of Plastic Surgery*, vol. 27, no. 4, pp. 311–317, 1974.

[51] V. J. Anselmo and B. E. Zawacki, "Effect of evaporative surface cooling on thermographic assessment of burn depth," *Radiology*, vol. 123, no. 2, pp. 331–332, 1977.

[52] A. Renkielska, A. Nowakowski, M. Kaczmarek et al., "Static thermography revisited—an adjunct method for determining the depth of the burn injury," *Burns*, vol. 31, no. 6, pp. 768–775, 2005.

[53] A. Renkielska, A. Nowakowski, M. Kaczmarek, and J. Ruminski, "Burn depths evaluation based on active dynamic IR thermal imaging-A preliminary study," *Burns*, vol. 32, no. 7, pp. 867–875, 2006.

[54] J. Hardwicke, R. Thomson, A. Bamford, and N. Moiemen, "A pilot evaluation study of high resolution digital thermal imaging in the assessment of burn depth," *Burns*, vol. 39, no. 1, pp. 76–81, 2013.

[55] A. A. Altintas, M. Guggenheim, M. A. Altintas, P. Amini, T. Stasch, and G. Spilker, "To heal or not to heal: predictive value of in vivo reflectance-mode confocal microscopy in assessing healing course of human burn wounds," *Journal of Burn Care and Research*, vol. 30, no. 6, pp. 1007–1012, 2009.

[56] K. Mihara, H. Shindo, M. Ohtani et al., "Early depth assessment of local burns by videomicroscopy: 24 h after injury is a critical time point," *Burns*, vol. 37, no. 6, pp. 986–993, 2011.

[57] K. Mihara, H. Shindo, H. Mihara, M. Ohtani, K. Nagasaki, and N. Katoh, "Early depth assessment of local burns by

videomicroscopy: a novel proposed classification." *Burns*, vol. 38, no. 3, pp. 371–377, 2012.

[58] R. E. Goans, J. H. Cantrell Jr., and F. B. Meyers, "Ultrasonic pulse echo determination of thermal injury in deep dermal burns," *Medical Physics*, vol. 4, no. 3, pp. 259–263, 1977.

[59] A. Kalus, J. Aindow, and M. Caulfield, "Application of ultrasound in assessing burn depth," *The Lancet*, vol. 414, pp. 188–189, 1979.

[60] J. H. Cantrell Jr., "Can ultrasound assist an experienced surgeon in estimating burn depth?" *Journal of Trauma*, vol. 24, no. 9, pp. S64–S70, 1984.

[61] T. L. Wachtel, G. R. Leopold, H. A. Frank, and D. H. Frank, "B-mode ultrasonic echo determination of depth of thermal injury," *Burns*, vol. 12, no. 6, pp. 432–437, 1986.

[62] S. Iraniha, M. E. Cinat, V. M. VanderKam et al., "Determination of burn depth with noncontact ultrasonography," *Journal of Burn Care and Rehabilitation*, vol. 21, no. 4, pp. 333–338, 2000.

[63] D. J. McGill and I. Taggart, "Tattoos: a confounding issue in laser Doppler imaging of burn depth," *Burns*, vol. 31, no. 5, pp. 657–659, 2005.

31

The Effect of Different Topical Agents (Silver Sulfadiazine, Povidone-Iodine, and Sodium Chloride 0.9%) on Burn Injuries in Rats

Emir Burak Yüksel,[1] Alpagan Mustafa Yıldırım,[2] Ali Bal,[3] and Tuncay Kuloglu[4]

[1] *Department of Plastic, Reconstructive & Esthetic Surgery, Elbistan State Hospital, Kahramanmaras, Turkey*
[2] *Department of Plastic, Reconstructive & Esthetic Surgery, Afyon Kocatepe University, Afyon, Turkey*
[3] *Department of Plastic, Reconstructive & Esthetic Surgery, Malatya State Hospital, Malatya, Turkey*
[4] *Department of Histology & Embryology, Firat University, Elazıg, Turkey*

Correspondence should be addressed to Ali Bal; alibal69@hotmail.com

Academic Editor: Nicolo Scuderi

It was aimed to comparatively evaluate the effects of dressing methods with silver sulfadiazine, povidone-iodine, and saline which have a common use in routine practices for burn injuries. Twenty-eight Sprague Dawley adult female rats were used in this study. All the rats were divided into 4 groups: the control group, the povidone-iodine group, the saline group, and the silver sulfadiazine group. On each rat, a second degree burn which covered less than 10% of the body surface area was created under general anesthesia by a metal comb including four probes with 2×1 cm area. The control group did not have any treatment during the experiment. Povidone-iodine, saline, and silver sulfadiazine administrations were performed under ether anesthesia every day. On 0, 7th, 14th, and 21st days of the study, tissue samples were taken for histological analyses. The sections taken from the paraffin blocks were stained and avidin-biotin-peroxidase method was used for collagen immune-reactivity. In the light microscope analyses, number of inflammatory cells, vascularization, fibroblast proliferation, collagen formation and epithelialization were evaluated histologically in all groups and analysed statistically. The agents that we used for injury healing in the treatment groups did not show any significant better results in comparison with the control group. In conclusion, further studies with the use of sodium chloride, silver sulfadiazine, and povidone-iodine by creating deeper and/or larger burn injury models are needed in order to accept these agents in routine treatment.

1. Introduction

Many types of medications have been used for burn injuries so far [1]. The common characteristics of these medications are that they all have antimicrobial effects. There are many studies conducted on the effects of these medications, which demonstrates that they insert their effects through various mechanisms. In this study, the effects of the most frequently used medications, that is, the silver sulfadiazine cream, antiseptic solution povidone-iodine, and 0.9% NaCl serum physiologic on the process of healing of the burn injuries, have been compared and examined [2–4].

2. Material and Method

Twenty-eight female adult Sprague-Dawley rats obtained from Firat University Experimental Researches Center (FÜDAM) have been used in the study.

The rats were separated into 4 groups each one consisting of 7 rats: the control group, 10% povidone-iodine group, 0.9% sodium chloride (Sf) group, and 1% silver sulfadiazine group. In all groups, second degree burns were induced on the shaved backs of the rats by pressing 4 metal plates (2×1 cm) after being kept in boiling water for 30 seconds. The metal plates were kept for 10 seconds on the backs of the rats, and

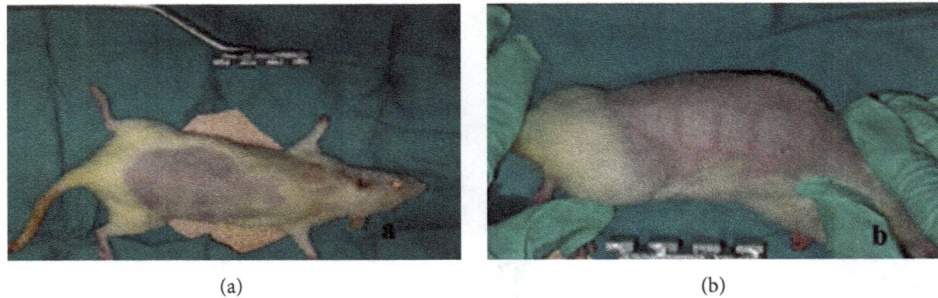

(a)

(b)

FIGURE 1: (a) The shaved view of the rats before the burn injury (b) and the view after the burn injury.

the burns did not exceed 10% of the body surfaces (Figures 1 and 2). 2 mg/kg paracetamol was added to their drinking water as analgesic. In the control group, the burn injury was covered with sterile gauze bandage in day 0, after the burn injury was performed. No treatments were applied during the experiment. Only the medical dressing was changed during the days of biopsy.

In the "10% povidone-iodine" group, 10% povidone-iodine was applied to the burn injury every day under ether aesthesia. The injury area was covered with sterile gauze bandage and this process continued for 21 days.

In the "1% silver sulfadiazine" group, silver sulfadiazine was applied to the burn injury every day under ether aesthesia. The injury area was covered with sterile gauze bandage and this process continued for 21 days.

In the "0.9% sodium chloride" group, the injury area was moisturized with serum physiologic twice everyday under ether aesthesia, and the injury area was covered with sterile gauze bandage, and this process continued for 21 days.

On the 0, 7th, and 21st day of the experiment, tissue samples were taken under anesthesia from predetermined areas from all subjects in all groups.

Histological study: the tissue samples taken from each group were stained with Hematoxylin-eosin (H&E) and Masson trichrome and assessed in light microscopy. For the assessment of the recovery with immunohistochemical study, the collagen I immune-reactivity was performed using the avidin-biotin-peroxidase complex method.

2.1. Statistical Analysis. The histological assessment results were analysed with one sample Kolmogorov-Smirnov test. Since the groups showed normal distribution, the parametric statistics methods were used for the analysis of the data. The one-way ANOVA test was applied, and the Bonferroni test was used for the post hoc comparisons. The value $P < 0.05$ was accepted as statistically significant. The SPSS 12.0 statistical package program was used for the analysis of the data.

3. Findings

In the light microscopy examinations of control group, it was observed on day 0 that there were no significant changes in

fibroblast proliferation, collagen formation, vascularization, epithelisation, and inflammatory cell density. On the other hand, it was observed that the epidermis layer was damaged due to the burn injury (Figures 2(a1), 3(a1), and 4(a1)). On the 7th day of the control group, severe inflammatory cell increase was observed, and in some subjects a slight increase in fibroblast proliferation, vascularization, and epithelisation was observed (Figures 2(b1), 3(b1), and 4(b1)). On the 14th day of the control group, a decrease was observed in the inflammatory cell density; and the fibroblast proliferation, vascularization, and collagen formation were obvious. Moreover, the epithelisation level was detected at medium level (Figures 2(c1), 3(c1), and 4(c1)). On the 21st day of control group, a decrease in the vascularization and an increase in inflammatory cell number were determined and the epithelisation, fibroblast proliferation, and collagen formation were observed (Figures 2(d1), 3(d1), and 4(d1)).

On day 0 of the 10% povidone-iodine group no changes were observed in fibroblast proliferation, collagen formation, vascularization, epithelisation, and inflammatory cell density; and the epidermis layer was observed to be severely damaged (Figures 2(a2), 3(a2), and 4(a2)). On the 7th day of the 10% povidone-iodine group, severe inflammatory cell infiltration was observed, and in some subjects, a slight increase was observed in fibroblast proliferation, vascularization, and epithelisation (Figures 2(b2), 3(b2), and 4(b2)). On the 14th day of the 10% povidone-iodine group, a decrease was observed in the inflammatory cell infiltration, and the fibroblast proliferation, vascularization, and collagen formation were obvious. The epithelisation was detected at medium level (Figures 2(c2), 3(c2), and 4(c2)). On the 21st day of the 10% povidone-iodine group, a decrease was observed in vascularization and inflammatory cell infiltration, and the epithelisation, fibroblast proliferation, and collagen formation were observed as severe (Figures 2(d2), 3(d2), and 4(d2)). No significant difference was observed between the treatment groups and control group.

On day 0 of the 1% silver sulfadiazine group, no difference was observed in fibroblast proliferation, collagen formation, vascularization, epithelisation, and inflammatory cell infiltration, and the epidermis layer was observed as damaged due to the burn injury (Figures 2(a3), 3(a3), and 4(a3)). On the 7th day of the 1% silver sulfadiazine group, a severe inflammatory cell infiltration was observed, and in some subjects a

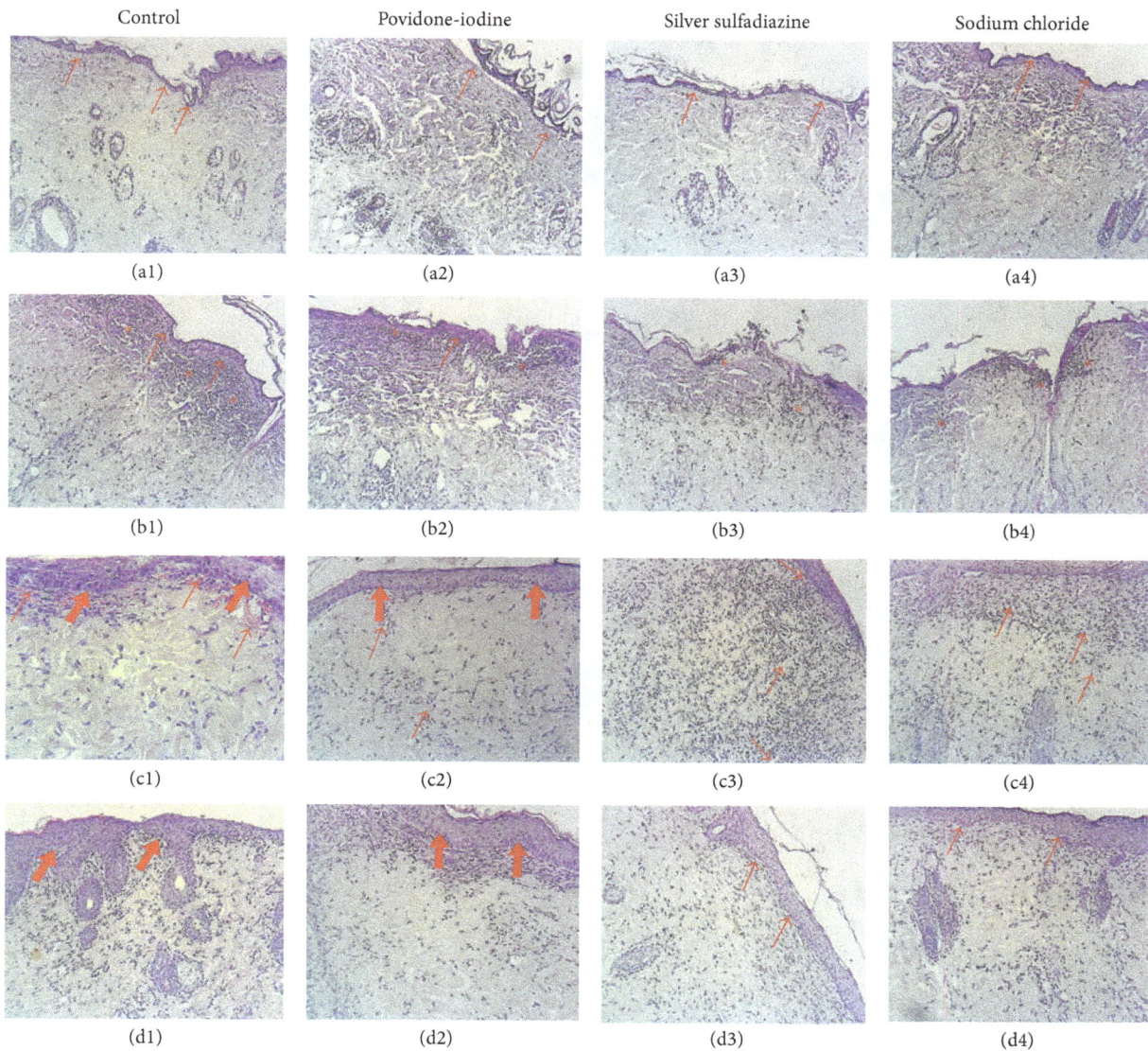

FIGURE 2: Day 0 ((a1), (a2), (a3), and (a4)), day 7 ((b1), (b2), (b3), and (b4)), day 14 ((c1), (c2), (c3), and (c4)), and day 21 ((d1), (d2), (d3), and (d4)) of hematoxylin and eosin staining. The arrows in (a1), (a2), (a3), and (a4) show the epidermis damage. The arrows in (b1), (b2), (b3), and (b4) show slight epithelisation, the star (∗) shows inflammatory cell infiltration. The thin arrows in (c1), (c2), (c3), and (c4) (→) show the vascularization; the thick arrows show the epithelisation. The thick arrows in (d1), (d2), (d3), and (d4) show the epithelisation. (×100).

slight increase in fibroblast proliferation, vascularization, and epithelisation occurred (Figures 2(b3), 3(b3), and 4(b3)). On the 14th day of the 1% silver sulfadiazine group, a decrease was observed in inflammatory cell infiltration and the fibroblast proliferation, vascularization, and collagen formation were obvious. The epithelisation was detected at medium degree (Figures 2(c3), 3(c3), and 4(c3)). On the 21st day of the 1% silver sulfadiazine group, a decrease in vascularization and inflammatory cell infiltration was observed, and severe fibroblast proliferation and collagen formation were observed (Figures 2(d3), 3(d3), and 4(d3)). No significant difference was observed between the treatment groups and control group.

On day 0 of the 0.9% sodium chloride group, no changes were observed in fibroblast proliferation, collagen formation,

vascularization, epithelisation, and inflammatory cell infiltration, and the epidermis layer was observed as damaged due to the burn injury (Figures 2(a4), 3(a4), and 4(a4)). On the 7th day of the 0.9% sodium chloride group, a severe inflammatory cell infiltration was observed and in some subjects there were slight increases in fibroblast proliferation, vascularization, and epithelisation (Figures 2(b4), 3(b4), and 4(b4)). On the 14th day of the 0.9% sodium chloride group, there was a decrease in the inflammatory cell increase, and the fibroblast proliferation, vascularization, and collagen formation were obvious. The epithelisation was detected at medium degree (Figures 2(c4), 3(c4), and 4(c4)). On the 21st day of the 0.9% sodium chloride group, a decrease was observed in vascularization and inflammatory cell infiltration, and there were severe epithelisation, fibroblast proliferation, and

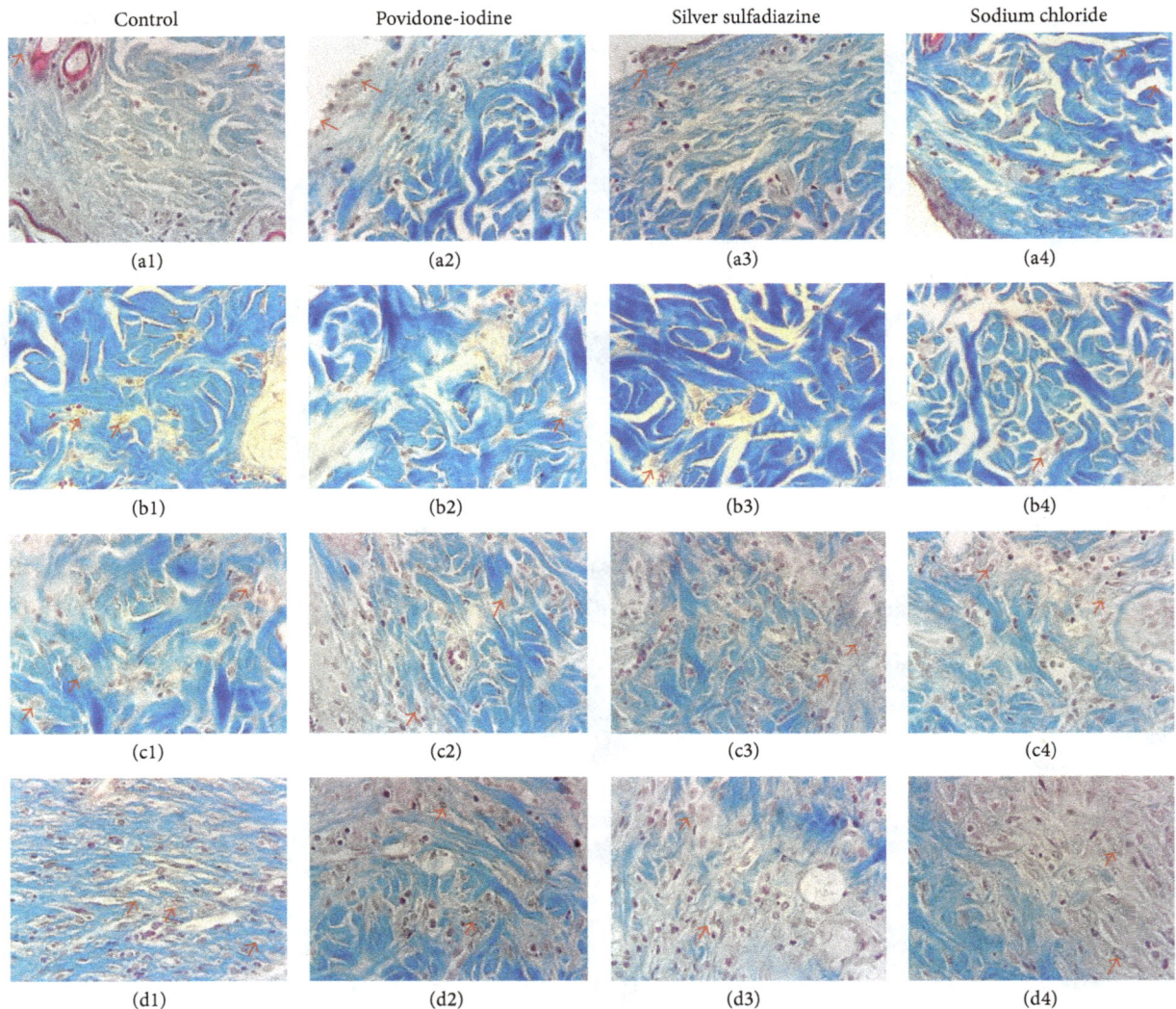

Control	Povidone-iodine	Silver sulfadiazine	Sodium chloride
(a1)	(a2)	(a3)	(a4)
(b1)	(b2)	(b3)	(b4)
(c1)	(c2)	(c3)	(c4)
(d1)	(d2)	(d3)	(d4)

FIGURE 3: Day 0 ((a1), (a2), (a3), and (a4)), day 7 ((b1), (b2), (b3), and (b4)), day 14 ((c1), (c2), (c3), and (c4)), and day 21 ((d1), (d2), (d3), and (d4)) of Masson trichrome staining. The arrows in (a1), (a2), (a3), and (a4) (→) show epidermis damage. The arrows in (b1), (b2), (b3), and (b4) show the fibroblasts which are few in number. The arrows in (c1), (c2), (c3), and (c4) (→) show a clear fibroblast increase and collagen formation. The arrows in (d1), (d2), (d3), and (d4) show a severe fibroblast increase and collagen formation. (×400).

collagen formation (Figures 2(d4), 3(d4), and 4(d4)). No significant difference was observed between the treatment groups and control group.

4. Discussion

Different surface agents are used in burn injury treatments. The basic purpose is to speed the epithelial healing up and to choose the methods that will prevent the formation of a scar in a wise manner [5]. The method in topical burn injury treatments depends on the depth of the injury and on the treatment targets [6].

While growth hormones and cytokines considerably support the healing of burn wound, suppressor hormones affect the healing of burn wound negatively [7–11]. Therefore, growth hormones, cytokines, and also pharmacological agents that influence receptors of target tissue positively are used for effective treatment of wound healing [12].

Maghsoudi et al. [13] have suggested the use of silver in wound healing, since it has antimicrobial effects on wound infections; silver has negative effects on wound healing though.

Povidone-iodine plays an indirect role in wound healing through controlling the infection. But it is disputable in the cases where iodine is absorbed excessively, which may cause systemic complications. Use of iodine is suggested only in the cases where iodine absorption is limited [14, 15].

Khorasani et al. [16] conducted a study in which they formed an experimental burn injury and showed that the use of saffron gives better results when compared with the use of silver sulfadiazine.

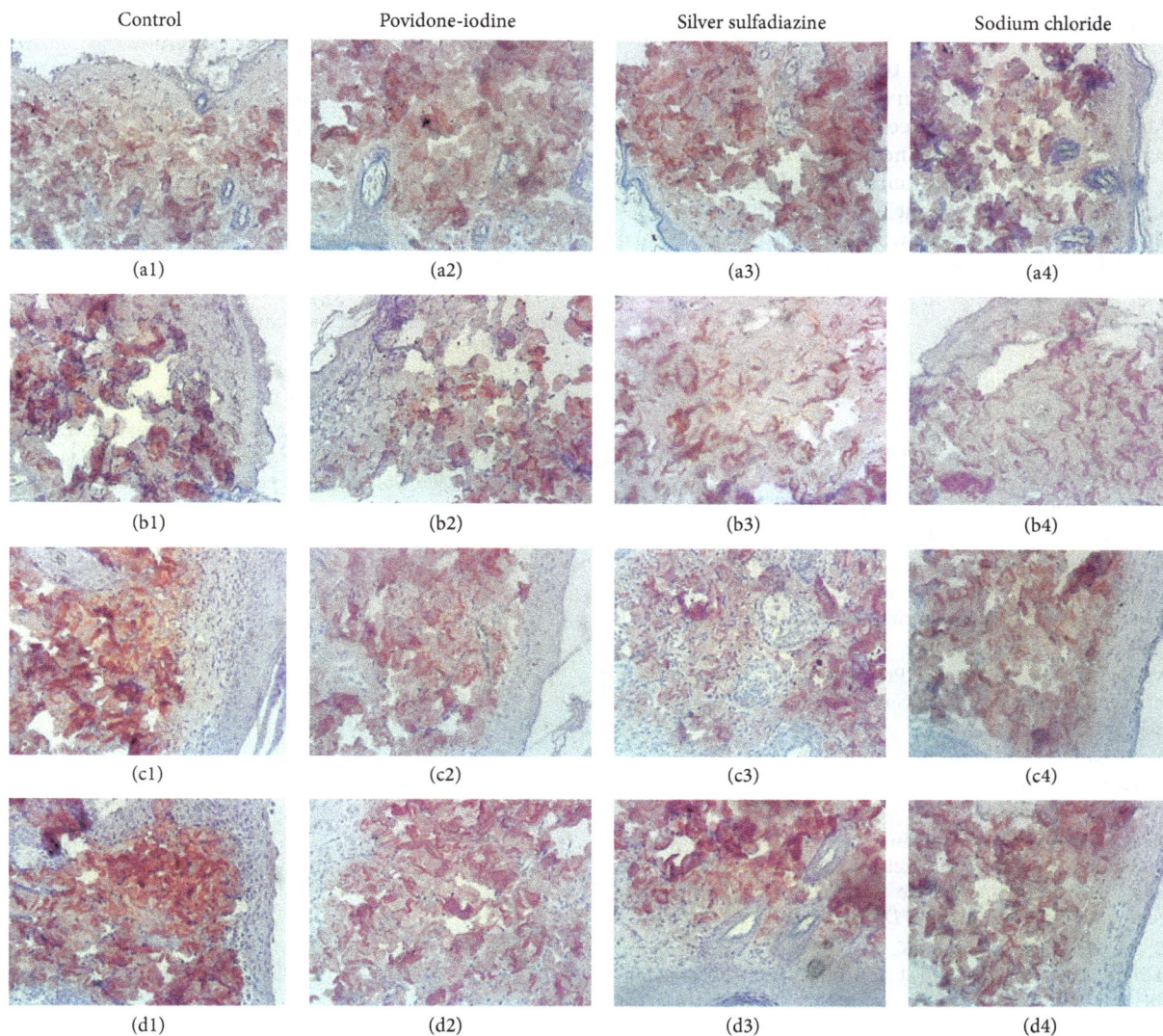

FIGURE 4: Day 0 ((a1), (a2), (a3), and (a4)), day 7 ((b1), (b2), (b3), and (b4)), day 14 ((c1), (c2), (c3), and (c4)), and day 21 ((d1), (d2), (d3), and (d4)) of type I collagen immune-reactivity (×200).

In the study conducted by Eski et al., they performed experimental burn injuries and compared the use of cerium nitrate and saline. They showed that the systemic increase in neutrophil, indicating that the inflammation did not change in the group receiving saline and decreased in the group receiving cerium nitrate [17].

In the study by Sezer et al., they performed experimental burn injuries and performed the assessment of the use of fucoidan-containing pharmaceutical agents in burn injuries treatment. They examined the fibroblast proliferation, inflammatory cell infiltration, epithelisation, and collagen increase in the burn injuries which were similar to those of our study on the 7th, 14th, and 21st days of their experiments. They showed that the inflammatory cell increase was severe on the 7th day and that the fibroblast and collagen increase was at maximum levels on the 14th and 21st days [18].

In our study we compared the effects of the sulfadiazine cream, antiseptic solution povidone-iodine, and 0.9% NaCl serum physiologic on the recovery process of the burn injuries. This comparison was not performed before. In the study we performed second degree burns and determined that there was inflammatory cell infiltration on the 7th day; vascularization, fibroblast proliferation, and collagen increase on the 14th day; and fibroblast proliferation on the 21st day. We also determined that there were no statistically significant differences between the groups in which the collagen increase was the highest.

No statistically significant differences were determined between the healing effects of the agents used in treatment groups in this study. The finding that there are no differences might be related with the depth and/or width of the burn injury or there might not be any differences between the treatment groups in fact.

5. Conclusion

In the current study, although these agents have different mechanisms of action, it has been determined that there were no significant differences between the effects of the silver sulfadiazine, povidone-iodine, and sodium chloride 0.9% on healing process of 2nd degree burns. The determination of this effect according to the model created in this study does not mean that the same effect will occur in different burn injury models, and it might be deduced that generally there will not be a clear difference in 2nd degree burns.

References

[1] G. Majo, *The Healing Hand*, Harvard University Press, Cambridge, Mass, USA, 1973.

[2] K. Yorgancı and Ö. Z. Yanıklar, *Temel Cerrahi*, Edited by I. Sayek, Güneş Kitabevi, Ankara, Turkey, 3rd edition, 2004.

[3] Y. Noda, K. Fujii, and S. Fujii, "Critical evaluation of cadexomer-iodine ointment and povidone-iodine sugar ointment," *International Journal of Pharmaceutics*, vol. 372, no. 1-2, pp. 85–90, 2009.

[4] E. M. Bulger and R. V. Maier, "Prehospital Care of the injured: what's new," *Surgical Clinics of North America*, vol. 87, no. 1, pp. 37–53, 2007.

[5] J. W. Richard III, B. A. Spencer, L. F. McCoy et al., "Acticoat versus Silverlon: the truth," *Journal of Burns and Surgical Wound Care*, vol. 1, p. 11, 2002.

[6] O. Çetinkale, O. Çizmeci, F. Ayan, C. Şenyuva, S. Büyükdevrim, and A. Pusane, "Early wound excision and skin grafting restores cellular immunity after severe burn trauma," *Türk Plastik, Rekonstrüktif ve Estetik Cerrahi Derneği*, vol. 1, pp. 1–5, 1993.

[7] B. S. Atiyeh, C. A. Al-Amm, K. A. El-Musa, A. Sawwaf, and R. Dham, "The effect of moist and moist exposed dressings on healing and barrier function restoration of partial thickness wounds," *European Journal of Plastic Surgery*, vol. 26, no. 1, pp. 5–11, 2003.

[8] B. S. Atiyeh, K. A. El-Musa, and R. Dham, "Scar quality and physiologic barrier function restoration after moist and moist-exposed dressings of partial-thickness wounds," *Dermatologic Surgery*, vol. 29, no. 1, pp. 14–20, 2003.

[9] K. Breuing, E. Eriksson, P. Liu, and D. R. Miller, "Healing of partial thickness porcine skin wounds in a liquid environment," *Journal of Surgical Research*, vol. 52, no. 1, pp. 50–58, 1992.

[10] A. J. Tonks, R. A. Cooper, K. P. Jones, S. Blair, J. Parton, and A. Tonks, "Honey stimulates inflammatory cytokine production from monocytes," *Cytokine*, vol. 21, no. 5, pp. 242–247, 2003.

[11] H. Mani, G. S. Sidhu, A. K. Singh et al., "Enhancement of wound healing by shikonin analogue 93/637 in normal and impaired healing," *Skin Pharmacology and Physiology*, vol. 17, no. 1, pp. 49–56, 2004.

[12] A. Jurjus, B. S. Atiyeh, I. M. Abdallah et al., "Pharmacological modulation of wound healing in experimental burns," *Burns*, vol. 33, no. 7, pp. 892–907, 2007.

[13] M. Maghsoudi, N. Nezami, and M. Mirzajanzaden, "Enhancement of burn wounds healing by platelet dressing," *International Journal of Burns and Trauma*, vol. 3, pp. 96–101, 2013.

[14] M. Steen, "Review of the use of povidone-iodine (PVP-I) in the treatment of burns," *Postgraduate Medical Journal*, vol. 69, supplement 3, pp. S84–S92, 1993.

[15] P. M. Vogt, J. Hauser, O. Robbach et al., "Polyvinyl pyrrolidone-iodine liposome hydrogel improves epithelialization by combining moisture and antisepsis. A new concept in wound therapy," *Wound Repair and Regeneration*, vol. 9, no. 2, pp. 116–122, 2001.

[16] G. Khorasani, S. J. Hosseinimehr, P. Zamani, M. Ghasemi, and A. Ahmadi, "The effect of saffron (*Crocus sativus*) extract for healing of second-degree burn wounds in rats," *Keio Journal of Medicine*, vol. 57, no. 4, pp. 190–195, 2008.

[17] M. Eski, F. Ozer, C. Firat et al., "Cerium nitrate treatment prevents progressive tissue necrosis in the zone of stasis following burn," *Burns*, vol. 38, no. 2, pp. 283–289, 2012.

[18] A. D. Sezer, E. Cevher, F. Hatipoğlu, Z. Oğurtan, A. L. Baş, and J. Akbuğa, "Preparation of fucoidan-chitosan hydrogel and its application as burn healing accelerator on rabbits," *Biological and Pharmaceutical Bulletin*, vol. 31, no. 12, pp. 2326–2333, 2008.

32

Implementing the Brazilian Database on Orofacial Clefts

Isabella Lopes Monlleó,[1,2] **Marshall Ítalo Barros Fontes,**[1]
Erlane Marques Ribeiro,[3] **Josiane de Souza,**[4] **Gabriela Ferraz Leal,**[5] **Têmis Maria Félix,**[6]
Agnes Cristina Fett-Conte,[7] **Bruna Henrique Bueno,**[8] **Luis Alberto Magna,**[8]
Peter Anthony Mossey,[9] **and Vera Gil-da Silva-Lopes**[8]

[1] *Medical Genetics Sector, State University of Alagoas (UNCISAL), Brazil*
[2] *Clinical Genetics Service, Federal University of Alagoas (UFAL), Brazil*
[3] *Medical Genetics Sector, Hospital Infantil Albert Sabin (HIAS), Brazil*
[4] *Medical Genetics Sector, Assistance Center for Cleft Lip and Palate (CAIF), Brazil*
[5] *Medical Genetics Sector, Facial Deformity Care Center (CADEFI), Brazil*
[6] *Medical Genetics Service, Hospital de Clínicas de Porto Alegre (HCPA), Brazil*
[7] *Molecular Biology Department, Medicine School of São José do Rio Preto (FAMERP/FUNFARME), Brazil*
[8] *Department of Medical Genetics, Faculty of Medical Sciences, University of Campinas, 13083-887, Brazil*
[9] *Dundee University Dental School, UK*

Correspondence should be addressed to Vera Gil-da Silva-Lopes; vlopes@fcm.unicamp.br

Academic Editor: Renato Da Silva Freitas

Background. High-quality clinical and genetic descriptions are crucial to improve knowledge of orofacial clefts and support specific healthcare polices. The objective of this study is to discuss the potential and perspectives of the Brazilian Database on Orofacial Clefts. *Methods.* From 2008 to 2010, clinical and familial information on 370 subjects was collected by geneticists in eight different services. Data was centrally processed using an international system for case classification and coding. *Results.* Cleft lip with cleft palate amounted to 198 (53.5%), cleft palate to 99 (26.8%), and cleft lip to 73 (19.7%) cases. Parental consanguinity was present in 5.7% and familial history of cleft was present in 26.3% subjects. Rate of associated major plus minor defects was 48% and syndromic cases amounted to 25% of the samples. *Conclusions.* Overall results corroborate the literature. Adopted tools are user friendly and could be incorporated into routine patient care. The BDOC exemplifies a network for clinical and genetic research. The data may be useful to develop and improve personalized treatment, family planning, and healthcare policies. This experience should be of interest for geneticists, laboratory-based researchers, and clinicians entrusted with OC worldwide.

1. Introduction

Accurate and detailed phenotype description of orofacial clefts (OC) is crucial to produce good etiological and epidemiological studies. In this regard, attention should be given to subphenotypic features of the lip (completeness of the cleft, presence of pits/prints, dental and orbicularis oris muscle anomalies), and palate (completeness of the cleft, submucous defects, bifid uvula, and ankyloglossia). Similarly important is the screening of minor and major associated defects which has prevalence rate that ranges from 8% to 75%. Although

there are true population differences, methodological factors such as sample source and size, method of ascertainment, case definitions, inclusion criteria, coding system, and case classification account for much of this wide variation [1–13].

In the postgenomic era capturing and processing information on human genetic variation, gene-environment interactions, and genotype-phenotype correlations are essential to develop personalized interventions. This has been reinforced by the Human Variome Project (HVP), an international effort launched in 2006. The HVP aim is to develop and make knowledge housed within linked databases on genes, mutations, and variants accessible to the research and medical communities [14, 15].

Databases may also serve as tools in educating health professionals, policymakers, and the general public towards prevention of unnecessary suffering, improvement of health-care, and elimination of erroneous beliefs that still remain in some cultures. On humanitarian and ethical grounds, these should be ultimate reasons for birth defects research [16–19].

Recognizing the impact of OC, the World Health Organization assigned the coordination of the International Perinatal Database of Typical Orofacial Clefts (IPDTOC) to the International Clearinghouse for Birth Defects Surveillance and Research (ICBDSR), in 2002 [18–20].

As stated in the report *Global Registry and Database on Craniofacial Anomalies* [18], the quality of recorded data should be of more concern than completeness of ascertainment in this kind of system. The IPDTOC was launched in 2003 and has collected and analysed case-by-case clinical and epidemiological information OC from birth defects registries worldwide using a standard definition and system for case classification [12].

Care for people with OC in Brazil has been funded by the government through the Unified Health System (Sistema Único de Saúde, SUS) since 1993. In 1998, the National Health Ministry (NHM) created the Brazilian Reference Network for Craniofacial Treatment (RRTDCF). These measures, however, were not preceded or followed by assessment of specific characteristics and impact of OC on the Brazilian population. Currently the RRTDCF numbers 21 units, but just five of them count with geneticist/dysmorphologist in the team [17, 21, 22].

Brazil is a continental country of more than 180 million inhabitants with diverse genetic background and multicultural profile. There is still a shortfall in epidemiological data on overall birth defects in the country. Similar to other parts of the world, data recorded through birth certificates has been criticized on the grounds of ascertainment, sensitivity, reliability, completeness, and consistence of the reports [23–25].

According to the Latin-American Collaborative Study of Congenital Malformations (ECLAMC), the Brazil's birth prevalence of cleft lip (CL) is 49/10,000, cleft lip with cleft palate (CLP) is 116/10,000, and cleft palate (CP) is 58/10,000 [26]. ECLAMC is a hospital-based register which covers only 2% of all Brazilian births [25]. Despite this limitation, the high quality of ECLAMC's data and the fact that OC are among the best ascertained birth defects probably make these figures representative of Brazil's prevalence.

Besides ECLAMC, some cleft services and hospitals linked or not to the RRTDCF record data according to their research field of interest. Therefore, they may include epidemiological, morbidity, mortality, clinical, genetic, and outcome issues. Information gathered, however, is not standardized [17].

High quality of clinical and genetic descriptions is crucial to improve knowledge on OC and support specific healthcare polices. The development and implementation of the Brazilian Database on Orofacial Clefts (BDOC) reported here is a pioneer nationwide initiative to fill in the gap on clinical and genetic information on OC in the Brazilian population.

2. Aim

The aims of this study are to report the implementation, to describe preliminary clinical and familial characteristics and to discuss the potential, and perspectives of the BDOC.

3. Methods

3.1. Database Design. BDOC is a nationwide, hospital-based, voluntary and primary database. Initially, a 10-year schedule was planned to run as a continuous and flexible system in which new aims and tools can be aggregated according to the experience gained. General planning of activities started in 2006 and the validation of the tools started in 2008 in voluntary hospitals with clinical geneticists. According to the strategy originally proposed, after this phase, other hospitals without geneticists could be invited to participate. Clinical and laboratory data are updated during the follow-up of each subject. The database was approved by the local Institutional Review Boards and the National Research Ethics Committee (CONEP # 14733). All subjects provided informed consent.

Standardized individual and familial information forms the core database. It is complemented by other five satellite protocols designed to cover the following issues: (1) genetic (Biobank of DNA); (2) morbidity and mortality; (3) services' structure and dynamics; (4) professionals' education characteristics and protocols; and (5) subject/parent satisfaction.

Core database was initiated in eight sites comprising three units of the RRTDCF, two multiprofessional non-RRTDCF centres, and three genetic services. These sites were invited because they all have geneticists with clinical experience in dysmorphology. All of them were personally visited by the coordinators (ILM and VLGSL) before starting the collection of data.

3.2. Target Population, Inclusion Criteria, and Work Definitions. Individuals with typical OC and Pierre-Robin sequence in isolated and nonisolated presentation were included. Data on abortuses, stillbirths, cleft uvula, median, oblique, and submucous clefts were not included.

Typical OC (CL, CLP, and CP) and Pierre-Robin sequence were defined according to the International Classification of Diseases 10th Edition. Terms *isolated* and *associated* were used to refer to additional minor or major defects regardless of the cause or mechanism involved while *syndromic* and *nonsyndromic*, to refer to the underlying aetiology [13].

Case classification was based on the definitions of the IPDTOC Working Group (2011) which defines three phenotype categories: isolated clefts, recognized syndrome, and multimalformed cases (MMC). Accordingly, cases of known nonrandom association (e.g., VACTERL) are included into the category of recognized syndromes. Cases with random combination of major unrelated defects with evidence of distinct aetiological factors are included in the group of MMC. Deformities were considered minor defects [12]. A list of minor defects was reviewed along with ICBDSR in May 2007 and is available at http://www.icbdsr.org/.

TABLE 1: Distribution of subjects according to participant site, geographic origin, age, and birth weight.

	RRTDCF	Multidisciplinary non-RRTDCF	Genetic service	Total
Number of cases n (%)	141 (38)	107 (29)	122 (33)	370 (100)
Geographic origin				
Northeast n (%)	62 (44)	86 (80)	86 (70)	234 (63.2)
South n (%)	79 (56)	21 (20)	—	100 (27)
Southeast n (%)	—	—	36 (30)	36 (9.7)
Age (years, mean)[#]	2.7	1.5	8.5	4.3*
Birth weight (grams, mean)[†]	3,057	3,152	2,932	3,055**

[#]Mann-Whitney test: RRTDCF × non-RRTDCF, $P = 0.049$; RRTDCF × genetic services, $P < 0.0001$; non-RRTDCF × genetic services, $P < 0.001$; *Kruskal-Wallis test, $P = .000$; [†]LSD test: RRTDCF × non-RRTDCF, $P = 0.230$; RRTDCF × genetic services, $P = 0.136$; non-RRTDCF × genetic services, $P = 0.014$; **ANOVA, $P = 0.047$.

3.3. Collection, Storage, and Processing of Data.

Data were collected using a paper-based record form specifically designed for this database according to the operating manual. These tools were based on the "US National Birth Defects Prevention Study" and ESF "common core protocols" for cleft research and developed as part of a previous study [27].

The record form comprises 80 questions which cover the following information: (1) obstetric, birth, neonatal, and medical history; (2) socioeconomic status; (3) family history where possible (1st-, 2nd-, and 3rd-degree relatives); (3) type of cleft according to topography (lip, alveolus, hard, and soft palate), severity (unilateral or bilateral) and laterality (left and right sided), (4) morphological assessment (including verbatim description of dysmorphic features); (5) laboratory tests (standard cytogenetics, fluorescence in situ hybridization— FISH) and/or molecular analysis, biochemical tests, ultrasound, X-ray images, and so forth; and (5) diagnosis and its evidences.

Operating manual includes the following content: (1) diagram for phenotype categorization, (2) operating definitions, (3) clinical descriptors, (4) list of related defects, (5) list of minor defects, (6) examples of twinning, (7) examples of toxic and occupation-related substances, (8) examples of consanguineous relationships, (9) instructions for taking standard photographs, and (10) examples on how to fill the form.

All subjects were personally interviewed and examined by the participant geneticist during routine genetic evaluation from November 2008 to December 2010. As the major proposal of this database is to collect clinical and familial information, there were no restrictions regarding age and existence of previous cleft surgery at the time of enrolment.

Forms were sent by post or delivered in person for data reviewing and coding at Unicamp where the BDOC is seeded. The data manager checked all the information received and sought for clarifications when needed. Before entering data into the electronic database, all record forms were manually reviewed and coded by the coordinators.

3.4. Pretest of the BDOC Tools and Strategy for Group Management.

Record form and operating manual were pretested by seven geneticists throughout a six-month period. A total of 143 record forms and 10 assessment questionnaires were included. Mean time spent to complete the record form at the end of this phase was 20 minutes (SD = 4.57) [28].

All geneticists asked for revision of wording, spacing, and ordering of some questions. Coordinator centre asked for further information and clarification of some responses in 28 record forms. Despite this, record form and operating manual were assessed as useful and reliable tools [28].

At the end of this phase a unit of the RRTDCF ceased its participation and, a new site, a genetic service, was included. All participants attended biannual meetings to exchange experience, discuss data, and plan the next stages.

3.5. Statistical Methods.

The electronic database was built using Microsoft Access version 2007. Data processing and analysis were performed using two statistical packages (SPSS for Windows version 15.0 and EpiInfo versions 3.5.1 and 3.04d). Categorical variables were analysed using chi-square test. Numerical variables were tested for normality using one-sample Kolmogorov-Smirnov test. Variables with normal distribution were tested using ANOVA and Student's t-test, while variables with nonnormal distribution were tested using Kruskal-Wallis and Mann-Whitney tests. The significance level of 5% ($P < 0.05$) was adopted for all tests.

4. Results

Demographic, clinical, and familial information of 370 individuals with OC was prospective and systematically recorded in the sites identified in Figure 1. As only minor amendments were recommended after the testing phase, respective record forms were included into the sample. Figure 2 summarizes how the BDOC worked throughout the studied period.

Majority of subjects (63.2%) were living in the northeast of Brazil. Males amounted to 219 (59.2%) while females to 151 (40.8%). Birth weight was available in 324 cases. It ranged from 1195 g to 4900 g (mean = 3100; mode = 2800; median = 3100; and SD = 606.6). Age ranged from 0 to 50 years (mean = 4.3; mode = 0; median = 0.5; and SD = 7.3).

Table 1 shows the distribution of patients according to participant site, geographic origin, age, and birth weight at the time of enrolment in the database. Ratio of patients seen at units of the RRTDCF, cleft multidisciplinary non-RRTDCF centres, and genetic services was 1.3 : 1.0 : 1.1. Patients seen at genetic services were significantly older ($P < 0.001$) and had lower birth weight ($P = 0.047$) than those seen elsewhere.

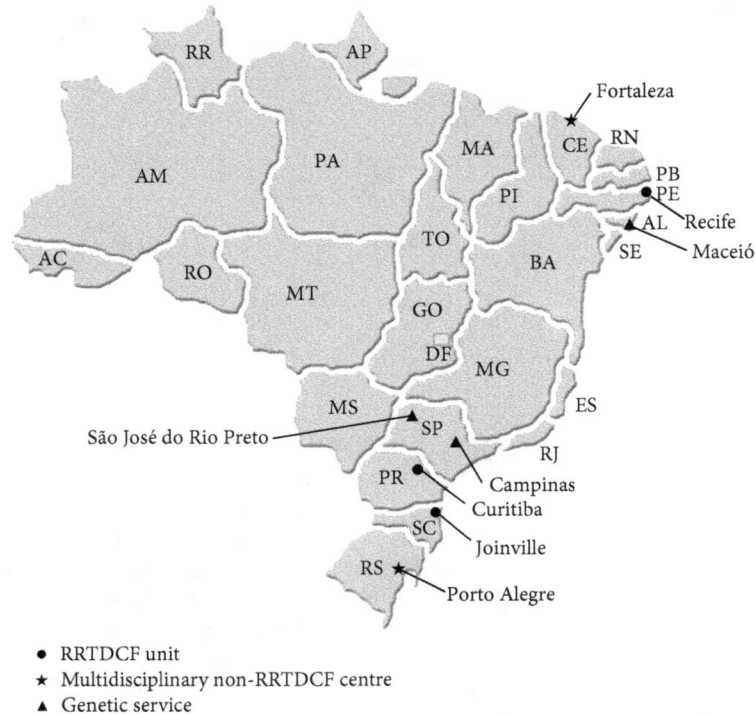

FIGURE 1: Map of Brazil showing localization of cities and sites participating in the Brazilian database on orofacial clefts (BDOC).

TABLE 2: Distribution of subjects according to type of clefts with regard to gender, cleft's severity and laterality, and presence of additional defects.

Variable	CLP	CL	CP	Total	$P^{\#}$
Number of cases (%)	198 (53.5)	73 (19.7)	99 (26.8)	370 (100)	
Gender					0.0001
Male	137 (69)	39 (53)	43 (43)	219 (59)	
Female	61 (31)	34 (47)	56 (57)	151 (41)	
Severity					0.0002
Unilateral	120 (60)	62 (85)	—	182 (67)	
Bilateral	78 (40)	11 (15)	—	89 (33)	
Laterality					0.0001
Unilateral left	85 (70)	41 (66)	—	126 (69)	
Unilateral right	35 (30)	21 (34)	—	56 (31)	
Additional minor defects					0.193
Yes	87 (44)	26 (36)	49 (49)	162 (44)	
No	111 (56)	47 (64)	50 (51)	208 (56)	
Additional major defects					0.003
Yes	41 (21)	6 (8)	29 (29)	76 (21)	
No	157 (79)	67 (92)	70 (71)	294 (79)	

$^{\#}$Chi square.

Distribution of subjects according to type of cleft (CL, CLP, and CP) with regard to gender, severity, laterality, and presence of additional defects is shown in Table 2. CLP prevailed over CP and CL, unilateral over bilateral, and left-over right-sided clefts.

Chi-squared contingency table revealed significant differences among all groups of clefts. There was an excess of males among individuals with CLP + CL (male : female ratio = 1.85, $P = 0.0001$) and of females among those with CP (female : male ratio = 1.30, $P = 0.0001$). Bilateral clefts were

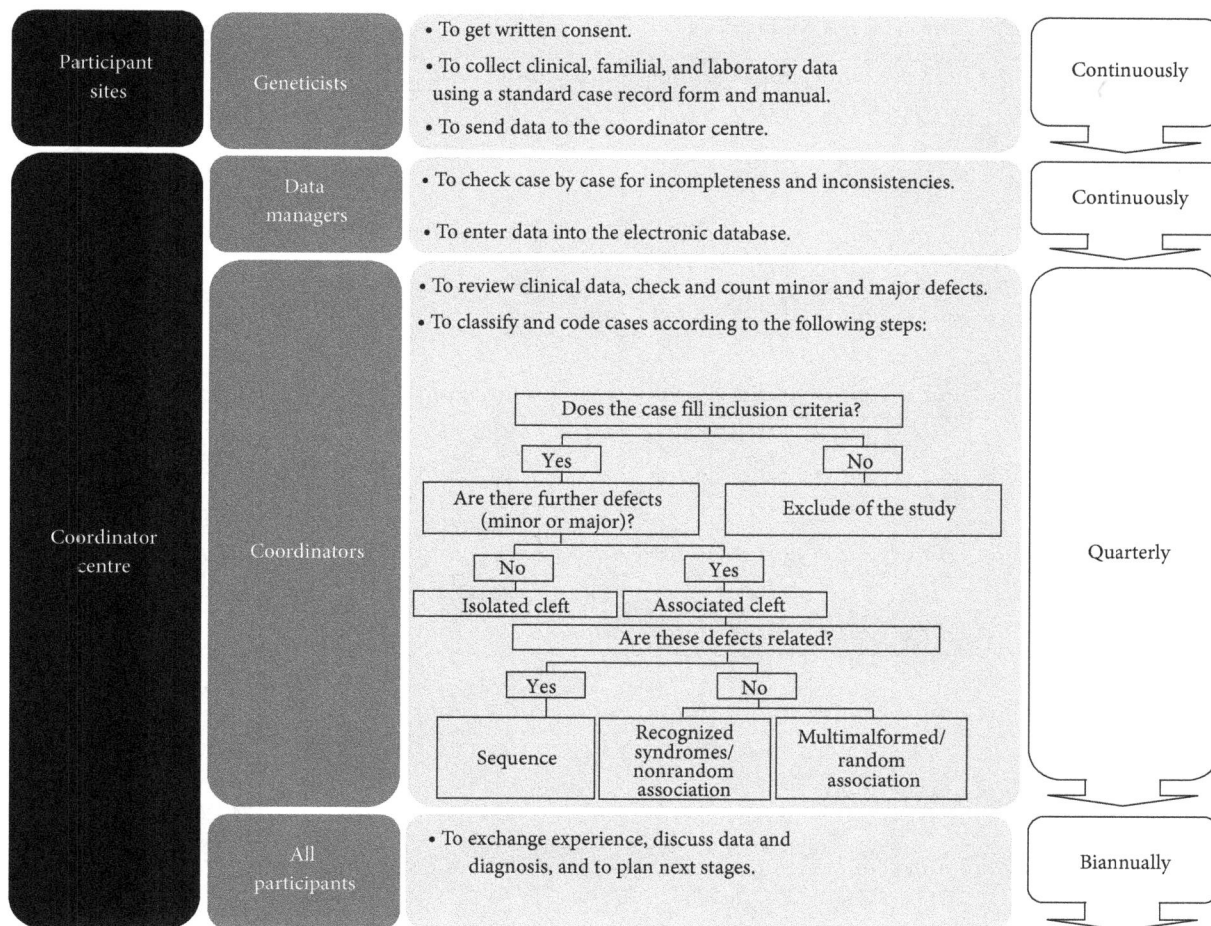

FIGURE 2: A summary of the process of recording cases through the Brazilian database on orofacial clefts (BDOC). Please refer to text for details.

more frequent for subjects with CLP than for those with CL ($P = 0.0002$).

Parental consanguinity was present in 21/368 (5.7%) cases, 10 of which were first cousins. Consanguineous marriages were not statistically associated with geographic origin ($P = 0.425$), type of cleft ($P = 0.451$), and phenotype category (i.e., if isolated versus syndromes and MMC) ($P = 0.381$).

Excluding 12 individuals from whom familial data were not available, familial history of cleft was found in 94/358 (26.3%) cases. First-degree relatives were affected in 18 (19.4%), second degree in 12 (12.9%), and third degree and above in 63 (67.7%) families. There was an excess of affected relatives in the CLP subgroup in comparison with CP ($P = 0.005$) but not with CL ($P = 0.183$).

Global rate of associated defects (minor plus major) was 179 (48.4%). Fifty-nine (15.9%) subjects showed both minor and major, 103 (27.8%) had only minor and 17 (4.6%) had only major-associated defects. As shown in Table 2, there was no statistically significant difference among subgroups of cleft with regard to rate of minor defects ($P = 0.193$). On the other hand, major defects were more likely to be found in the groups of CLP and CP and unlikely in the group of CL ($P = 0.003$).

Ninety-three (25%) subjects were classified as having syndromic clefts. Comparisons between nonsyndromic and syndromic cases are presented in Table 3. There were no statistically significant differences between these groups with regard to gender and severity of the cleft.

Syndromic cases were more likely to be found at genetic services ($P = 0.006$) and statistically more associated with CP ($P = 0.000$). These cases also showed lower birth weight in both categorical ($P = 0.001$) and quantitative analyses ($P = 0.000$) and higher mean of *minor* defects ($P = 0.000$).

Subjects were regrouped according to the number of minor defects into two categories (1–3 and ≥ 4 defects). There was a predominance of syndromic cases in the subgroup with four and above *minor* defects ($P = 0.000$). Anatomic distribution of *minor* and *major* defects is shown in Figures 3 and 4, respectively.

Based on verbatim description, the following phenotype categories were identified: 277 (75%) isolated clefts, 47 (12%) recognized syndromes or associations, and 46 (13%) multiple

TABLE 3: Distribution of syndromic and nonsyndromic cases according to several variables.

Variables	Nonsyndromic	Syndromic	Total	$P^{\#}$
Number of cases (%)	277 (75)	93 (25)	370 (100)	
Category of site				0.006
RRTDCF unit	111 (40)	30 (33)	141 (38)	
Non-RRTDCF centre	87 (31)	20 (21)	107 (29)	
Genetic services	79 (29)	43 (46)	122 (33)	
Gender				0.324
Male	168 (61)	51 (55)	219 (59)	
Female	109 (39)	42 (45)	151 (41)	
Birth weight (grams)				
≤2500	27 (11)	22 (26)	49 (21)	0.001
>2500	212 (89)	63 (74)	275 (79)	
Mean	3,145	2,800	3,055	0.000
Type of cleft				0.000
CLP	152 (55)	46 (49)	198 (53)	
CL	65 (23)	8 (9)	73 (20)	
CP	60 (22)	39 (42)	99 (27)	
Severity				0.167
Unilateral	150 (69)	32 (59)	182 (67)	
Bilateral	67 (31)	22 (41)	89 (33)	
Minor defects				0.000
0	192 (69)	16 (17)	208 (56)	
1–3	57 (21)	31 (34)	88 (24)	0.141
≥4	28 (10)	46 (49)	74 (20)	0.000
Mean	2.97	5.09	3.98	.000
Major defects (OC excluded)				
0	277 (100)	19 (20)	296 (80)	—
1–3	—	69 (74)	69 (19)	—
≥4	—	5 (6)	5 (1)	—
Mean	—	1.59	—	—
Phenotype category				
Isolated cleft	277 (100)	—	277 (75)	—
Syndrome and association	—	47 (51)	47 (13)	—
Multimalformed case	—	46 (49)	46 (12)	—

$^{\#}$Chi square.

malformed cases (Table 3). Eighteen (40%) individuals with recognized syndromes had not additional *major* defects.

The 47 clinical recognized syndromes and associations were categorized according to aetiology. Mendelian syndromes were in the lead (n = 21; 45%), followed by chromosomal (n = 18; 38%), heterogeneous (n = 6; 13%), and teratogenic categories (n = 2; 4%).

5. Discussion

The BDOC was designed to gather detailed, high-quality, and continuing updated information on clinical and familial characteristics of OC in the Brazilian population. This is crucial to set a solid basis for future genotype-phenotype studies in which accuracy and consistency of the collected data are issues of much concern than level of ascertainment [18, 19].

In this study, information was prospectively collected by experienced geneticists during their ordinary activities. Data was recorded and processed following a standard method and a strictly defined protocol.

The database was regularly updated with new clinical or laboratory data of patients registered. If on one hand these are strengths of our database, on the other hand they make the process of record taking lengthy. Moreover, complementary investigation and genetic tests are not equally available in different regions of Brazil. These issues have direct implications on the number of cases we are able to record and follow per year and should be borne in mind when interpreting our results.

More than 84.3% of the Brazilian population lives in the three regions from which our data were collected. Among them, southeast is the most densely inhabited area followed by northeast and south [29]. These regions host 17 out of 21

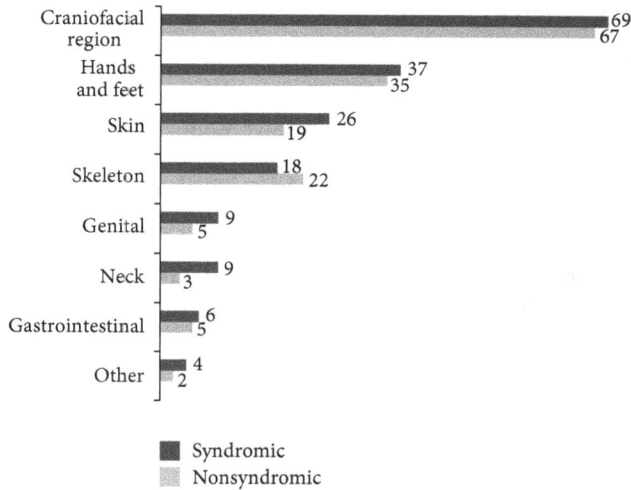

FIGURE 3: Distribution of minor defects according to anatomic region between nonsyndromic and syndromic cases.

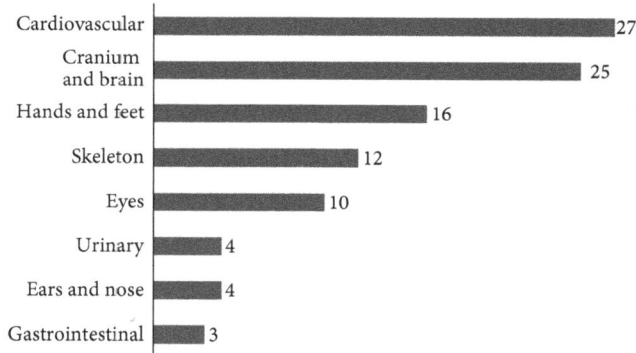

FIGURE 4: Distribution of major defects according to anatomic region among syndromic cases.

units of the RRTDCF, 18 out of 22 multidisciplinary non-RRTDCF sites [17], and 47 out of 56 clinical genetic services [30] of the country.

Subjects of this study were predominantly from northeast, followed by south and southeast. This result does not reflect differential prevalence of OC but specificities of the participant sites. Southeast region is represented by two genetic services in which individuals attend with various birth defects, OC included. South is represented by three sites specifically dedicated to cleft care (two RRTDCF units plus a multidisciplinary non-RRTDCF site). The northeast region counts with a site of each category of service (genetic, RRTDCF, and multidisciplinary non-RRTDCF). The genetic service from the last-mentioned region was conducting a parallel study on OC which justifies its high amount of subjects [31]. Taking these specificities into account, participant sites were proportionally represented in the study.

Study design allowed a wide range of subjects' age at enrolment. Younger individuals were preferentially seen in

multidisciplinary non-RRTDCF and RRTDCF sites. Subjects enrolled at genetic units were among the oldest, suggesting that the subjects primarily refer to surgery treatment instead of genetic evaluation. In addition, previous studies [22, 31] have showed that there is high level of inequality to access genetic evaluation and counselling in Brazil.

The overall results on type of cleft, gender ratio differences, severity (unilateral and bilateral) and laterality (left and right sided) of the lip defects corroborate the literature [2, 11, 13, 32, 33].

Prevalence of consanguinity in this sample was higher than that reported for the Brazilian population [34–36] and did not show preferential geographic distribution. It has been suggested that there is a greater genetic component in the aetiology of CL based on the observation of an excess of individuals with CL over CLP in the offspring of consanguineous parents [37]. We did not find statistically significant association between type of cleft and parental consanguinity. This result, however, should be confirmed in the future using a larger sample.

In the present study, more than one in four subjects showed family history of OC and almost one in five had an affected individual among their first degree relatives. In this subgroup, CLP was the most prevalent followed by CL and CP. A population-based study conducted in Denmark showed that anatomical severity does have an effect on recurrence in first-degree relatives and the type of cleft is predictive of the recurrence type. Third-degree relatives also have an increased recurrence risk compared to the background population [38].

In our sample, global rate of associated defects was around 48% and predominated among subjects with CP. Minor defects were more prevalent in craniofacial region, while cardiovascular and central nervous systems were mainly and almost equally affected by major defects. One out of four individuals was assigned as a syndromic case. Proportion of syndromic cases was higher among individuals with CP and lower among those with CL.

Methodological differences regarding case definition, inclusion or exclusion of minor defects, and anomalies/syndromes grouping-system hinder comparisons with many published data. Despite this, our results on global rate of associated defects and anatomic regions involved are similar to those reported by previous studies [9, 13, 32].

Among more than 20 investigated genes, IRF6, VAX1, and 8q24 locus have a confirmed role in nonsyndromic OC. Environmental factors, lifestyle, and the preventive role of vitamin supplements have been also investigated. Maternal smoking during pregnancy is consistently linked with increased risk of OC. Findings on the other risk factors and gene-environment interactions, including folic acid, have been inconclusive due to methodological issues [1–4, 39]. Besides these factors, a meta-analysis approach showed that parents of 40 years or older have higher probability of having a child with OC [40].

Despite important advances in the understanding of nonsyndromic OC, around 50% of patients with syndromic pictures remain as cases of multiple congenital anomalies without an identifiable aetiological factor. Laboratory facilities have improved the rate of specific diagnosis so that more than 600 syndromes involving OC have been already recognized. Chromosomal aberrations are the most frequent aetiological group, followed by Mendelian/heterogeneous abnormalities and teratogenic factors [8, 13, 32, 41, 42].

Numeric and structural chromosomal abnormalities, including 22q11 deletion, were detected in 13 cases. Mendelian, heterogeneous, and teratogenic conditions were diagnosed on the basis of clinical evidences.

Limited laboratory facilities are challengeable and the Brazilian database may be helpful to define which tests are critical to our population. Collaboration to make these tests available into the network would be economically advantageous. This is an important strategy for healthcare planning [15, 43–45].

As knowledge of genetics and of gene-environment interaction in the aetiology of OC improves, clinical genetics is becoming increasingly important specialty to ensure accurate diagnosis and allow appropriate genetic counselling [3]. Therefore, clinical genetic approach improves accuracy, consistency, and reliability of clinical descriptions and aetiological assessment which are critical to genotype-phenotype correlations. Understanding these imbricate mechanisms using modern technologies is important to improve therapy and prevention.

The process of interpreting clinical data to determine whether an individual has the defect of interest as syndromic or nonsyndromic defect is complex and involves some degree of subjectivity [4, 46]. Methods and terminology should be as well-defined as possible in order to make process uniform. In this regard, adoption of a stepwise approach is much advantageous [4].

The experience reported here shows how a group of geneticists has developed, implemented, and maintained a network suitable for clinical and genetic research on OC. Strengths of this study are that (1) information is prospectively collected by geneticists experienced in dysmorphology following a standard method and strictly defined protocol; (2) data is centrally storage and processed following a defined stepwise approach which uses IPDTOC/ICBDMS definitions, descriptors, and code system; (3) case record form and operating manual are user-friendly tools and may be incorporated in the routine in other cleft centres, these tools are available to interested researchers through contact with the Cranio-Face Brazil Project (cranface@fcm.unicamp.br); (4) experience gained throughout the process is shared among participants in face-to-face biannual meetings which improve enthusiasm and cohesiveness of the group.

Approaches with new technologies such as Genome Wide Association Studies (GWAS) and open array using accurate clinical data probably would bring interesting results to improve knowledge on the aetiology of OC. Besides research applications, information gathered in the BDOC may be useful to develop and improve personalized treatment, family planning, and public health policies on clinical and laboratory genetic investigation. This should be of interest not only for geneticists and laboratory-based scientists but also—and perhaps especially—for policymakers and clinicians entrusted with OC worldwide.

Acknowledgments

The authors thank Professor Pierpaolo Mastroiacovo, Director of the International Clearinghouse for Birth Defects Surveillance and Research (ICBDSR), Rome, Italy, Professor Eduardo Enrique Castilla, Director of the Estudio Colaborativo Latinoamericano de Malformaciones Congénitas (ECLAMC), Professor John Clark, Lead Clinician of the National Managed Clinical Network for Cleft Service in Scotland (CleftSis), for their expert opinion on the design of the BDOC, Romulo Mombach, Clinical Geneticist, for his collaboration during the test stage of the BDOC, and Mailme de Souza Oliveira and Renata Barbosa, Cranio-Face Brazil Project grantees, for technical assistance. This study was supported by Coordenação de Aperfeiçoamento de Pessoal de Nível Superior (CAPES no. 2854/06-6); Conselho Nacional de Desenvolvimento Científico e Tecnológico (CNPq nos. 408820/2006-3, 502438/2010-0, and 471422/2011-8); Fundação de Amparo a Pesquisa do Estado de Alagoas (FAPEAL no. 809 60030-700/2009), Fundação de Amparo à Pesquisa do Estado de São Paulo (FAPESP nos. 2008/50421-4 and 2008/09657-4; 2009/08756-1). V. G. Silva-Lopes is supported by CNPq 304455/2012-1.

References

[1] M. J. Dixon, M. L. Marazita, T. H. Beaty, and J. C. Murray, "Cleft lip and palate: understanding genetic and environmental influences," *Nature Reviews Genetics*, vol. 12, no. 3, pp. 167–178, 2011.

[2] P. A. Mossey, J. Little, R. G. Munger, M. J. Dixon, and W. C. Shaw, "Cleft lip and palate," *The Lancet*, vol. 374, no. 9703, pp. 1773–1785, 2009.

[3] P. A. Mossey, W. C. Shaw, R. G. Munger, J. C. Murray, J. Murthy, and J. Little, "Global oral health inequalities: challenges in the prevention and management of orofacial clefts and potential solutions," *Advances in Dental Research*, vol. 23, pp. 247–248, 2011.

[4] A. J. M. Luijsterburg and C. Vermeij-Keers, "Ten years recording common oral clefts with a new descriptive system," *The Cleft Palate-Craniofacial Journal*, vol. 48, no. 2, pp. 173–182, 2011.

[5] R. J. Shprintzen, V. L. Siegel-Sadewitz, J. Amato, and R. B. Goldberg, "Anomalies associated with cleft lip, cleft palate, or both," *American Journal of Medical Genetics*, vol. 20, no. 4, pp. 585–595, 1985.

[6] J. Milerad, O. Larson, C. Hagberg, and M. Ideberg, "Associated malformations in infants with cleft lip and palate: a prospective, population-based study," *Pediatrics*, vol. 100, no. 2, pp. 180–186, 1997.

[7] L. A. Croen, G. M. Shaw, C. R. Wasserman, and M. M. Tolarova, "Racial and ethnic variations in the prevalence of orofacial clefts in California, 1983–1992," *American Journal of Medical Genetics*, vol. 79, pp. 42–47, 1998.

[8] M. M. Tolarova and J. Cervenka, "Classification and Birth prevalence of orofacial clefts," *American Journal of Medical Genetics*, vol. 75, pp. 126–137, 1998.

[9] S. Beriaghi, S. Myers, S. Jensen, S. Kaimal, C. Chan, and G. B. Schaefer, "Cleft lip and palate: association with other congenital malformations," *Journal of Clinical Pediatric Dentistry*, vol. 33, no. 3, pp. 207–210, 2009.

[10] D. F. Wyszynski, A. Sárközi, and A. E. Czeizel, "Oral clefts with associated anomalies: methodological issues," *The Cleft Palate-Craniofacial Journal*, vol. 43, no. 1, pp. 1–6, 2006.

[11] A. E. Genisca, J. L. Frías, C. S. Broussard et al., "Orofacial clefts in the national birth defects prevention study, 1997–2004," *American Journal of Medical Genetics A*, vol. 149, no. 6, pp. 1149–1158, 2009.

[12] P. Mastroiacovo, A. Maraschini, E. Leoncini et al., "Prevalence at birth of cleft lip with or without cleft palate: data from the International Perinatal Database of Typical Oral Clefts (IPDTOC)," *The Cleft Palate-Craniofacial Journal*, vol. 48, no. 1, pp. 66–81, 2011.

[13] M. Rittler, V. Cosentino, J. S. López-Camelo, J. C. Murray, G. Wehby, and E. E. Castilla, "Associated anomalies among infants with oral clefts at birth and during a 1-year follow-up," *American Journal of Medical Genetics A*, vol. 155, no. 7, pp. 1588–1596, 2011.

[14] J. Kaput, R. G. Cotton, L. Hardman et al., "Planning the human variome project. The spain report," *Human Mutation*, vol. 30, pp. 496–510, 2009.

[15] G. P. Patrinos, J. A. Aama, A. A. Aqeel et al., "Recommendations for genetic variation data capture in developing countries to ensure a comprehensive worldwide data collection," *Human Mutation*, vol. 32, pp. 2–9, 2010.

[16] L. D. Botto, E. Robert-Gnansia, C. Siffel, J. Harris, B. Borman, and P. Mastroiacovo, "Fostering international collaboration in birth defects research and prevention: a perspective from the International Clearinghouse for Birth Defects Surveillance and Research," *American Journal of Public Health*, vol. 96, no. 5, pp. 774–780, 2006.

[17] I. L. Monlleo, P. A. Mossey, and V. L. Gil-da-Silva-Lopes, "Evaluation of craniofacial care outside the brazilian reference network for craniofacial treatment," *The Cleft Palate-Craniofacial Journal*, vol. 46, no. 2, pp. 204–211, 2009.

[18] World Health Organisation (WHO), *Global Registry and Database on Craniofacial Anomalies*, WHO, Geneva, Switzerland, 2003.

[19] World Health Organisation (WHO), *Addressing the Global Challenges of Craniofacial Anomalies*, WHO, Geneva, Switzerland, 2006.

[20] W. Shaw, "Global strategies to reduce the health-care burden of craniofacial anomalies: report of WHO meetings on International. Collaborative Research on Craniofacial Anomalies," *The Cleft Palate-Craniofacial Journal*, vol. 41, no. 3, pp. 238–243, 2004.

[21] I. L. Monlleó and V. L. Gil-da-Silva-Lopes, "Anomalias craniofaciais: descricao e avaliacao das caracteristicas gerais da atencao no Sistema Unico de Saude," *Cad Saude Publica*, vol. 22, pp. 913–922, 2006.

[22] I. L. Monlleó and V. L. Gil-Da-Silva-Lopes, "Brazil's Craniofacial project: genetic evaluation and counseling in the reference network for craniofacial treatment," *The Cleft Palate-Craniofacial Journal*, vol. 43, no. 5, pp. 577–579, 2006.

[23] A. L. C. Righeto, J. Huber, J. C. Machado, and D. G. Melo, "Anomalias congênitas: validade das informações das declarações de nascido vivo em uma maternidade de Ribeirão Preto, São Paulo," *Pediatria*, vol. 30, pp. 159–164, 2008.

[24] A. L. Geremias, M. F. Almeida, and M. P. O. Flores, "Avaliação das Declarações de Nascido Vivo como fonte de informações

sobre defeitos congênitos," *Revista Brasileira de Epidemiologia*, vol. 12, pp. 60–68, 2009.

[25] D. V. Luquetti and R. J. Koifman, "Quality of reporting on birth defects in birth certificates: case study from a Brazilian reference hospital," *Cadernos de Saude Publica*, vol. 25, no. 8, pp. 1721–1731, 2009.

[26] World Health Organization (WHO), "Programmes and projects," http://www.who.int/genomics/anomalies/americas_registry/en/index.html.

[27] I. L. Monlleó, *Atenção a pessoas com anomalias craniofaciais no Brasil: avaliação e propostas para o Sistema Único de Saúde*, Unicamp, Campinas, Brazil, 2008.

[28] I. L. Monlleó, P. A. Mossey, and V. L. Gil-da-Silva-Lopes, "The Brazilian database on orofacial clefts: preliminary validation," in *Proceedings of the 11th International Congress on Cleft Lip and Palate and Related Craniofacial Anomalies*, Fortaleza, Brazil, 2009.

[29] Instituto Brasileiro de Geografia e Estatistica (IBGE), Censo 2010, http://www.censo2010.ibge.gov.br/sinopse/index.php?dados=4&uf=00.

[30] D. D. G. Horovitz, J. C. Llerena, and R. A. Mattos, "Atenção aos defeitos congênitos no Brasil: características do atendimento e propostas para formulação de políticas públicas em genética clínica," *Cadernos de Saúde Pública*, vol. 22, pp. 2599–2609, 2006.

[31] M. I. B. Fontes, L. N. Almeida, G. O. Reis Jr. et al., "Local strategies to address health needs of individuals with orofacial clefts in Alagoas, Brazil," *The Cleft Palate-Craniofacial Journal*, 2012.

[32] D. R. FitzPatrick, P. A. M. Raine, and J. G. Boorman, "Facial clefts in the west of Scotland in the period 1980–1984: epidemiology and genetic diagnoses," *Journal of Medical Genetics*, vol. 31, no. 2, pp. 126–129, 1994.

[33] G. M. Shaw, S. L. Carmichael, W. Yang, J. A. Harris, and E. J. Lammer, "Congenital malformations in births with orofacial clefts among 3.6 million California births, 1983–1997," *American Journal of Medical Genetics*, vol. 125, no. 3, pp. 250–256, 2004.

[34] N. Freire-Maia, "Inbreeding in Brazil," *American Journal of Human Genetics*, vol. 9, no. 4, pp. 284–298, 1957.

[35] N. Freire-Maia, "Genetic effects in Brazilian populations due to consanguineous marriages," *American Journal of Medical Genetics*, vol. 35, no. 1, pp. 115–117, 1990.

[36] N. Freire-Maia, "Consanguinity marriages in Brazil," *Revista Brasileira de Biologia*, vol. 50, no. 4, pp. 863–866, 1990.

[37] E. W. Harville, A. J. Wilcox, R. T. Lie, H. Vindenes, and F. Åbyholm, "Cleft lip and palate versus cleft lip only: are they distinct defects?" *American Journal of Epidemiology*, vol. 162, no. 5, pp. 448–453, 2005.

[38] D. Grosen, C. Chevrier, A. Skytthe et al., "A cohort study of recurrence patterns among more than 54000 relatives of oral cleft cases in Denmark: support for the multifactorial threshold model of inheritance," *Journal of Medical Genetics*, vol. 47, no. 3, pp. 162–168, 2010.

[39] F. Rahimov, M. L. Marazita, A. Visel et al., "Disruption of an AP-2α binding site in an IRF6 enhancer is associated with cleft lip," *Nature Genetics*, vol. 40, no. 11, pp. 1341–1347, 2008.

[40] A. P. Herkrath, F. J. Herkrath, M. A. Rebelo, and M. V. Vettore, "Parental age as a risk factor for non-syndromic oral clefts: a meta analysis," *Journal of Dentistry*, vol. 40, pp. 3–14, 2012.

[41] R. P. Strauss and H. Broder, "Children with cleft lip/palate and mental retardation: a subpopulation of cleft-craniofacial team

patients," *The Cleft Palate-Craniofacial Journal*, vol. 30, pp. 548–556, 1993.

[42] Online Mendilian Inheritance in Man (OMIM), "Syndromes with cleft lip and or cleft palate," http://www.ncbi.nlm.nih .gov/omim.

[43] World Health Organization (WHO), *Medical Genetic Services in Developing Countries. the Ethical, Legal and Social Implications of Genetic Testing and Screening*, Human Genetics: Chronic Diseases and Health Promotion, WHO, Geneva, 2006.

[44] A. S. Daar, K. Berndtson, D. L. Persad, and P. A. Singer, "How can developing countries harness biotechnology to improve health?" *BMC Public Health*, vol. 7, article 346, 2007.

[45] M. R. Kohonen-Corish, J. Y. Al-Aama, A. D. Auerbach et al., "Human Variome Project Meeting. How to catch all those mutations—the report of the third Human Variome Project Meeting, UNESCO Paris, May 2010," *Human Mutation*, vol. 31, no. 12, pp. 1374–1381, 2010.

[46] S. A. Rasmussen, R. S. Olney, L. B. Holmes, A. E. Lin, K. M. Keppler-Noreuil, and C. A. Moore, "Guidelines for case classification for the National Birth Defects Prevention Study," *Birth Defects Research A*, vol. 67, no. 3, pp. 193–201, 2003.

33

Surgical Correction of Unicoronal Craniosynostosis with Frontal Bone Symmetrization and Staggered Osteotomies

Seyed Esmail Hassanpour,[1] **Masoumeh Abbasnezhad,**[2]
Hamidreza Alizadeh Otaghvar ⓘ**,**[3] **and Adnan Tizmaghz** ⓘ[4]

[1] *Professor of Plastic Surgery, Department Of Plastic Surgery, 15 Khordad Educational Hospital, School of Medicine,*
  Shahid Beheshti University of Medical Sciences, Tehran, Iran
[2] *Resident of Plastic Surgery, Department of Plastic Surgery, 15 Khordad Educational Hospital, School of Medicine,*
  Shahid Beheshti University of Medical Sciences, Tehran, Iran
[3] *Associate Professor of General Surgery, Iran University of Medical Sciences, Resident of Plastic and Reconstructive Surgery,*
  Shahid Beheshti University of Medical Sciences, Trauma & Injury Research Center, Tehran, Iran
[4] *Assistant Professor of General Surgery, Iran University of Medical Sciences, Tehran, Iran*

Correspondence should be addressed to Adnan Tizmaghz; adnan_ti@yahoo.com

Academic Editor: Hirohiko Kakizaki

Background. Craniosynostosis is the premature fusion of one or more cranial sutures that produce abnormal head shape. Plagiocephaly is a general term that describes unilateral flattening of the anterior or posterior quarter of the cranium. Anterior plagiocephaly is almost always due to unilateral coronal synostosis. Early surgical treatment is the best option for these patients. The aim of this study was to investigate the surgical correction results of unicoronal craniosynostosis with frontal bone symmetrization and staggered osteotomies. *Methods.* All unicoronal craniosynostosis cases treated surgically from 2013 to 2016 at our hospital, with frontal bone symmetrization and staggered osteotomies and fronto-orbital advancement, were reviewed. The following variables were analyzed: sex, age, weight, hospital stay time, ICU stay time, per os (PO) starting time, anesthetic time, estimated blood loss volume (ml), estimated blood loss as percentage of total volume, surgical complication, follow-up time, and Whitaker grade. All data were analyzed with SPSS. *Results.* The study consisted of 33 patients (19 females, 14 males). Average age was 10.24 months, average weight was 8.97 Kg, average hospital stay time was 7.84 days, average ICU stay time was 1.69 days, average PO starting time was 1.24 days after surgery, average anesthetic time was 397.72 minutes, average estimated blood loss was 213.78 ml, and estimated blood loss as percentage of total volume was 31.69%. One case (3.03%) needed reoperation and two cases had postoperative seizure. No mortality was seen. *Conclusion.* It is supposed that surgical correction of unicoronal craniosynostosis with frontal bone symmetrization and staggered osteotomies results in lower blood loss, lower complication rate and reoperation, and more durable results.

1. Introduction

Craniosynostosis is the premature fusion of one or more cranial sutures that produce an abnormal head shape. Non-syndromic craniosynostosis is an isolated condition without associated genetic syndromes. It occurs in approximately 1 in 1800-2500 births. In nonsyndromic forms, usually only one suture is involved and is specified as simple, but occasionally two or more sutures are involved and this condition is specified as complex [1]. Plagiocephaly is a general term

denoting the unilateral flattening of the anterior or posterior quarter of the cranium. Anterior plagiocephaly is always due to unicoronal synostosis. Female to male ratio is 68%. Unicoronal synostosis produces regional growth restriction and compensatory expansion of adjacent regions and obvious fronto-orbital dysmorphology [2]. Since the 1960s and disclosure of craniofacial surgery by Tessier, different techniques for craniosynostosis have been developed, such as fronto-parietal suturectomy, lateral canthal advancement, and bilateral fronto-orbital advancement [2]. One of the problems in

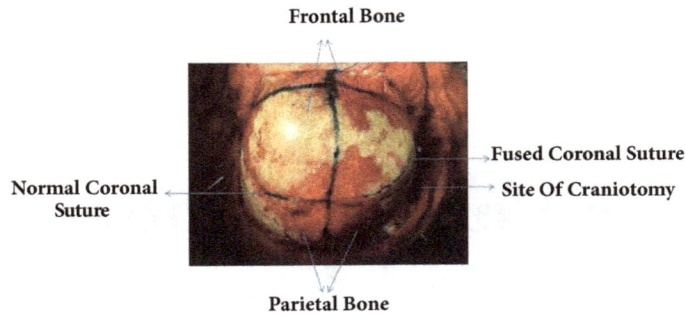

FIGURE 1: Craniotomy in unicoronal craniosynostosis was done posterior to the fused coronal suture producing bilateral frontal fragment symmetry.

patients with unicoronal synostosis is frontal bone deficiency in the affected side. To resolve this problem, we use the frontal bone symmetrization method with craniotomy in the posterior aspect of the fused coronal suture. The site of craniotomy in the affected side is determined by measuring the distance in the midline, lateral, and mid-way point in the unaffected side. We used staggered osteotomies in both sides for cranial rearrangement. Fronto-orbital osteotomy was done for fronto-orbital advancement. The aim of this study is to investigate surgical correction results in 33 patients who had been treated with this method.

2. Patients and Method

All unicoronal craniosynostosis cases that were treated surgically from 2013 to 2016 at our hospital with frontal bone symmetrization and staggered osteotomies were reviewed. Informed consents were obtained. The following variables were analyzed: sex, age, weight, hospital stay time, ICU stay time, PO starting time, anesthetic time, estimated blood loss volume (ml), estimated blood loss as percentage of total volume, surgical complications (e.g., bleeding, infection, wound dehiscence, seizure, need for reoperation, etc.), follow-up time, and Whitaker grade. Diagnosis is based on history, physical examination, and CT-scan. Genetic testing was not carried out in our study, due to financial reasons. A team composed of a plastic and reconstructive surgeon, a neurosurgeon, a pediatrician, an ophthalmologist, and anesthesiologist visited the patient before the operation. CBC, Cr, electrolytes, and blood cross-match were checked preoperatively. All procedures were done by the same plastic and reconstructive surgeon and neurosurgeon. All patients received prophylactic antibiotics. Under GA and after skin preparation and draping, in supine position, bicoronal incision was done. The flap was elevated to the superior orbital roof with preservation of supra-orbital bundle. Frontal craniotomy was performed in both sides, but in the affected side, craniotomy was done posterior to the fused coronal suture to produce bilateral frontal fragment symmetry. The craniotomy site in the affected side is determined by measuring the distance in the midline, lateral, and mid-way points in

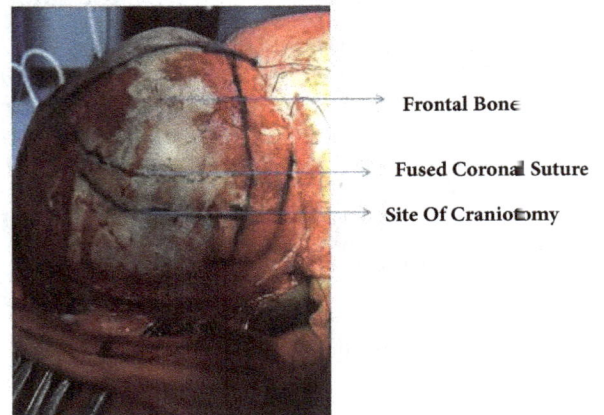

FIGURE 2: Craniotomy posterior to fused coronal suture in unicoronal craniosynostosis can add some parts of the parietal bone to the frontal bone segment.

the unaffected side. We added some parts of the parietal bone to the frontal bone segment (Figures 1 and 2).

In both sides, staggered osteotomies for remodeling and anterior cranial symmetry were done (Figure 3).

We corrected the orbital deformity by creating the orbital bandeau, advancing it anterior to the cornea (according to the severity of deformity) and symmetrizing both orbits with fronto-orbital advancement. Postoperative management was done in a pediatric ICU as routine and then in the pediatric ward.

3. Results

From 2013 to 2016, 33 patients (19 females, 14 males) with unicoronal craniosynostosis were operated on in our hospital with frontal symmetrization method and staggered osteotomies. Their average age was 10.24 months (range, 4–37 months), average follow-up time was 23.42 months (range, 5–44 months), and average weight at the time of surgery was 8.97 Kg (range, 5.8–17 Kg). Average hospital stay was 7.84 days (range, 6–18 days) and average ICU stay time was

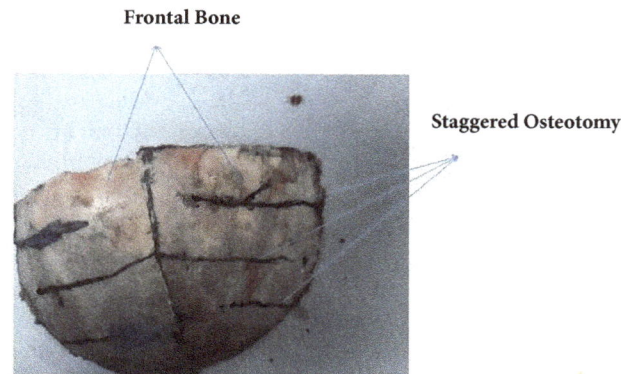

FIGURE 3: In both sides of unicoronal craniosynostosis, staggered osteotomies for remodeling and anterior cranial symmetry were done.

1.69 days (range, 1–5 days). Average PO starting time was 1.24 days after surgery (range, 1–5 days). Average anesthetic time was 397.72 minutes (range, 270–465 minutes). Average blood loss (intra- and postoperative from drain) that was estimated according to volume of packed cell transfused to the patient intra- and postoperative was 213.78ml (range, 60–500 ml), and average estimated blood loss as percentage of total volume was 31.69% (range 9.52-77.58%). Two cases developed postoperative seizure that was controlled with pharmacotherapy. They did not have any intracranial hemorrhage. One case (3.03%) needed reoperation 4 days postoperative, due to frontal flap dislocation and depression. No infection, wound dehiscence, or mortality was seen in our series. According to the Whitaker scale, 1 case (3.03%) was of grade IV and needed reoperation. Also, 1 case (3.03%) had forehead bony irregularity (grade III) that was proposed to be repaired, but the parents did not give consent. In total, 31 cases (93.93%) were grade I and did not need any further surgical intervention.

4. Discussion

Treatment goals of the craniosynostosis are adequate intracranial volume, enough for brain expansion and to minimize cognitive sequels and achieve normal cranial shape. The ideal time of surgery is controversial. Most surgeons operate on the patient as soon as possible. In nonsyndromic cases, surgery is done at around 6 months [3]. Surgical protocol involves a staged approach: (1) suture release, cranial vault decompression, and supra orbital region reshaping and advancement in infancy (6–12 months), (2) reconstructive surgery for midface abnormality in childhood (6-12 years), and (3) orthognathic surgery in adolescence (14–18 years). Exact timing and sequence of the surgical procedures are contingent upon functional and psychological aspects [3]. The categories of surgical procedure are as follows: (1) Strip craniectomy: the procedure involves cranial reshaping with fused suture removal. This method depends on the brain growth for cranial reshaping and does not treat hypoplasia or compensatory

cranial changes. (2) Cranial vault remodeling technique: that is accompanied by fused suture release with direct correction of hypo plastic and compensatory cranial changes. The cranium is reshaped with different techniques including burring of the bone, rotating and reattaching the remodeled segments; bone bending, separation and barrel stave osteotomies. (3) Distraction cranioplasty: in this approach, the cranium is reshaped based on distraction osteogenesis (new bone formation) and histogenesis (new soft tissue formation) with external and internal devices. (4) Posterior release: in this method, osteotomy in the posterior cranial portion is done. This technique often is associated with distraction osteogenesis and brain expansion that induces anteroposterior diameter growth of the cranium before the fronto-orbital advancement [4]. Each technique has different results. Different craniosynostosis series are reported in the literature. G.M. Zakhary et al. reported that 100 patients were undergoing open transcranial vault reshaping with barrel-stave and orbital bandeau advancement from 1997 to 2011. Average age of the patients was 8.9 months, average weight was 9.51 Kg, and average surgical time was 216.7 minutes. Complications included 2 hematomas, 2 wound infections, 1 subgaleal abscess, 6 dural tears, 3 reoperations due to residual deformity, 4 cases requiring coronal scar revision, 1 sagittal sinus bleeding, and 1 intraoperative death [5].

Zhilin Guo et al. reviewed 165 cases over a 20-year period that were operated on with fronto-orbital advancement. Average age was 12.1 months. In 165 cases, there were 38 cases of unilateral coronal synostosis, 127 cases of bilateral deformity, and 45 cases of Crouzon syndrome. Moreover, there was one postoperative death due to intracranial bleeding and five cases of CSF leaks. In a follow-up period from 3 months to 5 years, no reoperations were needed [6].

M.P. Ferreira et al. reviewed 120 craniosynostosis cases. Average age was 7.08 months, mean surgical time was 186 minutes, and mean hospitalization time was 6.8 days. Mortality rate was 2.6%. Six patients had cardio respiratory arrest in the perioperative period, hypovolemic shock, seizure, CSF fistula, extradural hematoma, and partial wound dehiscence.

Seven cases had complications such as pulmonary edema, respiratory obstruction, urinary tract infection, orbital cellulitis, and septic shock [3].

Jess-A Taylor et al. reviewed 238 nonsyndromic unicoronal craniosynostosis. These cases had undergone fronto-orbital advancement and cranial vault remodeling. They reviewed long-term aesthetic outcomes. Results showed that 55% had Whitaker class I, 6% had class II, 35% had class III, and 3% had class IV. Nasal root deviation and occipital bossing were the risk factors for Whitaker class III/IV. Bilateral cranial vault remodeling with extended unilateral bandeau had better results compared with strictly unilateral procedures. They noted traditional fronto-orbital advancement and cranial vault remodeling probably decreased the risk of intracranial hypertension, but as the patient grows, some aesthetic problems may appear [7].

Average anesthetic time in our series was 397.72 minutes. That is longer than the mentioned studies. This can be due to the time for venous and arterial line insertion, urinary catheterization, and time of intubation and extubation. We had less blood loss in our series in comparison with the mentioned studies, so less complication was seen. We had no mortality, infection, wound dehiscence, or hematoma. We had 1 case (3.03%) of reoperation due to frontal flap dislodgement. One case (3.03%) had forehead bony irregularity and was candidate for reoperation, but the parents did not give consent. Two cases (6.06%) had postoperative seizure that was controlled with pharmacotherapy.

5. Conclusion

It is supposed that unicoronal craniosynostosis correction with frontal bone symmetrization and staggered osteotomies can minimize bleeding, complications, and reoperation. This can be a more effective method for surgical correction of unicoronal craniosynostosis, although more studies with more cases and longer follow-up are required.

Ethical Approval

The study was performed in accordance with the ethical standards of the 1964 Declaration of Helsinki and its later amendments. Written ethical committee approval was obtained from the research committee at 15 Khordad Hospital, Tehran, Iran. All patients gave consent for treatment and the use of their data in education and research. No further formal consent was required because the study protocol included retrospective, epidemiologic evaluation of anonymous and routine patient data, and procedural and outcome parameters.

Disclosure

Level of Evidence V. This journal requires that authors assign a level of evidence to each article. For a full description of these Evidence-Based Medicine ratings, please refer to the Table of Contents or the online Instructions to Authors www.springer.com/00266.

Acknowledgments

This article has been extracted from the thesis written by Ms. Masoumeh Abbasnezhad in School of Medicine Shahid Beheshti University of Medical Sciences (Registration No:474) [8]. We would like to thank clinical Research Development Unit of 15 Khordad Hospital for their special support.

References

[1] E. D. Rodriguez, J. E. Losee, and P. C. Neligan, *Plastic Surgery E-Book: Volume 3: Craniofacial, Head and Neck SurgeryPediatric Plastic Surgery (Expert Consult-Online)*, Elsevier Health Sciences, 2012.

[2] G. Silav, G. Avci, M. Akan, G. Taylan, I. Elmaci, and T. Akoz, "The surgical treatment of plagiocephaly," *Turkish Neurosurgery*, vol. 21, no. 3, pp. 304–314, 2011.

[3] M. P. Ferreira, M. V. Collares, N. P. Ferreira, J. L. Kraemer, A. A. Pereira Filho, and G. A. Pereira Filho, "Early surgical treatment of nonsyndromic craniosynostosis," *World Neurosurgery*, vol. 65, pp. S22–S26, 2006.

[4] O. Kirmi, S. J. Lo, D. Johnson, and P. Anslow, "Craniosynostosis: A Radiological and Surgical Perspective," *Seminars in Ultrasound, CT and MRI*, vol. 30, no. 6, pp. 492–512, 2009.

[5] G. M. Zakhary, D. M. Montes, J. E. Woerner, C. Noarianni, and G. E. Ghali, "Surgical correction of craniosynostosis. A review of 100 cases," *Journal of Cranio-Maxillo-Facial Surgery*, vol. 42, no. 8, pp. 1684–1691, 2014.

[6] Z. Guo, M. Ding, X. Mu, and R. Chen, "Operative treatment of coronal craniosynostosis: 20 years of experience," *World Neurosurgery*, vol. 68, no. 6, pp. S18–S21, 2007.

[7] J. A. Taylor, J. T. Paliga, A. M. Wes et al., "A critical evaluation of long-term aesthetic outcomes of fronto-orbital advancement and cranial vault remodeling in nonsyndromic unicoronal craniosynostosis," *Plastic and Reconstructive Surgery*, vol. 135, no. 1, pp. 220–231, 2015.

[8] M. Abbasnezhad, *A survey of the surgical correction results of unicoronal synostotic plagiocephaly in the patients referring to Mofid Hospital in 1392-1395, Plastic surgery [MD thesis]*, School of Medicine Shahid Beheshti University of Medical Sciences, Tehran, Iran, 2018.

34

Risk Factors for Postoperative Complications among the Elderly after Plastic Surgery Procedures Performed under General Anesthesia

Kiyoko Fukui (ID),[1] **Masaki Fujioka,**[1,2] **Kazumi Yamasaki,**[3,4]
Sho Yamakawa,[1] **Haruka Matsuo,**[1] **and Miho Noguchi**[1]

[1] *Department of Plastic and Reconstructive Surgery, National Hospital Organization Nagasaki Medical Center, Nagasaki, Japan*
[2] *Department of Plastic and Reconstructive Surgery, Nagasaki University, Nagasaki, Japan*
[3] *Department of Liver Internal Medicine, National Hospital Organization Nagasaki Medical Center, Nagasaki, Japan*
[4] *Department of Clinical Research Center, National Hospital Organization Nagasaki Medical Center, Nagasaki, Japan*

Correspondence should be addressed to Kiyoko Fukui; k.ku.r@hotmail.co.jp

Academic Editor: Nicolò Scuderi

Background. The frequency of surgery involving elderly patients has been increasing. The use of free tissue transfers in the elderly has been examined previously (Howard et al., 2005, Hwang et al., 2016, Grammatica et al., 2015, Serletti et al., 2000, and Sierakowski et al., 2017), whereas there have not been any such studies of plastic surgery procedures. We evaluated the risk factors for complications after plastic surgery procedures performed under general anesthesia in patients aged ≥75 years. *Methods.* The cases of patients aged ≥75 years who underwent plastic surgery procedures under general anesthesia at the Department of Plastic and Reconstructive Surgery, National Hospital Organization Nagasaki Medical Center, between 2009 and 2016 were reviewed retrospectively. Multiple logistic regression analysis was used to identify the risk factors for postoperative complications. *Results.* Two hundred and sixty-three cases were reviewed. Complications were seen in 137 patients. Age was not predictive of complications. The risk factors included a serum albumin level of <2.8 g/dl (odds ratio (OR): 2.96), an operative time of ≥120 min (OR: 6.22), and an American Society of Anesthesiologists performance status of ≥3 (OR: 2.39). *Conclusions.* Age is not contraindication for surgery in the elderly. It is important to assess comorbidities and perform surgical procedures as soon as possible to shorten the surgical period.

1. Introduction

The populations of developed countries have been aging progressively, and Japanese society is aging especially rapidly [1]. The feasibility of performing surgery in elderly patients has increased, but this has resulted in a greater frequency of postoperative complications because the functional capacity of such patients' organs is impaired [2]. Thus, it is important to clarify the risk factors for postoperative complications in elderly patients.

The complications of free flap reconstruction after oncological surgery in elderly patients have recently been discussed [2–6]. However, the risk factors for complications after plastic surgery procedures in the elderly have not been reported. The aim of this study is to evaluate the

risk factors for postoperative complications after surgery performed under general anesthesia in patients aged over 75 years.

2. Materials and Methods

The cases of patients aged over 75 years who underwent plastic surgery procedures under general anesthesia at the Department of Plastic and Reconstructive Surgery, National Hospital Organization Nagasaki Medical Center, between 2009 and 2016 were evaluated retrospectively. Various preoperative and intraoperative variables were recorded, including age, gender, disease type, laboratory parameters (the levels of hemoglobin, albumin, and C-reactive protein and the white blood cell count), the subjects' preoperative ability to perform activities of daily living (ADL), the surgical procedure, the duration of general anesthesia, and the operative time. The subjects' preoperative ability to perform ADL was assessed based on two categories, i.e., whether or not the subjects maintained the ability to walk without support.

Comorbidity status was evaluated using the American Society of Anesthesiologists (ASA) performance status (PS) and the Charlson comorbidity index (CCI). The ASA PS is a scoring system that is used to define anesthesiological risk. The CCI is a grading system based on 16 medical conditions, and it is considered to be related to survival in hospitalized patients [3].

Postoperative complications and mortality were recorded, and overall complications were divided into two categories, i.e., into complications that were directly due to surgical procedures (surgical complications) and other complications (medical complications). Operative mortality was defined as deaths that occurred within 30 days of surgery.

All statistical analyses were performed using the SPSS 24.0 software. Multiple logistic regression analysis was used to assess the risk factors for postoperative complications, and p-values of <0.05 were regarded as statistically significant. Receiver operating characteristic (ROC) curves were used to estimate the optimal cut-off points for the serum albumin level and operative time.

3. Results

3.1. Patients. A total of 309 patients that were older than 75 years underwent surgery at our institution during the study period. Thirty-one patients were excluded because they underwent reconstruction after oncological surgery, including for laryngeal, oropharyngeal, or cervical esophageal cancer, and 15 patients were excluded because their preoperative laboratory data were insufficient. Thus, the cases of 263 patients were finally reviewed.

The subjects' median age at the time of surgery was 82 years (range: 75–99 years). There were 124 males (47.1%) and 139 females (52.9%). In total, 203 (77.2%) and 60 patients (22.8%) had ASA PS of ≤2 and ≥3, respectively. Moreover, 138 patients (52.3%) and 125 patients (47.5%) exhibited CCI scores of ≤2 and ≥3, respectively. The median operative time was 60 min (range: 11–451 min) (Table 1). In addition, 124 of 263 patients (47%) could not walk without assistance/a wheelchair or were bedridden before the operation.

3.2. Types of Disease. Thirty-five patients suffered peripheral arterial disease (PAD) with ulcers and/or necrosis; 47 patients had pressure ulcers; 19 patients had necrotizing fasciitis; and 31 patients developed ulcers caused by other diseases, such as diabetes, collagen disease, radiation, myelitis, or venous congestive disease. Twenty-six patients suffered traumatic injuries, such as facial fractures and hand injuries. Thirty-two patients suffered burns. Fifty-seven patients developed malignant tumors on their body surfaces. Two patients experienced scar contraction. Fourteen patients developed other conditions, such as blepharoptosis and facial nerve paralysis (Table 2).

TABLE 1: Baseline characteristics of all patients.

All patients	$n = 263$
Age (years)	
Median	82
Range	75–99
Males, n (%)	124 (47.1)
Females, n (%)	139 (52.9)
ASA PS	
≤2, n (%)	203 (77.2)
≥3, n (%)	60 (22.8)
CCI	
≤2, n (%)	138 (52.3)
≥3, n (%)	125 (47.5)
Operative time (min)	
Median	60
Range	11–451

TABLE 2: Types of disease.

Conditions	No of patients
Peripheral arterial disease	35
Pressure ulcers	47
Necrotizing soft tissue infections	19
Other ulcers	31
Traumatic injuries	26
Burns	32
Tumors	57
Scars	2
Others	14
Total	263

TABLE 3: Surgical procedures.

Surgery	No. of patients
Amputation	49
Pedicled flap transfer	76
Skin graft	59
Free flap transfer	3
Debridement	26
Fracture repair	15
Tumor resection	20
Others	15
Total	263

3.3. Surgical Procedures. Forty-nine, 76, 59, and 3 patients underwent amputation, pedicled flap transfer, skin grafts, and free flap reconstruction, respectively. Twenty-six, 15, 20, and 15 patients underwent debridement, fracture repair, tumor resection, and other surgical procedures, respectively (Table 3). There were 133 surgical procedures in which the operative time was ≥60 min (pedicled flap transfer: 51, skin graft: 26, amputation: 22, fracture repair: 11, debridement: 6, free flap transfer: 3, and others: 14) (Table 4).

TABLE 4: Surgical procedures involving operative times of ≥60 min.

Surgery	No. of patients
Pedicled flap transfer	51
Skin graft	26
Amputation	22
Fracture repair	11
Debridement	6
Free flap transfer	3
Others	14
Total	133

TABLE 5: Complications.

Complications	No. of patients
Overall	137 (52.1%)
Medical	87 (33.1%)
Surgical	80 (30.4%)

TABLE 6: Medical complications.

Medical complications	No. of patients
Delirium	73
Pneumonia, atelectasis	9
CHF*, arrhythmia, pulmonary edema	3
Others	4

CHF: congestive heart failure.

TABLE 7: Surgical complications.

Surgical complications	No. of patients
Skin necrosis	36
Loss of skin graft	23
Hematomas/seromas	11
Infection	9
Lymphorrhea	1

TABLE 8: Frequencies of medical and surgical complications according to the Clavien-Dindo classification.

Complication type	Clavien-Dindo grade						
	I	II	IIIa	IIIb	IVa	IVb	V
Medical	3	78	1	0	5	0	5
Surgical	19	11	36	13	0	0	1

TABLE 9: Overall complications.

Variables	OR	95% CI	p-values
Alb (g/dl)			
≥2.8	1 (ref)		
<2.8	2.96	1.68–5.19	0.00
Operative time (min)			
<60	1 (ref)		
≥60, <120	1.95	1.09–3.50	0.03
≥120	6.22	2.71–14.26	0.00
ASA PS			
≤2	1 (ref)		
≥3	2.39	1.24–4.63	0.01

the most complications, followed by skin grafts (12 patients) and then amputations (7 patients).

Six patients died after surgery (2.28%). Three patients died of pneumonia, 2 patients died of sepsis (1 patient suffered necrotizing fasciitis caused by a group G beta-hemolytic streptococcus, and another patient developed sepsis caused by necrosis of the small bowel), and 1 patient died due to an advanced malignant fibrous histiocytoma.

The frequency of each type of complication is shown according to the international Clavien-Dindo classification in Table 8.

3.5. Risk Factors for Postoperative Complications

3.5.1. Overall Complications. Age, gender, the preoperative levels of hemoglobin and C-reactive protein, the preoperative white blood cell count, the surgical procedure, the duration of general anesthesia, and the CCI score were not predictive of the overall frequency of overall complications. Conversely, the preoperative serum albumin level, the operative time, and the ASA PS were found to be associated with the overall frequency of overall complications (Table 9). Specifically, a serum albumin level of <2.8 g/dl (odds ratio [OR]: 2.96 [95% confidence interval [CI]: 1.68–5.19]; p < 0.001), an operative time of ≥60 min and <120 min (OR: 1.95 [95% CI: 1.09–3.50]; p = 0.03), an operative time of ≥120 min (OR: 6.22 [95% CI: 2.71–14.26]; p < 0.001), and an ASA PS of ≥3 (OR: 2.39 [95% CI: 1.24–4.63]; p < 0.001) were identified as risk factors for overall complications.

3.5.2. Medical Complications. The preoperative serum albumin level, operative time, and the subjects' preoperative ability to perform ADL were found to be associated with medical complications (Table 10). Specifically, the risk factors for medical complications were shown to include a serum

3.4. Complications.
Overall complications were seen in 137 patients (52.1%). Surgical complications occurred in 80 patients (30.4%), and medical complications arose in 87 patients (33.1%) (Table 5).

The most common medical complication was delirium, which was seen in 73 patients. Pneumonia or atelectasis occurred in 9 patients, and 3 patients were affected by congestive heart failure, cardiac arrhythmia, or pulmonary edema. Other medical complications (renal failure, cholecystitis, and sepsis) occurred in 4 patients (Table 6).

Regarding surgical complications, 36 patients developed skin necrosis, 23 suffered skin graft loss, 11 developed hematomas/seromas, 9 contracted infections, and 1 developed lymphorrhea (Table 7).

Surgical and medical complications occurred in 54 and 55 patients, respectively, who underwent procedures longer than ≥60 min. Among the surgical procedures that took ≥60 min, pedicled flap transfers for pressure ulcers (26 patients) caused

TABLE 10: Medical complications.

Variables	OR	95% CI	p-values
Alb (g/dl)			
≥2.8	1 (ref)		
<2.8	2.49	1.36–4.55	0.00
Operative time (min)			
<62	1 (ref)		
≥62	1.92	1.10–3.33	0.02
Preoperative ADL			
Walk without support	1 (ref)		
Physical assistance*	2.03	1.10–3.72	0.02

*Physical assistance: patients who cannot walk without assistance/a wheelchair or were bedridden.

TABLE 11: Surgical complications.

Variables	OR	95% CI	p-values
Operative time (min)			
<62	1 (ref)		
≥62	3.20	1.83–5.61	0.00
Types of disease			
Ulcers*	1 (ref)		
Others**	0.45	0.25–0.78	0.01

*Ulcers: PAD, pressure ulcers, necrotizing fasciitis, other ulcers (those associated with diabetes, collagen, radiation, etc.)
**Others: traumatic injuries, tumors, or scars.

albumin level of <2.8 g/dl (OR: 2.49 [95% CI: 1.36–4.55]; p < 0.001), an operative time of ≥62 min (OR: 1.92 [95% CI: 1.10–3.33]; p = 0.02), and the subjects' preoperative ability to perform ADL (patients who cannot walk without assistance/a wheelchair or were bedridden (OR: 2.03 [95% CI: 1.10–3.72]; p = 0.02)).

3.5.3. Surgical Complications. The operative time and type of disease were found to be associated with surgical complications (Table 11). Specifically, the risk factors for surgical complications included an operative time of ≥62 min and ulcers, including PAD, pressure ulcers, necrotizing fasciitis, and other ulcers.

4. Discussion

The proportion of the elderly has been increasing in Japan. The Japan Geriatrics Society defines 65- to 74-year-old people as "pre old", 75- to 89-year-old people as "old", and people aged over 90 years as "oldest-old" [7]. In total, 12.5% of the Japanese population is over 75 years old [1]. Chronic ulcers caused by PAD and pressure ulcers are particularly common in elderly people [8], and these wounds are associated with discharges, infection, foul smells, and severe ischemic pain and require frequent dressing changes. In order to improve the quality of life of patients with such conditions, it is expected that the frequency of surgery involving elderly patients will increase. Thus, it is important to evaluate the risk

factors for postoperative complications in the elderly after surgery performed under general anesthesia.

Recently, the use of free tissue transfers after oncological surgery in elderly patients has been examined [2–6], and a relationship was reported to exist between age and postoperative complications. Hwang et al. reviewed 41 studies about complications in the elderly after free flap surgery and reported that the overall and surgical complications rates increased with age [2]. On the other hand, Howard et al. reported that the frequency of medical complications was increased in the over 80 years age group, but not the 70 to 79 years age group; however, no age-related increase in the frequency of surgical complications was detected [3]. Grammatica et al. reported that microvascular reconstruction resulted in medical complications more frequently in the elderly, but the frequency of surgical complications was not affected by age [4]. Therefore, we considered that it would be useful to study the risk factors for postoperative complications in elderly patients who underwent surgery performed under general anesthesia. In our study of plastic surgery procedures, neither the overall frequency of complications nor the frequencies of medical or surgical complications increased with age.

As for other risk factors for postoperative complications, Serletti et al. reported that in microvascular surgery patients with higher ASA PS suffered medical complications more frequently, but the frequency of surgical complications was not increased in this group. Furthermore, a longer operative time was found to be associated with an increased frequency of surgical complications [5]. On the other hand, Howard et al. reported that alcohol consumption and coronary artery disease are risk factors for medical and surgical complications [3]. In our study of plastic surgery procedures, a longer operative time was associated with an increased frequency of complications, including both medical and surgical complications, and it appeared that the operative time had the strongest influence on the risk of postoperative complications. Of the procedures that took longer than 60 min, many involved pedicled flap transfers for pressure ulcers, skin graft transfers for ulcers or burn wounds, or major amputation for PAD (Table 4). It would be difficult to shorten the operating times of such procedures. However, improving the skill of the operator or treating patients with negative pressure wound therapy to cause their wounds to contract before they are resurfaced might help to shorten the operating time of such procedures to <60 min. In addition, a lower serum albumin level was demonstrated to be associated with increased frequencies of both overall and medical complications. The patients with ulcers (pressure ulcers, PAD, necrotizing fasciitis, or other ulcers) developed postoperative complications more frequently than the other patients, and these patients were also malnourished. In each of these cases, we consulted the nutritional support team and attempted to alleviate the patient's malnutrition.

Moreover, a higher ASA PS was shown to be associated with an increased frequency of overall complications. Concerning the patients' ability to perform preoperative ADL, patients who needed physical assistance suffered medical complications more frequently. It appeared that patients' preoperative medical status, for example, their nutritional status and their ability to perform ADL, had a greater influence on their risk of postoperative complications than age.

As for the patients' preoperative and postoperative functional status, 124 of 263 patients (47%) could not walk without assistance/a wheelchair or were bedridden before the operation. For example, some patients suffered from PAD or pressure ulcers, and many were bedridden or confined to a wheelchair before the operation. Therefore, their ability to perform ADL did not change very much after surgery because they were already bedridden before the operation. The remaining 139 patients (53%) were able to move independently before the operation, and 104 patients were suffering from conditions other than ulcers (facial fractures, hand injuries, malignant tumors, etc.). These patients were discharged shortly after the operation, and so their ability to perform ADL did not change very much.

The patients suffering from ulcers, including pressure ulcers and PAD, experienced postoperative surgical complications more frequently than the other patients. Bamba et al. reported that the surgical complications rate after pressure ulcer reconstruction was 58.7% (162 out of 276 patients) [9]. Keys et al. reported that 110 out of 231 flap transfer procedures (49%) for pressure ulcers resulted in postoperative dehiscence [10]. Regarding PAD, Beaulieu et al. found that readmission (because of infection, nonhealing wounds, or ischemia) was necessary in 13.9% of patients that underwent minor amputations for PAD [11]. Curran et al. reported that the complications rate was 43% (among 5732 patients) after amputation for PAD [12]. In our study, surgical complications occurred in 80 patients (30.4%), which is a similar frequency to those reported previously.

In conclusion, age is not a contraindication for plastic surgery procedures performed under general anesthesia in the elderly. In cases involving elderly patients, it is important to assess preoperative medical conditions and comorbidities carefully and to perform surgical procedures as soon as possible in order to shorten the surgical period.

References

[1] Statistics Bureau, Ministry of Internal Affairs and Communications website [Internet], http://www.stat.go.jp/data/topics/topi1031.htm.

[2] K. Hwang, J. P. Lee, S. Y. Yoo, and H. Kim, "Relationships of comorbidities and old age with postoperative complications of head and neck free flaps: a review," *Journal of Plastic, Reconstructive & Aesthetic Surgery*, vol. 69, no. 12, pp. 1627–1635, 2016.

[3] M. A. Howard, P. G. Cordeiro, J. Disa et al., "Free tissue transfer in the elderly: incidence of perioperative complications following microsurgical reconstruction of 197 septuagenarians

and octogenarians," *Plastic and Reconstructive Surgery*, vol. 116, no. 6, pp. 1659–1668, 2005.

[4] A. Grammatica, C. Piazza, A. Paderno, V. Taglietti, A. Marengoni, and P. Nicolai, "Free flaps in head and neck reconstruction after oncologic surgery: expected outcomes in the elderly," *Otolaryngology—Head and Neck Surgery*, vol. 152, no. 5, pp. 796–802, 2015.

[5] J. M. Serletti, J. P. Higgins, S. Moran, and G. S. Orlando, "Factors affecting outcome in free-tissue transfer in the elderly," *Plastic and Reconstructive Surgery*, vol. 106, no. 1, pp. 66–70, 2000.

[6] A. Sierakowski, A. Nawar, M. Parker, and B. Mathur, "Free flap surgery in the elderly: experience with 110 cases aged ≥70 years," *Journal of Plastic, Reconstructive and Aesthetic Surgery*, vol. 70, no. 2, pp. 189–195, 2017.

[7] The Japan Geriatrics Society [Internet], 2017, http://www.jpn-geriat-soc.or.jp/proposal/pdf/definition_01.pdf.

[8] D. Bergqvist, M. Delle, I. Eckerlund et al., *Peripheral Arterial Disease–Diagnosis and Treatment: A Systematic Review*, Swedish Council on Health Technology Assessment, 2008.

[9] R. Bamba, J. J. Madden, A. N. Hoffman et al., "Flap reconstruction for pressure ulcers: an outcomes analysis," *Plastic and Reconstructive Surgery–Global*, vol. 18, Article ID e1187, 2017.

[10] K. A. Keys, L. N. Daniali, K. J. Warner, and D. W. Mathes, "Multivariate predictors of failure after flap coverage of pressure ulcers," *Plastic and Reconstructive Surgery*, vol. 125, no. 6, pp. 1725–1734, 2010.

[11] R. J. Beaulieu, J. C. Grimm, H. Lyu et al., "Predictors for readmission and reamputation following minor lower extremity amputation," *Journal of Vascular Surgery*, vol. 62, pp. 101–105, 2015.

[12] T. Curran, J. Q. Zhang, R. C. Lo et al., "Risk factors and indications for readmission after lower extremity amputation in the american college of surgeons national surgical quality improvement program," *Journal of Vascular Surgery*, vol. 60, no. 5, pp. 1315–1324, 2014.

35

Therapeutic Options of Chondrodermatitis Nodularis Helicis

Lea Juul Nielsen,[1] **Caroline Holkmann Olsen,**[2] **and Jørgen Lock-Andersen**[1]

[1]*Department of Plastic Surgery and Breast Surgery, Roskilde Hospital, 4000 Roskilde, Denmark*
[2]*Department of Pathology, Roskilde Sygehus, Denmark*

Correspondence should be addressed to Lea Juul Nielsen; yuppielea@hotmail.com

Academic Editor: Nicolo Scuderi

Chondrodermatitis Nodularis Helicis is a benign inflammatory process affecting the skin and cartilage of the ear. It typically presents as a painful nodule surrounded by an area of erythema and often prevents the patient from sleeping on the affected side. Many treatments have been described in the literature, but the condition is prone to recurrence. A literature search was performed in order to identify the best possible treatment. Fifty-eight articles were included, describing and investigating nonsurgical as well as surgical treatment modalities. Large prospective, controlled, and randomised long-term studies are lacking, but based on the available literature, we recommend starting with a conservative approach using decompression devices. Simple surgical procedures should only be used if conservative measures fail.

1. Introduction

Chondrodermatitis Nodularis Helicis (CNH) is an inflammatory process affecting the skin and cartilage of the ear. Typically, it presents as a painful nodule of the helix and to a lesser extent the antihelix of the ear. Therefore, some have suggested changing the name to chondrodermatitis nodularis auricularis, as lesions are seen both on the helix and on the antihelix [1] and have even been reported on the posterior ear and in the external auditory canal [2, 3].

The condition was first described by the dermatologist Winkler in 1915 [4], who reported eight cases and soon afterwards by Foerster, who reported a further four cases [5]. Foerster later defined the condition in 1925 [6], with an additional eight cases, describing the clinical and microscopic features and the treatment of the condition.

The anatomy of the ear is unique, because the skin of the anterior and posterior surface is adherent to the perichondrium and is devoid of subcutaneous fat. The blood supply is provided by a rich subdermal plexus of vessels lying in the fascial layer between the skin and the perichondrium. The arterial supply to the auricle is derived from branches of the superficial temporal artery and the postauricular artery, so that the lateral surface of the ear has a dual arterial supply [7].

2. Method and Material

This paper is presented as a literature review. A PubMed search was performed on the 18th of December 2015 using the search term "chondrodermatitis", identifying 134 articles. Primarily, abstracts of articles from 1996 onwards were reviewed leading to a full article review according to relevance. Articles with special focus on treatment modalities were included. Reference lists of selected articles were reviewed for other relevant articles.

3. Results

Fifty-eight articles were included: 13 prospective studies [8–20], 16 retrospective studies [1, 21–35], 4 case series [36–39], 13 case reports [2, 3, 40–50], 8 descriptions of treatment methods [7, 51–57], and 4 reviews [58–61].

In general, the literature on CNH is of fairly low quality, as it includes many case reports and retrospective studies. The 13 prospective studies are neither randomised, blinded

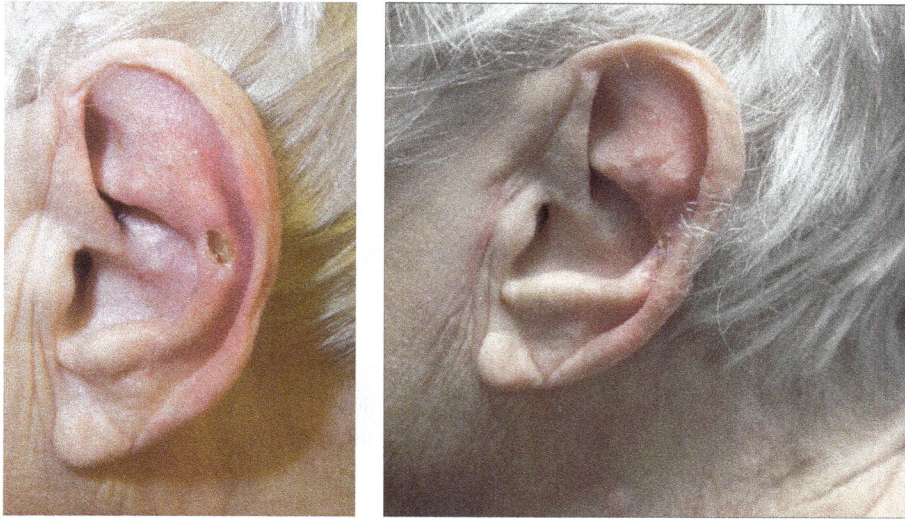

FIGURE 1: Pre- and postoperative pictures of a patient with CNH. 79-year-old woman with recurrence of CNH on the left antihelix. Two years prior to referral the patient was treated surgically (unknown method) for CNH in the same location. Recurrence occurred 3 months before referral and was initially treated with topical sodium fusidate with no effect. Treated with excision of skin and underlying cartilage and coverage of the defect with full thickness skin graft, all symptoms resolved and an acceptable cosmetic outcome was obtained at 3-month follow-up.

nor controlled, although one histopathological study, investigating nerve hyperplasia, did include other tumours of the ear as controls. Most of the prospective studies involve only small cohorts of patients ranging from 5 to 99. Many articles lack information on anamnesis, symptoms, clinical signs, or length of follow-up as well as a clear definition of outcome (i.e., is a successful outcome reduced pain, absence of pain, reduction in size of nodule, or complete resolution of the nodule?). The follow-up period is generally short, ranging from 2 to 12 months, although a few studies report on follow-up intervals of up to 41–96 months. Another weakness in most of the studies is the presence of confounding treatment modalities: many patients had previously tried other treatments, some were subjected to more than one treatment, and many were advised to decompress the lesion in conjunction with the investigated treatment.

3.1. Clinical Presentation.

CNH typically presents with an oval shaped nodule with elevated edges and a central crust or depression, usually 4–6 mm in diameter and frequently surrounded by an area of erythema. The nodule is usually firm to touch and bound to the underlying cartilage. It is characterised by exquisite tenderness, which often prevents the patient from sleeping on the affected side. Typically, the nodule is located on the outer ear (for men often on the helix and for women often on the antihelix) but locations on the posterior ear [2] and in the external auditory canal [3] have also been reported (see Figure 1). The lesions are typically located on the ear of the preferred sleeping-side, the right side being predominant, and are typically unilateral, although bilateral lesions have also been reported [8, 40–42]. Nocturnal pain is by far the most common symptom, with only few complaints of pain during the day, except when

touched. Other features associated with the nodules include crusting, bleeding, and exudate, which can make it difficult to exclude skin malignancy.

3.2. Gender and Age Distribution.

Historically, the literature describes a striking preponderance of males (10 : 1). In this review, 27 studies reported on the gender distribution, including a total of 628 males and 452 females, resulting in a male to female ratio of 1 : 0.7. As the exact cause of CNH is unknown, any discussion on the reasons for the gender difference is speculative.

CNH most commonly presents in patients over 40, although there have been isolated reports of children also affected [43–45]. Excluding all case reports and including only studies where a mean age is reported, 21 studies reported a mean age from 43 to 76 years.

Studies on incidence and prevalence were not identified, but anecdotally, our pathology department reports that the incidence is common.

3.3. Pathogenesis.

The pathomechanism of CNH has not yet been fully uncovered. The striking and repeated observation that CNH is usually unilateral and usually affects the ear of the preferred sleeping-side suggests that pressure damage, predominantly from the weight of the head during sleep, is the most important aetiological factor. CNH arising from pressure due to hearing aids and other headgear has also been described [9, 21, 42, 44, 46]. Other aetiological factors such as trauma from cold (frostbite) and actinic damage have also been suggested [9, 21–23, 40, 42–47, 58].

It is possible that anatomical features of the individual (e.g., a grossly protruding helix or antihelix) predispose to the condition, but in most cases, the cartilage does not

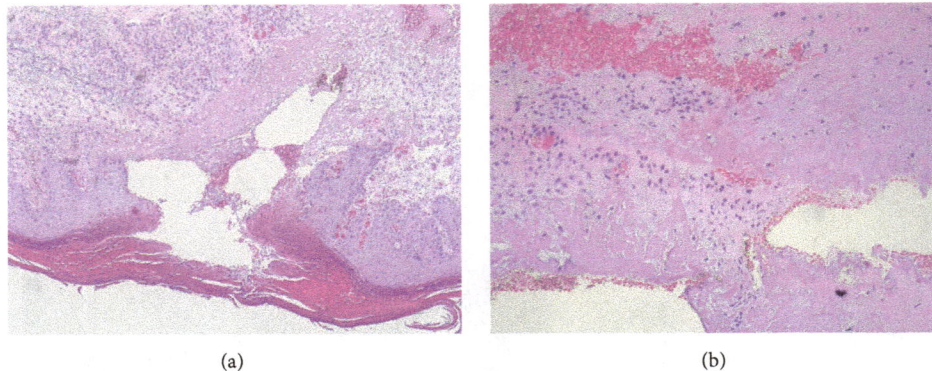

(a)   (b)

FIGURE 2: Classical histopathology of CNH. (a) shows the classical findings of hyperkeratosis, parakeratosis, adjacent hyperplasia of the epithelium, and substantial destruction of the dermal tissue lined by sclerosis and proliferation of small vessels. (b) shows the destruction of cartilage.

have to be grossly abnormal to initiate the disease. As the ear-shape does not change much during adult life, other factors must cause development of the disease in an otherwise unaffected ear. This could be due to distortion or calcification due to injury or simply because the cartilage becomes less flexible with increasing age and hence more vulnerable to pressure damage. It is also possible that the difference in site distribution between men and women is explained by the presence of a more protuberant helix in men and a more protuberant antihelix in women [24].

It has been suggested that pressure or repeated trauma may lead to ischemia of the cartilage and the auricular perichondrium. This arises because of the lack of protection of a thick subcutaneous tissue and changes in the perichondrial arterioles. Although dated, this vasculitis/inflammatory theory, first proposed by Halter in 1936 [62], is still the most widely accepted explanation for CNH. More recently, it was supported by Upile et al. in 2009 [23], with a histopathological review of 16 cases. Upile et al. confirmed the previous findings of epidermal acanthosis associated with a horny, partly parakeratotic, plug or ulceration and scale crust, superficial debris with fibrin, sclerosis, perichondrial fibrosis, and a varying degree of cartilage degeneration closely associated with areas of granulation tissue (see Figure 2). Upile et al. also confirmed the presence of consistent arteriolar narrowing in the part of the perichondrium most remote from the arterial blood supply, that is, the helix. This leads to ischemic changes and death of the metabolically active underlying cartilage with necrosis and extrusion and to severe local inflammation secondary to a foreign body reaction [23]. Furthermore, nerve hyperplasia is present in CNH, though often masked by the intense vascular and inflammatory reactions, which may explain the characteristic exquisite tenderness [10].

A possible association with systemic disease, such as dermatomyositis and systemic sclerosis, has also been suggested [11]. However, it is more likely that immobility caused by these diseases, and hence the inability to alter sleeping position, could be the true cause of a correlation between CNH and systemic disease.

3.4. Differential Diagnosis. The differential diagnosis depends on the clinical presentation, but the location of the lesion in combination with exquisite tenderness helps to differentiate CNH from other diagnoses. Gouty tophi may be suspected, when there are multiple lesions, not only on the ear, but also on fingers and toes. The nodular appearance with a central ulceration can mimic a basal cell carcinoma, while larger and more inflamed lesions may look like a squamous cell carcinoma, one of the most common misdiagnoses of CNH. Keratoacanthoma usually exhibits much faster growth, resulting in a larger tumour volume and with the classic resolution over months. When keratosis is the predominant clinical feature, an actinic or seborrheic keratosis may be suspected. However, only histopathological examination of a deep biopsy can secure the diagnosis and definitely rule out malignancy.

3.5. Treatment. In general, the scientific work on the treatment of CNH lacks large, randomised, controlled studies. Historically, surgical excision (Table 3) has been more frequently investigated and the preferred treatment modality [1, 8, 22, 24, 26, 32–35, 39, 50]. Recently, however, more conservative methods have been investigated in an effort to avoid the discomfort of surgery, the risk of postoperative infections, and problems with wound healing and deformity (Table 1).

3.5.1. Pressure Relieving Padding. The repeated observation that CNH usually affects the ear on the preferred sleeping-side suggests that pressure on the ear is an important aetiological factor. This leads to the logical conclusion that relieving pressure on the ear will be a successful treatment. Seven studies, including 148 patients treated with pressure-relieving padding alone, were identified (Table 1). Many of the studies on other treatment modalities also recommend decompression of the ear after treatment, making this a major confounding factor. Half of the studies on pressure relieving padding were prospective, but none were randomized or

TABLE 1: Topical treatment.

First author and year	Number of patients	Method	Cure rate	Follow-up (mean)	Recurrence rate	Pros and cons
Pressure relieving padding						
Travelute 2013 [25]	10	Self-adhering foam	90%	Not reported	0	Retrospective. Follow-up not reported.
Naqash 2013 [59]	1	Ear-padding	Pain resolved	6 weeks	0	Case report. Short follow-up.
Kuen-Spiegl 2011 [9]	12 (18)	Bandage + foam plastic	92%	41–61 months	25% (but discontinued treatment)	Prospective. 6 did not comply.
Durrant 2011 [12]	75	Customized ear prosthesis	74%	52 months	31%	Prospective. Confounder with topical steroid.
Sanu 2007 [13]	23	Doughnut pillow	57%	12 months	0	Prospective. 7 did not comply.
Moncrieff 2004 [26]	15	Foam-padding strapped to head	87%	18 weeks	0	Retrospective. Short follow-up.
Timoney 2002 [14]	12	Different decompression methods	92%	24 months	8%	Prospective. Used several methods.
Topical nitroglycerin						
Sanz-Motilva 2015 [27]	29	0,2% topical nitroglycerin	93%	5,9 months	0,03%	Retrospective. Confounder with decompression.
Colmenero 2014 [15]	11	Transdermal nitroglycerin patch	64%	3 months	0	Prospective. Lack of histology.
Yélamos 2013 [48]	1	2% nitroglycerin gel	Good effect	4 months	0	Case report.
Flynn 2011 [28]	12 pt/13 lesions	2% topical nitroglycerin	92%	2–13 months	0 (within follow-up period)	Retrospective. Wide range of follow-up.
Glucocorticoid injection						
Cox 2002 [29]	60	1x triamcinolone intralesionally	40% 3 months/33% long-term	3–96 months	6%	Retrospective.

TABLE 1: Continued.

First author and year	Number of patients	Method	Cure rate	Follow-up (mean)	Recurrence rate	Pros and cons
Lawrence 1991 [8]	44	Triamcinolone, 0,2–0,5 mL intralesionally + topical betamethasone ×2 daily + lidocaine gel 2% before bed for 8 weeks	27% at 8 weeks	16 months (4,5–34)	Non-respondents went on to surgery. Respondents had 0 recurrence after 14 months	Prospective. Confounding therapies.
Schmidt 1984 [36]	3	Local infiltration with Prednisolon-crystal-suspension, 3–6 inj.	67%	1 week after last treatment	Not reported	Case series. No follow-up after last treatment.
Wade 1979 [16]	8	Intralesional inj. with triamcinolone	100%	0–12 months	0	Prospective. Unsure follow-up.
Injectable collagen						
Greenbaum 1991 [17]	5	Collagen inj. over perichondrium	100%	16 months	0	Prospective.

controlled. Several methods were described, including self-adhering foam behind the ear, foam bandages strapped to the head, and sleeping on a doughnut-shaped pillow. All aimed to provide a means for relieving the pressure on the affected area of the ear. The cure rate reported in the pure decompression studies was as low as 57% and as high as 92%. In 2011 Durrant et al. published a prospective study on 75 patients treated with a customised ear prosthesis [12] where 47% experienced complete resolution and 27% improvement. After more than 6 months, 31% experienced recurrence, but overall 91% of the patients avoided surgery [12]. Considering all the studies on pressure relieving padding, we conclude that this conservative treatment-approach is inexpensive and cost-effective but that the result depends very much on the compliance of the patient.

3.5.2. Topical Nitroglycerin.

As CNH may result from chondrial ischemia arising from perichondrial arteriolar narrowing and nitroglycerin causes relaxation and vasodilation of the arteriolar smooth muscle, this treatment may restore adequate blood flow to reverse the ischemic changes [15]. Four studies totalling 53 patients treated with topical nitroglycerin were identified (Table 1). Forty-two patients were treated with nitroglycerin gel applied once or twice daily for up to three months and 11 patients were treated with a transdermal nitroglycerin patch, 12 hours a day for two months. Of the latter, two patients stopped the treatment due to moderate headaches and one patient only had a partial response and later underwent surgery, leaving 64% who had a complete response. Of the former, a 93% and 92% cure rate was reported. Topical nitroglycerin is usually used in the treatment of angina pectoris or chronic anal fissures and the most common side effect is transient headaches. Skin irritation has also been reported. Due to the low systemic absorption from the ear, topical treatment should not cause any major side effects [15]. We conclude that this treatment modality shows promising results, but further studies, with larger numbers of patients, are needed.

3.5.3. Glucocorticoid Injection.

As explained above, the aetiology of CNH probably includes local inflammation secondary to a foreign body reaction. Glucocorticoids are potent anti-inflammatory agents and should be able to stop the local inflammation. Three studies on intralesional injection of glucocorticoid were identified, one prospective (Table 1). A study by Lawrence from 1991 was actually a study of the effectiveness of surgery, but 44 patients first received intralesional steroid injections and those who had not responded after 8 weeks (73%) were then offered surgery [8]. Also noteworthy is the study by Cox and Denham from 2002 [29], who retrospectively reported the outcomes of 60 patients treated with one dose of 0,1 mL of intralesional triamcinolone, demonstrating a 40% response at three months. Four patients later required a second injection and were then symptom-free. Another four patients had late recurrence, decreasing the long-term success rate to 33%, after follow-up of up to eight years [29]. Although this treatment is easy, fast, and

inexpensive, we do not feel it should be recommended as first line treatment, due to the low cure rates.

3.5.4. Injectable Collagen.

Greenbaum reported on the outcome of treatment for 5 patients in 1991, who received injections of collagen over the perichondrium to relieve pressure on the cartilage (Table 1). The cure rate was reported to be 100% after a follow-up period of 0–16 months [17]. However, such results are inconclusive due to the small number of patients and relative short period of follow-up.

3.5.5. PDT.

It is thought that PDT acts on several pathways involved in CNH: it has an anti-inflammatory and immunomodulatory action, an effect on vascularisation and on collagen and it may also have a chondroprotective effect [30]. Treatment with aminolevulinic acid- (ALA-) PDT seems to slow the inflammatory reaction in the skin, because of the death of the resident macrophages and mast cells and the slow recovery to cytokine responsiveness of the surviving cell population. Although it is generally accepted that PDT causes acute inflammation, it can also interrupt the process of chronic inflammation and stimulate healing [30]. It has been shown that blood perfusion is increased immediately after irradiation and this persists for up to one week. It has also been shown that chondrocytes are not destroyed, but that PDT modulates in vitro cartilage metabolism, activating a chondroprotective effect in photosensitized cartilage in the context of osteoarthritis [30]. Two studies, involving only seven patients treated with PDT, were identified (Table 2). Gilaberte et al. reported on five patients treated with PDT, after preparing the site with curettage to scrape away crusts, and so forth. The cure rate was reported to be 80%, although the period of follow-up was not reported [30]. These results should be considered inconclusive because of the very small numbers of patients treated and the limited follow-up.

3.5.6. CO_2 and Argon Laser.

Only two studies, comprising 14 patients, were identified [19, 38] (Table 2). Patients received treatment with a CO_2 laser and their wounds were allowed to heal by secondary intention. However, they were also instructed to decompress their ears for 3-4 weeks. The cure rate was reported as 100%, after a follow-up period of 2–24 months. One study reported on the outcomes of nine patients treated with argon laser, with a 56% cure rate [18]. The small number of patients in these studies makes it difficult to form any definite conclusion, though the high cure rates warrant further studies.

3.5.7. Curettage/Electrocauterization.

Kromann et al. published the most comprehensive study of a nonsurgical treatment for CNH in 1983 [21] (Table 2). They reported the outcomes of 142 cases during a 15-year period who were treated with curettage followed by electrocauterization. Fifteen patients also underwent treatment with radiotherapy after curettage. A further five patients were treated with radiotherapy alone, with no effect, and then proceeded to curettage with electrocauterization. An unknown number

TABLE 2: Physical therapies.

First author and year	Number of patients	Method	Cure rate	Follow-up (mean)	Recurrence rate	Pros and cons
		Photodynamic therapy (PDT)				
Pellegrino 2011 [37]	2	PDT	100%	9 months	0	Case report.
Gilaberte 2010 [30]	5	PDT + curretage	80%	Not reported	Not reported	Retrospective, confounder with curettage, follow-up not reported.
		Cryotherapy				
Senel 2010 [47]	1	Cryotherapy ×2	100%	12 months	0	Case report.
		Argon laser				
Hesse 1994 [18]	9 pts/16 lesions	Biopsy + argon laser for surface and underlying cartilage	56%	3–16 months	"No real recurrence" (4 patients with recurrence after 3–16 months, retreated)	Prospective.
		CO₂ laser				
Taylor 1991 [19]	11 pts/12 lesions	CO$_2$ laser to vaporize the cutaneous nodule and involved cartilage + decompression for 3-4 weeks	100%	2–15 months	0	Prospective. Confounder with decompression.
Karam 1988 [38]	3	CO$_2$ laser at 15 W	100%	24 months	0	Case series.
		Curettage/electrocauterization				
Kromann 1983 [21]	142	Curettage followed by electrocauterization	69%	7,1 years (average)	31%	Retrospective. Confounder with many other therapies.

received treatment with intralesional triamcinolone injections and freezing with carbon dioxide in addition to curettage. Seventy-eight patients were reexamined after an average of 7.1 years and 31% were found to have relapsed. An overall recurrence rate of 25% was reported, but after an unknown follow-up [21]. Although curettage appears to have an acceptable cure and recurrence rate, there are many confounding variables, making it difficult to know with certainty whether curettage alone was responsible for the "cures" achieved. Moreover, there have been no other studies of this treatment since 1983.

3.5.8. Surgery. Many techniques have been described and most agree that a simple approach, with primary excision and meticulous trimming of the cartilage, is the preferred method [8, 11, 22, 24, 26, 32–35, 39, 43, 50].

Seventeen surgical studies, including more than 500 patients, were reviewed (Table 3). The surgical techniques described include wide excision with reconstruction of the ear using local flaps, skin grafts, excision of the affected skin and underlying cartilage, and skin-sparing techniques with excision of the cartilage only.

The cure rates reported range from 66% to 100% with a recurrence rate of up to 38%. In this review, recurrences were most frequent at the edges of the cartilage defect. Therefore, later studies advised greater attention to careful trimming of all affected cartilage.

In 1991, Lawrence [8] described a surgical technique to remove only the affected cartilage under a skin flap. With a cure rate of 88% and a recurrence rate of 12% this technique proved to be as efficient as any other at the time and has since been described in various modifications in an effort to simplify the procedure [8].

In 2014, Kulendra et al. described a method used to treat 59 patients [31]. On the helix, a skin incision was made which was 2-3 times the diameter of the nodule, 1-2 mm wide, and tapered to a point. The nodule and adjacent area were excised and sent for histology. The exposed, raised cartilage was gradually removed at the centre, using a surgical blade, sharp-pointed-scissors, or a diamond burr. The wound was then closed directly with interrupted sutures. On the antihelix, access to the nodule was achieved through an anterior interhelical and inferior releasing incision, elevating a skin flap with perichondrium to expose the cartilage. The nodule and surrounding cartilage were excised, avoiding

TABLE 3: Surgical treatment.

First author and year	Method	Patients	Follow-up	Cure rate (%)	Recurrence rate	Pros and cons
Kulendra 2014 [31]	Excision of nodule + rim shave + direct suture + decompression	59 pt/65 lesions	85 months	88% for the helix and 89% for the antihelix	12% for the helix, 11 for the antihelix	Retrospective. Confounder with decompression.
Magliulo 2014 [3]	Excision + skin graft	1	12 months	100%	No recurrence	Case report. No history, no picture.
Feldman 2009 [1]	Wedge resection/circumferential excision of skin + underlying cartilage + skin graft	55 pt/62 lesions	Not reported	89%/96%	11% (infection) only 30% of these needed reexcision	Retrospective. No report of follow-up.
Hussain 2009 [22]	No skin excision, only nodule + trimming of cartilage	34	4 months	94%	0 (6% did not respond)	Retrospective.
Chan 2009 [49]	Surgically excised	2	12 months	100%	0	Case report.
Dreiman 2007 [7]	Wedge-incision w Antia Buch reconstruction.	1	8 months	100%	0	Case report.
Rajan 2007 [32]	Punch and graft technique	22 pt/23 lesions	1–86 months	83%	18%	Retrospective.
Tsung-Hua 2007 [43]	Excision of nodule + decompression	1	6 months	100%	0	Case report. Confounder with decompression.
Grigoryants 2007 [44]	Exc. of skin + cartilage + skin graft + decompression	1	6 months	100%	0	Case report. Confounding treatment modalities.
Rex 2006 [33]	Narrow elliptical skin excision + cartilage shaving	74	Helix: 54 (14–90) months Antihelix: 50 (11–78) months	Helix: 90% Antihelix: 63%	Helix: 11% Antihelix: 38%	Retrospective.
Jacob K 2005 [50]	Excision of cartilage (+ necrotic muscle)	1	6 months	100%	0	Case report surgical procedure not well described.
Moncrieff 2004 [26]	Excision biopsy of nodule, paring the underlying cartilage, foam-padding	41	77 (15–150) weeks	66%	34%	Retrospective review, confounding treatment modalities.
De Ru 2002 [34]	Skin-sparing cartilage resection. All previously treated with Kenacort inj.	34 pt/37 lesions	31 months (3–111)	92%	3%	Retrospective. Confounding treatment modalities.

Table 3: Continued.

First author and year	Method	Patients	Follow-up	Cure rate (%)	Recurrence rate	Pros and cons
Hudson-Peacock 1999 [24]	Punch biopsy + cartilage resection + shaving + suture of skin	77	52 (helix) + 55 (antihelix) months	84% (helix) 75% (antihelix)	Helix: 16% Antihelix: 25% (all in excision margin)	Retrospective.
Zuber 1999 [39]	Modified shave-technique followed by electrosurgical feathering	4	Not reported	Not reported	Not reported	No relevant information available.
Munnoch 1996 [35]	Minimal skin excision and extensive cartilage resection	50	37 months (18–78)	100%	0	Retrospective.
Lawrence 1991 [8]	Intralesional steroid therapy/excision of cartilage without skin excision	46	16 months	88%	12% (at excision margins)	Confounding treatment modalities.

sharp edges and removing any of the remaining antihelix to a height lower than the helix. The skin flap was then scarified and sutured back in place. These techniques resulted in a cure rate of 88% for the helix and 89% for the antihelix after a follow-up of 85 months [31].

Some authors stress the importance of sending material, including skin, for histology to confirm the diagnosis and rule out malignancy. Rajan and Langtry, 2007 [32], support this argument and recommend their "punch and graft technique" used on 22 patients with a cure rate of 83% after a follow-up of 1–86 months. A punch biopsy instrument, with a diameter large enough to encompass the lesion, was used to cut the skin and the underlying cartilage. The specimen was then excised with scissors or blade and sent for histology. The same punch tool was used to harvest a full thickness skin graft from the postauricular area and the graft fixed in place with 6-0 interrupted sutures [32].

4. Conclusion

Even though CNH is not life threatening, it can impair quality of life. The incidence and prevalence is not known, but the disease appears to be common. Historically, a preponderance for males has been reported but in this review, we found a more equal gender distribution.

The vasculitis/inflammatory theory is most widely supported and explains the development of the lesion by arteriolar narrowing in the perichondrium leading to ischemic changes in the cartilage, followed by necrosis and extrusion of the necrotic material. This theory is further supported by the effectiveness of therapies aimed at improvement of the blood supply and/or dilation of blood vessels. One such therapy is topical nitroglycerin, which shows promising results, but larger studies are still warranted.

Much attention has recently been paid to decompression therapy and this seems to be a cost-effective therapy with acceptable cure rates but obviously depends on the compliance of the patient.

Multiple other therapies have been investigated, but in order to establish guidelines for the best treatment of CNH, larger, prospective, controlled, and randomised long-term studies are still required.

Based on the available literature however, we suggest first-line treatment with decompression devices and only if these are not effective surgical treatment. The surgical method recommended should be with minimal skin excision, primarily for histology, excision of the affected cartilage with careful trimming of the cartilage edges, and when possible direct skin closure, otherwise a skin graft.

References

[1] A. L. Feldman, C. H. Manstein, M. E. Manstein, and A. Czulewicz, "Chondrodermatitis nodularis auricularis: a new name for an old disease," *Plastic and Reconstructive Surgery*, vol. 123, no. 1, pp. 25–26, 2009.

[2] N. H. Cox, "Posterior auricular chondrodermatitis nodularis," *Clinical & Experimental Dermatology*, vol. 27, no. 4, pp. 324–327, 2002.

[3] G. Magliulo, G. Iannella, V. Moretti, and M. Re, "Chondrodermatitis nodularis chronica and external auditory canal," *Otology and Neurotology*, vol. 35, no. 4, pp. e157–e158, 2014.

[4] M. Winkler, "Knötcehnformige Erkrankung am helix. Chondrodermatitis nodularis chronic helicis," *Archiv für Dermatologie und Syphilis*, vol. 121, no. 2, pp. 278–285, 1915.

[5] O. H. Foerster, "A painful nodular growth of the ear," *The Journal of Cutaneous Diseases*, vol. 36, pp. 154–156, 1918.

[6] O. H. Foerster, "Painful nodular growth of the ear," *Archives of Dermatology and Syphilology*, vol. 11, no. 2, pp. 149–165, 1925.

[7] B. B. Dreiman, "Chondrodermatitis nodularis chronica helicis treated with antia-buch reconstruction: review and case report," *Journal of Oral and Maxillofacial Surgery*, vol. 65, no. 7, pp. 1378–1382, 2007.

[8] C. M. Lawrence, "The treatment of chondrodermatitis nodularis with cartilage removal alone," *Archives of Dermatology*, vol. 127, no. 4, pp. 530–535, 1991.

[9] M. Kuen-Spiegl, G. Ratzinger, N. Sepp, and P. Fritsch, "Chondrodermatitis nodularis chronica helicis—a conservative therapeutic approach by decompression," *Journal der Deutschen Dermatologischen Gesellschaft*, vol. 9, no. 4, pp. 292–296, 2011.

[10] B. Cribier, Y. Scrivener, and B. Peltre, "Neural hyperplasia in chondrodermatitis nodularis chronica helicis," *Journal of the American Academy of Dermatology*, vol. 55, no. 5, pp. 844–848, 2006.

[11] C. M. Magro, G. E. Frambach, and A. N. Crowson, "Chondrodermatitis nodularis helicis as a marker of internal syndromes associated with microvascular injury," *Journal of Cutaneous Pathology*, vol. 32, no. 5, pp. 329–333, 2005.

[12] C. A. T. Durrant, H. Lloyd-Hughes, R. Worth, D. L. Allen, and J. Pereira, "Auricular pressure-relieving cushions for treatment of chondrodermatitis nodularis helicis: a series of 75 cases and a review of the literature," *European Journal of Plastic Surgery*, vol. 34, no. 1, pp. 41–44, 2011.

[13] A. Sanu, R. Koppana, and D. G. Snow, "Management of chondrodermatitis nodularis chronica helicis using a 'doughnut pillow'," *Journal of Laryngology and Otology*, vol. 121, no. 11, pp. 1096–1098, 2007.

[14] N. Timoney and P. M. Davison, "Management of chondrodermatitis helicis by protective padding: a series of 12 cases and a review of the literature," *British Journal of Plastic Surgery*, vol. 55, no. 5, pp. 387–389, 2002.

[15] C. G. Colmenero, E. M. García, G. B. Morente, and J. T. Sánchez, "Nitroglycerin patch for the treatment of chondrodermatitis nodularis helicis: a new therapeutic option," *Dermatologic Therapy*, vol. 27, no. 5, pp. 278–280, 2014.

[16] T. R. Wade, "Chondrodermatitis nodularis chronica helicis. A review with emphasis on steroid therapy," *Cutis*, vol. 24, no. 4, pp. 406–409, 1979.

[17] S. S. Greenbaum, "The treatment of chondrodermatitis nodularis chronica helicis with injectable collagen," *International Journal of Dermatology*, vol. 30, no. 4, pp. 291–294, 1991.

[18] G. Hesse, C. Schmoeckel, and A. Wichmann-Hesse, "Argon laser therapy for chondrodermatitis nodularis chronica helicis," *Hautarzt*, vol. 45, no. 4, pp. 222–224, 1994.

[19] M. B. Taylor, "Chondrodermatitis nodularis chronica helicis: successful treatment with the carbon dioxide laser," *Journal of Dermatologic Surgery and Oncology*, vol. 17, no. 11, pp. 862–864, 1991.

[20] C. Wettlé, F. Keller, F. Will, F. Lefebvre, and B. Cribier, "Chondrodermatitis nodularis chronica helicis: a descriptive study of 99 patients," *Annales de Dermatologie et de Venereologie*, vol. 140, no. 11, pp. 687–692, 2013.

[21] N. Kromann, H. Høyer, and F. Reymann, "Chondrodermatitis nodularis chronica helicis treated with curettage and electrocauterization: follow-up of a 15-year material," *Acta Dermato-Venereologica*, vol. 63, no. 1, pp. 85–87, 1983.

[22] W. Hussain and R. J. G. Chalmers, "Simplified surgical treatment of chondrodermatitis nodularis by cartilage trimming and sutureless skin closure," *British Journal of Dermatology*, vol. 160, no. 1, pp. 116–118, 2009.

[23] T. Upile, N. N. Patel, W. Jerjes, N. U. Singh, A. Sandison, and L. Michaels, "Advances in the understanding of chondrodermatitis nodularis chronica helices: the perichondrial vasculitis theory," *Clinical Otolaryngology*, vol. 34, no. 2, pp. 147–150, 2009.

[24] M. J. Hudson-Peacock, N. H. Cox, and C. M. Lawrence, "The long-term results of cartilage removal alone for the treatment of chondrodermatitis nodularis," *British Journal of Dermatology*, vol. 141, no. 4, pp. 703–705, 1999.

[25] C. R. Travelute, "Self-adhering foam: a simple method for pressure relief during sleep in patients with chondrodermatitis nodularis helicis," *Dermatologic Surgery*, vol. 39, no. 2, pp. 317–319, 2013.

[26] M. Moncrieff and E. M. Sassoon, "Effective treatment of chondrodermatitis nodularis chronica helicis using a conservative approach," *British Journal of Dermatology*, vol. 150, no. 5, pp. 892–894, 2004.

[27] V. Sanz-Motilva, A. Martorell-Calatayud, C. G. García-Rodrigo et al., "The usefulness of 0.2% topical nitroglycerin for chondrodermatitis nodularis helicis," *Actas Dermo-Sifiliográficas*, vol. 106, no. 7, pp. 555–561, 2015.

[28] V. Flynn, C. Chisholm, and R. Grimwood, "Topical nitroglycerin: a promising treatment option for chondrodermatitis nodularis helicis," *Journal of the American Academy of Dermatology*, vol. 65, no. 3, pp. 531–536, 2011.

[29] N. H. Cox and P. F. Denham, "Intralesional triamcinolone for chondrodermatitis nodularis: a follow-up study of 60 patients," *British Journal of Dermatology*, vol. 146, no. 4, pp. 712–718, 2002.

[30] Y. Gilaberte, M. P. Frias, and J. B. Pérez-Lorenz, "Chondrodermatitis nodularis helicis successfully treated with photodynamic therapy," *Archives of Dermatology*, vol. 146, no. 10, pp. 1080–1082, 2010.

[31] K. Kulendra, T. Upile, F. Salim, T. O'Connor, A. Hasnie, and D. E. Phillips, "Long-term recurrence rates following excision and cartilage rim shave of chondrodermatitis nodularis chronica helicis and antihelicis," *Clinical Otolaryngology*, vol. 39, no. 2, pp. 121–126, 2014.

[32] N. Rajan and J. A. A. Langtry, "The punch and graft technique: a novel method of surgical treatment for chondrodermatitis nodularis helicis," *British Journal of Dermatology*, vol. 157, no. 4, pp. 744–747, 2007.

[33] J. Rex, M. Ribera, I. Bielsa, C. Mangas, A. Xifra, and C. Ferrándiz, "Narrow elliptical skin excision and cartilage shaving

for treatment of chondrodermatitis nodularis," *Dermatologic Surgery*, vol. 32, no. 3, pp. 400–404, 2006.

[34] J. A. De Ru, P. J. F. M. Lohuis, H. A. Saleh, and H. D. Vuyk, "Treatment of chondrodermatitis nodularis with removal of the underlying cartilage alone: retrospective analysis of experience in 37 lesions," *Journal of Laryngology and Otology*, vol. 116, no. 9, pp. 677–681, 2002.

[35] D. A. Munnoch, K. J. Herbert, and A. M. Morris, "Chondrodermatitis nodularis chronica helicis et antihelicis," *British Journal of Plastic Surgery*, vol. 49, no. 7, pp. 473–476, 1996.

[36] C. Schmidt, H. Heise, and H. Flegel, "Treatment of chronic nodular chondrodermatitis helicis with a suspension of prednisolone crystals," *Dermatologische Monatsschrift*, vol. 170, no. 3, pp. 181–182, 1984.

[37] M. Pellegrino, P. Taddeucci, S. Mei, C. Peccianti, and M. Fimiani, "Chondrodermatitis nodularis chronica helicis and photodynamic therapy: a new therapeutic option?" *Dermatologic Therapy*, vol. 24, no. 1, pp. 144–147, 2011.

[38] F. Karam and T. Bauman, "Carbon dioxide laser treatment for chondrodermatitis nodularis chronica helicis," *Ear, Nose and Throat Journal*, vol. 67, no. 10, pp. 757–763, 1988.

[39] T. J. Zuber and E. Jackson, "Chondrodermatitis nodularis chronica helicis," *Archives of Family Medicine*, vol. 8, no. 5, pp. 445–447, 1999.

[40] R. R. Kaur, A. D. Lee, and S. R. Feldman, "Bilateral chondrodermatitis nodularis chronica helicis on the antihelix in an elderly woman," *International Journal of Dermatology*, vol. 49, no. 4, pp. 472–474, 2010.

[41] S. Oelzner and P. Elsner, "Bilateral chondrodermatitis nodularis chronica helicis on the free border of the helix in a woman," *Journal of the American Academy of Dermatology*, vol. 49, no. 4, pp. 720–722, 2003.

[42] U. Khurana, L. S. Solanki, and M. Dhingra, "A man with painful nodules on both ears," *JAMA Otolaryngology-Head & Neck Surgery*, vol. 141, no. 5, pp. 481–482, 2015.

[43] T. Tsung-Hua, L. Yang-Chih, and C. Hsiu-Chin, "Infantile chondrodermatitis nodularis," *Pediatric Dermatology*, vol. 24, no. 3, pp. 337–339, 2007.

[44] V. Grigoryants, H. Qureshi, J. W. Patterson, and K. Y. Lin, "Pediatric chondrodermatitis nodularis helicis," *Journal of Craniofacial Surgery*, vol. 18, no. 1, pp. 228–231, 2007.

[45] N. E. Rogers, P. K. Farris, and A. R. Wang, "Juvenile Chondrodermatitis Nodularis Helicis: a case report and literature review," *Pediatric Dermatology*, vol. 20, no. 6, pp. 488–490, 2003.

[46] A. Ortiz, P. Martín, J. Domínguez, and J. Coneo-Mir, "Cell phone-induced chondrodermatitis nodularis antihelicis," *Actas Dermo-Sifiliográficas*, vol. 106, no. 8, pp. 675–676, 2015.

[47] E. Senel, "Chondrodermatitis nodularis chronica helicis," *Clinical Medicine Insights: Dermatology*, vol. 3, pp. 11–13, 2010.

[48] O. Yélamos, J. Dalmau, and L. Puig, "Chondrodermatitis nodularis helicis: successful treatment with 2% nitroglycerin gel," *Actas Dermo-Sifiliográficas*, vol. 104, no. 6, pp. 531–532, 2013.

[49] H. P. Chan, I. M. Neuhaus, and H. I. Maibach, "Chondrodermatitis nodularis chronica helicis in monozygotic twins," *Clinical and Experimental Dermatology*, vol. 34, no. 3, pp. 358–359, 2009.

[50] J. Jacob K, S. Satheesh, P. Menon, and K. G. Saju, "Winkler's disease," *Indian Journal of Otolaryngology and Head and Neck Surgery*, vol. 57, no. 4, pp. 323–324, 2005.

[51] P. K. Jain and S. Jain, "Use of disposable curette in the treatment of Chondrodermatitis Nodularis Helicis," *Clinical Otolaryngology*, vol. 30, no. 1, pp. 75–76, 2005.

[52] P. Ormond and P. Collins, "Modified surgical excision for the treatment of chondrodermatitis nodularis," *Dermatologic Surgery*, vol. 30, no. 2, pp. 208–210, 2004.

[53] D. Long and M. E. Maloney, "Surgical pearl: surgical planing in the treatment of chondrodermatitis nodularis chronica helicis of the antihelix," *Journal of the American Academy of Dermatology*, vol. 35, no. 5, pp. 761–762, 1996.

[54] B. M. Coldiron, "The surgical management of chondrodermatitis nodularis chronica helicis," *Journal of Dermatologic Surgery and Oncology*, vol. 17, no. 11, pp. 902–904, 1991.

[55] N. M. Bruns, S. Hessam, K. Valavanis, L. Scholl, and F. G. Bechara, "Surgical treatment of chondrodermatitis nodularis helicis via a retroauricular incision," *Journal der Deutschen Dermatologischen Gesellschaft*, vol. 13, no. 10, pp. 1049–1051, 2015.

[56] M. M. C. Yaneza and S. Sheikh, "Chondrodermatitis nodularis chronica helicis excision and reconstruction," *Journal of Laryngology and Otology*, vol. 127, no. 1, pp. 63–64, 2013.

[57] A. B. Cognetta Jr., C. M. Wolfe, W. H. Green, and H. K. Hatfield, "Triangular window technique: a novel approach for the surgical treatment of chondrodermatitis nodularis helicis," *Dermatologic Surgery*, vol. 38, no. 11, pp. 1859–1862, 2012.

[58] V. N. Sehgal and N. Singh, "Chondrodermatitis nodularis," *The American Journal of Otolaryngology—Head and Neck Medicine and Surgery*, vol. 30, no. 5, pp. 331–336, 2009.

[59] M. M. Naqash and S. A. Salati, "Chondrodermatitis nodularis chronica helicis—a review," *Journal of Pakistan Association of Dermatologists*, vol. 23, no. 3, pp. 320–326, 2013.

[60] G. Wagner, J. Liefeith, and M. M. Sachse, "Clinical appearance, differential diagnoses and therapeutical options of chondrodermatitis nodularis chronica helicis Winkler," *Journal of the German Society of Dermatology*, vol. 9, no. 4, pp. 287–291, 2011.

[61] M. Singh, A. Wilson, and S. Parkinson, "Two non-surgical treatments for chondrodermatitis nodularis helicis," *British Journal of Oral and Maxillofacial Surgery*, vol. 47, no. 4, pp. 327–328, 2009.

[62] K. Halter, "Zur Pathogenese der Chondrodermatitis nodularis chron. helicis," *Dermatology*, vol. 73, no. 5, pp. 270–284, 1936.

36

Bilateral Breast Reconstruction with Abdominal Free Flaps: A Single Centre, Single Surgeon Retrospective Review of 55 Consecutive Patients

Peter McAllister,[1] Isabel Teo,[1] Kuen Chin,[1] Boikanyo Makubate,[2] and David Alexander Munnoch[1]

[1]Department of Plastic and Reconstructive Surgery, Ninewells Hospital and Medical School, Dundee DD1 9SE, UK
[2]Department of Public Health, Faculty of Medicine, University of Botswana, Gabarone, Botswana

Correspondence should be addressed to Peter McAllister; pmcallister2@nhs.net

Academic Editor: Nicolo Scuderi

Breast reconstruction using free tissue transfer is an increasingly utilised oncoplastic procedure. The aim was to review all bilateral breast reconstructions using abdominal free flaps by a single surgeon over an 11-year period (2003–2014). A retrospective review was performed on all patients who underwent bilateral breast reconstruction using abdominal free flaps between 2003 and 2014 by the senior author (DAM). Data analysed included patient demographics, indication for reconstruction, surgical details, and complications. Fifty-five female patients (mean 48.6 years [24–71 years]) had bilateral breast reconstruction. The majority (41, 74.5%) underwent immediate reconstruction and DIEP flaps were utilised on 41 (74.5%) occasions. Major surgical complications occurred in 6 (10.9%) patients, all of which were postoperative vascular compromise of the flap. Failure to salvage the reconstruction occurred on 3 (5.5%) occasions resulting in a total flap failure rate of 2.7%. Obesity (>30 kg/m^2) and age > 60 years were shown to have a statistically increased risk of developing postoperative complications ($P < 0.05$). Our experience demonstrates that abdominal free flaps for bilateral breast reconstruction fares well, with a flap failure rate of 2.7%. Increased body mass index and patient age (>60 years) were associated with higher complication rates.

1. Introduction

In recent years, the number of bilateral breast reconstruction procedures has been increasing. This is a reflection of advancements in breast cancer screening and diagnosis supplemented by a desire for prophylactic surgery on the contralateral side. Positive genetic markers for BRCA confer an 85% lifetime risk of breast cancer, making this group of patients highly suitable for prophylactic mastectomies and reconstruction [1–4].

The options for reconstructing a breast mound following mastectomy include implants with or without autologous tissue flaps and can be performed at the time of the mastectomy (immediate) or at a later stage (delayed). Expanders and implants are a popular choice of breast reconstruction; however, the aesthetic outcomes are known to deteriorate with time, particularly in the context of radiation therapy [5–8].

The 2011 National Mastectomy and Breast Reconstruction audit, in which 8,159 women were sent patient satisfaction questionnaires, identified superior reported outcomes in patients who had received autologous tissue reconstruction compared to those with implant only reconstruction.

There are various choices of flaps for both pedicled and free flap breast reconstruction. Common pedicled options include the latissimus dorsi flap and the pedicled transverse rectus abdominis myocutaneous (TRAM) flap. The former is a reliable and robust flap but often requires an implant to augment the breast mound. The pedicled TRAM has traditionally been the workhorse for autologous breast reconstruction but is associated with higher rates of fat necrosis and abdominal wall hernia compared to free abdominal flap surgery. The free TRAM (where a small amount of muscle between the perforators and main pedicle is taken with flap harvest) has a role in certain patients but is known to have poorer outcomes compared to the muscle-preserving DIEP perforator technique which is associated with minimal functional loss and less postoperative pain [5–8]. The superficial inferior epigastric artery (SIEA) flap supplies less skin and fat abdominal tissue than the DIEP flap and is not always present [9].

The DIEP flap is currently widely regarded as the gold standard for breast reconstruction. It preserves the underlying musculofascial layer which reduces postoperative pain, duration of hospital admission, and long term donor site morbidity [10–12].

The superior cosmetic outcomes and acceptable morbidity rates of abdominal free flaps for unilateral breast reconstruction have been well published; however, the literature on bilateral procedures is limited.

The aim of this study was to review our experience with bilateral abdominal free flap reconstruction, analyse patient demographic and surgical data, and identify potential risk factors which may predispose to postoperative complications.

2. Materials and Methods

A retrospective case note review was performed of patients who had undergone free abdominal tissue transfer for bilateral breast reconstruction between August 2003 and February 2014. The list of patients was identified through a contemporaneous logbook of the senior author.

Patient demographic information including age, medical history, tobacco use, weight (body mass index (BMI) (kg/m^2)), and family and genetic history for breast cancer were recorded.

Surgical data included indication for breast resection (therapeutic or prophylactic), reconstructive timing, type of abdominal flap harvested, ischaemic time, recipient vessels, flap size, and hospital stay. Adjuvant radiotherapy and/or chemotherapy were also documented.

Data on complications of surgery were reviewed. Complications were classified as early (occurring within seven days of initial surgery) or late (occurring seven days after initial surgery).

The unit of investigation for data relating to the flap was the number of flaps (percentages). All other data were described as number of patients (percentages). Chi-squared tests for trend were used to compare 2 (two) groups. Chi-squared P values of less than 0.05 were considered significant. All statistical analyses were performed with IBM SPSS Statistics Version 22.0. (IBM Corp. (2013)) [13].

3. Surgical Technique

The majority of patients underwent standard DIEP flap reconstruction but the following may differ between units.

3.1. Preoperative. All patients are assessed at a preoperative anaesthetic assessment clinic approximately one month before surgery. They are admitted one day before surgery and seen by the senior author. A handheld Doppler probe is used to map potential perforators. We do not employ the routine use of CT-angiography. Preoperative low molecular weight heparin is not given and tamoxifen is not stopped prior to surgery.

3.2. Anaesthetic Considerations. Following intubation, all patients receive an arterial line and urinary catheter to monitor cardiovascular status. The abdominal flap edges are infiltrated with local anaesthetic and adrenaline. The mixture used is 60 mLs of 0.9% saline with 40 mLs of 0.5% levobupivicaine and 1 mL of 1 : 1000 adrenaline. Pneumatic compression stockings are utilised and patients receive intravenous Flucloxacillin on induction (clindamycin for patients with a Penicillin allergy).

3.3. Surgery. The patient is prepped with Betadine and a minimum of two surgeons operate simultaneously, the senior author and a trainee. In immediate cases, the contralateral flap is raised as the breast surgeon performs the mastectomy, with or without axillary node clearance. The mastectomies performed are commonly skin sparing. The superficial inferior epigastric vessels, if present, are routinely harvested prior to identifying DIEP perforators. Often two perforators are harvested and motor nerves preserved. The decision to use lateral or medial row perforators is made intraoperatively depending on location and size. The recipient vessels of choice, usually the internal mammary artery and vein, are exposed by removing the third intercostal cartilage. Anastomoses are performed end to end with 9/0 Ethilon. Venous couplers and intraoperative anticoagulants are not used. Two drains are placed in each breast pocket and one drain is placed on each side of the abdomen.

3.4. Postoperative Care. All patients return to a single room on the high dependency unit (HDU) and have hourly clinical flap observations overnight. All patients receive 24 hours of intravenous Flucloxacillin and 2500 units of low molecular weight heparin (LMWH) twice daily. Progressive mobilisation is encouraged and drains are kept until the patient is mobile with less than 30 mLs in 24 hours.

4. Results

The medical records of 55 consecutive patients (mean age 48 years, range 24–71 years) undergoing simultaneous bilateral breast reconstruction surgery with abdominal autologous free flaps ($n = 110$) were reviewed. The average follow-up to the time of this study was 46.1 (4–130) months. Patient demographics are provided in Table 1.

The majority of patients (41; 75%) underwent immediate reconstruction, 8 (15%) had a delayed reconstruction, and 6 (11%) had an immediate reconstruction unilaterally and a delayed reconstruction contralaterally. Surgical data are illustrated in Table 2.

Therapeutic surgery for unilateral or bilateral disease accounted for 45 (81.8%) patient breast resections. Invasive ductal carcinoma (22; 54%) and ductal carcinoma in situ (DCIS) (6; 15%) were most frequently encountered.

In this series, 12 (22%) patients were BRCA positive, and 12 (22%) had a strong family history of breast cancer

TABLE 1: Demographics of patients undergoing bilateral breast reconstruction.

Number of patients/flaps	*55/110*
Average age (years)	48.6 (24–71)
Average BMI (kg/m^2)	28.1 (21–37)
Patients with medical comorbidities* (%)	16 (29)
Previous abdominal surgery (%)	25 (45)
Smokers (%)	7 (13)
Ex-smokers (%)	8 (15)
No family history of breast cancer** and BRCA negative with disease	31 (56)
Family history of breast cancer (BRCA negative) (%)	12 (22)
Family history of breast cancer with known disease (%)	7 (13)
Family history of breast cancer with no known disease (%)	5 (9.1)
BRACA gene positive (%)	12 (22)
BRACA positive with known disease	7 (13)
BRACA positive with no known disease	5 (9.1)

* As per American Society of Anaesthesiology (ASA) II classification.
** First-degree relative.

(disease affecting a first-degree female relative) but were BRCA negative and 31 (56%) had no known familial or genetic risk factors.

Of the BRCA positive patients, 7 (13%) underwent unilateral therapeutic and contralateral prophylactic resection and 5 (9%) had bilateral prophylactic (risk reducing) mastectomies. Of the patients with a strong familial history (BRCA negative), 7 (13%) underwent unilateral therapeutic and contralateral prophylactic surgery and 5 (9%) patients requested bilateral prophylactic resection of breast tissue in the absence of identifiable pathology (Table 1).

Complications were classified as early (occurring within seven days of initial surgery) or late (occurring more than seven days after initial surgery). Forty-two patients (76%) experienced one or more early or late complications of flap, donor site, or both. All early complications ($n = 6$) were vascular problems of the free flap and all of these underwent immediate surgical exploration (Table 3). Three flaps were salvaged and three eventually failed and required surgical debridement. The most common late complication in the breast/flap site was native breast skin necrosis 12 (11%) and the most common late complication of the donor site was wound dehiscence 23 (41%). This is shown in Table 4.

We performed analysis of risk factors to identify potential predisposing features that may increase risk of complications. Specifically we analysed smoking, raised BMI, previous abdominal surgery, age, flap weight, and ischaemic time and adjuvant radiation therapy.

There were 15 patients who were active or ex-smokers, and this risk factor was not found to statistically increase the risk of overall complications ($P = 0.118$).

Obese patients were found to have increased risk of complications. Of 19 (35%) patients with a BMI greater than

TABLE 2: Surgical data for patients undergoing bilateral breast reconstruction.

	n (%)
Therapeutic surgery (known disease)	45 (82)
Prophylactic surgery (no known disease)	10 (18)
Immediate reconstruction	41 (75)
After prophylactic mastectomy	8 (15)
After therapeutic mastectomy	33 (60)
Delayed reconstruction, mean delay (years)	8 (15)
After prophylactic mastectomy	2 (3.6)
After therapeutic mastectomy	6 (11)
Immediate/delayed	6 (11)
Abdominal donor	55 (100)
DIEP	41 (75)
TRAM	7 (13)
SIEA	1 (1.8)
Combination	6 (11)
Average ischaemic time (mins)	68.57
Recipient vein	
Internal mammary	100 (90)
Serratus	4 (3.6)
Thoracodorsal	2 (1.8)
Additional perforator	4 (3.6)
Recipient artery	
Internal mammary	106 (96)
Serratus	2 (1.8)
Thoracodorsal	2 (1.8)
Average flap size (g)	692.25
Peri/post-op blood transfusion	8 (15)
Average hospital stay (days)	7.5
Average follow-up (months)	46.1
Adjuvant chemotherapy only	8 (15)
Adjuvant radiotherapy only	6 (11)
Adjuvant chemoradiotherapy	23 (42)

TABLE 3: Early complications requiring unplanned surgical intervention.

	Number (%)
Total	*6/110*
Vascular complications	6 (5.4)
Anastomotic venous complication	5
Anastomotic arterial complication	1
Partial flap failure	1
Total flap failure	3 (2.7)

or equal to 30 kg/m^2, 15 (78.9%) ($P = 0.019$) experienced flap complications, donor site complications, or both. This is in contrast to the group of patients with a BMI < 30 kg/m^2 where flap/and or complication rate was 19 (53%).

Increasing age was associated with increased complications. The majority of patients (47; 85%) were under 60 years of age, and, of eight patients older than 60 years, 6 (75%)

TABLE 4: Late complications.

	Number (%)
Breast/flap complications	18/110 (16.4)
Native breast necrosis	12 (11)
Fat necrosis	4 (3.6)
Seroma	1 (0.9)
Haematoma	1
Donor site complications	23/55 (42)
Dehiscence	13 (24)
Seroma	5 (9.1)
Hernia	1 (1.8)
Hypertrophic scarring	2 (3.6)
Lymphedema	1 (1.8)
Late donor site complications requiring surgery	1 (1.8)
Recurrence/metastasis	3 (5.4)

experienced flap and/or abdominal complications postoperatively. There was a statistically increased risk of abdominal wound dehiscence (2/8, 25%, $P = 0.02$) and native breast skin necrosis (2/8, 25%, $P = 0.039$) in this >60-year-old subgroup.

The weight of the flaps did not appear to affect complication rates and ranged in size from 280 g to 1200 g. Of 21 patients (38%) who had at least one flap exceeding 700 g in weight, 15 (71%, $P = 0.078$) experienced flap and/or abdominal complications of surgery but this was not regarded statistically significant.

In addition, flap ischaemic time did not appear to statistically affect complication rates. Ischaemic time, greater than 90 minutes for one or both sides, occurred in 17 (31%) patients, of which 12 (71%) ($P = 0.143$) encountered early or late flap complications.

Previous abdominal surgery did not have an effect on complication rates. Previous abdominal surgery was documented on 12 (22%) occasions and 4 (33%, $P = 0.388$) of these developed a degree of wound dehiscence postoperatively.

Radiation therapy was utilised in 29 (53%) patients (Table 2). Chest wall radiotherapy predating breast reconstruction was used in 15 (27%) patients. Time delay following radiotherapy to reconstruction varied from six months to 16 years and two (4%) patients experienced vascular complications of the venous anastomoses, one intraoperatively and one postoperatively. On surgical exploration, one was reanastomosed to the internal mammary vessels with no complications. One flap was anastomosed to the lateral chest wall vessels due to a concern regarding the original recipient chest wall vessel; this flap underwent partial flap failure.

Adjuvant radiotherapy after reconstruction was used in 14 (25%) patients with a mean duration of nine weeks following surgery. One patient experienced a significant loss of breast volume as a consequence of radiation treatment and underwent lipofilling to restore breast bulk. There were no other complications reported in this patient group.

Flap complications, abdominal complications, and associated risk factors are demonstrated in Tables 5 and 6, respectively. No patient encountered systemic complications as a consequence of reconstructive breast surgery. There were no pulmonary emboli, deep vein thrombosis, or sepsis events.

At the most recent follow-up, 30 (55%) patients had underwent further elective surgery, with nipple tattoo or nipple reconstruction accounting for half of these procedures. Three (5.4%) patients had been diagnosed with recurrent or metastatic disease and one (1.8%) was recently deceased secondary to fulminant heart failure.

5. Discussion

The use of abdominal donor perforator free flaps for breast reconstruction is widely advocated, with the DIEP flap heralded as the gold standard for breast reconstruction. This technique preserves the abdominal musculofascial system and is recognised as providing a favourable aesthetic outcome with low donor site morbidity (Figure 1) [14, 20]. The use of the DIEP flap in unilateral breast reconstruction is accepted and known to provide excellent cosmetic results and an acceptable morbidity profile. However, the literature on bilateral DIEP procedures is limited. A literature search identified only six similar publications reporting a bilateral DIEP series (Table 7). As illustrated, our early complications associated with flap vascularity (11%) (0%–12.5%), partial flap failure (1.8%) (0%–3.6%), and total flap failure (5.4%) (0%–9.6%) are comparable with previous studies [14–19].

In our study, 42 patients (76%) experienced one or more early or late complications of flap, donor site, or both.

All early complications ($n = 6$) involved vascular compromise of the flap and all of these required immediate surgical intervention; five of these underwent reanastomosis and three were salvaged. One patient's anastomosis was found to have active flow during reexploration and reanastomosis was not carried out. Anastomotic venous complication occurred in all but 1 case. Of the failed flaps, two were venous and one was arterial in origin and all of these had a failed reanastomosis (Table 3). Venous anastomotic compromise occurred more commonly than those of arterial origin, a finding in keeping with similar literature [21, 22].

TABLE 5: Flap complications and associated risk factors.

	Native breast necrosis n (%)	P value	Fat necrosis n (%)	P value	Corrected vascular problem n (%)	P value	Partial/total flap failure n (%)	P value
Smoker/ex-smoker	7/15 (47)	0.774	2/15 (13)	1.000	0/3	0.250	2/15 (13)	1.000
Nonsmoker	5/40 (13)		2/40 (5)		3/3 (100)		2/40 (5)	
High BMI	8/19 (42)	0.388	1/19 (5.2)	0.625	1/19 (5.2)	1.000	2/19 (11)	1.000
Normal BMI	4/36 (11)		3/36 (8.3)		2/36 (5.6)		2/36 (5.6)	
Age > 60	2/8 (25)	0.039	0	0.125	0	0.250	0	0.125
Age < 60	10/47 (21)		4/47 (8.5)		3/47 (6.4)		4/47 (8.5)	
Flap > 700 g	4/21 (19)	0.388	2/21 (9.5)	1.000	2/21 (9.5)	1.000	2/21 (9.5)	1.000
Flap < 700 g	8/34 (24)		2/34 (5.9)		1/34 (2.9)		2/34 (5.9)	
Ischaemic time > 90 (mins)	5/17 (29)	0.774	1/17 (5.9)	0.625	2/17 (12)	1.000	2/17 (12)	1.000
Ischaemic time < 90 (mins)	7/38 (18)		3/38 (7.9)		1/38 (2.6)		2/38 (5.3)	

TABLE 6: Donor site (abdomen) complications and associated risk factors.

	Dehiscence n (%)	P value	Seroma n (%)	P value
Smoker/ex-smoker	5/15 (33)	0.581	1/15 (6.7)	0.375
Nonsmoker	8/40 (20)		4/40 (10)	
High BMI	7/19 (37)	1.000	4/19 (21)	0.375
Normal BMI	6/36 (17)		1/36 (2.8)	
Previous abdominal surgery	4/12 (33)	0.267	0	n/a
No previous abdominal surgery	9/43 (21)		0	n/a
Age > 60	2/8 (25)	0.022	1/8 (13)	0.375
Age < 60	11/47 (23)		4/47 (8.5)	
Flap > 700 g	8/21 (38)	0.581	2/21 (9.5)	1.000
Flap < 700 g	5/34 (15)		3/34 (8.8)	

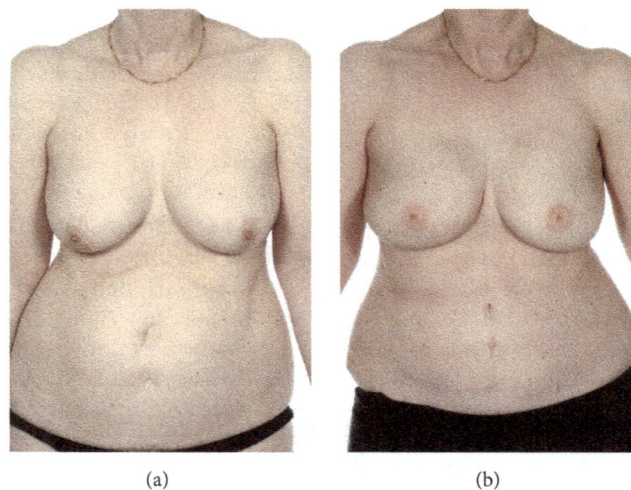

(a)   (b)

FIGURE 1: ((a) Preoperative; (b) postoperative breast and nipple reconstruction) 56-year-old with invasive ductal carcinoma underwent bilateral mastectomy and immediate bilateral DIEP reconstruction and delayed nipple reconstruction (consent obtained to use photographs).

TABLE 7: Complication rates in comparative bilateral breast reconstruction literature [1].

Study	N	TFF n^* (%)	PFF n^* (%)	VC n^* (%)	FN n^* (%)	H n^* (%)	AS n (%)	AH n (%)
Guerra et al. [14]	140	0	5 (3.6)	7 (5)	30 (21.4)	—	30 (21.4)	3 (2.1)
Scheer et al. [15]	32	2 (6.3)	1 (3.1)	4 (12.5)	12 (37.5)	3 (9.4)	0	4 (12.5)
Hofer et al. [16]	44	1 (2.3)	1 (2.3)	2 (4.6)	4 (9.1)	2 (4.6)	—	—
Drazan et al. [17]	55	0	—	0	2 (3.6)	4 (7.3)	2 (3.6)	—
Rao et al. [18]	114	11 (9.6)	—	—	—	—	—	—
Schaverien et al. [19]	10	0	0	0	1 (10)	—	0	0
Our study	55	3 (5.4)	1 (1.8)	6 (10.9)	4 (7.3)	1 (1.8)	5 (5.4)	0

TFF: total flap failure; PFF: partial flap failure; VC: vascular complications; FN: fat necrosis of flap; H: haematoma of flap; AS: abdominal seroma; and AH-abdominal hernia.
*Unit of investigation is the "patient" and not the "flap" as per previous tables.

Factor V Leiden (FVL) genetic mutation was subsequently identified in one patient with total flap failure following haematological investigation. Reports of free flap thrombosis in this group of patients leading to total or partial flap loss have previously been published [23, 24]. FVL is the most common inherited cause of hypercoagulability and leads to resistance of activated protein C leading to an increased risk of thrombotic events [25]. The prevalence of FVL is between 2% and 10% in the Caucasian population [26]. A personal or family history of unexplained thrombosis should raise the suspicion of FLV. It has been suggested that a preoperative thrombophilia screen in high risk patients should be carried out and consideration should be given for pedicled rather than free flap reconstruction in this group of patients [25, 26].

Our first total flap failure (2005) precluded routine haematological investigation for thrombophilia which is now routine following vascular compromise of the flap. However, the substantial size of flap (1200 g) may have contributed to its vascular compromise and failure. A negative thrombophilia screen was noted in the third patient and no obvious cause of flap failure has subsequently been identified.

In similar works, late complications are inconsistently defined and variably reported which makes comparison difficult [1]. Our late complication rate may be attributed to frequent outpatient follow-up over a long period of time (mean 46.1 months). Previous comparable studies had a shorter follow-up period (mean 14.6–32.1 months) [14, 16, 18]. Another possible contributing factor which may account for the late complications observed is the higher mean BMI ($28.1 \, \mathrm{kg/m^2}$) and/or increased active or recent tobacco usage (27.2%) in our cohort of patients compared with analogous literature on bilateral breast reconstruction [14–19].

Active or recent tobacco use was associated with late complications of the flap, including native breast skin necrosis, fat necrosis, and flap failure.

Guerra et al. [14] did not find a significant increased risk of fat necrosis or flap loss in smokers but did report an increased risk of breast wound dehiscence in this group of patients. Gill et al. [27] reviewed 758 unilateral and bilateral DIEP flaps and identified an increased risk of donor site complications in patients using tobacco. In contrast, our study donor site complication rates were not statistically significant among the smoking patient cohort.

Obesity is associated with an almost 12-fold increased risk of postoperative complications after breast surgery. Obese women often have bigger breasts which require a larger abdominal donor graft to be harvested. Further complications include delayed wound healing and longer postoperative recovery periods [28, 29].

The link between patient obesity and flap size is reflected in the observed rate of flap and/or abdominal complications in flaps exceeding 700 grams which was increased although not statistically significant ($P = 0.078$). Interestingly, a similar correlation between BMI, increased flap size, and overall complication rates was not identified by previous research on bilateral breast reconstruction [14].

The most common late complications of flap and donor site were native breast skin necrosis (12/110; 11%) and abdominal wound dehiscence (13/55; 24%), respectively (Figure 2). Patients aged 60 years or older were noted to have a statistically increased risk of developing these postoperative complications (Tables 5 and 6). Concomitant disease and decreased physical function are associated with higher levels of surgical morbidity in elderly patients undergoing breast surgery [30] and this is endorsed by the findings of this study.

Complications associated with radiotherapy in the context of autologous breast reconstruction are a topic of debate [31–35].

In our series of bilateral free tissue reconstructions, two patients with preoperative chest wall irradiation experienced vascular problems of the flap, one salvaged with no complications and one salvaged with partial flap failure. Overall complication rate in this patient cohort was not statistically significant. This finding is in keeping with Berry et al. [31] who on multivariate analysis identified no statistical difference in rates of complications between patients receiving preoperative radiation therapy and those who did not.

In those patients undergoing postoperative radiotherapy, only one patient was observed to have a reduction in breast volume following adjuvant therapy. No other complications were observed. This is similar to work by Chatterjee and coworkers [32] who concluded that postoperative radiotherapy did not significantly affect breast volume after reconstruction.

Overall complication rate in patients who had chest wall irradiation after autologous breast reconstruction in our

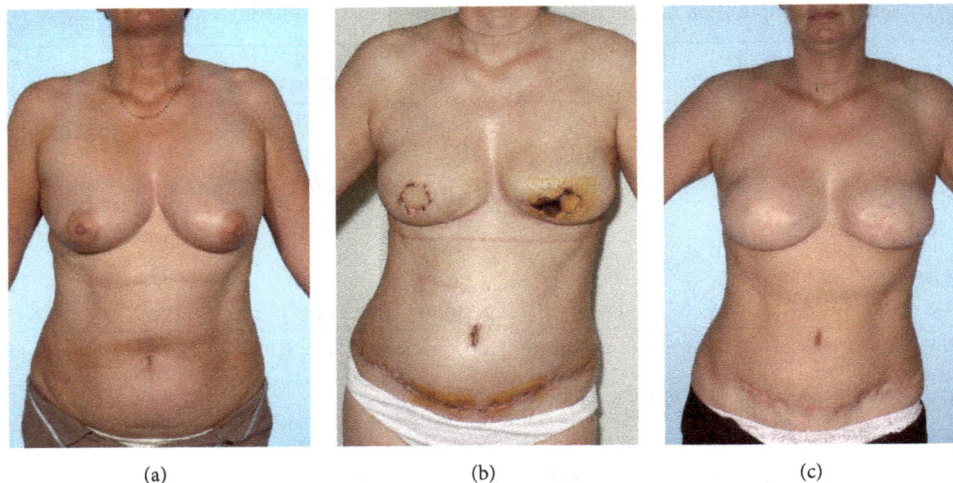

FIGURE 2: ((a) Preoperative; (b) 4 weeks after reconstruction; and (c) 6 months after reconstruction) 42-year-old smoker with family history of breast and ovarian cancer (BRACA negative) underwent risk reducing bilateral mastectomy and immediate DIEP reconstruction and delayed nipple reconstruction. Note native breast necrosis and abdominal wound dehiscence (consent obtained to use photographs).

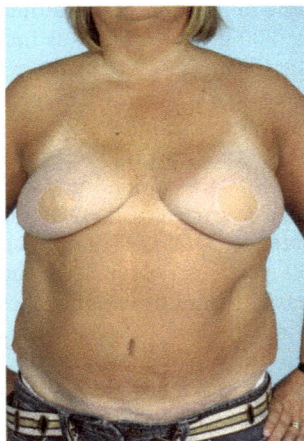

FIGURE 3: 43-year-old immediate bilateral DIEP reconstruction for DCIS. Photograph taken after recent holiday abroad. Note skin paddle pigmentation in response to abdominal sun exposure (consent obtained to use photographs).

series was not significant, a finding consistent with some literatures [34] and contradictory to others [33, 35].

The behaviour of autologous transplanted tissue and its genetic tendency to mimic donor site are illustrated in Figure 3. The phenomenon of unexposed reconstructed breast skin paddles changing pigmentation in response to abdominal sun exposure is not described in the literature reviewed [5, 11, 12, 14–20].

Abdominal free flaps are unique as the use of this flap in a unilateral setting precludes future use for the contralateral side. In a recent publication, Wormald et al. [1] performed a systematic review comparing the risks of unilateral versus bilateral DIEP reconstructions and observed bilateral DIEP reconstructions to be associated with a significantly higher

risk of total flap failure (RR 3.31, P = 0.003) and breast seroma (RR 7.15, P = 0.03), while other outcomes were comparable. At present, in non-BRCA patients with unilateral malignancy, bilateral mastectomies are not advocated as the risks of developing breast cancer in the contralateral side are comparable to the general female population. At our centre, all patients with a positive family history are sent for genetic testing, and lifetime risk estimates are provided for the patient to make an informed decision on the appropriateness of a contralateral prophylactic procedure. In this series, 12 (21.8%) patients were BRCA positive and 12 (22%) had a strong family history of breast cancer. Of these, 14 (26%) had identified breast pathology and underwent therapeutic surgery and 10 (18%) opted to have bilateral prophylactic (risk reducing) mastectomies.

Thirty-one (56%) patients with unilateral disease and no identifiable genetic or familial predisposition underwent bilateral mastectomy and reconstructive surgery. The decision to offer contralateral prophylactic mastectomy in a non-BRCA patient with no family history is controversial. However, in certain patients where there is a specific request for contralateral risk reducing procedure, a joint decision can be made with the breast surgeons, geneticist, oncologist, and plastic surgeon.

Limitations of the study must be considered. Retrospective case series studies are at risk of selection and reporting bias which reduce the reliability of results obtained. Prospective observational cohort studies to review objective and patient associated outcomes and reduce bias are considered preferable [1]. In addition, the relatively small size ensures that the study is insufficiently powered to accurately detect and predict uncommon but serious outcomes such as total flap failure. Moreover, utilising "the flap" as the unit of investigation for flap-associated data as opposed to "the patient" underestimates the clinical adverse outcomes. It has been suggested that using "the flap" as a data unit in bilateral breast reconstruction studies does not take into account "the patient" who ultimately has suffered from the complication that has arisen [1]. Finally undefined parameters pertaining to observer descriptions of complication presentations are a limitation of this study and similar studies.

6. Conclusion

Our experience demonstrates that abdominal free flaps for bilateral breast reconstruction fare well, with a flap failure rate of 2.7%. On analysis, smoking status, radiotherapy, flap weight, previous abdominal surgery, and ischaemic time were not associated with increased postoperative risks. We have found that an increased BMI and increasing age (>60 years) were associated with higher complication rates. This is useful information to help clinicians in decision making and counselling of future patients. Abdominal free flap surgery for bilateral breast reconstruction will continue to rise and the increasing popularity is a reflection of the natural evolution of breast reconstruction techniques to obtain maximal patient satisfaction and outcome.

Competing Interests

There is no conflict of interests.

References

[1] J. C. R. Wormald, R. G. Wade, and A. Figus, "The increased risk of adverse outcomes in bilateral deep inferior epigastric artery perforator flap breast reconstruction compared to unilateral reconstruction: a systematic review and meta-analysis," *Journal of Plastic, Reconstructive & Aesthetic Surgery*, vol. 67, no. 2, pp. 143–156, 2014.

[2] A. Abbott, N. Rueth, S. Pappas-Varco, K. Kuntz, E. Kerr, and T. Tuttle, "Perceptions of contralateral breast cancer: an overestimation of risk," *Annals of Surgical Oncology*, vol. 18, no. 11, pp. 3129–3136, 2011.

[3] M. A. Crosby, P. B. Garvey, J. C. Selber et al., "Reconstructive outcomes in patients undergoing contralateral prophylactic mastectomy," *Plastic and Reconstructive Surgery*, vol. 128, no. 5, pp. 1025–1033, 2011.

[4] E. Han, N. Johnson, M. Glissmeyer et al., "Increasing incidence of bilateral mastectomies: the patient perspective," *The American Journal of Surgery*, vol. 201, no. 5, pp. 615–618, 2011.

[5] R. O. Craft, S. Colakoglu, M. S. Curtis et al., "Patient satisfaction in unilateral and bilateral breast reconstruction," *Plastic and Reconstructive Surgery*, vol. 127, no. 4, pp. 1417–1424, 2011.

[6] W. M. Rozen and M. W. Ashton, "Improving outcomes in autologous breast reconstruction," *Aesthetic Plastic Surgery*, vol. 33, no. 3, pp. 327–335, 2009.

[7] G. R. D. Evans, M. A. Schusterman, S. S. Kroll et al., "Reconstruction and the radiated breast: is there a role for implants?" *Plastic and Reconstructive Surgery*, vol. 96, no. 5, pp. 1111–1115, 1995.

[8] S. S. Kroll, "Why autologous tissue?" *Clinics in Plastic Surgery*, vol. 25, no. 2, pp. 135–143, 1998.

[9] P. D. Butler and L. C. Wu, "Abdominal perforator vs. muscle sparing flaps for breast reconstruction," *Gland Surgery*, vol. 4, no. 3, pp. 212–221, 2015.

[10] R. J. Allen and P. Treece, "Deep inferior epigastric perforator flap for breast reconstruction," *Annals of Plastic Surgery*, vol. 32, no. 1, pp. 32–38, 1994.

[11] M. Hamdi, E. M. Weiler-Mithoff, and M. H. C. Webster, "Deep inferior epigastric perforator flap in breast reconstruction: experience with the first 50 flaps," *Plastic and Reconstructive Surgery*, vol. 103, no. 1, pp. 86–95, 1999.

[12] A. Keller, "The deep inferior epigastric perforator free flap for breast reconstruction," *Annals of Plastic Surgery*, vol. 46, no. 5, pp. 474–480, 2001.

[13] IBM Corporation, *IBM SPSS Statistics for Windows. Version 22.0*, IBM Corporation, Armonk, NY, 2013.

[14] A. B. Guerra, S. E. Metzinger, R. S. Bidros et al., "Bilateral breast reconstruction with the Deep Inferior Epigastric Perforator (DIEP) flap: an experience with 280 flaps," *Annals of Plastic Surgery*, vol. 52, no. 3, pp. 246–252, 2004.

[15] A. S. Scheer, C. B. Novak, P. C. Neligan, and J. E. Lipa, "Complications associated with breast reconstruction using a perforator flap compared with a free TRAM flap," *Annals of Plastic Surgery*, vol. 56, no. 4, pp. 355–358, 2006.

[16] S. O. P. Hofer, T. H. C. Damen, M. A. M. Mureau, H. A. Rakhorst, and N. A. Roche, "A critical review of perioperative complications in 175 free deep inferior epigastric perforator flap breast reconstructions," *Annals of Plastic Surgery*, vol. 59, no. 2, pp. 137–142, 2007.

[17] L. Drazan, J. Vesely, P. Hyza et al., "Bilateral breast reconstruction with DIEP flaps: 4 years' experience," *Journal of Plastic, Reconstructive and Aesthetic Surgery*, vol. 61, no. 11, pp. 1309–1315, 2008.

[18] S. S. Rao, P. M. Parikh, J. A. Goldstein, and M. Y. Nahabedian, "Unilateral failures in bilateral microvascular breast reconstruction," *Plastic and Reconstructive Surgery*, vol. 126, no. 1, pp. 17–25, 2010.

[19] M. V. Schaverien, C. N. Ludman, J. Neil-Dwyer et al., "Contrast-enhanced magnetic resonance angiography for preoperative imaging in DIEP flap breast reconstruction," *Plastic and Reconstructive Surgery*, vol. 128, no. 1, pp. 56–62, 2011.

[20] P. N. Blondeel, G. G. Vanderstraeten, S. J. Monstrey et al., "The donor site morbidity of free DIEP flaps and free TRAM flaps for breast reconstruction," *British Journal of Plastic Surgery*, vol. 50, no. 5, pp. 322–330, 1997.

[21] N. V. Tran, E. W. Buchel, and P. A. Convery, "Microvascular complications of DIEP flaps," *Plastic and Reconstructive Surgery*, vol. 119, no. 5, pp. 1397–1405, 2007.

[22] P. N. Blondeel, M. Arnstein, K. Verstraete et al., "Venous congestion and blood flow in free transverse rectus abdominis myocutaneous and deep inferior epigastric perforator flaps," *Plastic and Reconstructive Surgery*, vol. 106, no. 6, pp. 1295–1299, 2000.

[23] A. E. Handschin, M. Guggenheim, M. Calcagni, W. Künzi, and P. Giovanoli, "Factor v leiden mutation and thrombotic occlusion of microsurgical anastomosis after free TRAM flap," *Clinical and Applied Thrombosis/Hemostasis*, vol. 16, no. 2, pp. 199–203, 2010.

[24] I. Khansa, S. Colakoglu, D. C. Tomich, M.-D. Nguyen, and B. T. Lee, "Factor V leiden associated with flap loss in microsurgical breast reconstruction," *Microsurgery*, vol. 31, no. 5, pp. 409–412, 2011.

[25] K. Segers, B. Dahlbäck, and G. A. F. Nicolaes, "Coagulation factor V and thrombophilia: background and mechanisms," *Thrombosis and Haemostasis*, vol. 98, no. 3, pp. 530–542, 2007.

[26] D. C. Rees, M. Cox, and J. B. Clegg, "World distribution of factor V Leiden," *The Lancet*, vol. 346, no. 8983, pp. 1133–1134, 1995.

[27] P. S. Gill, J. P. Hunt, A. B. Guerra et al., "A 10-year retrospective review of 758 DIEP flaps for breast reconstruction," *Plastic and Reconstructive Surgery*, vol. 113, no. 4, pp. 1153–1160, 2004.

[28] C. L. Chen, A. D. Shore, R. Johns, J. M. Clark, M. Manahan, and M. A. Makary, "The impact of obesity on breast surgery complications," *Plastic and Reconstructive Surgery*, vol. 128, no. 5, pp. 395e–402e, 2011.

[29] L. Setälä, A. Papp, S. Joukainen et al., "Obesity and complications in breast reduction surgery: are restrictions justified?" *Journal of Plastic, Reconstructive and Aesthetic Surgery*, vol. 62, no. 2, pp. 195–199, 2009.

[30] N. A. De Glas, M. Kiderlen, E. Bastiaannet et al., "Postoperative complications and survival of elderly breast cancer patients: a FOCUS study analysis," *Breast Cancer Research and Treatment*, vol. 138, no. 2, pp. 561–569, 2013.

[31] T. Berry, S. Brooks, N. Sydow et al., "Complication rates of radiation on tissue expander and autologous tissue breast reconstruction," *Annals of Surgical Oncology*, vol. 17, no. 3, pp. S202–S210, 2010.

[32] J. S. Chatterjee, A. Lee, W. Anderson et al., "Effect of postoperative radiotherapy on autologous deep inferior epigastric perforator flap volume after immediate breast reconstruction," *British Journal of Surgery*, vol. 96, no. 10, pp. 1135–1140, 2009.

[33] N. V. Tran, G. R. D. Evans, S. S. Kroll et al., "Postoperative adjuvant irradiation: effects on tranverse rectus abdominis muscle flap breast reconstruction," *Plastic and Reconstructive Surgery*, vol. 106, no. 2, pp. 313–317, 2000.

[34] M. Y. Halyard, K. E. McCombs, W. W. Wong et al., "Acute and chronic results of adjuvant radiotherapy after mastectomy and transverse rectus abdominis myocutaneous (TRAM) flap reconstruction for breast cancer," *American Journal of Clinical Oncology: Cancer Clinical Trials*, vol. 27, no. 4, pp. 389–394, 2004.

[35] N. E. Rogers and R. J. Allen, "Radiation effects on breast reconstruction with the deep inferior epigastric perforator flap," *Plastic and Reconstructive Surgery*, vol. 109, no. 6, pp. 1919–1924, 2002.

37

Does the Use of Intraoperative Breast Sizers Increase Complication Rates in Primary Breast Augmentation? A Retrospective Analysis of 416 Consecutive Cases in a Single Institution

Lee Seng Khoo, Henrique N. Radwanski, Vasco Senna-Fernandes, Nsingi Nsosolo Antônio, Leonardo Luiz Fernandes Fellet, and Ivo Pitanguy

Instituto Ivo Pitanguy, Rua Dona Mariana 65, 22280-020 Botafogo, RJ, Brazil

Correspondence should be addressed to Lee Seng Khoo; khooleeseng@hotmail.com

Academic Editor: Selahattin Özmen

Background. Is the use of intraoperative breast sizers beneficial for plastic surgeons or do they result in higher complication rates? *Methods.* This is a retrospective study of 416 consecutive cases of primary breast augmentation with silicone implants at the Plastic Surgery Service of Professor Ivo Pitanguy at the 38th Infirmary Santa Casa Misericórdia Hospital, Rio De Janeiro, from January 2011 to March 2014. 212 cases (51%) were carried out with use of intraoperative breast sizers with 204 cases (49%) without the use of implant sizers. This study compares the outcome of cases that employed the use of intraoperative implant sizers versus those that did not in terms of infection, hematoma/seroma formation, and capsular contracture. *Results.* Of 416 primary breast augmentation cases, there were 5 cases of infection (1.2%), 4 cases of seroma (1%), 3 cases of hematoma (0.7%), and 7 cases of capsular contracture (Baker's Grade III/IV)(1.7%). Total complication rate limited to infection, seroma, hematoma, and capsular contracture was 1.15% (95% CI 0.96–1.93%). There was a significant difference in the scores for breast sizers (M = 4.3, SD = 1.4) and no breast sizers (M = 2.3, SD = 0.87) conditions, $t(8) = 2.79$, $p = 0.018$. The use of implant sizers was correlated with a higher complication rate. *Conclusion.* Good results could be obtained without the use of breast sizers in primary breast augmentation with use of a biodimensional tissue based planning system while eliminating risks of infection and reducing intraoperative time. Notwithstanding, in a residency program breast sizers can be an excellent training tool to shorten the learning curve in the novice surgeon.

1. Introduction

Many plastic surgeons utilize breast implant sizers in breast augmentation surgery to estimate the ideal implant volume after pocket dissection.

Intraoperative breast implant sizers are sterilizable and reusable and also provide a visual gauge of volume required to adequately fill the breast pocket.

However, the routine usage of these implant sizers may cause tissue trauma, augment contamination risks, and increase intraoperative time and may also be expensive. In the United Kingdom, implant sizers are mandated to be single use apparatus that must be discarded after one surgery [1].

Many sizers including tissue expanders do not accurately simulate the shape surface characteristics of the implant and therefore do not accurately reflect the visual appearance that a similar volume implant may produce [2, 3] (Figure 1).

The alternative to intraoperative breast sizers such as trial sizing with external breast sizers (Figure 2) or stockings filled with rice bags in the consultation room [4, 5] is also notoriously inaccurate in determining the ideal implant or visual representation.

Surgeons such as Tebbetts and Heden have developed mathematical preoperative breast tissue based planning to eliminate the use of implant sizers [2, 3].

Anecdotally, surgeons have been performing preoperative planning subjectively at best and often not even included prior to the surgical procedure. The premise of a tissue based preoperative algorithm such as the Akademikliniken method [3] and High Five system of Tebbetts [6] is to evaluate the

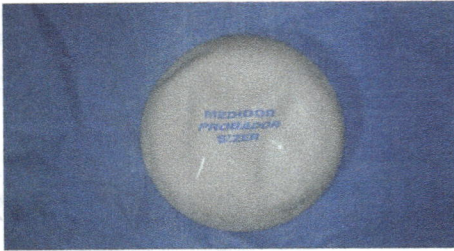

FIGURE 1: An example of an intraoperative sizer. Note that the sizer does not have the consistency of an implant.

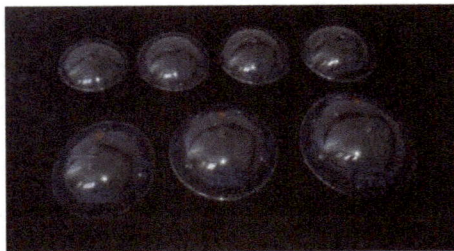

FIGURE 2: External breast sizers in various sizes.

patients' tissues and objectively match an implant specifically to what the tissues can accommodate.

Case series of 2500 primary breast augmentations performed with tissue based preoperative planning in the United States demonstrated a reoperative rate of 3% within 6 to 7 years' follow-up, compared to the reoperation rate of 15% to 20% in 3 years in all the PMA (Premarket Approval) implant case series [7–10].

Nonetheless, the use of breast implant sizers continues to be popular among surgeons [7–10]. Gore reported that less than 2% of patients in consecutive 200 case series developed complications such as hematoma, seroma formation, or infection [11]. Capsular contracture was noted in 7% of patients, but there were no visible or painful capsules [11]. A 5-year study detailing reoperative augmentation mammaplasty by Pitanguy et al. revealed complication rates of primary breast augmentation comparable to other studies [12]. Pitanguy described his preferred route for placing breast implants via a transareolopapilar incision [13] and utilized external breast sizers to determine the ideal volume necessary to obtain a satisfactory result [14].

The question therefore to be asked is whether the routine use of breast implant sizers is necessary in primary breast augmentation. Is there a higher rate of complications such as hematoma, seroma, infection, and capsular contracture in patients that undergo breast augmentation with sizers compared to those who did not?

2. Materials and Methods

We present a retrospective study of 416 consecutive cases of primary breast augmentation with silicone implants at the Plastic Surgery Service of Professor Ivo Pitanguy at the 38th Infirmary Santa Casa Misericórdia Hospital, Rio de Janeiro,

from January 2011 to March 2014. This study compares the outcome of cases that employed the use of intraoperative implant sizers versus those that did not in terms of infection, hematoma/seroma formation, and capsular contracture.

Inclusion criteria included all consecutive patients who underwent primary breast augmentation with or without the use of intraoperative implant sizers within the period of January 2011 to March 2014. Patients who also had simultaneous mastopexy (augmentation mastopexy), secondary augmentation mammaplasty, change of implants and reconstructive breast surgery with implants, and combined surgeries with other procedures were excluded from this study.

Accordingly we sought to measure complications that can be attributed to the use of intraoperative sizers per se such as infection, hematoma/seroma formation, and capsular contracture. We excluded technique/surgeon related complications such as inadequate size, breast asymmetry, implant malposition, implant palpability, and wrinkles, ripples, or folds seen in the breast tissue and the skin overlying the implant.

A list of all patients who underwent breast augmentation with implants from January 2011 to March 2014 was located from the archive database at the 38th Infirmary Santa Casa Misericordia Hospital. After applying the exclusion criteria we were left with a total of 416 patients that underwent primary breast augmentation from January 2011 to March 2014, 212 with intraoperative sizers and 204 without intraoperative sizers. Retrospective analysis of patient records was carried out with caution not to link any data to patient identifiers and the confidentiality of the patient records was maintained in all instances.

Patient records were thoroughly analyzed for the following data: (1) use of intraoperative sizers or none thereof (this was confirmed by operative notes and seal of proof of sterilization stamp of a breast sizer being utilized during surgery); (2) incision location: periareolar, inframammary, or axillary; (3) plane of placement of the implants: subglandular, submuscular (including dual plane), or subfascial; (4) type and volume of implant; (5) complications such as infection, hematoma/seroma formation, and grade of capsular contracture if any.

All the patients underwent either general anesthesia or high epidural anesthesia with sedation. The surgical approach used was either inframammary or periareolar incision for augmentation mammaplasty.

Intraoperatively, all surgical pockets were irrigated by an antibiotic solution containing 1 g of cefazolin, 80 mg of gentamicin, and 500 mL of normal saline. All implants were inserted via a no-touch technique with change of gloves prior to insertion. Meticulous hemostasis was achieved in all cases but no drains were used in 410 cases of primary breast augmentation except for 12 cases where it was judged necessary intraoperatively. All cases received preoperative antibiotic of 1 g cefazolin intravenously and antibiotics (500 mg Cephalexin three times a day) were continued for 7 days postoperatively in oral form.

Incisions were closed in 3 layers for inframammary approach with 3-0 Nylon sutures placed in the subcutaneous tissues, 4-0 Nylon deep subdermal sutures, and intradermal closure with 4-0 Nylon or 4-0 Monocryl suture. For the periareolar approach, incisions were closed with 3-0 Nylon for subglandular tissue, 4-0 Nylon for subdermal sutures, and 4-0 Nylon or 4-0 Monocryl for intradermal closure. Micropore strips (3M, St. Paul, Minn.) were placed and removed 2 weeks postoperatively in both approaches.

Patients were fitted with a surgical brassiere and instructions were given to wear the apparatus for 4 weeks postoperatively. In addition, patients were told to avoid wired brassieres, lifting heavy objects over head, and strenuous physical activity for 6 weeks after surgery.

The accompanying photographs in the immediate postoperative period and at 3 and/or 6 months were also evaluated. All 416 patients were contacted by telephone or seen in person at the clinics to enquire and ascertain if any complications arose in the postoperative period. The database of patients returning for complications was also obtained from the archives at the 38th Infirmary Santa Casa Misericórdia. Patients with noted complications were questioned to enquire if any further changes from their last evaluation occurred and the primary surgeon was contacted for further information. Those who had ongoing complications were seen and evaluated at the clinic. It is postulated that over 95% of patients do return to their original surgeon for early/immediate or intermediate period postoperative complications such as hematoma, seroma, infection, and early capsular contracture. The reason is that the institute covers all revisional surgery at minimal to no cost.

3. Statistics

Following a normal distribution curve in both groups that underwent primary breast augmentation (sizer versus no sizer), a Student t-test was used to appraise overall complication rates in both groups of patients. The Central Limit Theorem tells us that the sample means are approximately normally distributed with n number of 416 cases ($n = 416$).

As the collated results represent multiple surgeons collectively, the paired Student t-test compares the difference in the means from the two variables measured on the same set of subjects to a given number (n), while taking into account the fact that the scores are not independent (taking into account individual surgeon variability).

The software utilized was Statistical Package for Social Studies (SPSS) (IBM Corp. Released 2012; SPSS Statistics for Windows, Version 21.0 Armonk, NY: IBM Corp.).

4. Results

A total of 416 patients were subjected to primary breast augmentation carried out by surgical residents from January 2011 to March 2014. These results are representative of multiple surgeon teams of the 38th Infirmary Santa Casa Misericórdia Hospital Department of Plastic and Reconstructive Surgery.

The median implant volume was 300 cc and median age of patient was 38 years (standard deviation: 8.58 years). All implants were polyurethane coated cohesive silicone gel with either round or anatomic shape. One brand was used: Silimed (Silimed, Rio de Janeiro, Brazil). Mean follow-up time was 65.30 weeks (standard deviation: 37.92) (Table 1).

TABLE 1: Characteristics of breast implants used.

Type of implant	Number of cases	Percentage
Round, HI-profile	366	88.0%
Round, LO-profile	4	1.0%
Round, moderate profile	16	3.9%
Anatomic, HI-profile	17	4.0%
Anatomic, moderate profile	8	2.0%
Anatomic, LO-profile	5	0.1%
Total	**416**	**100.0%**

The majority of implants used were round and high profile for a total of 366 cases (88.0%) and 80% (332) of these round high profile implants had a volume range within 200–300 cc. The other patients received round low profile (4 cases (1%)), round moderate profile (16 cases (3.9%)), anatomical high profile (17 cases (4%)), anatomical moderate profile (8 cases (2%)), and anatomical low profile (5 cases (0.1%)). A total of 212 cases (51%) were carried out with use of intraoperative breast sizers with the remaining 204 cases (49%) without the use of implant sizers. The breast implants were placed via periareolar approach in 210 cases (50.48%) and inframammary in 206 cases (49.52%) with the majority being placed in the subglandular pocket, 402 cases (96.6%) and 14 (3.37%) in the submuscular pocket (including dual plane.) There were no documented cases of transaxillary and transumbilical approach and subfascial placement.

Out of these 416 primary breast augmentation cases, there were 5 cases of infection (1.2%), 4 cases of seroma (1%), 3 cases of hematoma (0.7%), and 7 cases of capsular contracture (Baker's Grade III/IV) (1.7%). Total complication rate limited to infection, seroma, hematoma, and capsular contracture was 1.15% (95% CI 0.96–1.93%). There was no documented implant rupture at time of study. A limitation of this study is the time frame where cases of delayed hematoma and capsular contracture may present in the future and were not included in the study (Figure 12).

It was noted that 4 of 5 cases that were complicated by infection involved the use of intraoperative breast sizers, and that 3 out of 5 of the afflicted infections were implants placed via the periareolar approach in the subglandular plane. The remaining 2 infected cases were placed in the subglandular plane via the inframammary approach. It is interesting to note that 2 out of the 5 infections also presented with recurring seroma.

Of the cases that presented with capsular contracture (Baker's Grade III/IV), 5 out of 7 involved use of intraoperative implant sizers. All were placed subglandularly with 3 out of 5 inserted via inframammary approach and the remaining 2 via periareolar approach.

The higher rate of infection and capsular contracture in cases of primary breast augmentation whereby intraoperative sizers were used (p value < 0.05) is statistically significant.

4.1. Case Report 1. This 37-year-old patient underwent primary breast augmentation in March 2014 with 285 cc moderate profile, round cohesive polyurethane coated silicone

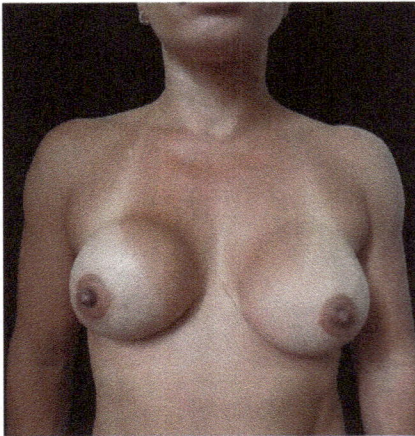

FIGURE 3: Baker Grade IV capsular contracture on right breast.

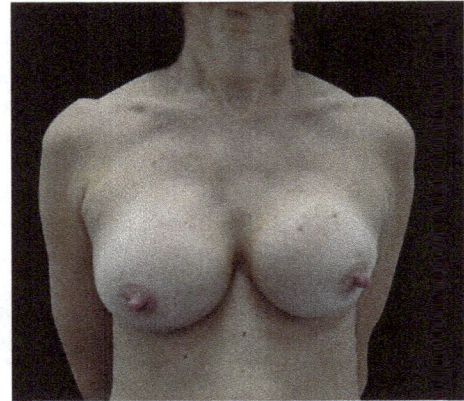

FIGURE 5: Baker Grade IV capsular contracture on left breast.

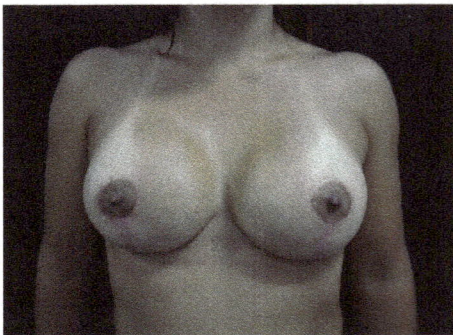

FIGURE 4: After removal of implants and augmentation mastopexy.

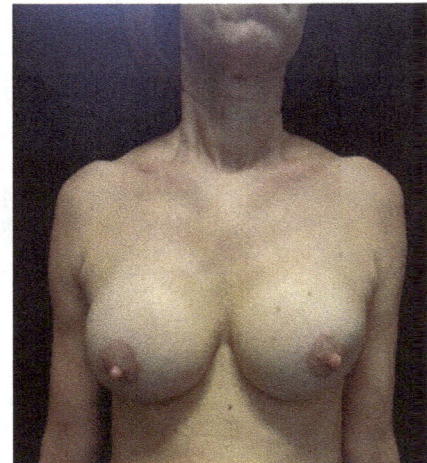

FIGURE 6: After capsulectomy and reinsertion of new 235 cc implant in subglandular plane.

implants inserted in the subglandular plane via an inframammary approach. Intraoperative breast sizers were utilized during surgery.

She returned in July 2014 with a Baker Grade IV capsular contracture on the right breast. The left breast was normal. The right breast was hard, painful, and grossly distorted (Figure 3).

In December 2014, bilateral implants were removed at the request of the patient and an augmentation mastopexy was performed with 305 cc moderate profile, anatomic cohesive polyurethane coated silicone implants (Figure 4). The postoperative results were satisfactory with no early recurrence of capsular contracture to date.

4.2. Case Report 2.

This 56-year-old lady underwent augmentation mammaplasty in September 2013 with 285 cc moderate profile, round cohesive polyurethane coated silicone implants placed in the subglandular region via the inframammary approach. Intraoperative breast sizers were used during surgery.

In February 2014, she noted a progressive distortion of her left breast which was painful on palpation (Figure 5). We assigned a Baker IV capsular contracture.

The left breast implant was removed and capsulectomy was carried out with reinsertion of 285 cc polyurethane

coated implants in the subglandular pocket in August 2014. Note that residual distortion is still evident postoperatively (Figure 6).

4.3. Case Report 3.

This 35-year-old patient underwent augmentation mammaplasty in March 2013 with 275 cc high profile, anatomic cohesive polyurethane coated silicone implants inserted in the subglandular plane via a periareolar approach with use of intraoperative breast sizers.

She returned on post-op day 20 with fullness and mild serous discharge at the suture line of the periareolar regions bilaterally. Ultrasonographic assisted drainage was carried out for seroma collection. There were no systemic or local signs of infection but drained material was sent for culture and sensitivity. No implicating organisms or bacteria were isolated on cultures. Patient was started on Ciprofloxacin 500 mg twice a day and Augmentin 875 mg twice a day for 14 days.

However, the patient continued to present with recurring seroma of minimal volume (about 3 to 5 ccs on each occasion) over the next 3 months. Although we recommended removal

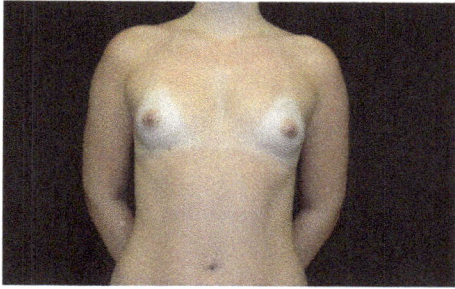

FIGURE 7: Pre-op frontal view.

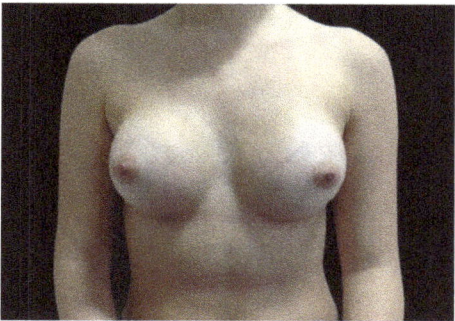

FIGURE 8: Immediate postoperative result.

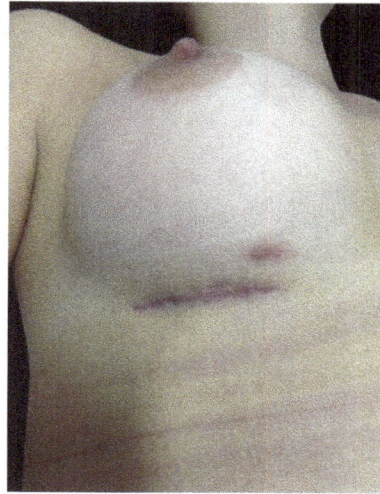

FIGURE 9: The residual fistula scar site medially.

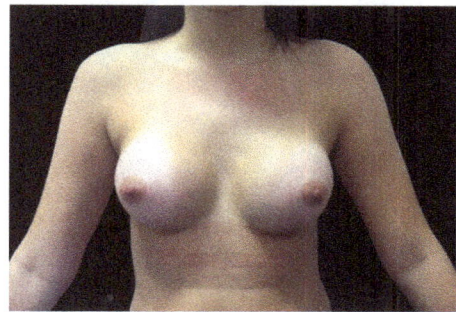

FIGURE 10: Final postoperative result.

on basis of subclinical infection, patient strongly opposed the removal. In the 3rd month, a trial of Diprospan (Betamethasone 7 mg per ampoule) was injected intramuscularly once a week for 2 weeks in an attempt to resolve inflammation. As the clinical picture improved with no more seroma, the breast implants were not removed as per request of patient. Again no particular organism was isolated on repeated culture including *Mycobacterium*.

Patient is still on 6-month follow-up and recent ultrasound scan is normal.

4.4. Case Report 4. This 23-year-old woman underwent primary breast augmentation in December 2013 (Figure 7). She had 280 cc high profile anatomic, cohesive polyurethane coated silicone implants inserted via the inframammary approach with intraoperative use of implant sizers. Implants were placed in the subglandular plane (Figure 8).

She returned in February 2014 (post-op day 52) complaining of redness and clear discharge from her right breast. On examination, she was hemodynamically stable and afebrile. A small fistula measuring 0.5×0.6 cm was noted medially with a 1 cm wound dehiscence at the lateral suture line. Antibiotic therapy with Ciprofloxacin 500 mg twice a day was initiated.

A swab was taken and 8 cc of seroma was drained via aseptic technique. The culture results returned a diagnosis of *M. abscessus*.

When reexamined at the clinic on post-op day 57, it was noted that more seroma had developed and the decision was made to remove the implants surgically with debridement and commence antibiotic therapy with Clarithromycin 500 mg twice a day for 4 months (Figure 9).

Culture results obtained during implant removal and debridement reconfirmed the *Mycobacterium* infection. Patient subsequently had reinsertion of implant after concluding the 4 months of antibiotic therapy with satisfactory results (Figure 10).

4.5. Case Report 5. This 35-year-old patient underwent breast augmentation surgery in July 2012 with 265 cc bilateral moderate profile, round, cohesive, polyurethane coated silicone implants placed in the subglandular plane via the periareolar approach. Intraoperative breast sizers were utilized during surgery.

The postoperative results were satisfactory but patient presented with a hematoma on post-op day 5. The right breast was grossly swollen and tense especially on the lower lateral region. This was drained aseptically and compression dressing was placed. The drain was removed 2 days later (Figure 11).

In August 2013, she returned with redness overlying the right breast at the previous suture line. No discharge was noted. She was prescribed Ciprofloxacin 500 mg twice a day for 7 days and the redness resolved. She has since been free of any complications and is happy with the postsurgical results.

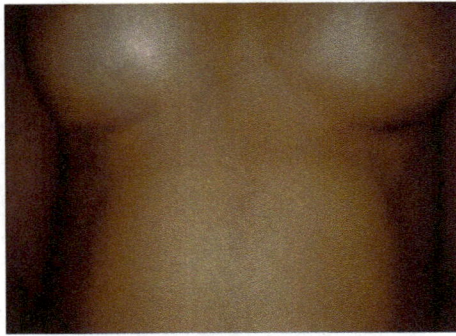

FIGURE 11: Appearance after removal of drain.

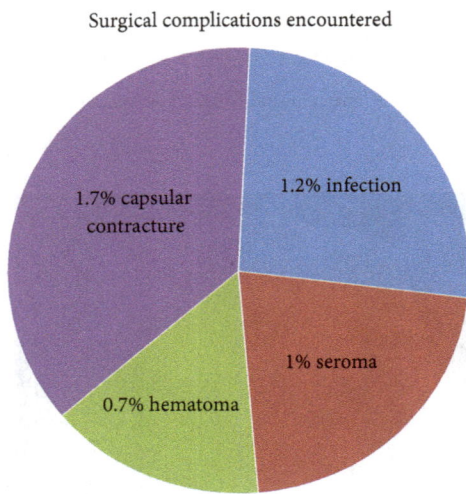

FIGURE 12: Pie chart of total percentage of surgical complications encountered.

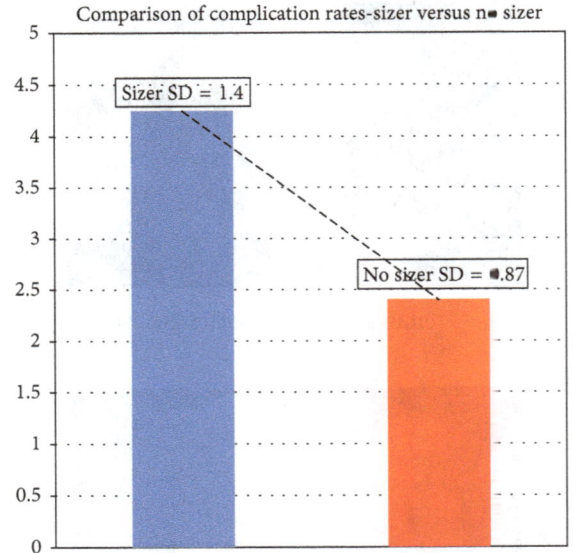

FIGURE 13: Comparison of complication rates: sizer versus no sizer. Note: $t(8) = 2.79$; $p = 0.018$.

5. Discussion

The exclusive use of polyurethane breast implants is both a strength and a limitation of this study. While this reduces the probability of the implant type being a confounding variable for postoperative results unrelated to the procedure, it may also account for the relative lower rates of capsular contracture among the patient group as a whole. Although selection bias was eliminated by including all patients who underwent primary breast augmentation without any other ancillary procedures within the time frame in a single institution, there would be technical variability as the cases recorded are not performed by a single surgeon.

Paired Student t-test was utilized to compare complication rate in surgeries with breast sizers and in those where no sizers were used. There was a significant difference in the scores for breast sizers (M = 4.3, SD = 1.4) and no breast sizers (M = 2.3, SD = 0.87) conditions, $t(8) = 2.79$, $p = 0.018$. These results suggest that the use of implant sizers is correlated with a higher complication rate in terms of infection, seroma, and capsular contracture (Figure 13).

Hence, while the results point toward a higher rate of infection, seroma, and capsular contracture in patients who

underwent augmentation mammaplasty with intraoperative implant sizers ($p < 0.05$), they do not address the variability in incision site selection, size of implant, and technical variability of the surgeon.

It is critical to address the controversy of not using intraoperative breast sizers instead of using them. Many proponents of using breast sizers intraoperatively cited that the sizers allowed them to pick an appropriate size for a patient while being able to simulate the end result. Intraoperative breast sizers are also a valuable tool in a training program to allow the novice surgeon to visualize and dissect an accurate breast pocket. The critics state that the use of these intraoperative breast implant sizers unnecessarily increases tissue trauma and augments possible infection rate while not actually reflecting the final result accurately as the projection, base diameter, and cohesivity of the sizer may not mimic the chosen implant.

Some surgeons advocate a biodimensional method of selecting appropriate breast implants for a particular individual [4–6]. This method involves an objective assessment to match an implant specifically to what the breast tissue can accommodate. In such instances, the decision for a specific sized implant, base diameter, height, and projection can be determined preoperatively without the need to resort to intraoperative sizers [4–6]. In published and peer-reviewed series, there are 2500 primary breast augmentations performed with similar concepts in tissue based preoperative planning, with reoperation rates of 3% with 6 to 7 years' follow-up compared to the reoperation rate of 15% to 20% in 3 years [7–10].

Implant sizers may augment contamination and infection risks, costs, tissue trauma, and operative time and are perhaps unnecessary in primary breast augmentation, if a surgeon is willing to quantitate tissue characteristics and use proved processes and biodimensional systems such as the High

Five™ System [6] during preoperative planning and implant selection.

Implants sizers may not accurately simulate the shape surface characteristics of the implant and in turn do not depict the appearance of a similar volume implant [4]. Sizer use can be habit forming, and surgeons who insist on using sizers rarely learn to use quantitative systems that are much more accurate and less traumatic to the soft tissues as the definite implant is only inserted once.

Notwithstanding, intraoperative breast implant sizers have their advantages as they can allow the novice surgeon to obtain an idea of an appropriate breast volume for picking an implant. They also free the surgeon from being rigid and having to learn and utilize a tissue based preoperative planning system. Proponents also claim that breast sizers are sterile, reusable, and readily available. However, health and safety regulations in the United Kingdom currently mandate that the sizers are for single use only, further increasing the cost of their use for estimating ideal implant size.

The controversy also arises if sizers do increase the rate of infection. An argument is made that biofilm accumulates on repeated use of implant sizers and this could be a problem for repeated usage [13]. Many surgeons in Asia, Latin America, and the United States resterilize their implant sizers for reuse. This may contribute to a higher probability of infection or subclinical infection.

Biofilm is a microbial community characterized by cells that are attached to a surface or to each other and that are embedded in a matrix they have produced. The biofilm possesses a highly effective defense barrier. Bacterial cells in the biofilm are protected from disinfectants, temperature changes, pH changes, antibiotics, and host defence in the form of the human immune system [15, 16].

Microorganisms suspended in liquid (water) are termed planktonic microorganisms. The various testing of the effects of different disinfection methods including autoclaving and use of ethylene oxide is carried out on planktonic microorganisms and not on established biofilm [17–19].

All antimicrobial activities will have the best effect on microorganisms in a planktonic phase before the biofilm will be established. Once the biofilm is well organized, it is more important to perform rigorous physical cleaning to destroy the biofilm [17, 18, 20]. Physical cleaning damages the biofilm, tears away parts of it, and removes the superficial layers of the biofilm. This will facilitate penetration of the bioburden by the disinfectants of which the most important is water, because water molecules finally will remove the bioburden from the breast sizer [17–20].

Thus, the mechanical removal of bacterial biofilms will therefore be more important than sterilization itself. Hence, while the breast sizer may be termed "sterile" on the surface after routine sterilization, once the surface material has been peeled or scraped off, biofilm may still be lying deep within the material itself. But by the same token, aggressive mechanical cleaning may damage the breast sizer and allow further deposition of biofilm between the microtears on the breast implant sizer itself that may serve as a nidus of infection if reused on another patient.

This hypothesis of biofilm on sizers may explain the outbreak caused by nontuberculous mycobacteria infection linked to breast augmentation surgery with implants in Campinas, Brazil [19]. The outbreak was caused by polyclonal strains of mycobacteria at different institutions, but no specific risk factors were found [19].

We recommend that breast sizers be mandated to single patient one-off use if used at all during breast augmentation surgery. Using breast sizers in this manner may not be economically feasible in many practices as multiple sizers may need to be placed into the breast pocket several times in order to determine the ideal volume necessitating that multiple sizers be purchased, stocked, and then discarded after a single patient surgery. Palmieri et al. reported an increase in operative time of an average of 10–15 minutes per case when using intraoperative sizing with graduated expander implant sizers [21]. This will have economic implications for the hospital and operating surgeon.

6. Conclusion

Although the infection rates and rates of capsular contracture remain low with the use of intraoperative breast sizers, we believe better results could be obtained without the use of breast sizers in primary breast augmentation with use of a biodimensional tissue based planning system while eliminating risks of infection and reducing intraoperative time. The advantage of not using an implant sizer may outweigh the advantage of using one provided the surgeon is willing to quantitate and measure breast tissue characteristics and utilize a proven biodimensional implant selection system in primary breast augmentation.

Notwithstanding, in a residency program breast sizers can be an excellent training tool. The sizers provided by implant manufacturers are helpful when it comes to determining the implant to be used particularly for a novice surgeon. Implants of various sizes can be simulated allowing the surgeon to dissect an accurate pocket for insertion of the implants. Another major advantage of the sizer is that it enables the surgeon to balance out differences in asymmetrical breasts with size discrepancy. When one is more experienced, one can begin to do so without using implant sizers but they still serve as a valuable adjunct for younger inexperienced surgeons.

Further studies need to be carried out to determine if subclinical infection and subsequently capsular contracture are indeed higher in patients undergoing primary breast augmentation with intraoperative sizers.

Competing Interests

The authors have no conflict of interests to declare.

References

[1] R. H. Caulfield and N. S. Niranjan, "Innovative techniques: a novel technique for intraoperative estimation of breast implant size in aesthetic and reconstructive breast surgery," *Aesthetic Plastic Surgery*, vol. 32, no. 1, pp. 126–129, 2008.

[2] J. B. Tebbetts, *Augmentation Mammaplasty—Redefining the Surgeon and Patient Experience*, Elsevier Health Sciences, Philadelphia, Pa, USA, 2009.

[3] P. Hedén, "Mastopexy augmentation with form stable breast implants," *Clinics in Plastic Surgery*, vol. 36, no. 1, pp. 91–104, 2009.

[4] J. H. James, "What size prosthesis for augmentation mammaplasty?" *Annals of Plastic Surgery*, vol. 19, no. 3, pp. 294–296, 1987.

[5] D. D. Dionyssiou, E. C. Demiri, and J. A. Davison, "A simple method for determining the breast implant size in augmentation mammaplasty," *Aesthetic Plastic Surgery*, vol. 29, no. 6, pp. 571–573, 2005.

[6] J. B. Tebbetts and W. P. Adams Jr., "Five critical decisions in breast augmentation using five measurements in 5 minutes: the high five decision support process," *Plastic and Reconstructive Surgery*, vol. 116, no. 7, pp. 2005–2016, 2005.

[7] W. P. Adams Jr., *Breast Augmentation—An Operative Atlas*, McGraw-Hill, 2010.

[8] B. Bengston, "Experience with 410 implant," in *Proceedings of the American Association of Aesthetic Plastic Surgery Meeting*, New Orleans, La, USA, 2005.

[9] M. Jewell, "S8 Breast education course," in *Proceedings of the American Association of Aesthetic Plastic Surgery Meeting*, New Orleans, La, USA, 2005.

[10] J. B. Tebbetts, "Achieving a zero percent reoperation rate at 3 years in a 50-consecutive-case augmentation mammaplasty. Premarket Approval Study," *Plastic and Reconstructive Surgery*, vol. 118, no. 6, pp. 1453–1457, 2006.

[11] S. M. Gore and B. G. H. Lamberty, "PERTHESE implant-identical cohesive-gel sizers in breast augmentation: a prospective report on 200 consecutive cases and implications for treatment of breast asymmetry," *Aesthetic Surgery Journal*, vol. 32, no. 3, pp. 310–318, 2012.

[12] I. Pitanguy, N. F. Amorim, A. V. Ferreira, and R. Berger, "Análise das trocas de implantes mamários nos últimos cinco anos na Clínica Ivo Pitanguy," *Revista Brasileira de Cirurgia Plástica*, vol. 25, no. 4, pp. 668–674, 2010.

[13] I. Pitanguy, *Aesthetic Plastic Surgery of Head and Body*, Springer, Berlin, Germany, 1981.

[14] I. Pitanguy, M. Vaena, H. N. Radwanski, D. Nunes, and A. F. Vargas, "Relative implant volume and sensibility alterations after breast augmentation," *Aesthetic Plastic Surgery*, vol. 31, no. 3, pp. 238–243, 2007.

[15] M. W. Mittelman, "Adhesion to biomaterials," in *Bacterial Adhesion: Molecular and Ecological Diversity*, M. Fletcher, Ed., pp. 89–127, Wiley-Liss, New York, NY, USA, 1996.

[16] I. Ofek and R. J. Doyle, *Bacterial Adhesion to Cells and Tissues*, Chapman & Hall, New York, NY, USA, 1994.

[17] M. Rosenberg and S. Kjelleberg, "Hydrophobic interactions in bacterial adhesion," *Advances in Microbial Ecology*, vol. 9, pp. 353–393, 1986.

[18] W. A. Corpe, "Microbial surface components involved in adsorption of microorganisms onto surfaces," in *Adsorption of Microorganisms to Surfaces*, G. Bitton and K. C. Marshall, Eds., pp. 105–144, John Wiley & Sons, New York, NY, USA, 1980.

[19] M. C. Padoveze, C. M. C. B. Fortaleza, M. P. Freire et al., "Outbreak of surgical infection caused by non-tuberculous mycobacteria in breast implants in Brazil," *Journal of Hospital Infection*, vol. 67, no. 2, pp. 161–167, 2007.

[20] M. M. Cowan, T. M. Warren, and M. Fletcher, "Mixed–species colonization of solid surfaces in laboratory biofilms," *Biofouling*, vol. 3, no. 1, pp. 23–34, 2009.

[21] B. Palmieri, P. Bosio, and M. A. Shiffmann, "Intraoperative assesment of breast prothesis volume using set of graduated expanders," in *Breast Augmentation*, M. A. Shiffmann, Ed., chapter 24, pp. 207–210, Springer, 2009.

Permissions

The contributors of this book come from diverse backgrounds, making this book a truly international effort. This book will bring forth new frontiers with its revolutionizing research information and detailed analysis of the nascent developments around the world.

We would like to thank all the contributing authors for lending their expertise to make the book truly unique. They have played a crucial role in the development of this book. Without their invaluable contributions this book wouldn't have been possible. They have made vital efforts to compile up to date information on the varied aspects of this subject to make this book a valuable addition to the collection of many professionals and students.

This book was conceptualized with the vision of imparting up-to-date information and advanced data in this field. To ensure the same, a matchless editorial board was set up. Every individual on the board went through rigorous rounds of assessment to prove their worth. After which they invested a large part of their time researching and compiling the most relevant data for our readers.

The editorial board has been involved in producing this book since its inception. They have spent rigorous hours researching and exploring the diverse topics which have resulted in the successful publishing of this book. They have passed on their knowledge of decades through this book. To expedite this challenging task, the publisher supported the team at every step. A small team of assistant editors was also appointed to further simplify the editing procedure and attain best results for the readers.

Apart from the editorial board, the designing team has also invested a significant amount of their time in understanding the subject and creating the most relevant covers. They scrutinized every image to scout for the most suitable representation of the subject and create an appropriate cover for the book.

The publishing team has been an ardent support to the editorial, designing and production team. Their endless efforts to recruit the best for this project, has resulted in the accomplishment of this book. They are a veteran in the field of academics and their pool of knowledge is as vast as their experience in printing. Their expertise and guidance has proved useful at every step. Their uncompromising quality standards have made this book an exceptional effort. Their encouragement from time to time has been an inspiration for everyone.

The publisher and the editorial board hope that this book will prove to be a valuable piece of knowledge for researchers, students, practitioners and scholars across the globe.

List of Contributors

Shkelzen B. Duci, Hysni M. Arifi, Zejn A. Buja, Vildane H. Ismajli, Adem N. Kllokoqi and Enver T. Hoxha
Department of Plastic and Reconstructive Surgery, University Clinical Center of Kosovo, Pristina, Kosovo

Mimoza E. Selmani
Dentistry Faculty, University Clinical Center of Kosovo, Pristina, Kosovo

Agon Y. Mekaj
Department of Neurosurgery, University Clinical Center of Kosovo, Pristina, Kosovo

Musli M. Gashi
Department of Emergency Center Kosovo, Pristina, Kosovo

Mitsuru Nemoto, Kenichi Kumazawa, Eiju Uchinuma, Natsuko Kounoike and Akira Takeda
Department of Plastic and Reconstructive Surgery, Kitasato University Hospital, 1-15-1 Kitasato, Minami-ku, Sagamihara, Kanagawa 252-0374, Japan

Michele Grieco, Eugenio Grignaffini, Francesco Simonacci and Edoardo Raposio
Department of Surgical Sciences, Plastic Surgery Division, University of Parma and Cutaneous, Regenerative, Mininvasive and Plastic Surgery Unit, Azienda Ospedaliero-Universitaria di Parma, Via Gramsci 14, 43126 Parma, Italy

Hani Sinno
Division of Plastic and Reconstructive Surgery, Department of Surgery, McGill University, Montreal, QC, Canada H3G 1A4
Biomedical Technology and Cell Therapy Research Laboratory, Department of Biomedical Engineering, Faculty of Medicine, McGill University, 3775 Rue University, Room 311, Lyman Duff Medical Building, Montreal, QC, Canada H3A 2B4

Sebastian Winocour, Anie Philip and Bruce Williams
Division of Plastic and Reconstructive Surgery, Department of Surgery, McGill University, Montreal, QC, Canada H3G 1A4

Meenakshi Malhotra, Justyn Lutfy, Barbara Jardin and Satya Prakash
Biomedical Technology and Cell Therapy Research Laboratory, Department of Biomedical Engineering, Faculty of Medicine, McGill University, 3775 Rue University, Room 311, Lyman Duff Medical Building, Montreal, QC, Canada H3A 2B4

Fadi Brimo
Department of Pathology, McGill University, Montreal, QC, Canada H3G 1A4

Lorne Beckman and Kevin Watters
Orthopedic Research Laboratory, McGill University, Montreal, QC, Canada H3A 1A1

Ferdinand Wanjala Nangole and Stanley Ominde Khainga
Department of Surgery (Plastic), University of Nairobi, Nairobi 00200, Kenya

Tiffany N. S. Ballard, Jennifer B. Hamill, Adeyiza O. Momoh and Edwin G. Wilkins
Section of Plastic Surgery, University of Michigan, Ann Arbor, MI 48109, USA

Yeonil Kim
Center for Statistical Consultation and Research, University of Michigan, Ann Arbor, MI 48109, USA

Wess A. Cohen and Andrea L. Pusic
Division of Plastic and Reconstructive Surgery, Memorial Sloan-Kettering Cancer Center, New York, NY 10065, USA

H. Myra Kim
Center for Statistical Consultation and Research, University of Michigan, Ann Arbor, MI 48109, USA
Department of Biostatistics, University of Michigan, Ann Arbor, MI 48109, USA

Carlos Alberto Torres-Ortíz Zermeño
Plastic and Reconstructive Surgery, General Hospital Dr. Manuel Gea González, Calzada de Tlalpan No. 4800, 14080 Mexico City, DF, Mexico

Javier López Mendoza
Hand and Microsurgery Clinic, General Hospital Dr. Manuel Gea González, Calzada de Tlalpan No. 4800, 14080 Mexico City, DF, Mexico

Percy Rossell-Perry
Faculty of Medicine, San Martin de Porres University, Lima, Peru
Outreach Surgical Center Program Lima Peru, ReSurge International, 120 Schell Street Apartment 1503 Miraflores, Lima 18, Peru

Carolina Romero-Narvaez
Outreach Surgical Center Program Lima Peru, ReSurge International, 120 Schell Street Apartment 1503 Miraflores, Lima 18, Peru

San Bartolome Children Hospital, Lima, Peru

Gabriel Djedovic, Johannes Jeschke and Hildegunde Piza-Katzer
Department of Plastic, Reconstructive and Aesthetic Surgery, Innsbruck Medical University, Anichstraße 35, 6020 Innsbruck, Austria

Florian Stefan Kamelger
Department of Plastic, Reconstructive and Aesthetic Surgery, Innsbruck Medical University, Anichstraße 35, 6020 Innsbruck, Austria
Department of Traumatology and Sports Medicine, Innsbruck Medical University, Anichstraße 35, 6020 Innsbruck, Austria

Panagiotis Zygouris, Adamantios Michalinos, Vassilis Protogerou, Evangelos Kotsiomitis, Antonios Mazarakis, Ioannis Dimovelis and Theodore Troupis
Department of Anatomy, National and Kapodistrian University of Athens, Mikras Asias 75 Street, Goudi, 11527 Athens, Greece

Satya Prakash
Division of Plastic and Reconstructive Surgery, Department of Surgery, McGill University, Montreal, QC, Canada H3A 2B4

Shehab Jabir
St. Andrews Centre for Plastic Surgery and Burns, Broomfield Hospital, Chelmsford, Essex CM1 7ET, UK

Sean Boutros
Hermann Memorial Hospital and Hermann Children's Hospital, Houston, TX 77030, USA
Houston Plastic and Craniofacial Surgery, 6400 Fannin Suite 2290, Houston, TX 77030, USA

Court Cutting
Institute for Reconstructive Plastic Surgery, New York University, New York, NY 10016, USA

Denis Souto Valente and Alexandre Vontobel Padoin
Graduate Program in Medicine and Health Sciences, PUCRS School of Medicine (FAMED), Avenida Ipiranga 6681, 90619-900 Porto Alegre, RS, Brazil

Luciano Silveira Eifler, Lauro Aita Carvalho, Gustavo Azambuja Pereira Filho and Vinicius Weissheimer Ribeiro
Mae de Deus Health System, Rua Soledade 569, 90470-340 Porto Alegre, RS, Brazil

Naveen Kumar and Satheesha Nayak Badagabettu
Department of Anatomy, Melaka Manipal Medical College, Manipal Campus, Manipal University, Manipal 576104, India

Pramod Kumar
Department of Plastic Surgery, King Abdul Aziz Hospital, Sakaka, Al-Jouf 42421, Saudi Arabia

Keerthana Prasad
Department of Information Science, Manipal School of Information Science, Manipal University, Manipal 576104, India

Ranjini Kudva
Department of Pathology, Kasturba Medical College, Manipal University, Manipal 576104, India

Raghuveer Coimbatore Vasudevarao
Department of Pathology, Yenepoya University, Deralakatte, Mangalore 575018, India

Wanjala F. Nangole, Stanley Khainga and Joyce Aswani
Department of Surgery (Plastic), University of Nairobi, Nairobi 00100, Kenya

Loise Kahoro and Adelaine Vilembwa
Kenyatta National Hospital, Nairobi 00202, Kenya

Imran Ahmad and Md. Sohaib Akhtar
Post Graduate Department of Burns, Plastic and Reconstructive Surgery, JNMC, AMU, Aligarh, Uttar Pradesh 202002, India

Felix J. Paprottka, Nils-Kristian Dohse and Detlev Hebebrand
Department of Plastic, Aesthetic, Reconstructive and Hand Surgery, Agaplesion Diakonieklinikum Rotenburg, Elise-Averdieck-Straße 17, 27356 Rotenburg (W¨umme), Germany

Nicco Krezdorn
Harvard Medical School, Brigham andWomen's Hospital, Department of Surgery, Division of Plastic Surgery, 75 Francis Street, Boston, MA 02115, USA

Heiko Sorg
Department of Plastic, Reconstructive, Aesthetic and Hand Surgery, Alfried Krupp Krankenhaus, Hellweg 100, 45276 Essen, Germany

Sören Könneker
Department of Plastic, Aesthetic, Hand and Reconstructive Surgery, Hannover Medical School, Carl-Neubergstraße 1, 30625 Hannover, Germany

Stiliano Bontikous
Department of Pathology, Agaplesion Diakonieklinikum Rotenburg, Elise-Averdieck-Straße 17, 27356 Rotenburg, Germany

Ian Robertson
Department of Surgery, Royal Brompton Hospital, Sydney St, London, UK

Christopher L. Schlett
Department of Diagnostic and Interventional Radiology, University Hospital Heidelberg, Im Neuenheimer Feld 110, 69120 Heidelberg, Germany

Meltem Ayhan Oral
İzmir Katip Celebi University, Ataturk Research and Training Hospital, Department of Plastic and Reconstructive Surgery, 35360 Izmir, Turkey

Kamuran Zeynep Sevim
Sisli Hamidiye Etfal Research and Training Hospital, Department of Plastic and Reconstructive Surgery, 34371 Istanbul, Turkey

Metin Görgü
Abant İzzet Baysal University, Department of Plastic and Reconstructive Surgery, 14280 Bolu, Turkey

Hasan Yücel Öztan
Private Practice, Plastic Surgeon, 35590 Izmir, Turkey

Adham Farouk and Saad Ibrahiem
Department of Plastic and Reconstructive Surgery, Faculty of Medicine, Alexandria University, Alexandria, Egypt

Akiko Sakakibara and Takahide Komori
Department of Oral and Maxillofacial Surgery, Kobe University Graduate School of Medicine, Kobe 650-0017, Japan

Kazunobu Hashikawa and Shunsuke Sakakibara
Department of Plastic Surgery, Kobe University Graduate School of Medicine, Kobe 650-0017, Japan

Satoshi Yokoo
Department of Stomatology and Maxillofacial Surgery, Gunma University Graduate School of Medicine, Gunma 371-8511, Japan

Shinya Tahara
Department of Plastic Surgery, Japanese Red Cross Kobe Hospital, Kobe 651-0073, Japan

Elaine Fung, Paul Hong and S. Mark Taylor
Department of Surgery, Dalhousie University, 5850 University Avenue, Halifax, NS, Canada B3H 2Y9
Department of Surgery, IWK Health Centre, 5850/5920 University Avenue, Halifax, NS, Canada B3K 6R8

Corey Moore
Department of Otolaryngology-Head and Neck Surgery, University of Western Ontario, London, ON, Canada N6B 2P2

Esko Veräjänkorva, Salvatore Giordano, Ilkka Koskivuo and Otto Savolainen
Department of Surgery, Division of Plastic Surgery, Turku University Hospital, Turku, Finland

Riitta Rautio
Department of Radiology, Turku University Hospital, Turku, Finland

Guillermo Ramos-Gallardo, Ana Pérez Verdin, Miguel Fuentes, Sergio Godínez Gutiérrez, Ana Rosa Ambriz-Plascencia, Ignacio González-García, Sonia Mericia Gómez-Fonseca, Rosalio Madrigal, Luis Iván González-Reynoso, Sandra Figueroa, Xavier Toscano Igartua and Déctor Francisco Jiménez Gutierrez
Plastic Surgery Department, Hospital Civil de Guadalajara Fray Antonio Alcalde, Calle Hospital 278, 44280 Guadalajara, JAL, Mexico

Adrian Ooi, Jonathan Ng, Christopher Chui, Terence Goh and Bien Keem Tan
Department of Plastic, Reconstructive and Aesthetic Surgery, Singapore General Hospital, Singapore 169608

David W. Grant, Alexei Mlodinow and John Y. S. Kim
Division of Plastic and Reconstructive Surgery, Feinberg School of Medicine, Northwestern University, Chicago, IL 60611, USA

Jon P. Ver Halen
Division of Plastic and Reconstructive Surgery, Baptist Cancer Center, Vanderbilt Ingram Cancer Center, St. Jude Children's Research Hospital, Memphis, TN 38139, USA

Debarati Chattopadhyay
Department of Plastic Surgery, IPGME&R, Kolkata, India

Souradip Gupta, Prabir Kumar Jash and Sandipan Gupta
Department of Plastic Surgery, Medical College Kolkata, 88 College Street, Kolkata, West Bengal 700073, India

Marang Buru Murmu
Department of Surgery, Midnapore Medical College, India

Jessica F. Rose, Sarosh N. Zafar and Warren A. Ellsworth IV
Division of Plastic Surgery, Department of Surgery, Houston Methodist Hospital, Medical Office Building, 118400 Katy Freeway, Suite 500, Houston, TX 77094, USA

Md. Sohaib Akhtar, Mohd Fahud Khurram and Arshad Hafeez Khan
Post Graduate Department of Burns, Plastic and Reconstructive Surgery, JNMC, AMU, Aligarh, India

Manaf Khatib, Shehab Jabir, Edmund Fitzgerald O'Connor and Bruce Philp
St. Andrews Centre for Plastic Surgery and Burns, Broomfield Hospital, Chelmsford CM1 7ET, UK

Emir Burak Yüksel
Department of Plastic, Reconstructive and Esthetic Surgery, Elbistan State Hospital, Kahramanmaras, Turkey

Alpagan Mustafa Yıldırım
Department of Plastic, Reconstructive and Esthetic Surgery, Afyon Kocatepe University, Afyon, Turkey

Ali Bal
Department of Plastic, Reconstructive and Esthetic Surgery, Malatya State Hospital, Malatya, Turkey

Tuncay Kuloglu
Department of Histology and Embryology, Firat University, Elazıg, Turkey

Marshall Ítalo Barros Fontes
Medical Genetics Sector, State University of Alagoas (UNCISAL), Brazil

Isabella Lopes Monlleó
Medical Genetics Sector, State University of Alagoas (UNCISAL), Brazil
Clinical Genetics Service, Federal University of Alagoas (UFAL), Brazil

Erlane Marques Ribeiro
Medical Genetics Sector, Hospital Infantil Albert Sabin (HIAS), Brazil

Josiane de Souza
Medical Genetics Sector, Assistance Center for Cleft Lip and Palate (CAIF), Brazil

Gabriela Ferraz Leal
Medical Genetics Sector, Facial Deformity Care Center (CADEFI), Brazil

Têmis Maria Félix
Medical Genetics Service, Hospital de Clínicas de Porto Alegre (HCPA), Brazil

Agnes Cristina Fett-Conte
Molecular Biology Department, Medicine School of São José do Rio Preto (FAMERP/FUNFARME), Brazil

Bruna Henrique Bueno, Luis Alberto Magna and Vera Gil-da Silva-Lopes
Department of Medical Genetics, Faculty of Medical Sciences, University of Campinas, 13083-887, Brazil

Peter Anthony Mossey
Dundee University Dental School, UK

Seyed Esmail Hassanpour
Professor of Plastic Surgery, Department Of Plastic Surgery, 15 Khordad Educational Hospital, School of Medicine, Shahid Beheshti University of Medical Sciences, Tehran, Iran

Masoumeh Abbasnezhad
Resident of Plastic Surgery, Department of Plastic Surgery, 15 Khordad Educational Hospital, School of Medicine, Shahid Beheshti University of Medical Sciences, Tehran, Iran

Hamidreza Alizadeh Otaghvar
Associate Professor of General Surgery, Iran University of Medical Sciences, Resident of Plastic and Reconstructive Surgery, Shahid Beheshti University of Medical Sciences, Trauma and Injury Research Center, Tehran, Iran

Adnan Tizmaghz
Assistant Professor of General Surgery, Iran University of Medical Sciences, Tehran, Iran

Kiyoko Fukui, Sho Yamakawa, Haruka Matsuo and Miho Noguchi
Department of Plastic and Reconstructive Surgery, National Hospital Organization Nagasaki Medical Center, Nagasaki, Japan

Masaki Fujioka
Department of Plastic and Reconstructive Surgery, National Hospital Organization Nagasaki Medical Center, Nagasaki, Japan
Department of Plastic and Reconstructive Surgery, Nagasaki University, Nagasaki, Japan

Kazumi Yamasaki
Department of Liver Internal Medicine, National Hospital Organization Nagasaki Medical Center, Nagasaki, Japan
Department of Clinical Research Center, National Hospital Organization Nagasaki Medical Center, Nagasaki, Japan

Lea Juul Nielsen and Jørgen Lock-Andersen
Department of Plastic Surgery and Breast Surgery, Roskilde Hospital, 4000 Roskilde, Denmark

Caroline Holkmann Olsen
Department of Pathology, Roskilde Sygehus, Denmark

Peter McAllister, Isabel Teo, Kuen Chin and David Alexander Munnoch
Department of Plastic and Reconstructive Surgery, Ninewells Hospital and Medical School, Dundee DD1 9SE, UK

Boikanyo Makubate
Department of Public Health, Faculty of Medicine, University of Botswana, Gabarone, Botswana

Lee Seng Khoo, Henrique N. Radwanski, Vasco Senna-Fernandes, Nsingi Nsosolo Antônio, Leonardo Luiz Fernandes Fellet and Ivo Pitanguy
Instituto Ivo Pitanguy, Rua Dona Mariana 65, 22280-020 Botafogo, RJ, Brazil

Index